The Correspondence of
Sigmund Freud and Sándor Ferenczi
Volume 1, 1908–1914

The Correspondence of

SIGMUND FREUD
and
SÁNDOR FERENCZI
Volume 1, 1908–1914

Edited by
Eva Brabant, Ernst Falzeder,
and Patrizia Giampieri-Deutsch
under the supervision of
André Haynal

Transcribed by
Ingeborg Meyer-Palmedo

Translated by
Peter T. Hoffer

Introduction by
André Haynal

The Belknap Press of Harvard University Press
Cambridge, Massachusetts
London, England
1993

This book has been supported by a grant from the National Endowment
for the Humanities, an independent federal agency.

This book is printed on acid-free paper, and its binding materials have
been chosen for strength and durability.

Library of Congress Cataloging-in-Publication Data

Freud, Sigmund, 1856–1939.
[Correspondence. English. Selections]
The correspondence of Sigmund Freud and Sándor Ferenczi/edited by Eva
Brabant, Ernst Falzeder, and Patrizia Giampieri-Deutsch, under the
supervision of André Haynal; transcribed by Ingeborg Meyer-Palmedo;
translated by Peter T. Hoffer; introduction by André Haynal.
p.   cm.
Includes bibliographical references and index.
Contents: v. 1. 1908–1914
ISBN 0-674-17418-6 (alk. paper)
1. Freud, Sigmund, 1856–1939—Correspondence. 2. Ferenczi, Sándor,
1873–1933—Correspondence. 3. Psychoanalysts—Correspondence.
4. Psychoanalysis. I. Ferenczi, Sándor, 1873–1933. II. Brabant, Eva.
III. Falzeder, Ernst. IV. Giampieri-Deutsch, Patrizia. V. Title.
BF109.F74A4 1993b
150. 19′52′0922—dc20
[B] 93-17479
CIP

Contents

Translator's Note

ALL TRANSLATIONS REQUIRE a compromise between a desire to retain the literal meaning and stylistic peculiarities of the original and the need to render it in acceptable, idiomatic English. Translations that are too literal are often cumbersome or stilted, whereas those that attempt to follow the norms of colloquial English run the risk of losing or distorting some essential meaning. In translating the letters of Freud and Ferenczi, an attempt has been made to retain, to the fullest extent possible, the style and meaning of the original. This entailed having to render many of Freud's idiosyncratic and imaginative metaphorical constructions in forms that have no exact English equivalent while retaining the otherwise precise yet uniquely intimate conversational tone of his epistolary prose style. In the case of Ferenczi, whose native tongue was Hungarian and whose German was flawed, obvious grammatical and stylistic errors have been silently corrected. But at the same time an effort has been made to translate certain peculiarities of Ferenczi's formal yet flowery, enthusiastic, and occasionally redundant prose into English. Correctness of style has thus, in some instances, been sacrificed for the sake of authenticity.

Certain conventions of translation have been adhered to throughout the volume. Salutations and closings have for the most part been standardized, except in a few instances where certain personal remarks were included. Abbreviations of names and terms regularly used by both writers have been silently spelled out, with the exception of the commonly used ΨA (ψα) for psychoanalysis and cs., pcs., and ucs. for conscious, preconscious, and unconscious, respectively. Original spellings of names and places have, for the most part, been retained.

Recent criticisms by Bruno Bettelheim, Darius Ornston, and others of James Strachey's translation in *The Standard Edition of the Complete Psychological Works of Sigmund Freud* have been taken into account in translating the correspondence. In instances where certain technical terms that have been called into question appear in the letters, I have chosen what I consider to be more appropriate alternative translations and have provided brief explanatory notes where the new translation is at variance with specific passages cited in the *Standard Edition*. In a few others I have elected to retain terms such as "libidinal cathexis" and "parapraxis" where the scientific context would make alternatives seem strange to the ear of a public which has grown accustomed to Strachey's terminology over the years. This would appear to be a prudent course to take until such time as a completely new translation of the *Standard Edition* is undertaken.

I gratefully acknowledge the support and assistance of Axel Hoffer, Otto Hoffer, Ernst Falzeder, Martin Stanton, Angela von der Lippe, and Amanda Heller in the preparation of the translation.

Peter T. Hoffer

Note on Transcription
of the Original Correspondence

THE TRANSCRIPTION of this correspondence was accomplished in several stages. Initially I worked with enlargements of microfilms of the manuscripts (typewritten versions). These reproductions were, however, so full of errors that it proved necessary to verify the texts systematically by referring to the originals preserved in the National Library of Austria, in Vienna. In addition, all the letters have been compared with the rough transcription prepared by Michael Balint in the 1960s. These various documents are discussed in the annotation, at the appropriate points. Passages that remain obscure or fragmentary, despite efforts to clarify them, are likewise pointed out in the notes.

The letters, postcards, telegrams, and notes have been numbered in chronological order. (The corresponding references from the catalogue of the National Library of Austria have been omitted in this edition.) The annotation discusses the physical characteristics of the letters, material that appears in the headings, missing elements, the conjectured dating of undated items, and passages that proved difficult to decipher. Corrections in the originals themselves have been noted only if they were made in a different hand, or could not be clearly deciphered, or are explicitly referred to in the text by the writer of the letter.

In his correspondence Freud almost always used one of two kinds of large-format letterhead which he would reorder from the stationer-engraver according to his needs, keeping the layout and typography essentially constant. It was his habit to write out the date by hand, just above the address. To avoid overscrupulous repetition of the same comment in item after item, a note mentioning this characteristic feature is appended only to his first letter (letter 2); in all the cases that follow, the preprinted line is transcribed without comment. Only the rare instances in which Freud departed from this general model are noted. Ferenczi used letterheads of many different sizes and formats: often paper without any preprinted heading, sometimes large sheets which he himself folded into smaller formats, and so on. For this reason, the notes appended to his letters contain a remark on each preprinted heading.

In general, anything that has been added to the original text to facilitate understanding appears in brackets. Inadvertent omissions, as well as errors in writing that may possibly have some sort of value as failed acts, have been either completed in brackets in the text or signaled in a note. Numbers that appear as numerals in the manuscript are, as a general rule, spelled out in the text. This is not the case for fractions, ordinal numbers, sums of money, weights and measures, days, months, and years, page numbers, hours of the day, tabular material, and groups of numbers, unless these were spelled out in the original.

At various points in the manuscript, proper names, place names, and other geographic designations were imprecise, illegible, or badly written. These have been verified and silently corrected in cases where no uncertainty existed; wherever the meaning was open to doubt, a note has been appended. Abbreviated proper names have been silently written out. An exception is "Frau G." (Mrs. G.)—for Gizella Pálos, who became Ferenczi's wife—since this abbreviation was used by the authors consistently throughout their correspondence. (But wherever the name was spelled out in the original, the complete spelling has of course been preserved.) Some characteristic abbreviations used by both Freud and Ferenczi have also been preserved.

Titles of books, journals, and contributions to books and journals, wherever these appear in the text of the letters, are in every case reproduced as in the original.

Postscripts always appear at the ends of letters, even if in the originals they were written in the margin.

Telegrams have been rendered throughout with a minimum of added punctuation.

Words underlined either once or twice have been reproduced in italics, as have terms that remain in German or other foreign languages. Other forms of emphasis have in each case been explained in a note.

The transcription of a correspondence as vast as this could not have been accomplished by one person. Many individuals have contributed to the realization of this project. Their efforts must be acknowledged here, since only the cooperation of all of them—whatever their field—could have made possible the completion of this transcription. To all these people I extend my personal thanks. They have earned the gratitude of this volume's readers.

First and foremost is Ilse Grubrich-Simitis, who, beginning with her collaboration with Michael Balint in the 1960s, made a major contribution to the project of publishing these letters. Not only did she apply her energies unstintingly and in numerous ways to the preparation of the transcription, but she also succeeded in raising funds for the project and in convincing other people of its importance. Throughout the lengthy task of transcription, she worked with me closely and sustained me with her advice and knowledge.

Those who donated funds played an essential role; without their support this project could never have been realized. They include Helga Breuninger and Horst Kächele of the Breuninger Foundation (S.A.R.L.) for Research in Psychoanalysis, in Essen, which financed the largest part of the work; Lotte Köhler of the René A. Spitz Society, Association for the Promotion of Psychoanalysis, in Munich, which helped make it possible to consult the original letters in Vienna; and Clemens de Boor of the Sigmund Freud Foundation in Frankfurt, which aided with part of the financing.

Also among these benefactors is Monika Schoeller, who at the outset generously placed at my disposition the technical, physical, and other facilities of Fischer Verlag in Frankfurt, including support for a substantial period of research at the National Library of Austria, in Vienna.

At the library itself, Eva Irblich and her colleagues in the Collection of Manuscripts and Incunabula extended an exceptionally gracious welcome. Owing to their cooperation, their specialized training, and the opportunity they gave me to devote sustained, intensive scrutiny to the originals, a great many baffling problems were resolved. Gerhard Fichtner gave readily and generously of his time, helping me at numerous points to decipher particularly difficult passages in the manuscripts. In the reading and translation of passages in Hungarian, Katarina Haeger and Inspector General István Nemeth of Vienna provided invaluable assistance. By helping me in a thousand ways, rendering those frequently underestimated services that may appear ancillary but are always indispensable, Barbara Mohr contributed enormously to the project.

A great many other people, too numerous to be mentioned here, provided me with encouragement, information, guidance, and suggestions.

For any errors remaining in the transcription, I of course assume sole responsibility.

Ingeborg Meyer-Palmedo

Abbreviations of Works Cited

Freud's works in the text are cited in conformity with the method used in the *Freud-Bibliographie mit Werkkonkordanz,* compiled by Ingeborg Meyer-Palmedo and Gerhard Fichtner (Frankfurt, 1989). The number following the date at the beginning of each citation of Ferenczi's works conforms to the numbering system of the bibliography in volume two of the *Schriften zur Psychoanalyse.*

Bausteine	Sándor Ferenczi. *Bausteine zur Psychoanalyse.* 4 vols. Bern: Verlag Hans Huber, 1984.
Binswanger, *Reminiscences*	Ludwig Binswanger. *Sigmund Freud: Reminiscences of a Friendship.* Trans. Norbert Guterman. New York: Grune & Stratton, 1957.
Brome, *Jones*	Vincent Brome, *Ernest Jones: Freud's Alter Ego.* London: Caliban Books, 1982.
C.	Sándor Ferenczi. *First Contributions to Psychoanalysis.* Trans. Ernest Jones. London: Hogarth Press, 1952. American ed., *Sex in Psychoanalysis.* New York: Basic Books, 1950.
Clark, *Freud*	Ronald W. Clark. *Freud: The Man and the Cause.* New York: Random House, 1980.
CW	*The Collected Works of C. G. Jung.* 19 vols. Ed. Gerhard Adler, Michael Fordham, and Herbert Read; executive ed. William McGuire. Trans. R. F. C. Hull. Princeton: Bollingen, 1953–.
Ellenberger, *Unconscious*	Henri F. Ellenberger. *The Discovery of the Unconscious: The History and Evolution of Dynamic Psychiatry.* New York: Basic Books, 1970.
F.C.	Sándor Ferenczi. *Further Contributions to Psychoanalysis.* Compiled by John Rickman. Trans. Jane Suttie et al. London: Hogarth Press, 1926 (2d ed., 1950).

Ferenczi/Groddeck, *Briefwechsel*	*Sándor Ferenczi/Georg Groddeck Briefwechsel, 1921–1933*. Frankfurt: S. Fischer, 1986.
Fin.	Sándor Ferenczi. *Final Contributions to the Problems and Methods of Psychoanalysis*. Ed. Michael Balint. Trans. Eric Mosbacher et al. New York: Basic Books, 1955.
Fliess Letters	*The Complete Letters of Sigmund Freud to Wilhelm Fliess, 1887–1904*. Trans. and ed. Jeffrey Moussaieff Masson. Cambridge, Mass.: Harvard University Press, 1985.
Freud/Abraham	*A Psycho-Analytic Dialogue: The Letters of Sigmund Freud and Karl Abraham*. Ed. Hilda Abraham and Ernst L. Freud. Trans. Bernard Marsh and Hilda C. Abraham. New York: Basic Books, 1965.
Freud, *Briefe*	Sigmund Freud. *Briefe, 1873–1939*. Ed. Ernst and Lucie Freud. Frankfurt: Fischer, 1960.
Freud, *Letters*	Letters of Sigmund Freud, 1873–1939. Ed. Ernst L. Freud. Trans. Tania Stern and James Stern. New York: Basic Books, 1960.
Freud/Arnold Zweig, *Correspondence*	*The Letters of Sigmund Freud and Arnold Zweig*. Ed. Ernst Freud. New York: Harcourt Brace, 1970.
Freud/Jung	*The Freud/Jung Letters: The Correspondence between Sigmund Freud and C. G. Jung*. Ed. William McGuire. Trans. Ralph Manheim and R. F. C. Hull. Princeton: Bollingen, 1974.
Freud/Pfister	*Psychoanalysis and Faith: The Letters of Sigmund Freud and Oskar Pfister*. Ed. Heinrich Meng and Ernst Freud. Trans. Eric Mosbacher. New York: Basic Books, 1963.
Gay, *Freud*	Peter Gay, *Freud: A Life for Our Time*. New York: Norton, 1988.
Hale, *Putnam*	*James Jackson Putnam and Psychoanalysis: Letters between Putnam and Sigmund Freud, Ernest Jones, William James, Sándor Ferenczi, and Morton Prince, 1877–1917*. Ed. Nathan G. Hale, Jr. Cambridge, Mass.: Harvard University Press, 1971.
Jahrbuch	*Jahrbuch für psychoanalytische und psychopathologische Forschungen*. Directed by Eugen Bleuler and Sigmund Freud under the general editorship of Carl Jung. Leipzig: Franz Deuticke, 1909–.

Jones, *Associations*	Ernest Jones. *Free Associations: Memories of a Psycho-Analyst.* London: Hogarth Press, 1959.
Jones	Ernest Jones. *Sigmund Freud: Life and Work.* 3 vols. New York: Basic Books, 1954–1957.
Jung, *Briefe*	C. G. Jung. *Briefe.* 3 vols. Ed. Aniela Jaffé, with Gerhard Adler. Olten: Walter Verlag, 1972.
Jung, *Letters*	*C. G. Jung: Letters.* 2 vols. Ed. Gerhard Adler, with Aniela Jaffé. Princeton: Bollingen, 1973, 1974.
Korrespondenzblatt	*Korrespondenzblatt der internationalen psychoanalytischen Vereinigung.* Ed. C. G. Jung and F. Riklin. Zurich, 1910–1911 (6 nos.); thereafter published as a section in occasional issues of the *Zentralblatt* and *Zeitschrift.*
Minutes	*Minutes of the Vienna Psychoanalytic Society.* 4 vols. Ed. Herman Nunberg and Ernst Federn. Trans. M. Nunberg. New York: International Universities Press, 1962–1975.
Nachtragsband	Supplementary volume (unnumbered) to *Freud's Gesammelte Werke, Texte aus den Jahren 1885 bis 1938.* Ed. Angela Richards, with Ilse Grubich-Simitis. Frankfurt: Fischer, 1987.
Schreber, *Memoirs*	Daniel Paul Schreber. *Memoirs of My Nervous Illness.* Trans. and ed. Ida Macalpine and Richard A. Hunter. Cambridge: Robert Bentley, 1955.
Schriften	Sándor Ferenczi. *Schriften zur Psychoanalyse.* 2 vols. Ed. M. Balint. Frankfurt: Fischer, 1970.
Schur, *Freud*	Max Schur. *Freud: Living and Dying.* New York: International Universities Press, 1972.
S.E.	*The Standard Edition of the Complete Psychological Works of Sigmund Freud.* 24 vols. Trans. James Strachey and Anna Freud, with Alix Strachey and Alan Tyson. London: Hogarth Press, 1953–1974.
Sophienausgabe	J. W. von Goethe. *Goethes Werke.* Weimar, 1887–.
Studienausgabe	*Sigmund Freud Studienausgabe.* 11 vols. Ed. A. Mitscherlich, A. Richards, and J. Strachey; supplementary vol. ed. Ilse Grubich-Simitis. Frankfurt: Fischer, 1969–1975.
Unbewusstes	Sándor Ferenczi. *Zur Erkenntnis des Unbewussten und andere Schriften zur Psychoanalyse.* Ed. Helmut Dahmer. Munich: Kindler, 1978.

Zeitschrift *Internationale Zeitschrift für ärztliche Psychoanalyse.* Vienna, 1913–.

Zentralblatt *Zentralblatt für Psychoanalyse; Medizinische Monatsschrift für Seelenkunde.* Wiesbaden, 1911–1913.

Introduction

by André Haynal

BEFORE WE SURVEY the eventful history of these letters, which are being published here for the first time, the people who played major roles should be introduced. Let me begin with the individuals who devoted their time and attention to this correspondence, and then present the two writers themselves.

Elma, the elder daughter of Sándor Ferenczi's wife, Gizella (she was the child of her mother's first marriage, to Géza Pálos), married an American named Hervé Laurvik. This union lasted only briefly, but it gave Elma American citizenship and enabled her to spend the years during the Second World War working at the U.S. embassy in Bern. After the war she persuaded her mother, now widowed, to move to Bern. At that time Anna Freud, who had accompanied her father into exile, was the director of the Hampstead Clinic in London. She worked jointly with Gizella as the representative of the Freud family's interests.

Michael Balint, a psychoanalyst originally from Budapest, and Sándor Ferenczi's most faithful and original disciple, emigrated to London in 1939. He brought with him the theories elaborated by the Budapest school, blended with his own ideas, and he strove to strengthen the reputation of his teacher, whose significance was at that time largely underrated.[1]

Sándor Ferenczi came from a family of Polish Jews who had emigrated to Hungary. His father, filled with enthusiasm for the liberal, progressivist, and nationalist revolution of 1848, had joined the insurgents and later, in 1879, had Magyarized his name from Fraenkel to Ferenczi. Owner of a bookstore in Miskolcz, a provincial town in northern Hungary which often served as the first stopping point for immigrants from the north, especially Poland, he was a publisher as well, and his commitment to the liberal and nationalist cause led him to become active in publishing the *samizdat* literature of his day—the literature of the underground resistance during the years of oppression that followed the revolution.

Sándor, born in 1873, the eighth of twelve children and his father's favorite, lost his father when he was fifteen. Stimulated by a family environment rich in books and music, he developed wide-ranging cultural interests: he wrote poems in the style of Heine and engaged in experiments in hypnosis when he was still a high school student in Miskolcz. He earned a medical degree at the University of Vienna. After moving to Budapest in 1897, he worked at St. Roch Hospital as an extern in a health service for prostitutes; then, in 1900, he joined the unit in neurology and psychiatry at St. Elizabeth's charity hospital; and in 1904 he joined the polyclinic of a cooperative health facility. Eventually he opened his own office as a general practitioner and neuropsychiatrist, and became a consultant in psychiatry to the courts.

In those days an extraordinary cultural efflorescence was taking place in the cities of the Austro-Hungarian empire. Ferenczi was a typical member of the intelligentsia of late nineteenth-century Budapest, a capital created in 1873 by the unification of Buda, the district containing the royal palace, and Pest, the city of commercial establishments, small workshops, and the university. That intelligentsia, which was as remote from provincial Hungary as the Left Bank of Paris is from rural France, consisted of émigrés from the empire's various territories; of ethnic Germans, commonly called Schwaben (Swabians), or more precisely Donauschwaben (Danube Swabians); of Jews from western Poland (which, since the reign of Maria Theresa, belonged to the Dual Monarchy); and of Hungarians from distant provinces (such as Transylvania, a multiethnic principality that had been independent for centuries). Ferenczi was a member of this Jewish-Hungarian intelligentsia, which played an immense role in transforming cultural life and which continued to make Budapest, like Vienna and Prague, one of the most important cultural centers of the late nineteenth century. The intellectuals of Budapest displayed a cosmopolitanism typical of central Europe. Georg Lukács, the Marxist philosopher, and Béla Balázs, author of the librettos for two celebrated works by Bartók, are among its best-known representatives.

As was characteristic of individuals in that milieu (Lukács did most of his writing in German, and Balázs used German and Hungarian interchangeably), Sándor Ferenczi, who had studied medicine in Vienna, was bilingual in Hungarian and German. He wrote even his personal diary in German. People who have difficulty imagining the cultural geography of the region may find it surprising that cities such as Prague and Budapest were permeated with Germanic culture. But even Count Széchenyi, the great reformer of early nineteenth-century Hungary, wrote in German. And Yiddish—the language spoken by Jews in Poland and Russia—is itself a

Germanic dialect. Although nationalist groups ultimately shattered the empire, the cosmopolitan culture of the great cities of central Europe, even after their collapse, continued to exert a profound influence on western culture of the twentieth century.

The poets, philosophers, thinkers, and men of letters gathered in cafés and various clubs, of which the most prestigious was the freethinking and antimilitarist Galileo Society, founded in 1901. In 1908 Hugó Ignotus and his friends founded the modernist review *Nyugat* (Occident). Members of the Nyugat movement, which coalesced around this periodical, included the writer Dezsö Kosztolányi, Georg Lukács (at that time closely associated with thinkers such as Søren Kierkegaard, Georg Simmel, and Stefan George), the great Hungarian poet Endre Ady, the composers Béla Bartók and Zoltán Kodály—and Sándor Ferenczi. As a result, psychoanalysis was to become inextricably linked with progressivist cultural movements—a relationship that was even stronger in Budapest than in the other cities where psychoanalysis was then coming into being. Certainly it was an important tie insofar as Ferenczi was concerned.

Upon his arrival in Budapest, Ferenczi made friends with Miksa Schächter and began writing essays for Schächter's medical journal, *Gyógyászat* (Art of Healing). He contributed articles on medical topics as well as on general problems, notably, in 1906, a work titled "Sexualis átmeneti fokozatokról" (On the Intermediate Sex), which protested the sociopolitical persecution of homosexuals and discussed the bisexuality of human beings. Endowed with insatiable curiosity, he was already a "restless spirit," as he would later describe himself—immersed in Darwinism and Lamarckism, in chemotherapy (using morphine), and in various literary notions that he believed might shed light on psychopathology. He readily cited Kant, Schopenhauer, and later Bergson, and took an interest in occultism. In sum, at the time he met Freud, in 1908, he was a man whose personality was firmly molded, who espoused broad cultural ideals, and who had acquired extensive experience in medical and therapeutic areas, including hypnosis—exactly like Freud.

As a young physician Ferenczi had read Freud's book *The Interpretation of Dreams.* Later he had had contact with Jungian experiments in word association—for example, during a visit to the Burghölzli clinic in Zurich in 1907 (see the letter of Jung to Ferenczi, October 1, 1907). On February 2, 1908, Freud and Ferenczi met for the first time; they were introduced by Dr. Fülöp Stein of Budapest, who, in order to bring this meeting about, had written to Carl Jung in Zurich. The first letter of the Freud-Ferenczi correspondence is a note in which Ferenczi tells Freud that he is looking forward to their imminent meeting. A mutual enthusiasm subsequently developed, along with an amity that Freud would later describe as a "fellowship of life, thoughts, and interests" (Freud to Ferenczi, January 11, 1933). They worked side by side in an intense exchange of ideas, in ongoing dialogue, in friendship, and also in disagreement. Regarding scientific matters, they always told each other of their respective theories and projects. Many of Ferenczi's notions and concepts reappear, often after an extended latency period, in works by Freud, mixed with Freud's own thoughts—on homosexuality, paranoia, phylogenesis, trauma, transference and countertransference, development of the ego, psychoanalytic technique, parapsychology, and other topics.

To these ties, based on scientific interests, were added others that were deeper and more complex: Freud's hope for a marriage between his daughter Mathilde and Ferenczi; the trip to America with Jung; numerous shared vacations, with their joys and difficulties; the visits they paid each other (for months preceding their trips they would study Baedekers, railway timetables, and ship schedules); Ferenczi's experimental analyses with Freud in 1914 and 1916; Ferenczi's relationship with his future wife, Gizella, and with her daughter Elma, a relationship in which Freud was involved in various ways, including a segment of analysis carried out with Elma in 1911–12. The relations of Ferenczi and Freud with other analysts (Carl Jung, Otto Rank, Ernest Jones, Georg Groddeck, Karl Abraham, Max Eitingon, Wilhelm Reich, and so on) likewise played a role in the contentious history of psychoanalysis, and the two men exchanged their ideas and feelings on the subject. It was natural that in these letters, which were not intended for the public, the two correspondents should express themselves spontaneously; they reveal their sensitivities and personal concerns, down to the details of their daily lives, as we see in their remarks about cigars, flour, and having to forgo morning showers (letter 22), as well as financial difficulties, lack of heating fuel, and worries about children and grandchildren during the winters that followed the war. Gizella and Sándor Ferenczi offered refuge to Ernst Freud in their home in Budapest (261).

The Faculty of Medicine at the University of Vienna was still a prestigious institution, but it was no longer at its zenith as it had been in the 1880s, when, along with the medical school at the University of Paris, it had dominated medical education on the Continent. Since then, German and Swiss-German universities had developed formidable reputations; in psychiatry the new figures included Emil Kraepelin in Munich and Eugen Bleuler at the Burghölzli.

During the years covered in this volume, Freud was a player of tarok (in German *Tarock*), a card game that was popular at the time. Just as Robert Musil had given the nickname "Kakania" to that "k.u.k." empire (*kaiserlich und königlich*, or imperial and royal), another, less well-known writer, Herzmanowsky-Orlando, dubbed his country "Tarockania," the land of tarok.[2] Fondness for the game even led Freud to cancel a visit by Ferenczi one Saturday evening (194, 195). It is interesting to note that Freud's tarok partners were not psychoanalysts; evidently this was one domain in which he temporarily separated himself from "the Cause" *(die Sache).*

Freud was not a habitué of cafés and salons, in contrast to Alfred Adler in Vienna and especially Ferenczi in Budapest, who, along with other intellectuals (journalists, writers, poets) of the empire's major cities, liked to gather in the cafés. Apparently he did not even visit the celebrated salon of Hugo Heller, his publisher. And yet, in keeping with the fashion of the day, he was often seen at Karlsbad, a Czech resort known today as Karlovy Vary. He was fond of outings in the mountains and of "study trips," especially in the Mediterranean countries, which many people, following Goethe, regarded as the cradle of western culture.

Contrary to the prevailing image of him, Freud was a lover of music, especially of opera. Once, when a patient canceled an appointment, he took advantage of the opportunity and went to see *Don Giovanni* (364); on another occasion, during a session with one of his analysands, instead of giving an interpretation he softly sang an air from the same opera.[3] Perhaps he affected a lack of interest in the philosophy and music that filled intellectual Vienna, for he never truly devoted himself to them, even though he attended the lectures of (among others) Franz Brentano, who had ties to his circle of friends.[4]

Freud kept his distance from the large newspapers, even from the distinguished *Neue Freie Presse,* which published articles by Stefan Zweig, Hugo von Hofmannsthal, Arthur Koestler, and Theodor Herzl; essays on psychoanalysis, in serial form, by Wilhelm Stekel; and announcements of happy events in Freud's own family (313). For a time Freud was close to *Die Fackel* and its editor, Karl Kraus ("There are so few of us, we ought to stick together," Freud wrote to Kraus.)[5] But around 1910 their relationship deteriorated, partly as the result of a harsh analysis of Kraus by Fritz Wittels, a member of Freud's circle (112). It was from this circle that Freud recruited most of his clients. Among these were "Little Hans" (the son of Max Graf) and Gustav Mahler, who was referred to Freud by Richard von Nepallek, one of the earliest members of the Wednesday Society (Jones II, 79).

Curiously, politics played a very minor role during the years covered by this volume of correspondence. There are discreet allusions to the anti-Semitism in the air; this was, after all, the era of Vienna's Christian-Socialist mayor Karl Lueger, who, despite his election, was four times denied appointment by Emperor Francis Joseph I because of his anti-Semitism.[6] Then there was the situation in the Balkans, where, after the gradual withdrawal of the Ottoman Empire, the Austro-Hungarian monarchy tried to seize power during that colonial period which was so redolent of gunpowder, and which would finally explode in 1914, engulfing the whole world. The Viennese response: "The situation is hopeless, but not serious."

The decision to ignore these problems seems also to have been the attitude adopted by our two correspondents.

Mail service in those days was faster than it is today; letters between Budapest, Vienna, Zurich, and Berlin would usually reach their destination within one day. Although people moved about the city streets of Vienna and Budapest in horse-drawn cabs, the railway system was already excellent, linking Vienna, Budapest, Prague, and Trieste. Freud and Ferenczi also exchanged numerous telegrams, and there are references to some telephone conversations (see, for example, 112, 159, 165, 463).

Residents of Vienna and Budapest could spend their vacations in the far-flung territories of the multinational empire, in regions as diverse as the Carpathians (which were then under the Hungarian crown but which, after the First World War, would become part of Slovakia), the Austrian Alps, or the Mediterranean and Adriatic coasts (today part of Italy and the former Yugoslavia). It is true that Francis Joseph took little advantage of this freedom of choice: with his well-known obsessive regularity he spent every summer at Bad Ischl, and it was in this region of northern Austria, called Salzkammergut, that fashionable Vienna, including most of its psychoanalysts, congregated during the summer.[7] The only country that was closed to Jews was Russia; hence Martin Freud's wish to go to Russia without having to change his *Konfession* (his religious denomination), that is, by the expedient of enlisting in the army (Jones II, 173).

With each successive letter Freud and Ferenczi become more human in our eyes, as they reveal to us their concerns and even, occasionally, their faults. For the relationship between them was not only a deep friendship but also a *controversy*, full of arguments, affronts, and misunderstandings. In 1910, in the course of a vacation they were spending together in Palermo, Ferenczi refused to take dictation for Freud when the latter was making notes on the Schreber case; for the rest of their trip the two men were unable to discuss this incident and its affective meaning. Freud then took to criticizing, openly or indirectly, Ferenczi's behavior in his relations with Gizella and Elma Pálos.

On July 14, 1911, Ferenczi informed Freud that he had begun an analysis of Elma, the daughter of his friend Gizella (at that time married to Géza Pálos), whom he had already analyzed (80). In October he wrote Freud that the analysis had been going well until one of Elma's despairing admirers had killed himself. In the course of the analysis Ferenczi fell in love with Elma Pálos, who "won" his heart (256). He repeatedly begged Freud to take over Elma's analysis. Reluctantly, Freud agreed. On this note Elma's psychoanalysis began, with many indiscretions between the two men, and with extreme oscillations in the attitude of Ferenczi, who at times declared a wish to marry her and at other times wanted to resume analysis with her in Budapest (even imposing this as a condition for eventual marriage), until, at Easter 1912, she came to the end of her analysis in Vienna with Freud, having reached the "narcissistic stage" (286). In short, we see the entire imbroglio, all the evidence (if any were needed) that Freud would later bring to bear in determining if the love involved in transference is a genuine love (see Freud 1915a [1914], p. 168).

Along the way Freud reported to Ferenczi the details of the treatment— above all the question of whether Elma's love for him was "holding up" in the face of the analysis. All the people involved committed indiscretions: Ferenczi sent Freud copies of Elma's letters, in which she "wants to know *positively* what you [Freud] have written to me about her" (268); Freud wrote confidentially to Gizella about Ferenczi (259)—and the letter fell into Ferenczi's hands (261).[8] But Ferenczi likewise asked Freud to say certain things to Gizella for him (see letter 658). Furthermore, Elma's father, to whom she conveyed all these details, wished to become involved. Ferenczi visited Freud in Vienna to speak with him about Elma. This meeting was kept secret from Elma herself, who was living in Vienna at the time.

When Elma had finished her segment of analysis with Freud, which ran from New Year's Day to Easter 1912, Ferenczi once again took her on as a patient—under circumstances that were, needless to say, quite delicate—in order to complete the analysis. It left him with a feeling of sadness to which he had difficulty resigning himself and which would perhaps never entirely fade. After all this Elma married her American suitor, Laurvik, but the marriage did not last long. Some years later, in 1919, Gizella married Sándor Ferenczi. They would remain together until his death.

A Man of Wholehearted Commitment

The fact that Ferenczi had violated his role as psychoanalyst and had created a triangle with Gizella (his mistress and future wife) and her daughter Elma (his analysand, then Freud's, then Ferenczi's again) allowed all those who considered Ferenczi's later ideas audacious to point to this episode, which was undoubtedly problematic in his professional and private life. Moreover, we know that, over the years, he suffered personal repercussions from the affair in the form of depression and hypochondriacal complaints ("Kränkeln"; 374), and that he had great difficulty recovering his inner equilibrium. His relations with Freud were likewise impaired: in a letter to Georg Groddeck, Ferenczi referred to Freud as the person "who . . . prevented my marriage" (Ferenczi/Groddeck, *Briefwechsel*, February 27, 1922, p. 41).

All this is characteristic of Ferenczi's temperament and testifies to the way in which he engaged himself wholeheartedly, without a backward

glance, in any therapeutic situation. It also shows that he made little clear
or defensive distinction between his professional life and his private life.
In his relations with others he committed himself not only as an analyst
but as a man, and he did so to the utmost of his abilities, with a courage
that was his strength and—in this episode—certainly also his weakness.

Not long afterward, before taking Ferenczi into analysis, Freud expressed
"concern about connecting the fate of our friendship with something else,
something indefinable" (294), and he spoke of the "danger of personal
estrangement [*Entfremdung*] brought about by the analysis" (392). Apparently he saw the danger clearly; nevertheless, after analyzing Elma, he also
analyzed Ferenczi.

This episode, the "Elma affair," did nothing to help Ferenczi become the
"equal" of Freud, as the latter had hoped (though this "request" was not
unambiguous): "I would have wished for you to tear yourself away from
that infantile role and take your place next to me as a companion with
equal rights, which you did not succeed in doing" (169). That Freud had
been Elma's analyst did not make relations between the two men any
easier. And Ferenczi wrote—in a single brief phrase—that he had "über-
standen" (gone through) the "period in which you [Freud] analyzed Elma
and I [Ferenczi] subsequently couldn't marry her" (394).

The ideas exchanged in this part of the correspondence are so rich that
to discuss them in detail would involve retracing the entire evolution of
psychoanalytic thought. This was the time of the Salzburg Congress at
Easter 1908, a completely informal gathering (which was only in retrospect
baptized a "congress"), and two years later, in 1910, of the Nuremberg
Congress and its change of atmosphere, with the founding of the International Psycho-Analytical Association, according to a proposal that Freud
had directed Ferenczi to make (109, 126). Ferenczi, in his speech on behalf
of the proposal, displayed a psychoanalytic clarity that was remarkable in
connection with this organization, which would pose so many problems
in the subsequent history of psychoanalysis: "I know the excrescences that
grow from organized groups, and I am aware that in most political, social,
and scientific organizations childish megalomania, vanity, admiration of
empty formalities, blind obedience, or personal egoism prevail instead of
quiet, honest work in the general interest" (Ferenczi 1911, 79, p. 302). But
he thought that the struggle to promote "the Cause" made such an association necessary, and that psychoanalysts were perhaps "the best adapted
to found an association which would combine the greatest possible personal liberty with the advantages of family organization. It would be a
family in which the father enjoyed no dogmatic authority, but only that to
which he was entitled by reason of his abilities and labours. His pronounce-
ments would not be followed blindly, as if they were divine revelations"

(ibid., p. 303). Freud, in his letter of April 3, 1910 (126), noted that Ferenczi's speech aroused little interest, that Ferenczi's "impassioned pleading" had had the unfortunate effect of inciting opposition; but he concluded nevertheless by thanking Sándor for his work and for their perfect agreement and for his "decidedly successful support." The following year the psychoanalysts met at a congress in Weimar, where, although tensions with Jung cast a shadow, he was unanimously reelected "by acclamation" to the presidency of the Association (*Freud/Jung*, p. 443). In Munich in 1913 two fifths of the members abstained from voting (twenty-two out of fifty-two, including Ferenczi); but all evidence suggests that Freud was still in favor of Jung's election (see the addendum to letter 430).

For Freud it was a time of difficulties with Adler, with Stekel, and then with Jung. Although this is not the place for details, we can at least follow the thread of one of Freud and Ferenczi's major preoccupations: the problem of the "psychoanalytic method." Here we are dealing with a basic historical continuity within the evolution of psychoanalytic practice. Freud discovered the importance of transference and the extraordinary impact of the emotional forces mobilized in psychoanalytic cures; reluctantly, and despite numerous difficulties, he confessed to Oskar Pfister, "The transference is indeed a cross" (*Freud/Pfister*, 5, VI, 1910, p. 39). After the triangle of Bleuler, Anna O., and himself, he was again involved—twice—in an analogous situation: with Sabina Spielrein and Carl Jung, and with Elma Pálos and Sándor Ferenczi. Because he was simultaneously enmeshed in these difficulties, the possibility of *understanding* emerged within him, leading him to the notion of countertransference and, in a more general way, to the problem of the psychoanalyst's emotional involvement in the treatment. These important communications take place, in part, outside consciousness, from unconscious to unconscious, "without passing through the *Cs.*" (Freud, 1915e, p. 194), a fact that motivated him to resume studying parapsychology and occultism with Ferenczi. It was in this mysterious sphere that they attempted to explore the active forces of nonverbal communication in psychoanalysis, although it was difficult for them to enter into these perplexing and forbidden domains. Freud wrote to Jung, saying that his (Freud's) essay on countertransference was one which he deemed essential, but that "we could not publish it, we should have to circulate copies among ourselves" (*Freud/Jung*, December 31, 1911, p. 476). A year earlier he had made a similar remark to Ferenczi (185).

All these reflections culminated, during late 1911 and the two and a half years that followed, in the publication of six works on technique (Freud 1911e, 1912b, 1912e, 1913c, 1914a, 1914g), which Freud viewed as constituting a series (in fact, in 1918 he had them reprinted together under the title *Zur Technik der Psychoanalyse* [On the Technique of Psychoanaly-

sis]). At no time, however, was there ever a systematic work on technique—
a sign, perhaps, that Freud never considered this a closed chapter.

Meanwhile, as we have seen, the triangular episode involving the two
protagonists and Elma, which is much discussed in this volume, played an
important role in the discoveries in this area. Only a few months after their
first meeting, Freud informed Ferenczi that he intended to write a book on
the psychoanalytic method (22). Ferenczi responded on November 29,
1908, "We have great need of it; it would spare us much effort and disappointment." They pondered the idea together, and it was thus that Freud
came to include Ferenczi's thoughts in his writings on technique (see, for
example, 332).

Freud had already acquired a great deal of experience and had developed
highly complex ideas regarding the forces at work in analytic treatment.
He had discovered the phenomenon of transference some while back: he
had spoken of it in 1895 as the "worst [*ärgste*] obstacle" by which "the
patient's relation to the physician is disturbed" (Freud 1895d, p. 301), but,
all the same, as being "in the special solicitude inherent in the treatment
[*therapeutischen Bekümmerung*]" (p. 302). At that time it still represented
"the worst obstacle that we can come across," which one can nevertheless
"reckon on meeting . . . in every comparatively serious analysis" (p. 301)
because "these drawbacks . . . are inseparable from our procedure" (p. 266).
Now, this transference and its counterpart, which in 1909 he named "countertransference," posed a problem. They were apparent not only in his own
practice but also, to all indications, in the experiences related by others.
The Freud-Jung correspondence and the material published on Sabina Spielrein testify to this. Freud increasingly recognized the importance of affective *experience* and its *repetitive character* (forming part of the transference—affectionate, erotic, hostile, and so on). He wrote to Jung that "the
cure is effected by love" (*Freud/Jung*, December 6, 1906, pp. 12–13). One
month later, on January 30, 1907, a statement similar to Freud's appeared
in the *Minutes* of the Vienna Psychoanalytic Society: "Our cures are cures
of love" ("Unsere Heilungen sind Liebesheilungen,") *Minutes* I, 101. On
January 19, 1908, he wrote to Abraham: "Back to technique. You are right,
that was the most taxing of all to acquire, and that is why I want to spare
those who follow in my footsteps part of the grind—and part of the cost"
(*Freud/Abraham*, p. 24). Easter 1908 was also the time of the Salzburg
Congress, where Freud presented his analysis of the "Rat-Man," speaking
for five hours without a break, moved by the desire to express the thoughts
that were engrossing him, as he wrote to Abraham: "I have to recuperate
from psycho-analysis by working, otherwise I should not be able to stand
it" (*Freud/Abraham*, July 3, 1912, p. 120); and to Ferenczi: "I was depressed
the whole time and anesthetized myself with writing—writing—writing"
(264).

"Slandered and Scorched by Love"

The suffering that preoccupied Freud stemmed from the affective mobilization of the analyst: "To be slandered and scorched by the love with which we operate—such are the perils of our trade, which we are certainly not going to abandon on their account. *Navigare necesse est, vivere non necesse.*[9] And another thing: 'In league with the devil, and yet you fear fire?'" (*Freud/Jung*, March 9, 1909, pp. 210–211). Thus, he wrote again to Jung:

> Such experiences, though painful, are necessary and hard to avoid. Without them we cannot know life and what we are dealing with. I myself have never been taken in quite so badly, but I have come very close to it a number of times and had a *narrow escape.*[10] I believe that only grim necessities weighing on my work, and the fact that I was ten years older than yourself when I came to ΨA, have saved me from similar experiences. But no lasting harm is done. They help us to develop the thick skin we need and to dominate 'countertransference,' which is after all a permanent problem for us; they teach us to displace our own affects to best advantage. They are a *blessing in disguise.*[11] (*Freud/Jung*, June 7, 1909, pp. 230–231)

It was in this letter that the word "countertransference" appeared for the first time and that Freud first suggested the concept, which he presented one year later in a published work (Freud 1910d).

The importance of the analyst's emotions became ever clearer to him. On December 26, 1908, he wrote to Abraham that it was precisely those cases in which he was most interested personally that failed because of the intensity of his feelings.[12] One month after Freud wrote to Jung of the risks of the trade, Abraham told him that once, while waiting for a patient's response during a session, he had been surprised to find himself gazing at a photograph of his parents with a certain feeling of guilt, wondering what they would think of him (*Freud/Abraham*, April 7, 1909, p. 77).

A few months later, in August 1909, Freud, Ferenczi, and Jung set out on their trip to America, where Freud gave his famous lectures on the occasion of the twentieth anniversary of the founding of Clark University, in Worcester, Massachusetts. By all accounts the problems he had been seeking to clarify over the years continued to absorb him and were the subject of intense exchanges throughout the trip. The three men analyzed their dreams and tried to fathom all that was unknown, unconscious, and obscure in the realm of the psyche. Was it Ferenczi's influence that led Freud and Jung to take renewed interest in occult phenomena (which had been the subject of Jung's doctoral thesis)? It was no doubt typical that the trip should end with a visit to Berlin, where Freud and Ferenczi met the clairvoyant Frau Seidler, seeking a better understanding of the *Gedanken-*

übertragung, the "transference" (or transmission) of thought.[13] And Ferenczi would take further exploratory steps: with a certain Frau Jelinek in Budapest (85), with Professor Alexander Roth (436), and with Professor Staudenmeier (308). Subsequently he directed his brother to pay another visit to Frau Seidler (76, 83). Meanwhile, Freud gave advice on the best ways to carry out these experiments (see, for example, 75, 78, 84). Ferenczi likewise conducted experiments using his patients (addendum to 160, 180), Gizella (see, for example, 182), and himself as medium. All of this "finally shattered," in Freud's mind, "the doubts about the existence of thought transference" (163).

In 1913 Freud immersed himself in an idea that culminated in *Totem and Taboo.* In this work Ferenczi immediately noted (406) the idea of the transmission of highly important psychic processes "For psychoanalysis has shown us that everyone possesses in his unconscious mental activity an apparatus which enables him to interpret other people's reactions, that is, to undo the distortions other people have imposed on the expression of their feelings" (Freud 1912–13a, p. 159).

By that time Ferenczi had already shown himself to be an expert clinician, gifted with a keen sense of the interactions that take place during treatment, of all that transpires, even fleetingly, in the analytic situation—an ability that is revealed in (among other works) his 1912 essay "On Transitory Symptom-Constructions during the Analysis." His brief clinical notes, such as "To Whom Does One Relate One's Dreams?" (1913, 105), "A Little Chanticleer" (1913, 114), "Falling Asleep during the Analysis" (1914, 139), and "The 'Forgetting' of a Symptom and Its Explanation in a Dream" (1914, 145), are real gems that give early glimpses of the theoretician who would develop a deep understanding of the forces of transference and countertransference, who would advocate interactive empathy and the use of regression. His theory of object relations, which would endure as his contribution to posterity, was adopted by virtually all of the psychoanalytic community, though he was not explicitly credited with the formulation of this interactive technique, which is based on direct experience and intersubjectivity.[14] How his role came to be obscured can be seen in the two volumes that will follow this one, which I shall refrain from previewing here.

Freud and Ferenczi did more work *together* than has sometimes been acknowledged. Later, in the mid-1920s, their views would diverge in ways that proved crucial to the history of psychoanalytic thought, an evolution that readers will be able to follow in the second volume of this correspondence. But on June 28, 1914, when the student Gavrilo Princip assassinated the heir to the throne, Francis Ferdinand, and his wife, the history of the empire in which our two correspondents lived was profoundly disrupted. Black clouds appeared on the horizon, foreshadowing the end of an era and, in large part, the destruction of their native community. The letters collected in subsequent volumes will show how they survived the war, the collapse, the revolution and counterrevolution in Hungary, and the rise of Hungarian protofascism.

THE LETTERS CLAIMED BY GIZELLA FERENCZI

Michael Balint writes: "When I left Budapest for England in January 1939, Mrs. Ferenczi gave me [Sándor Ferenczi's] *Diary*, with all the letters written by Freud to Ferenczi, and asked me to keep them until the time arrived when they could be published."[15] Shortly afterward, having just arrived in Bern, Gizella Ferenczi asked Anna Freud to send her all the letters that her husband had written to Freud. Anna immediately responded with a draft statement:

> We . . ., the heirs of Professor Sigmund Freud, transfer the entire property, consisting of all the letters written by Dr. Sándor Ferenczi to our testator, as well as other documents of a similar nature, to Mrs. Sándor Ferenczi, widow, and her two children.
>
> The delivery of the letters will take place through the mediation of Dr. Michael Balint . . ., who has them in his safekeeping . . . All other rights adhering to the property shall be transferred at the same time.

In a letter to Gizella of April 2, 1948, Anna wrote:

> I have just been discussing your letter with my brothers, and we all agree to let you have, for your daughters, the letters that your husband wrote to our father. With Dr. Balint, I shall try to find out how we can have them copied as quickly as possible. As soon as we have the copies here in London, with an eye toward their eventual *partial use*, the originals of your husband's letters shall enter into your possession. My brothers agree that there is no need to draw up a formal agreement between us on this matter. [emphasis added]

In her response (which was not precisely dated), Gizella expressed her great satisfaction:

> I was happy to learn from my faithful Dr. Balint that he is in full agreement with you, dear friend, on the manner in which the correspondence of Sándor and the Professor is to be catalogued and published . . . We shall see how many of the letters can be published, and in what form. These letters contain a great many personal details concerning me, and I wouldn't want them to fall into the hands of just anyone—anyone but you, that is.
>
> Throughout the remaining years of my life, which now are few, I would rejoice if I could leave Sándor's letters—especially the ones he sent the Professor—to my two children.

The letter continues, touchingly: "The fact that my husband maintained such an intimate intellectual and personal relationship with one of the greatest men of our time is of immense moral value. Since I have scarcely anything else of value left, it would be consoling and gratifying for me and my children to possess this document produced by two such remarkable men."

"Dr. Balint Didn't Want to Believe Me"

After these three swift acts came a hesitant minuet, full of reticences. A handwritten letter from Anna Freud to Gizella Ferenczi, dated April 26, 1948, reads:

> Dear *Frau Doktor:* My heartfelt thanks for your letter. I was absolutely sure that you and I were in agreement, but Dr. Balint didn't want to believe me and expressed some reservations. For this reason, it would be better if you communicated directly with him, to reiterate your point of view.
> He is so much younger than we are, and cannot know how closely our past—yours and mine—is bound together [*innig zusammengehört*, literally, "belongs together"].
> With best regards, your Anna.[16]

Negotiations followed. Should they publish the entire collection, or should they suppress certain parts, as was usually done in those days? It is true that many of the people concerned were still living, notably Gizella (who would die a year later, on March 14, 1949), and Elma (who would die in 1972 and who, like her sister Magda, would leave no children).[17]

Gizella received the letters that her husband had written to Freud. She was likewise in possession of his diary, but publication was delayed because of various reservations, among them the fact that Michael Balint wanted to publish the correspondence and the diary at the same time. At one point the fair-minded mediator Balint proposed to publish only the correspondence from carefully selected years, a procedure that would eliminate the need for excisions. But there were no years that would do. Matters dragged on.

"A Certain Selection Must Be Made"

In time the parties involved in the negotiations changed: after Gizella's death in the spring of 1949, Elma took her place in the dialogue with Michael Balint. The latter continued faithfully to send reports: "The cataloguing and copying are now in progress. All of Sándor's letters have already been copied. Anna has not yet finished with the Professor's letters—she is up to about 1914. According to the agreement we made with Aunt Gizella, it is I who will assume the costs."[18] He added: "Then there is the diary that Sándor wrote during the last two years of his life. I think that for now, we won't do anything with it. I hope that in the near future, however, we can look forward to preparing it for publication."

On November 12, 1951, Elma wrote back, "If only I could live to see the publication of this correspondence," adding sharply, "which I know has been delayed because of Anna." On December 15, 1953, Balint confirmed to Elma:

> I agree with you. It is vexing that we are unable to publish the letters as they are, but one must realize that they contain numerous remarks concerning people who are still living, comments of such frankness that neither the writer nor the recipient would ever have envisioned making them public. This means that a certain selection must be made, whether we like it or not. I think that the wisest course would be to wait and see what reactions the new volume evokes, and then decide on the most appropriate thing to do with the correspondence.[19]

In 1955 he was more pessimistic. He wrote to Elma:

> The correspondence between Professor Freud and Sándor poses a very difficult problem. As you'll recall, I had the letters typed, so that they are now ready for publication at some still unspecified time. Unfortunately, they contain so many personal references and allusions that they simply couldn't be published anytime soon, unless substantial excisions were made. So I propose that we leave things as they are for a few years, and then review the situation.
>
> Likewise with Sándor's scientific diary, which Gizella entrusted to me in Budapest. This is a document of major scientific importance, but because it contains references to individuals who are still living, it cannot yet be published in its entirety. My advice remains the same: let it sit for several years, and then reconsider it.

During the subsequent decade there was no further discussion of these problems in Michael Balint's letters. He avoided all reference not only to the Freud-Ferenczi correspondence but also to the diary.

The Agreement and Elma

More than ten years later, on April 28, 1966, Balint suddenly wrote to Elma:

> Once again, I have important news, namely, that after long, drawn-out discussions and negotiations, *I have reached an agreement* with Anna Freud so that the correspondence between Sándor and Freud can be published. Since the complete correspondence comprises about 2,500 letters,[20] we thought it would be unwise to publish it in its entirety, for it would amount to approximately five volumes, which scarcely anyone would

want to buy. After lengthy deliberations, we came to the conclusion that a good solution would be to use this material for two independent volumes. (a) The first volume would consist of selected letters, roughly 400 to 500 in all. The criterion for selection would be the general interest of their content. The selection itself would be made jointly: Anna Freud would choose from Freud's letters and I would choose from Sándor's. (b) A second volume, written by me, would present a historical account of the friendship between Freud and Sándor and its ultimate breakdown. Anna and Ernst [Freud] have given me permission to use the material contained in the correspondence as freely as I wish. This raises a very difficult problem, that of your relationship with Sándor. To write a biography of Sándor, particularly of the years that immediately preceded and followed the First World War, without mentioning the role that you played in his life, would be a falsification, or at least a *suppressio veri* [suppression of truth]. Moreover, as you can well imagine, a certain number of people know (by hearsay) an approximate version of that history, and if the official biography were to remain silent on this point, it would give rise to fresh gossip and new rumors.

T1.e work on the first volume of selected letters can begin immediately, to the extent that it can be done without your collaboration. What interests us are the letters containing important scientific material. For our part, the work on the other volume cannot begin without your permission. Thus, I would like to ask you to think about this very personal and delicate problem, and let me know your feelings on the matter. [emphasis added]

INTRICATE TIES BETWEEN COUCHES

What was the "very personal and delicate problem" to which Balint alluded? In 1911, when Sándor was involved with Elma's mother, he began an analysis of Elma, as I have noted. He very quickly fell in love with her and asked Freud to take over the analysis—among other things, to find out if she shared his feelings—then resumed analysis with her in 1912. The projected marriage between Elma and Sándor never took place (he blamed Freud for the failure). Elma married Laurvik, and Sándor later married her mother, in 1919. Of course, the correspondence between Freud and Ferenczi discussed this episode, which was especially delicate for Elma, her mother, and Sándor. Would she agree to let these letters appear in the volume? And with what conditions?

Elma's response, dated May 7, 1966, is an extraordinary document in its very simplicity.[21] She understood that her role in Sándor's life could not be passed over in silence, and she generously gave her consent to publish the letters because to do otherwise "would be unethical and because historical truth does not allow one to even think of it." She likewise realized that Ernest Jones's biography of Freud had already harmed Ferenczi and that any manipulation of history would only exacerbate this. She nevertheless placed confidence in Michael Balint's "tact"—a term that, as everyone knows, has profound Ferenczian resonances. "It was not easy to put these memories in writing," she admitted.

Balint answered her on May 11, 1966: "I was deeply touched by your prompt and understanding response. I can well imagine how many memories—some dear to you, others painful—my request must have awakened in you, and I greatly appreciate the way in which you responded." And further on: "You asked me how many and what sorts of people know about that episode. This is a question that is of course impossible to answer. Let me say simply that when I began my analysis in Berlin in 1921, I heard all kinds of gossip on the subject; and having begun another analysis with Sándor, I found myself in great difficulties during the first few weeks of sessions, because I felt a strong resistance to saying what I believed I knew about the matter."

How intricate the ties between couches can become!

A Pseudonym

On June 6, 1967, Michael Balint wrote to Elma: "I have in hand about 2,500 letters, of which more than half were written by Sándor, and the rest—about 1,100—by Freud. We plan to select 800 to 1,000, which would give an accurate picture of the relationship between the two men." He added: "It was agreed that I would write a kind of biography of their friendship, making use of all the information at my disposal—that is, including the letters that will *not* be published in this edition . . . I hope you find this acceptable."

Balint wrote again to Elma and Magda on July 16, 1968: "At present, I am engaged in correcting the transcription of Sándor's diary. The diary contains a great deal of extremely interesting material, but I am still not certain that the time has come to publish it. In any case, I shall get it all ready for publication and then try to find out what reactions it might evoke."

Later that year, on December 10, he wrote:

May I take this opportunity to pursue our discussion of the way in which I think we could approach the complex problem of your role in the Freud-Ferenczi correspondence? Having looked closely at the years 1908 to 1913—which encompass the greatest number of events that bear on this question—I would like to propose the following:

1. We give you a pseudonym that would conceal your identity but not your existence;

2. We say that you were closely related to Gizella but do not reveal that you were her daughter.

If these proposals are acceptable to you, please let me know what pseudonym you would like us to use.

On January 14, 1969, Balint wrote to Elma and Magda that he was very glad to have "your approval to use the pseudonym 'Sylvia' and to describe Sylvia as a close relation of Gizella's. I don't think it will be necessary to give any further details. This has effectively cleared the way, and I can proceed much more freely and easily with the task of making the selection." A draft preface for the diary reveals that at a certain point, in 1969, Balint thought publication of the two works was imminent.[22] But as we now know, he was still too optimistic.

After Michael Balint's death, in December 1970, at the age of seventy-four, Enid Balint, his widow, and Judith Dupont, the literary executor of Ferenczi's estate and the person to whom Elma granted the Ferenczi copyright, contacted Mark Paterson, director of Sigmund Freud Copyrights, who was in constant touch with the Freud family. They set up a committee for the publication of the correspondence and invited the participation of Ilse Grubrich-Simitis, who had already worked with Balint on the project (and who had close relations with Fischer Verlag, the publisher of most of Freud's original texts), and myself. Later, Arthur Rosenthal, former director of Basic Books and at that time director of Harvard University Press (prospective publisher of the English-language edition of this correspondence), joined our group. All obstacles were finally eliminated, as the publication of this first volume attests. Others will soon follow, and thus this treasury of more than 1,200 letters will be made available to a large, curious public and to the scrutiny of specialists. It is certain that, along with other collections of correspondence already in part accessible, these writings will change the image we have of Freud and his circle, revealing them as less inaccessible and more human than we have hitherto believed. We will be able to follow the private course of their thought and recognize its extraordinary creative potential.

Translated by Maria Louise Ascher

1. André Haynal, *Controversies in Psychoanalytic Method: From Freud to Ferenczi to Michael Balint* (New York: 1989).

2. F. von Herzmanowsky-Orlando, *Maskenspiel der Genien* (1928; reprint, Munich, 1957). If one had to devise a name typical of the *Völkergemisch* (blend of peoples) that inhabited the cities of the empire, one could scarcely do better than Herzmanowsky-Orlando. Its components are Germanic (*Herz-* and *Mann-*), Slavic (*-owsky*), and Italian (*Orlando*). Only the Hungarian element is missing.

3. J. M. Dorsey, *An American Psychiatrist in Vienna, 1935–1937* (London, 1980), p. 51. Throughout this introduction I use the term "analysand," a gerundive form proposed by Ferenczi, to refer to the person who is being analyzed.

4. Brentano's wife was the sister of a famous patient of Freud's, Anna von Lieben, whom Freud called his "Lehrmeisterin" (instructress). P. Herzog, "The Myth of Freud as

Anti-Philosopher," in P. E. Stepanski, ed., *Freud: Appraisals and Reappraisals*, vol. 2 (Hillsdale, N.J., 1988); P. J. Swales, "Freud, His Teacher, and the Birth of Psychoanalysis," ibid., vol. 1 (1986).

5. E. Hartl, "Karl Kraus und die Psychoanalyse," *Merkur* (February 1977).

6. W. M. Johnston, *The Austrian Mind: An Intellectual and Social History, 1848–1938* (Berkeley, 1972), p. 64.

7. Staying at Bad Goisern, for example, were István Hollós (who wrote his book there), Heinrich Meng, and Max and Olga Graf. Freud's mother spent summers at Bad Ischl. At Grundlsee one could often find psychoanalysts of the younger generation: Siegfried Bernfeld, Berta and Stefanie Bornstein, Wilhelm Reich, Willi Hoffer, and on one occasion Marie Bonaparte. (Information provided by Ernst Federn in a letter of July 31, 1990, to Ernst Falzeder.)

8. Later, in 1917, Gizella would show Ferenczi another letter from Freud (February 11, 1917): "My previous letter to you was intended for your eyes only. It was too frank for him."

9. "To navigate is necessary, to live is not" (in Latin in the original).

10. In English in the original.

11. In English in the original.

12. "It has often been my experience that just those cases in which I took an excessive personal interest failed, perhaps just because of the intensity of feeling" (*Freud/Abraham*, December 26, 1908, p. 63).

13. In German they are expressed by the same word.

14. André Green was referring to subsequent events when he wrote: "We know that between 1928 and 1932 Ferenczi would produce a series of works on these themes which make him the father of modern psychoanalysis." *Le complexe de castration* (Paris, 1990), pp. 60–61.

15. Michael Balint, Draft "Introduction," in Sándor Ferenczi, *The Clinical Diary of Sándor Ferenczi* (Cambridge, 1988), p. 220. In 1947 Gizella Ferenczi signed an authorization making Michael Balint Sándor Ferenczi's legal representative in literary matters.

16. It was customary in German, especially in central Europe, to address the holder of a doctorate, and even his wife, with the title *Doktor.* Mrs. Ferenczi often began her letters to Anna Freud with the phrase "Liebe Freundin" (Dear Friend), whereas Anna Freud used the more formal salutation "Liebe Frau Doktor." It is likewise touching to note that these two women, exchanging letters between Bern and London, wrote in Viennese German, the German of central Europe—that *Mitteleuropa* which, along with the Jewish culture of Vienna and Budapest, Hitler had just destroyed.

17. Magda had married Lájos Ferenczi, Sándor's younger brother.

18. In Hungarian, when speaking with relatives older than oneself, one addresses men as "uncle" *(bácsi)* and women as "aunt" *(néni).*

19. Balint was referring to the third and last volume of Ferenczi's works, which was just being published in English.

20. A curious error: he doubles the number of letters. Actually, only about 1,236 letters were preserved.

21. For the complete text, see André Haynal, "Brefs aperçus sur l'histoire de la correspondance Freud-Ferenczi, 'Les intrications des différents divans,'" *Revue internationale d'histoire de la psychanalyse* 2 (1989): 243–254.

22. Balint, Draft "Introduction," p. 219.

The Correspondence of
Sigmund Freud and Sándor Ferenczi
Volume 1, 1908–1914

1

Budapest, January 18, 1908
VII., Erzsébet-körút 54[1]

Dear Professor,

I am very grateful to you that you have declared yourself ready to receive me, unknown that I am, in the company of my colleague Dr. Stein.[2] Not only because I am eager to approach personally the professor whose teachings have occupied me constantly now for approximately a year, but also because this meeting promises much that is useful and instructive.

I need erudition more than ever, now that I am about to appear before a partly ignorant, partly misinformed medical audience.[3] In view of this I am keeping in mind your axiom that, in order to be true, one must be considerate of one's audience, and I therefore want for the moment to bring out only rather conspicuous, easily understandable facts. The task is very difficult at best; I would only do harm to the cause with a tactless surprise attack and want at least to turn out to be a master in my limitation.[4]

Forgive me if I get right *in medias res.* The subject easily overwhelms one.

I thank you again for your cordiality and remain in pleasant anticipation of February 2.

Your most obedient
Dr. Ferenczi

1. Ferenczi's letterhead identifies him as a neurologist and royal forensic expert. Erzsébet-körút - Elisabeth-Ring.

2. Philipp (Fülöp) Stein (1867–1918), Hungarian psychiatrist and neurologist; proponent of the antialcohol movement. His and Ferenczi's visit with Freud was arranged by C. G. Jung (*Freud/Jung,* pp. 65f). Stein had collaborated on the latter's association experiments at the Burghölzli clinic (see letter 2, n. 4), and Ferenczi had also been a guest there (unpublished letter of Jung to Ferenczi, January 10, 1907).

3. On March 28 Ferenczi gave a speech before the Budapest Society of Physicians, "Die Neurosen im Lichte der Freudschen Forschungen" [Actual- and Psycho-Neuroses in the Light of Freud's Investigations and Psycho-Analysis] (Ferenczi 1908, 60; *F.C.*, p. 30); see letter 5, n. 2, and letter 7).

4. "In der Beschränkung zeigt sich erst der Meister / Und das Gesetz nur kann uns Freiheit geben" (The master shows himself only in limitation / And only the law can

give us freedom). Johann Wolfgang von Goethe, "Natur und Kunst" [Nature and Art] (1802), in *Sophienausgabe* IV, 129.

2

Vienna, January 30, 1908
IX., Berggasse 19[1]

Dear colleague,

I will be very pleased to see you and your colleague Dr. Stein at my home on Sunday, February 2. Owing to illness in my family[2] my wife[3] is unfortunately unable to receive both of you as guests at table, as we were able to do in better times with Dr. Jung[4] and Dr. Abraham.[5] I can only ask you to visit me at approximately 3 o'clock in the afternoon and give me the day from then on.

Collegially yours,
Dr. Freud

Best regards to Dr. Stein.

1. This line of the letterhead is preprinted. See "Note on Transcription."
2. Several members of the family had influenza; Mathilde (1887–1978), Freud's eldest child, was suffering from an abdominal irritation after an appendectomy (*Freud/Jung*, January 25, 1908, p. 113), perityphlitis, an inflammation of the peritoneal lining of the appendix and vermiform appendix (letter of Karl Abraham, March 8, 1908, to Max Eitingon, in Hilde Abraham, *Karl Abraham* [Munich, 1976], p. 81). In 1909 Mathilde married Robert Hollitscher (1875–1959), a businessman. The couple died childless, having emigrated to London with Freud in 1938.
3. Martha Freud (1861–1951), daughter of Berman (1826–1879) and Emmeline Bernays, née Philipp (1830–1910). The Bernayses were a prominent Jewish family; Isaak, Martha's paternal grandfather (1792–1849), was appointed chief rabbi of Hamburg in 1821. Of his sons, Jacob (1824–1881) became a professor of philology, and Michael (1834–1897) became a professor of literary history. Berman Bernays, a merchant, moved to Vienna with his family in 1869 and there became secretary to the national economist Lorenz von Stein. Martha became engaged to Freud in 1882 in Vienna, but in 1883 she went to Wandsbek in Germany at the behest of her mother. During their separation the engaged couple maintained an almost daily correspondence (see a selection of Freud's letters in Freud, *Letters*, and in *Brautbriefe*, ed. Ernst L. Freud [Frankfurt, 1988]). The couple were married in 1886 in a Jewish ceremony. They had six children: Mathilde, Jean Martin, Oliver, Ernst, Sophie, and Anna.
4. Carl Gustav Jung (1875–1961) was at the time chief physician at the Cantonal Sanatorium and Psychiatric University Clinic of Burghölzli in Zurich. (At the Burghölzli, under the direction of Auguste Forel and his successor, Eugen Bleuler [see letter 18, n. 2], one of the most important and progressive institutions of Europe, many subsequently well-known personalities were then guests or co-workers. The group included, among others, Karl Abraham, Roberto Greco Assagioli, Ludwig Binswanger, Trigant Burrow, Abraham Arden Brill, Charles Macfie Campbell, Imre Décsi, Max Eitingon, Sándor Fer-

enczi, Johann Jakob Honegger, Smith Eli Jelliffe, Ernest Jones, Alphonse Maeder, Herman Nunberg, Johan H. W. van Ophuijsen, Nikolai J. Ossipov, Franz Riklin, Hermann Rorschach, Tatiana Rosenthal, Leonhard Seif, Eugenie Sokolnicka, Sabina Spielrein, Philipp Stein, Wolf Stockmayer, Johannes Irgens Stromme, Jaroslaw Stuchlik, and G. Alexander Young.) By 1906 Jung's investigations of word associations had already attracted Freud's attention. Jung subsequently became a pupil, collaborator, and friend to Freud, who saw in him his "dear son and successor" (*Freud/Jung*, August 10, 1910, p. 343). Jung became editor of the first psychoanalytic periodical, the *Jahrbuch für psychoanalytische und psychopathologische Forschungen* [Yearbook for Psychoanalytic and Psychopathological Research], founded in 1908, and served as the first president of the International Psychoanalytic Association (IPA) (1910–1914). In 1912 Jung began to develop theoretical constructs which deviated from those of Freud—especially in relation to the concept of libido—and founded analytical psychology. He was a pioneer in understanding the psychoses, and he investigated the archaic heritage of the human psyche. Many were offended by his statements about the "Jewish psyche" and by his activities during the Third Reich (in 1933 he became president of the Internationale Allgemeine Ärztliche Gesellschaft für Psychotherapie [International General Medical Society for Psychotherapy] and until 1939 editor of the *Zentralblatt für Psychotherapie und ihre Grenzgebiete* [Central Organ for Psychotherapy and Related Fields]).

5. Karl Abraham (1877–1925), German psychiatrist; had been working since 1904 under Jung at the Burghölzli. In close contact with Freud since 1907, he became one of his closest collaborators and, with Sándor Ferenczi, Ernest Jones, Otto Rank, and Hanns Sachs, a charter member of the secret Committee, founded in 1912 (see letter 320 and n. 5). In 1908 Abraham founded an unofficial psychoanalytic association in Berlin which in 1910 became the first branch society of the IPA and, after the First World War, a center for psychoanalytic training and instruction. He remained its president until his death. He and Eduard Hitschmann took over the editorship of the *Jahrbuch* from Jung. From 1919 on Abraham was editor of the *Internationale Zeitschrift für (ärztliche) Psychoanalyse* [International Journal for (Medical) Psychoanalysis]. In 1914 Abraham took over the presidency of the IPA from Jung, which he held until 1918. In 1924 he was elected in his own right to this office. His theoretical works, especially those about pregenital developmental stages and psychoses, are considered classic contributions to psychoanalysis.

3

Budapest, February 10, 1908

Dear Professor,

In the course of tomorrow a Frau Marton from Tapolcza (Hungary) will look you up. I examined her several days ago and diagnosed a still rather fresh paranoia with a predilection for delusions of jealousy. A rather lengthy conversation convinced me that the patient is still capable of transference, and I believe that this is a case where one could attempt analysis with some prospect of success. But before I made a decision about this I wanted to know your opinion and had the patient travel to Vienna. The treatment must—in my opinion—be carried out in an institution. Or do you think institutionalization can be dispensed with?

Last Sunday, which I was allowed to spend in your company, is constantly on my mind, and I cannot thank you enough for the kindness and ceaseless stimulation which you showed me.

For a few days I have been rummaging through collections of Hungarian proverbs, folk songs, "riddle-tales," etc. The interpretation of riddles is quite analogous to the interpretation of dreams. Every riddle contains—I believe—a sadistic element: reveling in the torment of the riddle's solver. People who like to solve riddles may also exhibit masochistic traits. The sexual allusions in folk riddles are remarkably numerous, and all the other motives and means of presentation of the joke[1] discovered by you find application in riddles.

Your theory about the origin of phobias (which, by the way, should no longer be called theory) finds its analogy in the Hungarian proverb: "It is better to fear than to be frightened."[2]

I believe that occupying oneself with riddles sharpens the mind for the interpretation of dreams.*

Kindest regards from

Your most obedient
Dr. Ferenczi

* and interpretation of symptoms

1. *Jokes and Their Relation to the Unconscious* (Freud 1905c).
2. "Es ist besser, sich zu fürchten, als zu erschrecken." The sense of this proverb depends on a subtle difference in the meaning of the two verbs [Trans.].

4

Vienna, February 11, 1908
IX., Berggasse 19

Dear colleague,

I saw Frau Marton today. It is a [case of] mature paranoia and probably beyond the limits of therapeutic intervention; still, she may be treated, and one can in any event learn something from her. Her brother-in-law, the physician who accompanies her, is an ass; he will probably advise her to do something other than what I have proposed. I asked that she go to the institution in Budapest and be treated there by you. To get her there we should employ the fiction, which has already been introduced, that her husband is the sick one, and that she should go along to look after him. After two days we could say that her husband was called away, and, as long as it works, we could keep her in an experiment to get to the bottom of her delusion. It is possible to influence her only in that way, not through logic.

From a theoretical point of view the case has confirmed what I already knew, namely, that in these forms of paranoia it is a case of detaching the homosexual component of the libido. In consequence of juvenile homosexual fixation, she is actually attracted to all the women with whom she suspects her husband of being involved. She struggles against this attraction and projects it onto her husband; her libido for her husband is strengthened by being detached from the women. By means of her jealousy she then realizes in her husband her youthful ideal of unheard-of potency, etc.[1]—

I was very happy about your interest in riddles. You know that the riddle advertises all the techniques which the joke conceals. A parallel study would actually be instructive. No one has followed me up on aesthetic aberrations such as jokes.

Kind regards,
Your Freud

1. Freud had already brought up the role of projection in paranoia in 1896 ("Further Remarks on the Neuro-Psychoses of Defence," 1896b). At the same time the problem of paranoia was a central theme in Freud's correspondence with Jung.

5

Budapest, March 18, 1908
VII., Erzsébet-körút 54

Dear Professor,

I am taking the liberty of reporting to you on the progress of the analysis of Frau Marton (paranoia).

For all of four weeks she has maneuvered around with unimportant heterosexual stories which she shoves conspicuously into the foreground and on account of which she pretends to reproach herself.

Meanwhile it comes out *without the slightest resistance* that in boarding school she had her "ideal" among her girlfriends and that she always preferred her "incomparable" mother (at her father's expense) and that at the age of two years she was repeatedly indecently touched by a slightly older girl. She ascribes no significance to all these things. She is "absolutely not perverse."

She seems to have completely succeeded in divesting the homosexual memories of affect and transposing her attraction to women onto her husband—as you so correctly recognized.

It is remarkable that the patient always suspected her husband of involvement with very old, very young, or socially prominent females. Where she could hide her attraction behind familial or amicable relations, she didn't need to implicate her husband.

In the institution she also became friendly with a few women of her own age. Once she was caught measuring these women, wanting to ascertain who had the thickest calves.

At the same time she "despises" her attendant and finds an elderly fellow patient (whom she saw undressed) "disgusting." The disgust here seems also (as always) to be a compromise feeling of pleasure and unpleasure. (One finds "bittersweet" to be disgusting.) One must also interpret the aversion of men toward old women in the same way.—

The prospect for therapeutic success in the case of Frau Marton = o [is equal to zero]. She has simply woven psychoanalysis into her delusional system and suspects that I have sounded her out in the service of her enemies.[1]

I have finished the lecture about "the Neuroses in Light of Freudian Research."[2] It was a difficult task. I will report to you about its effects soon after the lecture (March 28) and send you a copy in German.

Many thanks for the instructions regarding the analysis of Frau Marton. They greatly facilitated my task.

Kindest regards,
Dr. Ferenczi

1. Ferenczi described this case in "Introjektion und Übertragung" [Introjection and Transference] (1909, 67; *Schriften* I, 30; *C.*, pp. 65f).
2. Published under the title "Über Aktual- und Psychoneurosen im Lichte Freudscher Forschungen und über die Psychoanalyse" [Actual and Psycho-Neuroses in the Light of Freud's Investigations and Psychoanalysis] (1908, 60; *F.C.*, p. 30).

6

Vienna, March 25, 1908
IX., Berggasse 19

Dear colleague,

Severe disturbances at home have prevented me from answering your interesting letter earlier. Now some calm has returned and I have just received the notice of your lecture, for which I wish you the best of luck, which you need for this difficult undertaking.

Don't concern yourself about the lack of success in the case of Frau Marton's paranoia. Success is not possible there, but we need these analyses in order finally to reach an understanding of all neuroses. I believe that the case is typical, and you have comprehended it flawlessly. I have often seen it so: a woman unsatisfied by a man naturally turns to a woman and tries to invest her long-suppressed gynecophilic component with libido. But a resistance arises against it; she can no longer become homosexual, and for that reason she detaches her libido from the woman. In paranoia it often happens that the sublimations are destroyed by this projection and the homosexual component in particular comes to the fore.

—Today the program for Salzburg[1] arrived; I am very much looking forward to seeing you and Dr. Stein again there. Give him my warmest regards. We became very good friends in one day.

Yours truly,
Freud

1. The first international meeting of psychoanalysts, called the First Congress for Freudian Psychology by Jung in his printed invitation (*Freud/Jung*, ca. January 18–20, 1908, pp. 110f). It was held in Salzburg on April 27, 1908. According to Jung, the inspiration for the conference came from Ernest Jones (see letter 9, n. 3) and from the "Budapesters," Ferenczi and Stein (*Freud/Jung*, November 30, 1907, p. 101).

7

Budapest, March 28, 1908
9 P.M.

Dear Professor,

I have just come out of the Society of Physicians, where I gave the lecture which I announced to you. It was a "success," as they say;—the medical public listened to your teachings with great attentiveness and much applause.—Naturally, there were two neurologists who spoke against it, *Dr. Donat*[1] and *Dr. Sarbó*.[2] Both raised the most hackneyed objections. When I have the official transcript in my hands, I will communicate the discussion to you *in extenso*. It was easy for me to refute them. The discussion was rather heated, at times personal. But I believe most were on my side and had a sense of the scope of the questions that interest us.

I offered to psychoanalyze Messrs. D[onath] and S[arbó] a little—they *never* concern themselves with the cause (and I reproached them for that)—then, I said, they will certainly be on our side.

Donat is, by the way, a *conditional* adherent to the doctrine. He considers it valid for certain cases. *Sarbó* was at times outrageous; I didn't owe him the dignity of a reply. (No complex left behind.)

I must forward the compliments given to me to the right address and thank you for the opportunity to be the first to be able to interpret such important questions here.

Many thanks for your kind letter, and with obedient greetings to your family, I am

Thankfully yours,
Dr. Ferenczi

1. Gyula Donáth (1849–1945), since 1902 chief physician, St. Stephen's Hospital, Budapest. "Donat" is Ferenczi's spelling.
2. Artúr von Sarbó (1867–1943), chief physician in the neurological section of the Workers' Health Insurance Company and in St. Stephen's Hospital.

8

Vienna, March 30, 1908[1]

Esteemed colleague,

Very happy about your courageous step and its success. Would like to believe that you defended yourself capably. Carry on.

You will in the meantime have received "Anal Erotism."[2]

Cordially,
Freud

1. Postcard.
2. "Character and Anal Erotism" (Freud 1908b).

9

Budapest, May 9, 1908
VII., Erzsébet-körút 54

Dear Professor,

You were so kind as to empower me to write to you regarding my summer stay in Berchtesgaden.[1] Since I am also in an official position,[2] I must be clear about the time of my departure in order to arrange for someone to represent me. For that reason I am free to request that you inform me by means of a postcard when I can avail myself of your permission to spend some time with you in Berchtesgaden. I intend to spend four weeks there, but I would consider myself fortunate if I could spend only a few hours in your company and will by no means be a burden to you. If I could be of assistance to you in some work or other, I would do so with pleasure.

Messrs. Jones[3] and Brill[4] spent yesterday in Budapest. We spoke almost exclusively about psychological matters and about the splendid success of the Salzburg gathering.

Since my return home, the analytical work is going much more briskly, especially since I have become more aware of the important question of the transference to the physician.

I am reading Rank's excellent book (The Artist)[5] with much satisfaction.

In the April issue of the "Neuer Rundschau" I read the following lines by Gerhart Hauptmann[6] in a description of his travels in Greece:

And it becomes strangely vivid to me, how Greek culture is buried, but still not dead. It is buried very deeply, but only in the souls of living men; and only when one knows all the layers of marl and slag under which the Greek soul lies buried, as one knows the layers over the Mycenaean, Trojan, or Olympian sites of old cultural remains, of stone and ore, then perhaps the great hour of excavation will also come for the living heritage of Greece.[7]

I would like to call Hauptmann's attention to the extent to which the excavations have already progressed.

With kindest regards and with a renewal of my request, I remain

Your obedient
Dr. Ferenczi

1. During the Salzburg meeting Freud had invited Ferenczi to spend part of the summer with him and his family (see letter 11). In Salzburg Freud had spoken for more than four hours about the analysis of the "Rat-Man" (Freud 1909d). Ferenczi had spoken on the theme "Welche praktischen Winke ergeben sich aus den Freudschen Erfahrungen für die Kindererziehung?" [What Practical Tips for the Rearing of Children Come from Freudian Experiences?] ("Psychoanalyse und Pädagogik" [Psychoanalysis and Education], Ferenczi 1908, 63; *Fin.*, p. 280), the first work about education in the psychoanalytic literature. It was also decided to publish the *Jahrbuch* under the direction of Freud and Bleuler and the editorship of Jung.

2. Ferenczi was chief physician of the neurological-psychiatric outpatient department of the Budapest General Health Insurance Company (1904–1910) and neurological and psychiatric specialist for the court of Budapest (1905–1918).

3. Ernest Jones (1879–1958), Welsh psychiatrist. He had first been made aware of Freud by his friend Wilfred Trotter; in 1907 he met Jung at the Neurological Congress in Amsterdam, and shortly thereafter spent a short time at the Burghölzli. He met Freud for the first time in Salzburg, after which he and Brill visited Freud in Vienna. Jones played an extremely significant role in the psychoanalytic movement and its historiography. He was, along with Ferenczi, an initiator of the Committee, founder of the American and London (later British) psychoanalytic societies, president of the IPA from 1920 to 1924 and 1934 to 1949, and author of the well-known Freud biography (Jones I–III). Jones underwent an analysis with Ferenczi in 1913 and translated and edited a number of his writings; their later relationship was strained, however, and they differed on important organizational and theoretical issues. Among Jones's scientific writings are a

large number of works on the dissemination of psychoanalysis, as well as on specific themes (psychoanalysis and religion, *Hamlet*, and symbolism, among others). His writings on female sexuality gave rise to a number of controversies.

4. Abraham Arden Brill (1874–1948), psychiatrist of Hungarian-Jewish origin, emigrated alone at the age of fourteen to New York, where in 1903 he began a course of study in medicine. After a practicum at the Burghölzli and a brief analysis with Freud, he returned to the United States in 1908, where in 1911 he founded the New York Psychoanalytic Society and became its first president. Brill was professor of psychiatry at New York University and lecturer in psychoanalysis at Columbia University. He translated many of Freud's and some of Jung's works into English.

5. Otto Rank (originally Rosenfeld) (1884–1939), a learned trade school student, had introduced himself—by arrangement with his personal physician, Alfred Adler—to Freud and became one of his first students and closest collaborators. He was paid secretary and scribe for the Wednesday Psychological Society, the discussion group meeting in Freud's apartment which in 1908 became the Vienna Psychoanalytic Society. With Freud's support he undertook a course of study (Ph.D. 1912) and from 1912 to 1924 was, in close collaboration with Freud, editor of the periodicals *Imago* and *Internationale Zeitschrift für (ärztliche) Psychoanalyse* and from 1919 to 1924 head of the International Psychoanalytic Press. Around the time of publication of his book *Das Trauma der Geburt* [The Trauma of Birth] (Leipzig, 1924), he gradually became estranged from Freud and Ferenczi and distanced himself in his relations with them. Rank had been friendly with Ferenczi and had published *Entwicklungsziele der Psychoanalyse* (Leipzig, 1924) (*The Development of Psychoanalysis* [New York, 1925]) with him. In 1926 Rank moved to Paris and then in 1934 to the United States. Many of his works—especially those on the artist and on mythology—are regarded as classics. His writings of the 1920s about separation anxiety and psychoanalytic technique, which unleashed stormy controversy at the time, are viewed today as pioneering works which have exerted undeniable influence. His further development of an abbreviated therapy, however, which was based on the individual's ability to make decisions ("will therapy"), was likewise influential but can no longer be considered psychoanalytic. Ferenczi is referring here to Rank's book *Der Künstler, Ansatz zu einer Sexualpsychologie* [The Artist: An Approach to Sexual Psychology] (Vienna, 1907).

6. Gerhart Hauptmann (1862–1946), German poet and dramatist, representative of naturalism in the German-speaking countries. He received the Nobel Prize for literature in 1912.

7. "Und seltsam eindringlich wird es mir, wie das Griechentum zwar begraben, doch nicht gestorben ist. Es ist sehr tief, aber nur in den Seelen lebendiger Menschen begraben, und wenn man erst alle die Schichten von Mergel und Schlacke, unter denen die Griechenseele begraben liegt, kennen wird, wie man die Schichten kennt über den mykenäischen, trojanischen oder olympischen Fundstellen aller Kulturreste, aus Stein und Erz, so kommt auch vielleicht für das lebendige Griechenerbe die grosse Stunde der Ausgrabung." Gerhart Hauptmann "Aus einer griechischen Reise," 2d ser., in *Die neue Rundschau*, no. 19 of the *freie Bühne*, vol. 2 (Berlin, 1908), pp. 584–599; quotation on p. 599.

10

Vienna, May 10, 1908
IX., Berggasse 19

Dear colleague,

On July 15 we are going to Berchtesgaden, where we have rented a beautiful, isolated house called Dietfeldhof. I usually stay there with my family until around September 1 and then take a short trip, which this year will probably take me to Holland and England. You are welcome at any time, whether you spend the weeks of your vacation in Berchtesgaden or whether you want to spend part of the time on the trip with me. It is understood at the outset that you will not disturb me in my work and that I won't have to take any precautions against you, but I can only look forward to discussing various things with you and not completely dispensing with meaningful association.

We can easily find lodging for you in a boardinghouse or hotel once we are there. Now and then you will take a meal with us or climb a mountain with my boys.[1]

In expectation of hearing from you again,

Cordially,
Freud

1. Jean Martin (1889–1967), Oliver (1891–1969), and Ernst (1892–1970). Martin studied law, receiving his doctorate in 1913, and from 1932 on was business manager of the International Psychoanalytic Press. In 1919 he married Ernestine Drucker (1896–1980) and had two children, Anton Walter (b. 1921) and Sofie (b. 1924). Oliver became an engineer (1915) and in 1923 married Henny Fuchs (1892–1971). The couple had a daughter, Eva Mathilde (1924–1944). Ernst studied architecture; in 1920 he married Lucie Brasch (1896–?) and had three children, Stephan Gabriel (b. 1921), Lucian Michael (b. 1922), and Clement Raphael (b. 1924). Freud's sons all emigrated to London and died without returning to Vienna. An especially close relationship developed between Martin Freud and Ferenczi. See Martin Freud, *Sigmund Freud, Man and Father* (New York, 1958), p. 109.

11

Budapest, June 23, 1908
VII., Erzsébet-körút 54

Dear Professor,

Since I am not able to attend the meetings of the Vienna Freud Society, I would at least like to belong as a corresponding member, and I would like to initiate myself, as the strict statutes require,[1] with the enclosed short paper.[2] It is actually intended not only for this select circle but also for the medical public at large, and therefore contains much that would be of interest only to the latter. But such popularizing works are probably not yet superfluous. I beg your forgiveness for the lack of style.

In order to save you time I have not answered your last friendly letter, in which you were so kind as to renew in writing our conversation in Salzburg about our sojourn together this summer. I am using this opportunity to thank you kindly for the information.—Rarely have I so looked forward to the vacation as this year. I have only four weeks at my disposal.—I want to distribute them in such a way that I can spend fourteen days in Berchtesgaden and the other fourteen on the trip with you. Accordingly, I will arrive in Berchtesgaden on August 15. If you consider it necessary, I will accept your kind offer regarding lodging and inform you in a timely fashion of the exact time of my arrival.

I must also thank you for your kindness in recommending me to Dr. Bedö (a lawyer in Budapest). He spoke with me already. The treatment with his wife has not yet begun, however.

Your most obedient
Dr. Ferenczi

1. There were no statutes in the organizational sense in the Wednesday Society. New members were elected, and it was customary for them to introduce themselves with a lecture. Stricter criteria for membership—such as election by secret ballot with a two-thirds majority—were discussed on February 5 and 12, 1908, and finally rejected (*Minutes* I, 298–302, 315f).

2. "Analytische Deutung und Behandlung der psychosexuellen Impotenz des Mannes" [Analytic Interpretation and Treatment of Psychosexual Impotence in Men] (1908, 61; *C.*, p. 11).

12

Vienna, June 28, 1908
IX., Berggasse 19

Dear colleague,

Your idea of entering our Society as a corresponding member will probably meet with the approval of all the members. I will bring it up in the fall,[1] since our gatherings have been suspended until then. You will be assessed a small sum of money as a member's contribution, which, in addition to the honor, will give you the right to use the library, to vote with the membership, etc. In short, quite a cheerful story.

Your beautiful, clear work[2] should not lie around unused for so long, however. It is especially suited for publication, and I would like to request that you choose where you would like it to go. If you choose the *Zentralblatt für Geschlechtskrankheiten* [Central Periodical for Sexual Illnesses] like Steiner,[3] then I will send it back to you immediately after your decla-ration. But if you wish, I can send it myself to Bresler,[4] who will certainly not refuse to accept it for his monthly, as he does with other short works.

As to the matter itself, I would note the following: I share completely your views and experiences but wonder only about the following: since the family complex (Oedipus complex) is overemphasized in *all* neurotics, there is need for only one factor to determine that it is specifically the inhibition of potency that occurs instead of some other neurotic distur-bance.[5] Now what this factor is, whether constitutional or accidental (such as the association of unpleasure in the first attempt at sexual activity, punishment in childhood), requires clarification, and that actually contains the riddle of ψ impotence to begin with. But this is esoteric; for the public, your investigations, as well as Steiner's and Stekel's,[6] are sufficient.

The choice of time of your arrival in Berchtesgaden is quite agreeable to me. By then I will certainly be sufficiently restored from the travails of the past year that I will be able to have the desired pleasure of your company. I hope you won't say no to climbing the mountains with my youngsters, if this is on your agenda. We will find lodging for you.

The treatment of the young wife of the lawyer is not supposed to begin until fall; it will be a very interesting task. Of course with neurotics, everything is uncertain as soon as a postponement becomes unavoidable.

Cordially,
Your Freud

From July 15 on: Berchtesgaden, Dietfeldhof

1. Freud proposed Ferenczi as a new member on October 7, 1908. He was unanimously accepted (*Minutes* II, 1).

2. See letter 11, n. 2.

3. Maximilian Steiner (1874–1942), specialist in skin and sexual diseases and member of the Wednesday Society. In 1907 he had published a paper, "Die funktionelle Impotenz des Mannes und ihre Behandlung" [Functional Impotence in the Male and Its Treatment], in the *Wiener Medizinische Presse* (no. 48, col. 1535), not in the *Zentralblatt für Geschlechtskrankheiten.*

4. Johannes Bresler (1866–1936), psychiatrist; editor of the *Psychiatrisch-neurologische Wochenschrift* [Psychiatric-Neurological Weekly] (N.B.: not Monthly), in which Fer-enczi's paper was also published.

5. In his paper (1908, 61) Ferenczi had stressed the role of incestuous fixation as a cause of impotence.

6. Wilhelm Stekel (1868–1940), Viennese neurologist, originally from Bukovina. As Freud's analysand and one of his first students, he had prompted the founding of the Wednesday Society. Author of numerous popular articles and books about psychoanaly-sis, he was (initially with Adler) editor of the *Zentralblatt,* where, after his estrangement from Freud in 1912—probably owing to differences in temperament as well as Stekel's attempts at abbreviated therapy—he continued on his own until 1914. His numerous

contributions to the investigation of symbols were always viewed by Freud as fundamental and were integrated into *The Interpretation of Dreams* (Freud 1900a). Freud here cites Stekel's book *Nervöse Angstzustände und ihre Behandlung* [Conditions of Nervous Anxiety and Their Treatment] (Berlin, 1908), to which he had written a foreword (Freud 1908f).

13

Budapest, July 3, 1908
VII., Erzsébet-körút 54

Dear Professor,

I thank you cordially for your willingness to find accommodation for my little work. I prefer Bresler's *Wochenschrift* to a sexual periodical and permit myself to request that you send the article there.

To be sure, I am aware that this work does not get to the heart of the impotence question. That has to do with the question of the more precise pathogenesis of neuroses in general, the solution to which we are awaiting first from you. Adler's theory of inferiority is certainly not the last word on this contentious issue;[1] it is actually only a broader extension of your idea of "somatic compliance."[2] Adler's weighty hypothesis (somatic inferiority—psychic overachievement) should not achieve general validity; it is just as easily possible that organic superiority causes the overemphasis. In addition to a quantitative factor (deficit or surplus of substance), the *temporal* disposition of *one* specific *organ* (in the sense of Fliess's doctrine of periodicity)[3] could play a role, e.g., as *locus minoris resistentiae* [the path of least resistance] at the moment of a psychic insult. In any event, Fliess, to the best of my knowledge, knows only the periodic stress of body sectors and not of organs.

The vulnerability of organs may also come into consideration. The reflex function of copulation is probably the most complicated that the infracortical nervous system is capable of. No wonder it breaks down in so many neurotics.

We should perhaps approach the question of the constitutional factor by means of numerous *family analyses* and pay particular attention to cases where the family members were exposed to quite different influences of milieu.

The long and short of this lengthy discourse is, however, that I cannot say much about the essence of the pathogenesis of impotence; that is why I left these questions untouched. Perhaps I should have touched on them *as questions to be posed.*

I am looking forward to the Bavarian mountains no less than to Messrs. your sons. It will be a pleasure to go on excursions with them.

Dr. Campbell[4] and wife visited me yesterday. I devoted an evening to them. They send you their best regards, Professor.—Once again, with thanks for your kindness, I remain

Your obedient
Dr. Ferenczi

1. Alfred Adler (1870–1937), Viennese physician and psychologist, in contact with Freud since at least 1899 (see Freud to Adler, February 27, 1899, Library of Congress); had been a member of the Wednesday Society from its beginnings (1902). In 1910 he became presiding officer of the Vienna Psychoanalytic Society and (with Wilhelm Stekel) editor of the *Zentralblatt.* In 1911 he went his own way and founded the field of individual psychology, which views itself as a unique movement, different from psychoanalysis, which emphasizes, among other things, the role of aggression, of rivalry among siblings, and social factors. Adler's *Studie über die Minderwertigkeit von Organen* [Study on the Inferiority of Organs] (Berlin, 1907) was based on the premise that the "inferiority" of an organ (e.g., morphological phenomena of loss, anomalies of reflex capability or deformities) can lead to compensation in the motor, neurological, or psychic domain.

2. Freud coined the expression "somatic compliance" and first mentioned it in the case history of "Dora" ("Fragment of an Analysis of a Case of Hysteria," 1905e [1901]), by which he meant a "normal or pathological process in or connected with one of the bodily organs" (p. 40), which in hysteria "may afford the unconscious mental processes a physical outlet" (p. 41).

3. Wilhelm Fliess (1858–1928), Berlin physician and specialist in diseases of the ear, nose, and throat, and Freud's closest friend from 1887 to 1900 (see Freud's *Letters to Fliess*); had developed a comprehensive theory about the role of periods of twenty-eight and twenty-three days, to whose influence he believed the entire organic world to be subjected (*Der Ablauf des Lebens, Grundlegung zur exakten Biologie* [The Course of Life: Foundation for an Exact Biology], Leipzig, 1906). After the break in their relations—in which accusations of plagiarism played a role (see letter 163, n. 2)—Freud remained skeptical about these and other of Fliess's theories.

4. Charles Macfie Campbell (1876–1943), Scottish physician and co-founder of the *Review of Neurology and Psychiatry* (Edinburgh), visited Freud and Ferenczi at the beginning of July. He later moved to the United States, where he became a professor in Baltimore and at Harvard.

14

Vienna, July 14, 1908[1]

Dear colleague,
Bresler has just confirmed acceptance of your paper.

Cordially,
Freud

1. Postcard.

15

Budapest, July 17, 1908
VII., Erzsébet-körút 54

Dear Professor,
    Many thanks for your efforts in the interests of my work. My next project will be a commentary on Ibsen's works in the light of their psychology. It is astounding how much he has anticipated. The Lady from the Sea,[1] for example, could be compared with the psychoanalytic treatment of an obsessional idea.[2] The other works are also full of apt presentiments and allusions. Before I became acquainted with your work I never fully understood Ibsen, and I don't completely understand his previous commentators even now. To be sure, he didn't even understand *himself* completely. I am thinking of arriving in Berchtesgaden on August 25. I ask you to concern yourself with lodging only if you think it is necessary to make advance reservations. I don't want to burden you unnecessarily.

Your gratefully obedient
Dr. Ferenczi

1. In Henrik Ibsen's *Lady from the Sea* (1888), the heroine Ellida's husband, Dr. Wangel, helps her come to grips with her past and her fantasies. See also letter 114.
2. Ferenczi never did write a paper about Ibsen's works, but he did take up the idea he mentions here several times, for example in "Psychoanalyse und Suggestion" [Suggestion and Psychoanalysis] (1911, 94; *Unbewusstes*, pp. 198f; *F.C.*, p. 59), where he also briefly recapitulates the action of Ibsen's play.

16

Budapest, August 3, 1908
VII., Erzsébet-körút 54

Dear Professor,
    I have arranged for my vacation to begin two days earlier. Taking advantage of your gracious offer, I am taking the liberty of informing you that I

will arrive in Berchtesgaden on August 8. If you have made arrangements for me with a boardinghouse or hotel in the meantime, please be so kind as to notify them of my arrival.

I am quite exhausted from the efforts of the past year and am looking forward to the beauties of the mountainscape which I have missed for so long. I don't need to repeat the fact that I am anticipating this vacation with doubled joy.

With respectful greetings to you and your family, I remain

Your obedient
Dr. Ferenczi

I have taken the liberty of having my mail temporarily forwarded to your address.

17

Berchtesgaden, Dietfeldhof
August 4, 1908

Dear colleague,

I have just reserved a room for you at the Hotel Bellevue, not too far from us; it is impossible to be close by, because of the isolated location of our house. I may say that I am very much looking forward to your coming, although a change in circumstances has disrupted an anticipated pleasure. On September 1 I have to go to England, where my brother's family awaits me,[1] and I am unable to visit some of the cities of Holland in your company a week earlier, as I had planned.

I am swamped with the work of writing.[2] I find everything more difficult and wearying than I had imagined, and I hope that you will occasionally tear me away from it.

Until now I have had little vacation. My boys will be pleased if you are a mountaineer and are willing to make a planned tour of the Hochkönig.[3] Our house will remain open to you, but you should maintain your freedom, and you should not be surprised if I go about my business.

Auf Wiedersehen.

Cordially,
Freud

1. Freud's half-brother Emanuel (1833–1914), son of Jakob Freud (1815–1896) and his first wife, Sally Kanner (?-1852?); his wife, Marie (1836–1923); and their children Pauline (1856–1944), Bertha (1859–1940), and Solomon (Samuel) (1860–1945). The family lived in Manchester, where Emanuel ran a dry goods shop. The couple had already lost four children: John (b. 1855, missing after 1875), Matilda (1862–1868), Harriet Emily (1865–1868), and Henrietta (b. and d. 1866). See also letter 18, n. 1.

2. Freud was working on the final draft of "Little Hans" (Freud 1909b), and probably also on his analysis of the "Rat-Man" and his article "On the Sexual Theories of Children" (1908c); see *Freud/Jung*, June 21, July 18, and August 5, 1908, pp. 159, 165–166.

3. Alp in the vicinity of Berchtesgaden.

18

Vienna, October 7, 1908
IX., Berggasse 19

Dear colleague,

I am happy to be able to correspond with you uninterruptedly once again. My visit to Zurich was very satisfying.[1] Jung is making a complete break with Bleuler,[2] is going unreservedly with us, and arranged some very pleasant days for me.

On Friday, the 9th of this month, Bleuler and his wife, who are here for the Congress for the Treatment of the Insane,[3] will be our guests for the evening.[4] Would it be possible for you to be with us (8 P.M.) (or somewhat later)? They will all be pleased, as you know.

This afternoon is the first "Almtanz."[5]

Best regards,
Your Freud

In a hurry.

1. After his trip to England, Freud traveled by way of Berlin, where he visited relatives, to Zurich, and was Jung's guest in his house at the Burghölzli September 18–21. Subsequently he spent a few days with his sister-in-law Minna Bernays at Lake Garda (see letter 50, n. 3).

2. Eugen Bleuler (1857–1939), prominent Swiss psychiatrist, professor in Zurich; was the director of the Burghölzli and thus Jung's superior. He coined the terms *schizophrenia, autism*, and *ambivalence*. He was a champion of the antialcohol movement. This role, and above all his misgivings about taking part in the psychoanalytic movement, led to tensions with Freud (see Freud-Bleuler correspondence, Library of Congress; F. Alexander and S. T. Selesnick, "Freud-Bleuler Correspondence," *Archives of General Psychology* 12 [1965]: 1–9; and Jones II, 72f. Jung had a strained relationship with Bleuler and was about to give up his position in the clinic to open a private practice.

3. Third International Congress for the Treatment of the Insane, Vienna, October 7–11, 1908.

4. "They were very kind, insofar as his inaccessibility and her affectation permit," Freud reported to Abraham (*Freud/Abraham*, p. 54).

5. Traditional dance festival on the Alm (alpine meadow), often at the beginning or end of the Alm season. Here the term refers to the first gathering of the Wednesday Society after the summer break.

19

Budapest, October 12, 1908

Dear Professor,

Lately I have caught hold of *daydreams* in myself and in others and tried to explain them. The result was, naturally, the full confirmation of your theory of dreams. In your "Creative Writers and Day-Dreaming"[1] I find the *undistorted* wishful daydreams fully explained. In my experience, however, fantasies are often (usually) subjected to the same distortions as night-dreams. There are, for example, very many anxious dreams (imaginings of unpleasant eventualities or probabilities, often also pleasurable fantasies which are seemingly quite unjustified). Partly daydreams are impatient fantasies about unpleasant things that lie ahead. The "wish fulfillment" in this case is mainly the circumstance that the expected trouble is presented as immediate—one is therefore rid of the anxiety of expectation. This corresponds approximately to the frequently repeated wish, "If only I had already overcome it!"

Part of these fantasies goes further and adds to the anticipated unpleasant events in the fantasy less unfavorable ones, which signify finally a good outcome to the bad things which cannot be avoided. #[2] In both of these instances it could be—just as in the comical, in contrast to the joke—a case of the fulfillment of *preconscious* wishes (albeit ones that have perhaps been strengthened by the unconscious).[3]

There are, however, also anxious or horrible daydreams about whose meaning the preconscious can give no clarification. These can be explained only by means of strict dream analysis, and they then prove to be concealed realizations of *repressed*—therefore unconscious—wishes. (I mention for example an earthquake fantasy which I had in the Museo delle Terme;[4] it concealed selfish but completely unconscious wishes which could have been realized by an earthquake in the museum.)

Displacement, condensation, plays the same role in all fantasies of the latter sort as it does in night-dreams. With regard to indirect presentation, I found a difference between the healthy and the neurotic. In the latter, fantasy also comes close to dream in this regard; in the healthy person—whose criticism is much more active in the waking state—the symbolisms, the words of double meaning, etc. seem to achieve a lesser significance than in the night-dream.—The reverse relationship occurs with "secondary revision."[5] It occupies the greatest space in daydreams (in waking, one wants on no account to have thought something quite nonsensical or illogical). So-called normal people, however, manage to achieve this much better than psychoneurotics, whose daydreams much more frequently bear the character of the illogical and inexplicable.

The fantasies of the psychoneurotic are "symptom thoughts"; the relative potency of unconscious wishes whose repression failed "complicates" extraordinarily the otherwise easily understandable preconscious wishful impulses.

In the healthy person the ucs. is so completely layered over by the pcs. that in the waking state only a few and distant characters from the ucs. stray into the fantasies. The fantasies of the normal person are thus *usually* motivated by preconscious or sublimated wishes.—All kinds of possible transitions are available between both, however, according to individual character development. Even in one who otherwise fantasizes "meaningfully," some exciting external cause can disrupt the security of the repression and make possible temporary neurotic fantasies (as well as other "symptoms").

Musical people very often conceal their fantasies—according to content or mood—behind the same associable melodies.

Fantasies that are fragments or displacements of unconscious trains of thought are perhaps transitions to the "unconscious fantasies" of neurotics. "Unconscious fantasies" probably exist in all people during the course of their lives, however; but in normal people they make no or only slight complications in preconscious fantasies and in conscious thought.

I can show you this letter as an interesting example of how one can deceive oneself in fantasizing, as in the dream, so completely about the *value* of one's thoughts. As I was sitting down to write, I believed myself to be so full of the most valuable thoughts about fantasizing. Now I see that I have not gotten beyond banalities of Freudian psychology and dream theory (banalities, naturally, only for your adherents). I will overcome my vanity and send you this letter anyway. Nothing is totally unsuitable as an impetus to something better.

In overestimating my ideas about daydreams, it may have been a case of a small displacement. You see, I now have something to say about paranoia which could yield a minor confirmation of your conception of its essence. I was telling you that my maid's husband suffers from an insane alcoholic jealousy. Now, I established that his jealousy, which is directed against all men (more precisely, against his wife because of all men) rises and falls with his consumption of alcohol. During an abstinence lasting six weeks he acted quite calm; he has been drinking for four days—since then he has been incessantly reproachful and suspicious of everyone.—In my opinion that corresponds completely with your view, according to which the insane idea always comes to light in conjunction with a renewed flaring up of previously withdrawn libido. Alcohol is well known as a *pleasure-producing* medium; it makes one talkative, inclined toward tenderness, capable of sexual arousal. But in the case of previous disturbance (regressive formation) of object love, such a shot of libido must be extremely painful; it is therefore transposed in a different guise onto other persons—in fact, onto the original object of one's love. (In my maid's case, the libido was at some point disengaged from the *heterosexual* component.)

From all this it follows, however, that "alcoholic persecution, that is to say, jealousy mania," must be conceived of not as the specific effect of alcohol, but as an intensification and projection of libido caused by a pleasure-producing toxin in an individual who has already previously been autoerotic.

One can conceive of an analogy between the (actual) anxiety neurosis and the persecution anxiety in paranoia. In both cases it has to do with an excess of libido which has not been psychically mastered and has changed its sign. But I have no experience as to what influence consumption of alcohol has on an anxious person.

Observations of alcoholic paranoids will have a certain significance for a future "sexual chemistry."[6]

I hope I will have the opportunity to go over these questions in more detail;[7] I therefore ask you to send this letter back when you get a chance. Notes like these—right from the spigot—are later of a certain value.

I think back with much pleasure about the evening which, alas, flew by so quickly.[8] I feel lonely here, without someone to talk to. You will, I fear, have many letters wash over you from your very obedient

Dr. Ferenczi

Best wishes to your dear family.

I am sorry that in the few hours with you I was unable to find out the details of the conversation about paranoia you had with Jung.[9] I would especially like to have learned more about the recognition that in paranoia it is *always* a case of recrudescent homosexuality. Incidentally, I find it theoretically highly plausible that the failure of the detachment of libido consists precisely in the fact that the libido is actually detached from only one part of the objects (the heterosexual), whereby the homosexuality which had been repressed undergoes a sudden strengthening, that is to say, overemphasis, so that it must press forward into consciousness, but as a consequence of resistance it is presented with a negative sign and as a projection, if only symbolically. This applies to ordinary persecution mania (being persecuted by those of the same sex).

More complicated, however, is the case of jealousy mania. Here, not even the heterosexual libido appears to have been withdrawn; it returns as a "revenant" to the formerly beloved person, as a negative projection—at the same time, however, it is also projected onto those of the same gender, and both systems of projection are welded together into a unity, that of jealousy mania.

Normal jealousy of the male, for example,—the fear that the beloved person can be attracted to another man—*is already partly a projection of homosexual libidinal impulses onto the woman.* In some modern writers I found written down the observation that men conceal from themselves and from the world an unadmitted liking for and great interest in their rivals.

It is probable that in the end it will come out that the path from paranoia via paranoid dementia to dementia praecox is a continuous transition, and that the proportional relationship of autoerotism and projection can be different in every case of disturbance of object love. The content of the delusional ideas will also probably always be explicable if in each case one asks: From which libidinal tendencies could the patient completely withdraw cathexis, and which ones were projected by him to the outside?

———

[This insert was written on a loose single page which was enclosed.]

(The following reverse situation occurs more frequently: unconcealed fantasies of wish fulfillment with subsequent painful ones. The latter play the role of the censor—they are the punishment for having been caught in something forbiddingly egoistic, erotic, or fantastic-childish. They are logical or moral corrections of wish fantasies.)

[10]

1. Freud 1908e.

2. This symbol, as well as a similar one at the beginning of the final paragraph of the letter, was added in blue ink.

3. See Freud 1905c, pp. 174, 208.

4. The Roman National Museum, housed partly in the rooms of the Baths of Diocletian.

5. See Freud 1900a, pp. 488–508.

6. An allusion to Freud's idea of a chemism of sexual processes (see Freud 1905d, pp. 212–216, and 1906a, pp. 278f).

7. Many of the thoughts expressed here, as well as those about correcting fantasies, were later taken up by Ferenczi in "Über lenkbare Träume" [Dirigible Dreams] (1912, 83; *Fin.*, p. 313) and in "Gedanken über das Trauma" [Some Thoughts on Trauma] (1934, 296; included in *Notes and Fragments* [1920 and 1930–1933]; *Fin.*, pp. 216–278]; about temporary neurotic phenomena in "Über passagère Symptombildungen während der Analyse" [On Transitory Symptom Constructions during Analysis] (1912, 85; *C.*, p. 193); on musical associations in "Zur Deutung einfallender Melodien" [On the Interpretation of Tunes Which Come into One's Head] (1938 [1909], 299; *Fin.*, p. 175); and those about the role of alcohol and homosexual tendencies in paranoia in "Alkohol und Neurosen" [Alcohol and Neuroses] (1911, 81) and in "Über die Rolle der Homosexualität in der Pathogenese der Paranaoia" [On the Part Played by Homosexuality in the Pathogenesis of Paranoia" (1911, 89; *C.*, p. 161ff), where he also describes the case he talks about here (*Schriften* I, 77–78).

8. Ferenczi had evidently accepted Freud's invitation for October 9 (see letter 18).

9. He refers to Freud's visit with Jung in September.

10. The letter ends with a line drawn in blue ink.

20

Vienna, October 27, 1908
IX., Berggasse 19

Dear colleague,

If I answer your letters so late and inadequately, then one can justifiably conclude that this results from an external disruption, because internally nothing has changed between us. In fact, I can inform you that my daughter has become engaged to a young man of her own choosing, a young merchant, Robert Hollitscher, here in Vienna, with whom she became acquainted—or, at least, better acquainted—in Merano.[1] The mood is a very happy one, but there is naturally much more than usual that takes up one's free time.

I therefore refrain from answering your letter in more detail, but I do note already today that I regard your work on daydreams as very fruitful. I know the difficulties; one can monitor fantasies completely only in one's own person, and there one cannot share them.

Perhaps you have sought too anxiously to confirm me. If you abandon this intention, you will find rich material from whose investigation confirmation will certainly emerge in the end.

I would like to talk with you soon about your nice remarks about paranoia; I would like to see you soon in any case. I can say the inner as well as the outer circle of Berggasse 19 will be very happy about your visit.

Cordially,
Freud

1. Freud's convalescent daughter Mathilde (see letter 2, n. 2) had spent half a year recovering in Merano, in the Italian Alps. Her marriage to Robert Hollitscher (1876–1959) took place February 7, 1909 (see letter 37).

21

Budapest, November 22, 1908
VII., Erzsébet-körút 54

Dear Professor,

The second edition of your "Interpretation of Dreams," which you were kind enough to send me, is to me not only a valuable gift but also the symbol of last summer in Berchtesgaden, the most meaningful one that I have ever experienced. I have already hurriedly read once through the bracketed passages; the new chapter on typical dreams[1] brought me the solution to many heretofore unsolved dream problems. [2 A small contribution to tooth-pulling dreams: In the first and second grade we green boys applied our freshly learned Latin to school pornography (a not yet sufficiently appreciated chapter of juvenile sexuality). Among other things was the following bad Latin verse, which as far as I know had been going around for an incalculably long time:

"Inter pedes est figura,
Inde fluit aqua pura.
Barbam habet, sed non dentes,
Inde oriuntur gentes."[3]

It is noteworthy that in normal (not anatomical) Hungarian vernacular no distinction is made between foot (pes) and leg (crus). The comparison between external female genitals and the face, between vulva and mouth, seems to be deeply rooted in the popular consciousness. As an insult, on the other hand, the mouth is often referred to by the name of the female genital or the rectal opening. In Kleinpaul's Stromgebiet der Sprache[4] I have found numerous instances which speak for the generally human aspect of this identification.—

I am sorry that I have not yet had any tooth-pulling dreams to analyze (other than one of my own). The expression "sich einen herunterreissen"[5] has completely different analogs in Hungarian. Would the interpretation be different with Hungarians?[6]]

The analyses (4–5) are going very well now. Not always, to be sure; there are days when one experiences many unpleasant things. I am still taking my patients' affairs too much to heart.

The "Rundschau" and the *Psychiatrisch-neurologische Wochenschrift* have already sent me proofs.[7]

On November 7 I gave a lecture to the Society of Physicians about the analytical explanation of psychic impotence. The audience was very attentive, and they applauded. A neurologist who wants to cure all cases of impotence through prostate massage asked to speak.[8] Then Salgó[9] spoke very impertinently. I don't owe them any reply; I was especially ruthless and callous with Salgó, which I later almost regretted. The excitement made me incredibly eloquent, so much so that when I was finished, I was surprised by thunderous applause. The evening was not without significance for our cause here.

I have since reflected a great deal about paranoia and projection[10] and would like to speak with you very soon about a number of "freely emergent" ideas.

Please write me if it would be inconvenient for me to call on you next Sunday?

I am convinced that you would tell me frankly if you were otherwise disposed with your time.

Once again many thanks for your "Interpretation of Dreams"—and best regards to all the members of your dear family.

Your most obedient
Dr. Ferenczi

I would rather come on Sunday than on Wednesday. The minutes[11] tell me enough about the proceedings in the Society. I prefer an hour of conversation with you to Wednesday evening.

1. Freud 1900a, chap. 5, pp. 241–276.

2. This opening bracket is Ferenczi's, as is the concluding bracket at the end of the third paragraph.

3. "Between the feet [legs] is the figure; from it flows pure water. It has no teeth but a beard, and from it comes the species."

4. Rudolf Alexander Kleinpaul (1845–1918), *Das Stromgebiet der Sprache—Ursprung, Entwicklung und Physiologie* [The Watershed of Speech: Origin, Development, and

Physiology] (Leipzig, 1892). Freud had also referred to Kleinpaul, a noted philologist and linguist, among others, in the *Interpretation of Dreams*.

5. See Freud 1900a, p. 392. A literal translation of this phrase would be "to tear one down." Its closest English equivalent is "to jerk off" [Trans.].

6. Ferenczi may have been thinking of the vulgar Hungarian expression "kiverni a faszát" (to wag the tail). See also his contribution to the discussion of masturbation (1912, 100; *Schriften* I, 129; *C.*, pp. 191f).

7. The proofs to Ferenczi's paper on impotence (1908, 61; *C.*, p. 11) appeared in the *Psychiatrisch-neurologische Wochenschrift*; proofs to the paper on actual and psychoneuroses (1908, 60; *F.C.*, p. 30) appeared in the *Wiener Klinische Rundschau*.

8. Mor Pórosz (originally Moritz Popper) (1867–1935?), chief physician in a military hospital for sexual diseases; recommended massaging the prostate as a therapy for neuroses.

9. Jakab Salgó (1848–1918); in 1884 became director of the state institution for the insane, Lipótmezö.

10. See letter 4 and Ferenczi's thoughts about this question in his paper "Introjektion und Übertragung" [Introjection and Transference] (1909, 67; *C.*, p. 35), which he was writing at the time.

11. The minutes of the meetings of the Wednesday Society, compiled by Otto Rank (*Minutes* I–IV).

22

Vienna, November 26, 1908
IX., Berggasse 19

Dear colleague,

I regret having to turn you down for Sunday, which also reflects the sentiments of the corona,[1] and for that reason I must at least share with you the complex motivation for it. First, we have a bedridden patient; second, we are expecting an extensive visit from the new relatives;[2] and third, I am so tired out by having to do without my morning shower, which has kept me fresh for twenty-two years, that I am compelled to maintain complete rest on the Sabbath. But I would still like to converse with you for a few hours about our science. For that reason I suggest a postponement to one of the following Sundays, when everything will have improved. It should not be any later than Christmas, however, when we will certainly expect you for the holidays (I was just disturbed by a ten-year-old obsessive-compulsive from Budapest). I don't consider your cancellation for Wednesday definitive, either.

You don't have to make amends for your rudeness toward Salgó; I mean, misfortune doesn't come to him without justification. The applause that you had in the Society of Physicians certainly was for your personal appearance rather than for the cause, but it still does one good.

A book on dreams in a foreign language would be desirable and very

interesting. I constantly talk about this to the English. Up to now no one
wanted to bite. But it must one day be.

I am working now—if one can call it that, because I hardly get to it,
except on Sunday—on a general methodology of psychoanalysis,[3] of which
twenty pages are presently extant. I think that should become very meaningful to those who are already analyzing. Those who are still on the
outside won't understand a word of it.

Brill has published a nice analysis of a dementia praecox, dating from
the time he spent in Zurich, in Morton Prince's journal;[4] he, Jones, Abraham, and Jung are naturally in regular correspondence with me. I hope soon
to hear about the half-volume[5] which is supposed to appear in January but
will hardly be on time. Otherwise, the stream of work is flowing forth
evenly, without my having time to observe its effects. What I have learned
I usually don't experience until fall. Indifference toward my patients has
certainly been behind it for a long time, however. Jung has quite correctly
remarked that one must cure hysteria with a kind of dementia praecox.

Technique and mythology share the rudiment of interest that remains
to me in my few free hours. The meaningful summer lies behind me like
long years, and it seems positively incredible to me that another summer
will come again after this year of work.

Best regards,
Freud

1. Freud's family.
2. The Hollitschers.
3. Freud continued on this project until 1910 but then gave it up in this form and wrote
six shorter papers on techniques of treatment between 1911 and 1914 (1911e, 1912b,
1912e, 1913c, 1914g and 1915a [1914]); see the "Editor's Introduction" in *Studienausgabe*, Ergänzungsband [Supplement], pp. 145–148.
4. Brill's paper appeared under the title "Psychological Factors in Dementia Praecox"
in the *Journal of Abnormal Psychology* 3 (1908): 219ff, edited by Morton Prince (1854–
1929), psychiatrist and professor in Boston. Freud spoke about Brill's paper on December
9, 1908, at the Wednesday Society (*Minutes* II, 78f).
5. The first half-volume of the *Jahrbuch*, publication of which had been decided on in
Salzburg in 1908.

23

Budapest, November 29, 1908
VII., Erzsébet-körút 54

Dear Professor,

I thank you very much for your extensive letter, which pleased me very
much, although it meant a postponement of the trip to Vienna which I had
planned for tomorrow and was eagerly awaiting. I will not postpone carrying out these plans for long, however; perhaps I will use the Christmas

vacation to that end. I may make so free as to inquire still earlier (by telephone) whether there is no obstacle, and come still earlier.—The announcement of the *Technique* has very pleasantly surprised me; we have great need of it; it would spare us much effort and disappointment. There must, however, be something painful in simply yielding this knowledge, with such difficulty and so many sacrifices, to us youngsters. The greatness of the gift that you bestow upon us with this will certainly be appreciated by everyone who has up to now advanced in such a paltry fashion without this aid.

I hope that before my trip to Vienna I will finish a small paper[1] which will also touch on the technical side of the analyses and whose substance I have already put together, so that I will not come with empty hands. But I can't tell you this for certain; and if I do share it with you, it is only because in so doing I want to force myself to greater diligence.

I hope that the illness in your family is not serious and that this obstacle to my visit will soon be eliminated. (This wish is not to be understood as purely egoistic.)

Cordially,
Dr. Ferenczi

The matter of the Hungarian dream book is very close to my heart. I also want to speak to you about it in Vienna.[2]

1. Probably the first part of "Introjektion und Übertragung" (1909, 67; *C.*, p. 35).
2. On the remaining blank space on the page is written in someone else's handwriting, possibly Freud's: "11:30 Dr. Frank Lobkowitz, 1–3 sessions."

24

Budapest, December 10, 1908
VII., Erszébet-körút 54

Dear Professor,

I will probably postpone my trip to Vienna until Christmas vacation, all the more so that I might then spend not only one but two or even three days in Vienna. With your accustomed openness, with which I feel very comfortable, you will certainly tell me frankly if there is any obstacle to our meeting and whether this time I shouldn't stay longer than one day.

In the pleasant expectation of talking with you soon I will now refrain from inadequate written communication and remain, with cordial greetings to your dear family and thanks for the beautiful card from Miss Mathilde,

Obediently yours,
Dr. Ferenczi

25

Vienna, December 11, 1908
IX., Berggasse 19

Dear colleague,

Many thanks for your clever work.[1] A return mailing,[2] which is as familiar to you as your work was to me, is on the way to you. I am pleased to
accept your advance notice of arrival for Christmas and hope that no
untoward disturbance will interfere with it. Friday, Saturday, and Sunday
fit together well this time; that gives a more compact holiday than usual.

Just bring along everything that you have in mind; we will find time for
it. You know that the children are very much looking forward to your visit.

Technique will probably not be quite what you expect. Thirty-four pages
have been done up till now, and by Christmas we won't have more than
forty or fifty, which you can then read here in order to tell me your
impression of them. I hardly get to work, and right now I am not very
capable of accomplishing anything. I will be able to share something theoretically significant with you on the paranoia question.

I hear that your other essay is presently being printed by Kunn.[3] By
Christmas I am hopeful of having the final clarification of an extremely
severe case of ψ impotence, which I have been treating unsuccessfully since
spring and which is just now taking a surprising turn. So we will certainly
not be at a loss for material.

But I still hope to hear from you before then.

Best regards,
Freud

1. Probably Ferenczi's paper on impotence (1908, 61; *C.*, p. 11).
2. Probably "On the Sexual Theories of Children" (Freud 1908c).
3. Ferenczi's essay "Über Aktual- und Psychoneurosen" (1908, 60; *F.C.*, p. 30) appeared
in the *Wiener Klinische Rundschau*, edited by Karl Kunn (1862–1912).

26

Budapest, December 15, 1908
VII., Erzsébet-körút 54

Dear Professor,

So, it has been decided: I am coming to Vienna at Christmas and am very
much looking forward to it. It is self-explanatory that I will steal only as
much of your valuable time as you have in excess.

Many thanks for the "Sexual Theories of Children." In my most recent
reading I have again learned a great deal about this. In so doing it occurred

to me that I ought to go through the Interpretation of Dreams for a fourth time; when one understands something more, one gets much more from reading your works.

I call to your attention a typographical error in the article;[1] in the note on p. 771, instead of 1909, it reads: 1809. This would not be very noteworthy, were it not for the fact that the same typographical error occurs in the second edition of the "Interpretation of Dreams," on p. 181.[2] It could be a case of a writing error on your part. Besides the strangeness of the number 1909, I presume that *antedating* (dating of a work that has not yet been printed) also plays a role in this. In both cases one is requested to compare (cf.) a certain literary source, although this comparison is impossible, for the time being. The "wrongness" [*Verkehrtheit*] of such a request is expressed in reversing [*Verkehren*] the digits of the year 1908. A determining factor could also be your dissatisfaction with the all-too-slow publication of the "Schriften"[3] and especially of the "Jahrbuch."

With cordial regards to you and your dear family.

Dr. Ferenczi

1. In "On the Sexual Theories of Children" (1908c, p. 218) Freud refers to the case of "Little Hans" (1909b), which had not yet been published.
2. Freud 1900a, p. 250.
3. The second issue of Freud's *Sammlung kleiner Schriften zur Neurosenlehre* [Collected Papers on the Theory of the Neuroses], which was just being printed (*Freud/Jung*, December 11, 1908, p. 186).

27

Vienna, January 1, 1909
IX., Berggasse 19

Dear colleague,

My first writing of the new year goes to you amid hearty congratulations.

Marcuse[1] has replied with a refusal. He supposedly has so much material since the merger that he cannot commit himself to publication on a certain date. I had specified April as such.

Now, the question arises whether *you* want to try it with Marcuse by giving him a later date of May or June, or whether you wish for me to turn to Bresler on your behalf, or whether you renounce your well-deserved priority and even so prefer publication in the second half-volume along with my big paper. I await your decision.[2]

We are very well here. Jung sends his regards.

With the news from Messina[3] you must certainly have thought about

our plans for the summer. I would almost have given in to an invitation
to America in July.[4]

Best regards,
Freud

1. Max Marcuse (1877-?) Berlin physician for skin and sexual diseases and one of the
pioneers of scientific sexual research. Editor of, among others, the journal *Sexual-
Probleme,* in which two of Freud's works (1908c, 1908d) had appeared. It had just merged
with the *Zeitschrift für Sexualwissenschaft,* edited by Magnus Hirschfeld.

2. The discussion here and in the following letters is about the publication of Ferenczi's
article "Introjektion und Übertragung" (1909, 67; *C.,* p. 35), the manuscript of which
Ferenczi had brought along on his Christmas visit. The "well-deserved priority" refers
to Freud's project of a "general methodology of psychoanalysis," which was never realized (see letter 22, n. 3). Ferenczi's article was finally published along with Freud's
analysis of the "Rat-Man" (1909d) in the second half-volume of the *Jahrbuch.*

3. He refers to a catastrophic earthquake in Sicily and Calabria on December 28, 1908,
in which approximately 75,000 to 100,000 people died and the town of Messina was
almost totally destroyed.

4. In December 1928 Granville Stanley Hall (1844–1924), professor of psychology and
education and president of Clark University in Worcester, Massachusetts, had invited
Freud to give a series of lectures on the occasion of the twentieth anniversary of the
founding of the university. Freud declined, for the time being, for financial reasons. In
1911 Hall became a founding member of the American Psychoanalytic Association and
then turned to Adler's school (see letter 472).

28

Budapest, January 2, 1909
VII., Erzsébet-körút 54

Dear Professor,

First, heartfelt thanks for the many manifestations of your kindness with
which you have again allowed me to be blessed. If I didn't know that
gratitude always means also being guilty and that it more often than not
separates people rather than brings them together, I would uninhibitedly
give myself over to these feelings. Therefore I accept what you have offered
me simply as a gift of my favorable fate and think of your words in Berchtesgaden: "Man should also be able to accept gifts."

I am sorry that you have so much to do with my work. Certainly I would
like, if possible, to avoid having your work compared directly with mine.
I know all too well that this little paper can justify its existence only when
considered in and for itself, but it loses its justification after the publication
of your work. I will therefore attempt the following: I will write to Jung
about the matter and ask him if he couldn't manage to have the *Journal
für Psychologie und Neurologie*[1] bring out the article before the second

half-volume. At the same time I will ask him, if appropriate, to recommend another organ. If Jung declines, I will permit myself to come back to your kind offer regarding Bresler.

Incidentally, I have already revised the work but interpolated only a few sentences; otherwise I have left it unaltered. I especially guarded against using what I learned in your "methodology." I would not have been able to avoid that in a more thorough revision, so I preferred to leave it as is.

After the beautiful days in Vienna it was difficult to resume work. To be sure, I am presently at an extremely low ebb; the month of December was fateful. I lost—all too soon—three patients. At the moment I have only two, and they are at "reduced rates." But I am not depressed. I know it will come.

The local *"Ärzte Verein"* [physicians' association] (not the "Society of Physicians" [Gesellschaft der Ärzte], where I recently lectured)[2] asked me to give a lecture on the present state of the pathology of neuroses and, in particular, therapy.[3] The Association is very respectable; it pays 120 crowns for such a lecture. That would be the place where one could speak in somewhat greater detail about nonanalytic methods of treatment and their effectiveness. It would be inappropriate here to bring up a critique of the usual conception of neuroses. Otherwise I can offer the medical lay public only a repetition of my first, introductory work. After I proceed with the subject on my own I will allow myself to seek your opinion and ask if you would perhaps like to see me lecture on something else.

The catastrophe in Sicily has shaken me also; naturally, I immediately thought about our plans for the summer and wondered whether they might not be jeopardized by this. I am comforted by the fact that you only "almost" accepted the trip to America, although I am even "able" to follow you there. You see, you won't get rid of me so easily! (Now I notice that the joke about being "able" was also determined by pecuniary motives.)

Cordial New Year's greetings to the entire extended family from

Your very obedient
Dr. Ferenczi

1. Edited by Korbinian Brodmann (1868–1918), whom Jung did go on to ask about publishing Ferenczi's work.

2. See letter 7.

3. Ferenczi gave the lecture "Über die Therapie der Neurosen" [On the therapy of the neuroses] on February 15, 1909. See letters 31 and 42, n. 2.

29

Budapest, January 4, 1909

DR. FERENCZI SÁNDOR[1]

Dear Professor,

Here is a sample of the hard and painful work that I impose on myself.[2] You will certainly discover something in it which must have eluded me. Please, don't spare anything and say everything. I am determined to face the truth, no matter what it may look like.

Your very obedient
Ferenczi

1. Correspondence card with preprinted name.
2. This enclosure is missing.

30

Vienna, January 10, 1909
IX., Berggasse 19

Dear colleague,

Jung writes me today that he has contacted Brodmann about your paper. It deserves their efforts on its behalf. You can imagine why I did not favor presenting your ideas in the Wednesday Society.[1] The question of priority would have been confused thereby. I hope that you also know that I am making difficulties with the Jahrbuch only in your interest, and that only for the time being as well. I don't have the feeling of being the "benefactor" toward you and others and thus do [not] tie to my actions the otherwise justified fears of which you speak. I find that in consideration of my age I must keep space available for those who come after me, that is, that I do everything only for the cause, which, again, is basically my own; i.e., that I proceed thoroughly egoistically. There will certainly be a prominent place for you among my successors and proponents.

I was also sorry about declining to go to America, and if the trip does come about contrary to all expectation, I would also be in a position to ask you to accompany me. But I do find the presumption to sacrifice so much money in order to give lectures there much too "American." America should bring money, not cost money. By the way, we could soon be "up shit creek" the minute they come upon the sexual underpinnings of our psychology. Brill writes, alternating between hopefulness and misgiving, that he thinks he will soon find this very hard.

A work by Strohmayer[2] in Jena about anxiety is the most gratifying event these days. For the lecture at the Physicians' Association I would like to advise you to do nothing other than what you intend yourself. We will have to repeat ourselves often. For the time being you will naturally keep the therapeutic pessimism that has lately dominated you in your pocket.

I am trying to encourage Stein to stick it out in Budapest. It is not easy to find something suitable for him, and, above all, it cannot go as quickly as he wishes.

Best wishes for the new year. May it keep us all and carry us all forward.

Cordially,
Freud

1. See letter 27, n. 2. Questions of priority played a major role in the Wednesday Society (see, for example, the debate about "intellectual communism" on February 6, 1908; *Minutes* I, 302f).

2. Wilhelm Strohmayer (1874–1936), physician and Privatdozent (a German academic title, roughly the equivalent of assistant professor [Trans.]) and from 1910 professor of psychiatry and neurology in Jena; had published "Über die ursächlichen Beziehungen der Sexualität zu Angst- und Zwangszuständen" [On the Causal Relations of Sexuality to Anxiety and Compulsive States], *Journal für Psychologie und Neurologie* 12 (1908–9): 69–95.

31

Budapest, January 11, 1909

Dear Professor,

Jung's intervention proved to be effective. Dr. Brodmann just wrote me that he is accepting the paper for publication and that he also guarantees that it will come out before July. This matter is thus settled.

I will lecture on February 15 in the Physicians' Association on "The Therapy of the Neuroses."[1] The lecture will be a critique of pre-Freudian therapy and an acknowledgment of psychoanalytic and etiological therapy.

The local abstinents have asked me to lecture them on something having to do with the relation of nervous illness to sexuality. The lecture takes place today in a Good Templar Lodge.[2] I will tell them approximately the same as was contained in my first lecture[3] (only in a somewhat more popular fashion).

Jung writes me about a work by Strohmayer, with the remark that it is "an arrow that hits its mark." But since I don't know where the work was published, I haven't a clue as to whom the arrow hit.

With cordial greetings,

Your obedient
Dr. Ferenczi

Continued on January 12.

Have just received your friendly communication and thank you for it as a further sign of your interest in my activity. If you, Professor, don't at all want to be a benefactor, then you still practice the sublimest form of egoism; and if you claim that, when you support me, you are acting "in the interest of the cause," then you are again unwillingly my benefactor by lifting my often wavering spirit and my self-awareness. But despite much deliberation there is one sentence of your letter which I cannot understand; therefore I allow myself to quote it word for word. It says there: "I don't have the feeling of being the 'benefactor' toward you [and others] and thus tie to my actions the otherwise justified fears of which you speak." No matter how hard I try, I cannot now remember any fears that I expressed to you. I presume that the sentence is somehow garbled; perhaps a "not" or some other negation is missing there. As a true adherent to your teachings, however, I cannot consider an occasional writing error meaningless, just as the *total* forgetting on my part of those fears means something. In any event, I ask you to be willing to clarify the situation at the next opportunity.—

Yesterday I gave the lecture for the "Good Templars." The audience was very interested, and after the lecture a few women came to me and told me stories from the nursery that support your teachings. I asked them to send me such observations. I also made a characteristic slip of the tongue. I spoke about Möbius's[4] view that men have a longer active sex life, and got to speaking about cases where the man marries the daughter of his former lover. But instead of saying that such an action was justified, I said "unjustified." The conversation that I recently had with you will explain this parapraxis.

The trip to America also occupies my thoughts; from a material point of view I have no insurmountable difficulties. In a few years America will probably sooner pay money for your lectures; there everything depends on fashion.—As long as it doesn't stop quaking in Messina, I have no real desire to inquire about travel arrangements. My brother says the most comfortable thing is to make the voyage from Fiume with one of the big cruise ships of the Cunard Line.—

With most cordial greetings, to your family as well,

Your most obedient
Dr. Ferenczi

1. See letter 42 and n. 2.

2. The Lodge of the Order of the Good Templar, founded by Philipp Stein, played a prominent role in the Hungarian antialcohol movement. The order itself (the Association for Combating Alcoholism) was a creation of Auguste Forel.

3. On March 28, 1908, before the Society of Physicians (see letter 5, n. 2).

4. Paul Julius Möbius (1853–1907), doctor of philosophy and medicine, psychiatrist, and neurologist in Leipzig; known for his pathographies of famous men and his work *Über den physiologischen Schwachsinn des Weibes* [On the Physiological Feeble-Mindedness of Women] (Halle, 1900).

32

Vienna, January 17, 1909
IX., Berggasse 19

Dear colleague,

You are correct. The sentence lacks a negation. The letter was written on the eve of an inner earthquake, a bad migraine, and at such times I have the bad habit of directly contradicting myself. The attack certainly has no worse significance.

Look for Strohmayer's work where we will soon find yours. It is really good and perhaps all the more suited to making an impression in that it protests initially against belonging to the school—it is to be hoped out of diplomatic rather than arrogant motives.

I have heard nothing more from America, not even a reply to my inquiries of Brill. I have no trust, and fear the prudery of the new continent. If the trip should materialize, against all human expectation, then your participation is a matter of course. I am still missing the offprint of your first lecture at the Society of Physicians and have also not seen one in the archive of the Wednesday Society.

The work is now very difficult, hardly capable of getting accomplished. These demands on me should have come along a decade earlier.

Cordially,
Freud

33

[Budapest, undated][1]

Dear Professor,

I am sorry that I have to talk about my work again, because, although I cannot consider the little opus totally worthless—especially after your laudatory acknowledgment—I would have liked to see the case regarding it closed and it left to its fate. But Dr. Brodmann, to whom I sent the work, has decided otherwise. He sent the manuscript back to me immediately and wrote me that he can't publish it. That this refusal brought me twenty-four hours of depression was surely only the consequence of impulses of feelings of inferiority. Now I see clearly that rejection from an uninitiated, indeed hostile quarter should not shatter one's self-confidence. I am convinced that the article comes up to the normal, average level of articles otherwise published in the "Journal"; this gagging of the free expression of opinion in a scientific organ can therefore only have a "party-political" basis.

The following day brought me a patient whose analysis brought shining confirmation of your view of the double root of "erythrophobia."[2] It was a—naturally incomplete but very transparent—"quick analysis" in a culturally inferior person. Such forced analyses are—in my opinion—especially appropriate with less cultivated people and in this case also successful. A representative of the masses even at maturity remains much closer to the child, has sublimated less than educated people, and doesn't have such colossal defects of memory as we. Only a very great traumatic burden evokes psychoneuroses in simple people; these traumata are also not totally forgotten, or more correctly, they are capable of being reproduced relatively quickly. That they still determine symptoms can be explained by the fact that *in the present* all meaning is denied them and the actual significance can thus manifest itself only in conversion or substitutive symptoms as a sign of ucs. fantasizing.

That was also the case here. It had to do with a very well behaved agent, honorably married for eight years, who in three hours produced a plethora of sexual traumas. The cause of his erythrophobia is *shame* and *rage*. Shame on account of his repressed homosexuality and brutality; rage over a sadistic brother, a strict teacher, and a strict mother. As a child he was punished for every heterosexual attempt. At the age of eight he was beaten by his mother (who slept with him) because he rubbed his erect member against her leg. Soon thereafter—driven by curiosity—he looked at his mother's genitals, and to his disgust he saw at the location of the vulva "something big, red, hanging out" (evidently prolapse).[3] After seeing the prolapsed uterus, he condensed the vulgar Hungarian saying "the vulva bites" (naturally it was called something else) and the superstition that "worms hang out of the vulvas of bad girls" into the belief that his mother's genitals (i.e., of many or all women) are hanging, biting beings. All this is obviously only a modification of the "infantile sexual theory" of the female penis, probably blended with the idea of intestinal worms (ascarids).[4] Being frightened away by a female, especially by the mother, was here certainly the most important cause of the actual (half-unconscious) homosexuality. I don't want to go into the remaining incidents in more detail here; I intend to work out the case for a Wednesday evening.[5]—The patient had to depart in three days. My clarifications calmed him down greatly.

The correctness of the view of the role of "transference" in suggestion cures is proved by the enclosed letter, which I received from a Romanian hysteric after an eight-day suggestion cure. Neurologists have always received such letters. How could we have been so blind and not recognized that the patients only got well "for the sake of the doctor"!

Most cordial greetings to you and your dear family

Your truly obedient
Dr. Ferenczi

Please return the enclosed letter.[6]

1. This undated letter has been put into sequence based on its content.
2. On May 27, 1908, Freud had described unconscious shame and suppressed rage as the two roots of erythrophobia (the fear of blushing) (*Minutes* I, 402f).
3. Prolapse of the uterus.
4. Roundworms in the small intestine.
5. No details exist concerning such a lecture.
6. The enclosure is missing.

34

Vienna, January 18, 1909
IX., Berggasse 19

Dear colleague,

Be prepared to laugh at me. Today I looked at the first fourteen pages of our Jahrbuch and was delighted. Jung has done a magnificent job in bringing it out;[1] true revenge for Amsterdam.[2] It is something to be proud of.

And now something has made my heart heavy: that you are not represented in a volume that we will not soon see the likes of again in such a splendid and honorable form. Then I told myself it was my *fault*, because, out of misguided discretion, or God knows why, I prevented your beautiful paper about transference from being published in the second half-volume. I told myself you could easily write another paper for the second half-volume, but then it occurred to me that you would hardly be able to produce anything as significant in one year. In short, it is necessary for me to ask you to regard my earlier objection as rescinded and to reconsider whether you wouldn't rather withdraw the paper from Brodmann's journal and designate it for the Jahrbuch. That would appear to me now to be *far more correct*. You can lay the blame for inconsistency on me before Jung; you needn't be concerned about Brodmann. Give him any old reason. So, have a good laugh at me and take the advice I am giving you now.

Cordially,
Freud

1. As editor of the *Jahrbuch*.

2. From January 2 to 9, 1907, in Amsterdam, the Premier Congrès International de Psychiatrie, de Neurologie, de Psychologie et de l'Assistance des Aliénés [First International Congress of Psychiatry, Neurology, Psychology, and Care of the Insane] had taken place, at which Jung had read a paper, "Die Freudsche Hysterietheorie" [The Freudian Theory of Hysteria]. He ran over his allotted time, had to break off the lecture, and was sharply attacked in the discussion (see Jones II, 112f).

35

[Vienna] January 20, 1909[1]

Up, Brodmann! That is the best solution. A part of that power, etc.[2] Console yourself, he did the same thing to me with the Dora analysis.[3] Now, write Jung immediately, explain to him my bizarre reservations, and set it up there.

Cordially,
Freud

1. Postcard.

2. "Faust: 'Nun gut, wer bist du denn?' Mephisto: 'Ein Teil von jener Kraft, die stets das Böse will und stets das Gute schafft'" (Faust: "Who are you?" Mephistopheles: A part of that power that always wants evil and always creates good"). Johann Wolfgang von Goethe, *Faust*, pt. 1, vv. 1335f, quoted in *Sophienausgabe* XIV, 67.

3. In 1901 Freud had sent the Dora analysis ("Fragment of a Case of Hysteria," 1905e [1901]) to Brodmann, although Theodore Ziehen, the editor of the *Monatsschrift für Psychiatrie und Neurologie*, had already agreed to publish it. Brodmann had evidently sent the manuscript back under the pretext that it violated the physician's obligation to confidentiality (see the editor's preliminary remarks in *Studienausgabe* VI, 84f; Jones I, 362, and II, 255f).

36

Budapest, January 20, 1909

Dear Professor,

I don't want to let the day go by without answering your very kind letter.

You ask me if I am laughing at you because of your inconsistency.—Nothing could be further from the truth. On the contrary: my observation that you so often waste your precious time on my literary attempts causes me to reproach myself, and I often think of Lichtenberg's[1] words: "It is always better for an office to be lesser than its holder's capabilities."—Very often I am overcome by doubt whether in the long run I will be able to justify the trust that you have in my activities.

Your honorable invitation to have the work published in the first volume came at a very opportune time, almost simultaneous with Brodmann's rejection. Was it a coincidence?

I sent the manuscript to Jung right away and wrote him how happy I am to be able to introduce myself to such a pleasant company of comrades of similar attitude and conviction.

I call your attention to the fact that in the paper I have added, among other things, a few sentences in which I cite and briefly paraphrase your statements about transference ("we may treat a neurotic any way we like, he always treats himself psychotherapeutically, that is to say, with transference").[2]

With cordial greetings and thanks, again, for your great interest,

Your most obedient
Dr. Ferenczi

1. Georg Christoph Lichtenberg (1742–1799), German natural scientist and writer especially well known for his aphorisms.
2. "Introjektion und Übertragung" (1909, 67); *Schriften* I, 24; *C.*, p. 55.

37

Vienna, February 2, 1909
IX., Berggasse 19

Dear colleague,

I hope that your work is now in the safe haven of the Jahrbuch. Three days ago my behavior in this matter suddenly became understandable as completely rational, and the misleading trimmings of feeling fell away. I saw, apparently right away, that I cannot finish my paper on technique during the months of practice but must postpone it until July-August. Therefore, it can only get into the second volume of the Jahrbuch, which then makes room for your paper in the first. Perhaps I possessed this insight for a long time already and only learned its consequence earlier than its premise.

Colleague Stein was with me on Sunday and gave me very interesting insights into his *vita sexualis*. He is not an uninhibited homosexual, and his present suffering is a true anxiety hysteria. I decided to ask you to take him into analysis, on the one hand, to help him, but on the other, to take advantage of such a rare opportunity to get a lasting impression of the genesis of homosexuality. Certain of my reservations about this suggestion were dispelled by the realization that you are a constitutionally kind person and that you also usually act unselfishly (which you shouldn't do). I talked with him about this, but he explained that he wanted to get your opinion first.

Cordially,
Your Freud

Nothing new from the U.S.

[enclosure]¹
[*Inside left of page, folded over*]
    Professor Siegmund² Freud and wife
    hereby announce that the marriage of their daughter
    Mathilde to Mr. Robert Hollitscher
    will take place on Sunday, February 7.

[*Inside right of page*]
    Mrs. Emma Hollitscher
    hereby announces that the marriage of her son
    Robert to Miss Mathilde Freud
    will take place on Sunday, February 7.

[*Inside middle, bottom*]
    Vienna, February 1909
    Reception after the wedding from 3–4:30, IX., Berggasse 19.

    1. This printed wedding invitation contains no written additions. It is missing in the photostats as well as in the Balint folder. In the collection of the Austrian National Library in Vienna it is listed as an enclosure to letter 95, although chronologically it belongs before February 7 and was placed here for that reason. See Freud's thank-you note of February 7, 1909, letter 39.
    2. Spelled this way in the original.

38

Budapest, February 4, 1909
VII., Erzsébet-körút 54

Dear Professor,

Now the fate of my work has been decided. Jung wrote me about it already and fully endorses the content of the article. The motives for your change of mind in this matter have henceforth been completely clarified, and I can await the publication of the first half-volume with peace of mind. I am prepared for strong criticism on the part of exoteric medicine.

The fate of colleague Stein is also very close to my heart. With regard to the analysis to be taken on by me, however, I must note the following:—As I already mentioned to you verbally, our relationship has cooled considerably over the past year or so, and little is left of our earlier mutual honesty.—Naturally the fault lies with a competition complex!—I now want to confess to you quite honestly, even in the face of the danger that you will change your view of my constitutional kindness. I first noticed that he doesn't like the fact that I am becoming active in our cause to a certain extent. He has stayed away from both of my lectures—all the while making little excuses—so that I stood there in the Society of Physicians quite alone.

In the beginning I thought that such trivialities and others like them should not influence me; but more and more even I would frequently "forget" the Wednesday evenings when we met, and I had to admit that competitive feelings were also present in me. For a time I still forced myself to these encounters, but when I saw that it wouldn't work, I gave up trying; now we see each other only very rarely, and when we do meet there is never any question of a free exchange of views. You should not be surprised that it has come to this. Stein and I were complete strangers until two years ago; in the first—I should say, passionate—period of my psychoanalytic "renaissance" I was together with him a great deal; at the time I was fond of anyone with whom I could talk about our science.—Then came the hard work; it is still continuing. Stein didn't follow our movement sufficiently, hypnotized, talked about mneme, etc. And since he remained a stranger to me—apart from our common science—, only a few coincidences were necessary to cool our relationship.

Under these circumstances I cannot promise much about the treatment of our colleague. Or do you have a different opinion?

You have correctly surmised that money plays no role in this.—In asking you to consider this letter in strictest confidence and thanking you for your kind letter, I remain

Your most obedient
Dr. Ferenczi

Best regards to the entire dear household.

In the event that the trip to the U.S. does not materialize, I would like to recommend trying a trip to Egypt.

When the excitement and distractions of the wedding days are over, I request that you share with me your views about Stein's case.

39

Vienna, February 7, 1909
IX., Berggasse 19

Dear colleague,

Thank you for your kind telegram[1] and your splendidly beautiful gift. I can now admit to you that in the summer[2] I would have liked to have seen you in the place of the young man who, having since endeared himself to me, has now gone away with my daughter.

Your last letter sounded somewhat forced. I noticed you didn't reject my suggestion without a struggle. But, of course, if your relationship with Stein is not better, I cannot expect as much from you and will inform him to that effect today. Strange that most of these inverts are not complete human beings.

The wedding celebration was beautiful and warm. Both of the principal participants were in the most cheerful of moods. Now everything is quiet, and I am using the evening hours to make up for what I have neglected over the last few days.

As for America, probably nothing will come of it. Egypt has been my greatest desire for a long time, but I don't believe one can exist there in September. I will consult Baedeker.[3] Would you also inquire about it?

Kind regards,
Freud

1. This telegram is missing.
2. He refers to their vacation together in Berchtesgaden.
3. A well-known handbook for travelers.

40

[Budapest, ca.
February 8–11, 1909][1]

Dear Professor,

I am in a hurry to answer your letter of today. Stein's case forces me to hurry. You see, I have to know what reasons you gave our colleague Stein before I meet him—otherwise the matter could cause great embarrassment.

I must reiterate to you that I am extremely sorry for colleague Stein and fear that he will be hurt by this refusal—all the more so since our relationship up to now has seemingly been quite cordial, and there never has been any open exchange of views between us.

His latest sad experiences also pose the risk that he will misunderstand my refusal and will interpret it as a sign of disdain (because of his homosexuality).

Would you please, if possible, reassure me in this matter.

The idea that you had about me makes me proud, inasmuch as I gather that you consider me—worthy to assume a place in your family, whom I hold in such esteem.

With kindest regards,

Your most obedient
Dr. Ferenczi

1. Undated, but evidently written in reply to Freud's letter of February 7.

41

Vienna, February 12, 1909
IX., Berggasse 19

Dear colleague,

I told Stein that a certain indecision, a vacillation on your part, has alienated you from him in the matter of ΨΑ. This information was intended to counter his conviction that you disapprove of him because of his homosexuality. Nothing else.

Nothing pleasant can come out of the entire matter. But we want to prevent anything worse.

Cordially,
Your Freud

P.S. Muthmann[1] was our guest on Wednesday.

1. Arthur Muthmann (1875–1957), German psychiatrist, author of *Zur Psychologie und Therapie neurotischer Symptome, Eine Studie auf Grund der Neurosenlehre Freuds* [On the Psychology and Therapy of Neurotic Symptoms: A Study Based on Freud's Theory of Neurosis] (Halle, 1907), and one of Freud's first adherents in Germany, had been a guest of the Wednesday Society on February 10, 1909 (*Minutes* II, 145–152).

42

Budapest, February 16, 1909
VII., Erzsébet-körút 54

Dear Professor,

The case of Stein is still not settled! My impropriety toward him is now being avenged. Still, it occurs to me that he must now be judging me so strictly and unjustly because it outwardly appears as though I accused him in front of you of being an "apostate"—which was the last thing on my mind. I already sat down to write him—but I couldn't get the letter out. The matter oppresses me all the more, since I owe Stein a great debt of gratitude. It was he who called Jung's work to my attention and engaged in association experiments *before* me. (To be sure, he was stuck too long with the association game and Bettola[1] and only started with real psychoanalysis as a result of my explanations.)

You see how I am searching for excuses!

If you have an idea as to how to settle this matter in some fashion, you would do me a great service by communicating it to me.

Yesterday I gave the lecture in the "Physicians' Association."[2] Owing to unfavorable circumstances there were only a few people in the audience, but they listened very attentively and applauded. The lecture began with the assertion that for the time being we cannot get by without looking at the psychoneuroses from a dualistic perspective. Then came a general overview of the unfounded attempts to explain psychoneuroses and functional psychoses anatomically and physiologically, followed by the purely psychological explanation (hysteria, obsessional neurosis, paranoia, dementia praecox) in your sense, with a few critical remarks about experimental psychology to date. Finally, I went through the therapeutic methods to date (psychotherapy, sanatoria, medications, etc.) and cursorily explained the successes of psychoanalysis. The lecture concluded with an attack against professional colleagues who judge our science without examining it. The way in which they treated Abraham in Berlin gave me the motivation for this.[3]

Should I translate the lecture into German?

With kindest regards,

Your obedient
Dr. Ferenczi

1. Presumably Dumeng Bezzola (1868–1936), a Swiss psychiatrist who used a cathartic method.

2. The talk was given in the framework of a lecture series in the Budapest Physicians' Association and published in *Gyógyászat* 22/23 (1909): 360–362, 378–382; translated into German as "Zur analytischen Auffassung der Psychoneurosen" [The Analytic Conception of Psycho-Neuroses] (1909, 65; *F.C.*, p. 15).

3. A lecture of Abraham's in Berlin on November 9, 1908, before the Berlin Society for Psychiatry and Nervous Diseases, "Die Stellung der Verwandtenehe in der Psychologie der Neurosen" [The Significance of Intermarriage between Close Relatives in the Psychology of the Neuroses], had been strongly criticized (*Freud/Abraham*, November 10, 1908, pp. 55f; Jones II, 114).

43

Budapest, February 23, 1909
VII., Erzsébet-körút 54

Dear Professor,

To my pleasant surprise, today I received a letter from Stein in which he asks a favor of me. From this circumstance I saw that he doesn't take the situation as tragically as I had presumed. Cheerfully, I seized the opportunity to agree to do him a favor (to take over his office hours at the health service) and to ask him at the same time to give me an opportunity to talk things over. The prospect of a halfway satisfactory settlement of this affair has put an end to the depression which has been hanging over me since this matter worsened.

My improved mood as a result of this could have contributed to my having completed a little work (Contribution to Knowledge about the Triggering Causes of Neuroses)[1]—Jung wrote me[2] that he will be in Vienna in March and asked me to meet him in Vienna. I agreed.

Stein was just with me and has dispelled our misunderstandings through personal discussion. Certainly, after what has taken place, an analysis with him would be out of the question. In the aforementioned work I want to focus on two observations—on the basis of several cases.

1.) That often neurosis becomes manifest not through a further intensification or sharpening of repression but rather through a momentary slackening of censorship. Under the influence of a strong excitation of feeling, the complexes can seize dominance for themselves and impel the patient to an action (of a sexual or violent nature) that consciously strives against him. In a very large number of my cases (particularly in hysteria or anxiety hysteria) the lasting disturbance of equilibrium was the consequence of such a one-time discharge, which overcomes the inhibition.*[3]

* "—the black Furies in time \ When a man prospers in sin \ By erosion of life reduce him to darkness" (Aeschylus, Oresteia).[4]

2.) In two cases the manifestation of the symptoms emerged as a "scheduled action" [Terminhandlung] in the sense of suggestion psychology. In our terminology I would define the matter such that, in some patients, the maturation of the illness is the fulfillment of a forgotten (repressed) wish. (Ten years before his illness my patient had resolved to have himself pensioned—after he had served as an official for ten years—in order to be able to dedicate himself entirely to literary activity. His wish became fulfilled, even though he had long forgotten it. He fell ill with a severe obsessional neurosis whose content was determined by the Oedipus complex with masochistic components.)[5]

Such "scheduled actions" also play a role in the treatment. A patient (anxiety hysteria), who, up to February 9, could only be accompanied to my office with difficulty and effort, today, unaided, took a walk of two and a half hours (accompanied by her maid—otherwise she only went with her husband). She couldn't explain this to me; but I remembered having told her at the beginning of the analysis just three months earlier (November 9, 1908) that she would need ca. three months to be able to get around. This patient is certainly transferring thoroughly. One cannot preclude the possibility that the order for the deadline *inhibited* the first patient's falling ill and the second patient's cure up to the activation of the deadline.

———————

I hope you have good news from the young couple, to whom I send kind regards.

Your most obedient
Dr. Ferenczi

1. Unpublished; see Freud's reply (letter 44) and letter 45.
2. Unpublished letter of February 18, 1909.
3. Ferenczi also occupied himself further with the play of forces between complexes and censorship and their effects, especially in his work "Über passagère Symptombildungen während der Analyse" [On Transitory Symptom Constructions during the Analysis] (1912, 85; *C.*, p. 193).
4. Aeschylus, *Oresteia, Agamemnon*, vol. 1, *Norton Anthology of World Masterpieces*, 4th ed. (New York, 1979), p. 311.
5. Ferenczi published this case in "Introjektion und Übertragung" [Introjection and Transference] (1909, 67; *Schriften* I, 39f; *C.*, pp. 81f).

44

Vienna, February 28, 1909
IX., Berggasse 19

Dear colleague,

The following has occurred: as you recall, Clark University in Worcester near Boston invited me in December to give a series of lectures which are supposed to take place during the second week of July. I turned them down, because a great material loss would have been connected with a departure in June. Now, President Stanley Hall reports to me that the celebration that has occasioned the invitations has been postponed until the week beginning on September 6. This change, which is accompanied by an increase in the travel allowance, makes it possible, in fact convenient, for me to accept the invitation. I will therefore embark on August 20 or so and hope to return around October 1. In accordance with our earlier arrangement, I ask if you want to came along on this journey. It would be a great pleasure for me.

The Jahrbuch[1] and the second series of the *kleine Schriften* [*zur Neurosenlehre*][2] have been published. The latter will come to you in the next few days; the book will not be distributed before March 1.

I am very happy that the affair with Dr. Stein is taking a favorable turn, since I caused embarrassment through my ignorance of the relationship between the two of you. I am still not clear about your refusal to take him into treatment.

With regard to the first part of your intended work, I am of the opinion that it forms an important piece of a large context and should be left alone until the rest has materialized. The second part concerns a detail that is interesting but not in principle significant, and certainly allows for further interpretation. Particular motives are present when deadlines play such a large role.

The young couple arrived this morning in splendid condition, and they are very happy with their new home, which you will see in March.

Cordially,
Freud

1. The first half-volume of the *Jahrbuch*; see also letter 48, n. 5.
2. *Sammlung kleiner Schriften zur Neurosenlehre*, zweite Folge (Leipzig, 1909).

45

Budapest, March 2, 1909
VII., Erzsébet-körút 54

Dear Professor,

Last Saturday I went away to visit my mother[1] and didn't get back to Budapest until Monday, where I found your letter, which was followed today by the book you sent. I thank you very much for both. (In the process I must admit to you that through your gift you have robbed me of the satisfaction of "spending money for something valuable." That might sound somewhat neurotic to you; and it really is a "symptom feeling" [*Symptomgefühl*], as I have learned by closer self-analysis.)

I have the intention of making the trip to America with you. More correctly: I accept your kind invitation to travel along, and only unforeseen obstacles could hold me back. A certain preparation for overseas excursions would be very useful to me, by which I mean not only brushing up on my deficient English-language skills but also some reading about America. Along with this perfection of my education, studying the means of transport is a task in itself.—From my perspective we could travel significantly more cheaply with the big excursion ships from Fiume (Cunard Line)—but it would take much longer. I think we will decide upon a faster ship (Hamburg A.L., Cherbourg); the passage across shouldn't take up the main part of the entire journey, otherwise we will get to see too little of America.

Following your advice, I will let the work on the "triggering causes" be for the time being. It wouldn't really be much more than a modern transcription of the Breuer-Freud "Hysteria." Now that I see this book for the second time, I notice in it the kernel of everything that we now know.

Cordially,
Dr. Ferenczi

1. Rosa Ferenczi, b. Eibenschütz (1840–1921). She lived in Ferenczi's birthplace, Miskolcz, about 150 kilometers northeast of Budapest.
2. The *Studies on Hysteria* (Freud, with J. Breuer, 1895d) had been published in a second edition in 1909.

46

Vienna, March 9, 1909
IX., Berggasse 19

Dear colleague,

America is dominating the situation. Your acceptance has made me very happy. My brother, whom you know, has likewise decided to make the trip[1] and is busy preparing for it. We are thinking of the Austro-Americana (Trieste), from which a *very* beautiful ship, the *Laura*, leaves on August 21 for New York by way of Patras-Palermo. The longer passage should not be avoided, since it is an exquisite pleasure, at least in the Mediterranean. But we will see to all other details later on by word of mouth.

Jung wants to meet me on the 19th. I hope you will come over on the following Sunday. Everything will be ripe for decision making until then. I have also ordered works about America for myself and am looking for a teacher to polish my English. It appears to be shaping up to be a great experience.

Cordially,
Freud

1. Alexander Freud (1866–1943). Without an academic degree he became an expert witness at the Court of Commerce, an expert for the Ministry of Freight, Transport, and Tariff Affairs, and Imperial Counsel. He was a lecturer at the Consular Academy (across the street from Freud's apartment in the Berggasse) and editor of the periodical *Allgemeiner Tarif-Anzeiger*. Dispossessed by the Nazis, he died in exile in Canada. The brothers took many trips together, but their plans were not realized this time.

47

Vienna, March 19, 1909
IX., Berggasse 19[1]

Dear Doctor,

Jung has postponed coming here because he was called away to Berlin to attend to a patient. I will inform you of his further intentions.

Cordially,
Freud

1. Correspondence card.

48

Budapest, March 21, 1909
VII., Erzsébet-körút 54

Dear Professor,

Thank you for both communications. Jung also informed me of the postponement of his travel plans; I hope that he does come to Vienna in the not too distant future and that I will have occasion to visit you. I was very much looking forward to the planned trip to Vienna. I wanted to present you and Jung with a work which I finished in the meantime on "Suggestion and Hypnosis in Light of Psychoanalysis."[1]

This work has prevented me up to now from concerning myself seriously with the trip to America. Now I intend to read up with more enthusiasm on Dr. E. Deckert's North America (from the General Regional Studies of Prof. Sievers)[2] as well my English Baedeker.—

I am very comfortable with the fact that we are traveling by way of Patras-Palermo and that your brother will also come along.

The Jahrbuch is impressive. I find the most valuable thing (apart from the magnificent analysis of "clever Hans") to be Jung's total conversion to your views. Now he writes only about the "vicissitudes of the libido." Binswanger's[3] case is very nicely presented, and his uncle's testimonial is also of value. Abraham, as always, writes cleverly and convincingly. I haven't read Maeder's[4] article yet. It seems to be a meritorious, industrious piece of work.[5]

With cordial greetings to you and your dear family and in hopes of seeing you soon,

Your most obedient
Dr. Ferenczi

1. "Die Rolle der Übertragung bei der Hypnose und bei der Suggestion" [The Part Played by Transference in Hypnosis and Suggestion], published as the second part of "Introjektion und Übertragung" (1909, 67; C., p. 58).

2. The reference is to the chapter by Emil Deckert in Wilhelm Sievers, ed., *Amerika* (Leipzig, 1897).

3. Ludwig Binswanger (1881–1966), Swiss psychiatrist and nephew of Otto Binswanger, who was a professor and director of the psychiatric clinic at the University of Jena. Ludwig Binswanger had participated as an assistant physician in Jung's association experiments; in 1910 he was elected first president of the Zurich branch society of the IPA and from 1911 to 1956 headed the Bellevue Clinic in Kreuzlingen on Lake Constance. He was interested simultaneously in psychiatry, psychoanalysis, and philosophy, which in his opinion complemented one another. Despite their partly diverging views, Freud and Binswanger maintained a lifelong friendship. See the latter's book *Sigmund Freud: Reminiscences of a Friendship* (New York, 1957).

4. Alphonse Maeder (1882–1971), Swiss psychotherapist, temporary representative of the Zurich Association. He followed Jung after the latter's separation from Freud.

5. The contents of the second half of the volume were: Freud, "Analyse der Phobie eines fünfjährigen Knaben" [Analysis of a Phobia in a Five-Year-Old Boy]; Abraham, "Die Stellung der Verwandtenehe in der Psychologie der Neurosen" [The Significance of Intermarriage between Close Relatives in the Psychology of the Neuroses]; Maeder, "Sexualität und Epilepsie" [Sexuality and Epilepsy]; Jung, "Die Bedeutung des Vaters für das Schicksal des Einzelnen" [The Significance of the Father in the Destiny of the Individual]; and Binswanger, "Versuch einer Hysterieanalyse" [Attempt at an Analysis of a Case of Hysteria].

49

Vienna, March 23, 1909
IX., Berggasse 19

Dear Doctor,

At the same time as your letter there came a communication from Jung announcing his arrival in Vienna for Thursday evening.[1] I therefore repeat my invitation to you, which is not strictly tied to Sunday.

We will acknowledge your work[2] in the small committee. It must be the necessary continuation of the previous one[3] and will, I hope, coincide with the corresponding piece of my "Methodology." In addition, we will hold an America conference. My brother is *very* probably not coming along, because there is now complete turmoil at his work. The trip by way of Patras with the Austro-Americana would suit me very well, but the ship leaves on August 21, supposedly takes fourteen days, and we are in danger of arriving too late because of some chance occurrence.

The Jahrbuch also seems to me to be a shining accomplishment. It is at the same time an incarnation, and, for its part, it holds the cause together.

I will bring Jung to Deuticke so that he gets free rein in continuing the planned framework.[4]

From our little congress in the next few days I anticipate an elevation of mood that one needs from time to time, after one has suffered from indisposition and overwork.

Best regards,
Freud

1. Jung and his wife arrived March 25, as announced, and remained in Vienna until March 30. Ferenczi's planned Easter visit, however, evidently did not come about.

2. See letter 48 and n. 1.

3. The first part of "Introjection und Transference," "Introjection in the Neuroses."

4. Franz Deuticke (1850–1919) had published Freud's *Sammlung kleiner Schriften zur Neurosenlehre*, the *Schriften zur angewandten Seelenkunde* (taken over by the publisher Hugo Heller from volume three on), and the *Jahrbuch*. Freud and Jung subsequently negotiated with him about changing the *Jahrbuch* into a bimonthly journal and about publishing additional periodicals (*Freud/Jung*, April 12, 1910, pp. 305f).

50

Vienna, April 7, 1909
IX., Berggasse 19

Dear Doctor,

An eye inflammation necessitates my keeping this letter as brief as possible.

I thank you for the material,[1] which I will probably use, for the most part (under your name). The accompanying letter is being returned,[2] which probably corresponds most closely to your wishes.

I have not yet made a decision regarding the ship. I have just written to Brill as well as to Stanley Hall himself for information and will decide after I receive it—at the end of the month. If you have not said no by then, I will reserve a second cabin for you.

On Friday evening I intend to go to Venice over Easter. Brother and sister-in-law are already there.[3]

Cordially,
Freud

1. Probably Ferenczi's contributions to the third edition of *The Psychopathology of Everyday Life* (Freud 1901b); see letters 57 and 59.

2. This letter is missing.

3. Alexander Freud and Minna Bernays (1865–1941), Martha Freud's sister. After the death in 1886 of her fiancé, Ignaz Schönberg, a boyhood friend of Freud's, Minna had

worked as a companion. At the beginning of 1896, after the birth of Anna Freud, she had moved into the Freud household, where she remained until her death. She was interested in the subject of psychoanalysis and accompanied Freud on numerous trips.

51

Budapest, April 21, 1909
VII., Erzsébet-körút 54

Dear Professor,

I hope you have returned to Vienna in good shape and renewed yourself in Italy.

I am eagerly anticipating the news from America. Should Stanley Hall place a value on arriving punctually, we will, I think, have to renounce plans for the Mediterranean trip. A somewhat longer stay in America and perhaps an excursion to some of America's large cities will compensate us for giving up the blue Mediterranean sky.

I now have in my practice some very interesting cases, which capture my attention completely.

One is of a young, very intelligent "homosexual," who has almost been cured in twenty analytical hours. Cured at least *quoad libidinem sexualem.*[1]

Communicating the existence of his *colossally strong mother complex* produced a terrific reaction in him, which lasted three days. It was a reaction like in a test tube. I drilled a hole into the partition between cs. and ucs., whereby I ignited a fireworks display of motor and psychical affective discharges. After the "reaction" had run its course, I saw before me a changed man.—He had been homosexual for four years (at that time he had "discovered" himself); was minimally potent with women, and lately he could perform coitus only when he thought of men. Along with this, colossal remorse over every homosexual act.

According to what he has communicated to me up to now (and what is not suited for a brief letter), he became homosexual

1.) because he wanted to do something very forbidden (substitute for the Oedipus complex),
2.) and in so doing he looked for what was forbidden on the opposite pole. (He preferred tall, thin men; his mother is a rather small, plump woman.)

Despite the relatively great improvement in his condition, I will not discontinue his treatment until I have fundamentally cleared up the case.

With the young man's intelligence, I hope that the six months which I have anticipated for the treatment will suffice.

Next time I will report to you about an interesting but very complicated case of hypochondria.

With cordial greetings.

Yours,
Dr. Ferenczi

The local social science association[2] has asked me to give four lectures on psychological subjects next semester. I intend to lecture on the following four themes: 1.) psychopathology of everyday life, 2.) interpretation of dreams, 3.) sexual theory, 4.) psychological and pathological role of sexuality.—

I am very much looking forward to the promised visit of Mr. and Mrs. Hollitscher.[3] In order to be able to reserve a room, I request notification one to two days beforehand.—

1. "As regards sexual libido."

2. This at first liberal then increasingly radical association had been founded in 1901 by a group of economists, journalists, and lawyers. It was closely connected with the journal *Huszadik Század* [Twentieth Century], in which numerous articles about psychoanalysis appeared. In 1906, with the goal of popular enlightenment, it founded the Free School of Social Sciences, at which Ferenczi gave lectures.

3. The Hollitscher newlyweds' trip to Budapest did not take place because Mathilde had a recurrence of her abdominal abscess.

52

Vienna, April 25, 1909
IX., Berggasse 19

Dear colleague,

On Thursday my daughter[1] was operated on for the residues of her abscess from the year 1905; she has since been doing well, and we at last have hope that she will finally be restored to health.

Many thanks for your inquiries. I see there is not much doing with Cunard. The information about North German Lloyd cannot be correct. The George Washington leaves on August 21, just right for us. It takes eight days, so that we have about a week free for America before Worcester. I am firmly committed to decide that way; we can do the Mediterranean in any other year, but America will not come again so soon. Responses from America have not yet arrived, but in any case, if it's all right with you, I will reserve two cabins end of this week. I think it is more secure from Vienna and could cost 600–700 marks. It depends on whether the cabins are on the upper decks and outside. The deeper, the cheaper; the outside cabins, by the way, are usually for two, which we don't want. Incidentally, it doesn't make much difference, since, except for sleeping, all activity in a cabin is precluded, unless one has the royal suite. I ask once more for your consent.

I will not respond to your very interesting researches because we will have an opportunity to talk everything out. Aren't you coming to the Wednesday Society in the meantime?

I am just now awaiting two very interesting guests, Moll,[2] from Berlin, at 11:30, and Pfister,[3] from Zurich, at noon. Moll will be very badly received; Pfister, to the contrary.

My practice is at a peak, inversely proportional, naturally, to the condition of my strength and health. It is difficult to bear. It's pretty quiet in the literature. A paper by Bleuler[4] that completely accepts infantile sexuality. Rank's Birth of the Hero[5] has already appeared; it will interest you very much.

Cordially,
Your Freud

April 26

Moll was just here. I scolded him and almost threw him out. He is a disgusting, vicious, maliciously pettifogging individual. Then came Pfister, who is a charming fellow and flattered everyone to death, a warm-hearted dreamer, half Saviour, half Pied Piper. We parted good friends.

Fr.

1. Mathilde Hollitscher.

2. Albert Moll, German neurologist and, above all, sexual scientist, editor of the *Zeitschrift für Psychotherapie und medizinische Psychologie,* in which Freud's paper "Some General Remarks on Hysterical Attacks" (1909a [1908]) had appeared; and of *Abhandlungen aus dem Gebiete der Psychotherapie und medizinischen Psychologie.* Moll's book *Das Sexualleben des Kindes* (Berlin, 1909; English edition, *The Sexual Life of the Child* [New York: Macmillan, 1912]) had been discussed in the meeting of the Wednesday Society on November 11, 1908 (*Minutes* II, 43–52).

3. Oskar Pfister (1873–1956), Protestant minister in Zurich, in correspondence with Freud since January 1909 (Freud/Pfister, *Briefe 1909–1939,* ed. Ernst L. Freud and Heinrich Meng, Frankfurt, 1963; English edition, *Psychoanalysis and Faith: The Letters of Sigmund Freud and Oskar Pfister* [New York: Basic Books, 1963]). He was active as a psychoanalyst all his life and as a pioneer in the application of psychoanalysis to the ministry and to education. Pfister became and remained a close friend of the Freud family.

4. Eugen Bleuler, "Sexuelle Abnormitäten der Kinder," *Jahresbericht der schweizerischen Gesellschaft für Schulgesundheitspflege* 9 (1908): 623. Cited, among other works, by Freud in his American lectures (1910a [1909], p. 43) in support of his views.

5. Otto Rank, *Der Mythus von der Geburt des Helden, Versuch einer psychoanalytischen Mythendeutung* (Leipzig, 1909).

53

Budapest, [undated]¹
VII., Erzsébet-körút 54

Dear Professor,

Your letter of today has saddened me greatly, although I get the sense from the tone of your communication about your daughter's illness that there is no question of grave danger. When you are so worried, and on top of that still so busy, you really don't need to make the effort to answer my letters, although I will permit myself from time to time to send you mine.

Today I was at the local central ticket agency, where they could give out information only about *Cunard Line* and *North German Lloyd* because the schedules of the other steamship companies (Hamburg America Line, etc.) have supposedly not yet been set. (But that could also be a dodge; the agency only represents *Cunard* and *Lloyd*.)

The only ship of the *Cunard* with which we could travel is the *Carpathia*, which leaves from Fiume on *August 7* and lands in New York on *August 24*. (All other ships come too early or too late.) The passage costs 18 £ (432 crowns) and up, depending on location of cabin. So, very cheap— but for our purposes somewhat too early, and the passage (seventeen days!) too long. The stops are Palermo, Naples, Gibraltar.

We might further consider the Cunard liner *Campania*, which leaves *Liverpool* on August 21 and arrives in New York before September 1 (the ship already heads back on September 1). (Price of the trip 20 £ 10 s = ca. 500 crowns.) Better cabins probably somewhat more.

Of the *Lloyd ships* we could take the *Kronprinz Wilhelm*, which departs Bremen on August 24 and reaches New York in seven days. Price of a first class cabin: 480–1,800 marks,

I still want to ask an acquaintance who lives in Hamburg for information.

Cordially,
Dr. Ferenczi

1. This letter has been placed in sequence based on its content.

54

Vienna, April 27, 1909
IX., Berggasse 19

Dear colleague,

I am so busy that I am asking you to take something from me, namely, the responsibility for booking passage to America. The matter is as follows: the Austro-Americana has a ship leaving on August 21, the Laura, which takes at least fourteen days and thus does not land before September 4, and possibly takes a day longer, when we are supposed to be in Worcester on the 6th. Many advise against traveling on such a tight schedule. I wrote to Brill and Stanley Hall in order to get direct advice, expect a reply still in April, and will then decide; in any case have tickets on April 30 (with your help).

The Austro has two advantages: the Mediterranean trip and the low price for good cabins, 650 crowns, whereas on the Hamburg and the NG Lloyd the price could be double that. Perhaps you could inquire if the *dates and prices of the Cunard Line from Fiume offer the same advantages, and then put together an overview of the travel possibilities and price differentials.*[1] We must decide very soon, since from experience the good spots are soon taken. A great deal depends on the cabin, so we don't want to economize there. I am so busy that I would be happy if you could take the matter out of my hands. As soon as I get word from America I will ask you to make the reservations, perhaps by telegram. Here I can get them more easily *only with Austro*, where my brother has connections, in case you decide not to do it.

My daughter has fallen ill again (from the same remnant of the operation), which doesn't exactly make me more animated and should excuse my effort to impose on you for this.

Cordially,
Your Freud

1. Underlined in a different ink, presumably by Ferenczi.

55

Vienna, April 27, 1909[1]

americans make arrival possible after 4 sept if agreeable I will reserve space on laura 21 august austroamericana = Freud

1. Telegram.

56

Budapest, May 1, 1909
VII., Erzsébet-körút 54

Dear Professor,

Finally the great journey has been irrevocably decided upon. I am very happy about it, especially since the first—Mediterranean plan—is to be carried out. Please let me know the amount I owe so that I can send it to you with thanks.

I thank (I never get away from thanking) you as well as Martin[1] for your kind information about Mathilde's condition; I hope that she is now completely well and that I will soon be able to greet Mr. and Mrs. Hollitscher here.

I would like to spare you "researches," but a serious case necessitates my seeking your assistance. It has to do with the nephew of a busy doctor who underwent a syphilitic infection and has uneven and sluggishly reacting pupils with induced knee reactions. Other signs of tabes[2] or paralysis are not present. The psychic manifestations are: colossal talkativeness i———[several words are missing because part of the letter has been torn off] symptoms, indecisiveness, fear of every activity, lack of any self-confidence, fear of everything having to do with the court, exaggerated cleanliness, pensiveness, etc. (along with this, various paresthesias). All that would fit very well the diagnosis of "obsessional neurosis," and it is precisely these symptoms which encourage me to make a favorable prognosis. Unfortunately, a month has gone by already without my having accomplished anything. The patient is a frightful chatterer; he has no lack of ideas, but the things that he brings up don't amount to anything. I couldn't use the method of "letting him talk himself out" this time; by forcefully interrupting him and inquiring about the motivation for particulars, I brought out the fact that he is a *sperm hypochondriac* but represses this hypochondria and transforms it into symptoms. The court phobia has to do with the fact that he unconsciously fantasizes about divorce. Despite the fact that these things have come out, he maintains unshakably that he loves his wife, that he is not afraid of tabes, paralysis, etc.—There *is no trace* of transference. He behaves like a paranoiac. Even the small signs of megalomania (he thinks he is much smarter than I; he can be cured only by someone who impresses him) I relate not to paralysis but rather to paranoia and presume that he has a very strong but completely unconscious homosexual component that also can't be made conscious. (He is afraid of assassinations and always has a revolver on him.) His speech is rife with sexual, especially homosexual, symbolism. I would like to ask you: Is there really a hypochondriacal paranoia—or are all hypochondriacs actually paranoid? And what can one do with a hypochondriac?

Pardon me for this imposition; I only want to ask you to give me a few hints in a few words about similar cases. The question is, by the way, also significant in principle———[some words are missing, as earlier].

Yours,
Dr. Ferenczi

In two weeks [I] hold [words missing] "Interpretation of Dreams."[3]

1. Freud's eldest son.

2. Tabes dorsalis (consumption of the spinal chord), one of the consequences of final-stage syphilis.

3. Probably the announcement of the lecture in the Society of Physicians, which was then postponed until fall (see letter 61 and n. 1).

57

Vienna, May 2, 1909
IX., Berggasse 19

Dear colleague,

In the turmoil and also as a consequence of the little bodily pains of recent months I have appreciated your interesting letters less than they deserved. Today, on a happy, rainy, and guest-free Sunday I will attempt to repair something.

I also know cases like the one you describe, if I correctly judge the similarity. I now have a woman who is recovering from syphilis and every-thing connected with it, but who, because of her own inaccessibility, her distinct arrogance, her endless evasive chatter, reminds me of your patient and probably belongs to the same type. I took her into treatment at the time because of hysterical symptoms, which could all be reduced to light organ disturbances and sensitivities. Everything in her speaks a displeasing albeit similar language to the one with which we are familiar, something akin to what happens when someone who knows Spanish is displaced to Portugal, where he can't actually make himself understood.

I can't give you any certain information. With my patient there is a slight chance of resolution through identification with a crazy [*meschuggene*] mother; great it is not. It also seems to me that these cases of paranoia can be pursued and perhaps find their representation in the querulist type; you correctly refer to the commonality with hypochondria. We have distin-guished a paranoid subtype from the latter, hypochondria. The querulist would be a sublimated hypochondriac. We still know too little about this and must collect and learn, but there are certainly new, up to now misun-derstood forms. We should hold fast to the idea that what we call different *forms* of illness are actually only different outcomes of the same process of repression and substitutive formation.—

My brother, who knows Schenker[1] personally, has consulted with him regarding the cabins on the Laura and has received no answer as yet. I will report to you as soon as the matter is settled.

My daughter[2] is doing very well. She will leave the sanatorium in a few days. Then my wife is going to Karlsbad with Sophie,[3] who has gallbladder ailments. The summer problems, unresolved to date, are presently being discussed.

You will perhaps be happy to hear that yesterday Deuticke asked for the second edition of the Theory of Sexuality.[4] Your contributions[5] will provide the most valuable, perhaps the only enrichment to the third.

I greet you cordially and hope for news about your lecture.

Your
Freud

P.S. Brill is looking forward to your coming[6] in a truly amicable spirit.

1. Possibly Dr. August Schenker-Angerer (1866–1914) of the Schenker shipping agency, which still exists today.

2. Mathilde.

3. Sophie (1893–1920), Freud's second daughter. In 1913 she married the Hamburg photographer Max Halberstadt (1882–1940). The couple had two sons, Ernst Wolfgang (b. 1914) and Heinz Rudolph ("Heinerle") (1918–1923). Sophie died in the influenza epidemic after the First World War while pregnant with a third child.

4. *Three Essays on the Theory of Sexuality* (1905d), 2d. ed. (1910).

5. Freud thanked Ferenczi in the third edition of *The Psychopathology of Everyday Life* (1901b) for his numerous (pp. 19, 26f, 28ff, 39, 85, 125, 156f, 182f, 268) and "valuable" (p. 267) contributions.

6. That is, to the United States.

58

Budapest, May 5, 1909
Hotel Royal

Dear Professor,

In response to your kind letter, for which I am most grateful, I must first expand upon my last report about the supposed paranoiac. Strangely, *his* father (like the mother of *your* patient) was also mentally ill. He died of paralysis. Naturally, this circumstance (especially since the patient also underwent syphilis and is informed about the significance of syphilis for paralysis) very effectively supports his original sperm hypochondria.—I definitely want to observe the case for a while and report my impressions to you.

There is now a noticeable increase in my practice; and although the slump which I have endured for some months was not enough to depress me seriously, I do feel a certain satisfaction now that I see that better times seem to be breaking out.

The analysis of a homosexual, very intelligent young man brings me great satisfaction. He brought me interesting parapraxes; I am sending one of them to you enclosed.[1]

The thing with the "déjà vu" was *striking* with him![2] A few times he came with a fresh dream. Then he told me about the events of the day, about a "déjà vu," among other things; in the subsequent dream analysis a forgotten piece of a dream then came to the fore, which became comprehensible to him, either directly, or only after interpretation, through that feeling of being acquainted. The "other life many thousands of years ago" was the dream life of the previous night, closely associated, to be sure, with the long forgotten impressions of childhood.[3] Perhaps the very widespread belief in rebirth and metempsychosis permits the same explanation?

I will review Rank's "Hero" for the "Wiener Klinische Rundschau."[4]

As you can read on this letterhead, I am now living in the hotel[5] across from my home, where all kinds of workers (painters, plumbers) are at work. I am moving from the ground floor to the second floor, but am staying in the same house.—I hope to be able to go home tomorrow.

Urbantschitsch[6] was here not long ago, and we spent a few pleasant hours together.—

I very much look forward to seeing Brill again. I consider him one of the most honest and intelligent of your pupils; he is also very agreeable to me personally.

I close my rhapsodical reports and greet you as your

Obedient
Dr. Ferenczi

Kindest regards also to your family.

1. This enclosure is missing.
2. Ferenczi is referring to the view represented by Freud in *Everyday Life* that the sensation of déjà vu is a "recollection of an unconscious phantasy" (1901b, p. 266).
3. This example was cited by Freud in *Everyday Life* (1901b, p. 297) and was also used by Ferenczi in his communication "Ein Fall von déjà vu" [A Case of Déjà Vu] (1912, 86; *Fin.*, p. 319).
4. No record has been found of this review.
5. The Hotel Royal, still in existence today. In the ground-floor Café Royal (now the

Café and Restaurant Hungaria) Ferenczi used to meet with his friends, including the journalist Hugó Ignótus, the poet Dezsö Kostolanyi, the writers Gyula Krudy and Sándor Brody, the painter Robert Berény, and others.

6. Rudolf von Urbantschitsch (1879–1964), Viennese physician and author of popular psychoanalytic writings and belles lettres. In 1908 he founded the Cottage Sanatorium in Vienna, which he headed until 1920. In 1908 he became a member of the Wednesday Society but, with Freud's consent, kept his membership secret in order not to jeopardize the economic position of his clinic. In 1922 he underwent analytic training in Vienna and Budapest, but after 1924 he again distanced himself from psychoanalysis. He eventually emigrated to California.

59

Vienna, May 5, 1909
IX., Berggasse 19

Dear colleague,

When my brother availed himself of Schenker there was no more room to be had on the Laura (from Trieste, August 21). So, after overcoming my disappointment, I made a reservation with N[orth] G[erman] Lloyd. George Washington, August 21, a proud, new ship. Unfortunately, we have to be content with inside cabins; the outside cabins are without exception intended for two persons and would cost at least 1,000 marks per person. Now, that has well-known disadvantages, but they are otherwise well situated, right next to a bath. Price, 600 marks, 100 of which I have paid for you, and which I won't hold you to until Bremen. The numbers are 182 and 184. I let myself be guided by the consideration that you would be willing to accept a certain deprivation of fresh air and view of the sea at night if, instead, you can be undisturbed. I hope it will be bearable.

I will just add your contributions to the third edition of Everyday Life. You will permit my giving your full name?

My daughter is very well. With cordial regards,

Yours,
Freud

P.S. Diagram of the ship will follow.

60

Budapest, May 7, 1909
Hotel Royal

Dear Professor,

The same disappointment had a less depressing effect the second time.
I am very much looking forward to the trip and thank you for your efforts.
The choice of cabins also fits my intentions.

I feel very honored to be cited by name in Everyday Life.

Best regards from

Your obedient
Dr. Ferenczi

61

Budapest, May 18, 1909
VII., Erzsébet-körút 54

Dear Professor,

Finally my home is in order, and I wanted to sit down to finish the lecture
on the interpretation of dreams when I learned that the Society of Physicians is having its last meeting of the semester next week and that the
lecture has to be postponed until the fall series.[1] I breathed easily, because
such a lecture about dreams for the completely uninitiated proved to be
quite a difficult task.

The practical work of analysis is now going very smoothly; I am now
doing three to five analyses daily, among them a homosexuality, an impotence, an obsessional neurosis, the already mentioned querulist, an
erythrophobia—*nothing but* men. I evidently have more luck with men
than with women, although the transference of women has already given
me a lot to do.

Brill wrote me a very cordial letter, in which he pleads for us to stay
longer in America. I hardly think we can get into that.—

Jung also notified me that he has returned from his Italian trip[2] and wants
to dedicate himself totally to scientific work. He wants to conclude the
association work and immerse himself in the analysis of psychoses.

I have still not given up hope that Mr. and Mrs. Hollitscher will make
the postponed trip to Budapest a reality, after the patient's complete recov-

ery. This little diversion would be quite pleasant in the beautiful weather
which now prevails.

Kindest regards from your

Obedient
Ferenczi

1. Ferenczi gave the lecture on October 15, 1909 (see letter 77 and n. 1).

2. During the second half of April, Jung had taken a bicycle tour of northern Italy after
having relinquished his position at the Burghölzli (*Freud/Jung*, April 12, 1909, p. 215).

62

Vienna, May 23, 1909
IX., Berggasse 19

Dear colleague,

Our correspondence is doubtless suffering in expectation of the summer.
Everything is being unintentionally postponed until the days when we will
walk on the deck of the Washington and chat about the present and future
of ΨA. I can't do anything against this compulsion and am therefore confining myself to factual information.

I note with satisfaction that you have again reconciled yourself with ΨA,
and I also understand that you are not uncomfortable with postponing your
lecture. I am counting the weeks until the vacation, and there are still too
many. We have made reservations for the summer in the Hotel Ammerwald on the Tyrol-Bavaria border (region of the Bavarian royal castles).
There I hope to find the solitude of the forest [*Waldeinsamkeit*], for which
I yearn so much and which my body also needs so much. I will then depart
directly for Bremen on August 19. We will talk later about how we shall
meet.

My daughter is very well again. It is foreseeable that she will realize her
intention to visit Budapest, if not in the next few months, then certainly
in the fall. My wife is in Karlsbad with Sophie. (I never know if I have
already communicated a piece of news.) I will visit her over Whitsuntide.

The hard work at present naturally can't be made use of, but the impressions keep on accumulating and will probably yield something when I am
more tranquil. Have I written to you much about the third edition of
Everyday Life? I accepted the lion's share of your contributions but left out
some as being too fine for the elementary nature of the book; I know that
I can be very grateful to you for these things, and I am happy to be so. The
book won't come out until fall. Then the *second* edition of the Theory of
Sexuality will also materialize.

America will really be an experience. I am very happy that you are coming along. Clark University recently sent me its publication for its first Tenth Anniversary Celebration. We can conclude from it that the lectures will be printed and that the title of honorary "Doctor of Laws"[1] will be bestowed upon the European guests.

How is your English doing?

Cordially,
Freud

1. Written in English in the original [Trans.].

63

Budapest, June 10, 1909
VII., Erzsébet-körút 54

Dear Professor,

The enclosed excerpt from the "New York Medical Journal"[1] should interest you. It was gratifying at first to see that the spirits are so prepared to receive you. On the other hand, in America, the land of business, the apparent increasingly widespread tendency to rediscover and to "modify" your things is becoming evident. Since I also learned something similar about *Jones* from a reliable source, I was happy that it was he who seems to have mentioned your name at least *once*.

Aside from the sense of justice, such phenomena (along with these ethical ones) also seem to have a certain real significance for the future; they show whose hands your ideas are getting into. I am convinced that no progress is possible in psychoanalysis without honesty. But I find this attribute (among the Americans) only in *Brill*, who unfortunately didn't get to speak in New Haven.—

My little work about the interpretation of dreams has—I believe—come out so well that it deserves to be translated into German.[2] I will bring it along on the ship.

The lecture that I gave to the Physicians' Association has already been printed;[3] it was read with interest by many.

I sent the manuscript of the "introjection" and hypnosis paper[4] to Zurich,[5] after minor revision and inclusion of your theory of masochistic suggestion.[6] I left the two parts separate as two chapters of the work. The mood in which both were written is so different that a total amalgamation seemed unnatural to me.

America is occupying me, unfortunately, only theoretically. I could find time neither to learn English nor to read about America.—I hope everything is all right with you at home. Please give my regards to *all* the dear members of your family.

Best regards from

Your obedient
Ferenczi

I have a young *Rigorosant*[7] as a helper at the health service, a capable, honest chap. He will, I think, in time become an energetic collaborator. I learn from him that your ideas are very popular among students—although they learn nothing or only disparaging things from their professors.—

1. Correspondence, "Letter from New Haven: Recent Discussions on Psychotherapy: The New Haven Discussion," *New York Medical Journal*, May 29, 1909, pp. 1099–1101. Ernest Jones and James Putnam had spoken at the American Therapeutic Congress in New Haven, Connecticut, in May of that year; see Clark, *Freud*, p. 261; Nathan G. Hale, *Freud and the Americans* (New York, 1971), p. 147, and Jones, *Associations*, p. 189.

2. See letter 77 and n. 1.

3. See letter 42 and n. 2.

4. Part 1, "Introjection in the Neuroses," and part 2, "The Part Played by Transference in Hypnotism and Suggestion," of "Introjection and Transference" (1909, 67; *C.*, p. 35).

5. To Jung, the editor of the *Jahrbuch*.

6. Ferenczi cited Freud's view (see Freud 1905d, p. 150) that *"hypnotic credulity and pliancy take their root in the masochistic component of the sexual instinct"* (1909, 67; *Schriften* I, 39; *C.*, pp. 80f).

7. A student just short of terminating his studies (*Rigorosum* = oral doctoral examination).

64

Vienna, June 13, 1909
IX., Berggasse 19

Dear colleague,

Thanks for your letter and excerpt. The "modifications" are of no consequence. They are attempts to "adapt" to things [*sich die Dinge "anzueignen"*],[1] as our language states with such incisive double meaning; priority is of no consequence, and the whole matter has developed so much in the full light of day that obfuscations will not be able to endure for long. Otherwise, your judgment is certainly correct; honesty will not be any more frequent a phenomenon in America than it is in Europe; progress is also not to be expected from that quarter.

But we won't let ourselves be distracted from the pleasure of the beautiful vacation trip, which we won't otherwise take too seriously.

You already know from Jung himself that he has received an invitation to give three lectures at our celebration on a topic which has been given to him? Now, that elevates the whole business and will certainly enhance and enlarge everything for us. I don't know whether he will succeed in sharing the ship with us, but in any case we will stay together there.

I was very pleased about the notices concerning your works. I am now writing down the Salzburg Rat-Man[2] for the Jahrbuch. With America, things are going for me exactly the way they are for you. No talk of preparation. It is also too late in the year; during the few weeks of vacation I will be writing the paper on technique, and I would also like to get some enjoyment from the woods. Have I already told you that we have rented a place in Ammerwald, Post Reutte on the Bavarian-Tyrolian border? An isolated hotel in the middle of the most beautiful forest, region of the royal castles.

We are awaiting the return of wife and daughter (Sophie) from Hamburg[3] in the course of this week. Wouldn't you like to participate in our Wednesday farewell dinner on the *Konstantinhügel?*[4] Stegmann[5] is expected as a guest; Rank will already have sent you the invitation.

Kind regards,
Freud

1. The German verb *sich aneignen* literally means "to make one's own" [Trans.].
2. "Notes upon a Case of Obsessional Neurosis" (1909d); and see "Original Record of the Case of Obsessional Neurosis" (1955a).
3. The home of Freud's mother-in-law, Emmeline Bernays.
4. On June 16, 1909, at the end of the work year, the Wednesday Society organized a "social gathering on the Konstantinhügel [Hill of Constantine]" (*Minutes* II, 259), a popular tourist restaurant in the Prater, Vienna's amusement park.
5. Arnold Georg Stegmann (?–191?), court physician and psychiatrist in Dresden; participant in the Salzburg meeting (1908) and co-founder of the German Psychoanalytic Society. He was killed in the First World War.

65

Vienna, June 28, 1909
IX., Berggasse 19

Dear colleague,

? ? ?

Cordially,
Freud

66

Budapest, June 30, 1909
VII., Erzsébet-körút 54

Dear Professor,

I don't know if these lines have reached you in Vienna still, but I hope that the letter's contents will be forwarded to you.

I can make your question marks superfluous in a very calming manner. I knew that you were overloaded with work and that in addition you have to make all kinds of preparations for the trip, so I wanted at least to spare you the effort of answering my letters. Also, the things I could have written to you are mostly of a scientific nature, and we will be able to dispense with them in a much more comfortable and profitable fashion on the deck of the "Washington."

I am happy that you were able to withdraw for a time from the grinding work, and I wish you nice weather and good mood for your vacation and (if this wish doesn't do any harm in the hunt for vegetables) a rich harvest of mushrooms. You write me that the Hotel Post Reutte is situated on the Bavarian-Tyrolian border, only I don't know whether it is in Bavaria or Tyrol? Please be so kind as to let me know which. During the day I am constantly busy, have relinquished all "family practice," and busy myself (aside from the agendas of the court and my hours at the health service)[1] almost exclusively with analyses. The material side of this practice is gradually improving, especially since I no longer accept any new nonpaying patients.

In the evenings I am usually so tired that I don't feel any real desire for work. Then, caught between duty and desire, I grasp for the compromise of reading your works. I am now reading the last chapters of the "Interpretation of Dreams" for the nth time—each time I get new insights from it and clarifications which I had overlooked, or hidden, as it were. I believe that the "Interpretation of Dreams" contains the kernel of everything that we know and will have to work on for the foreseeable future.

Most cordial greetings to you and your dear family from your obedient

Dr. Ferenczi

How are you planning to put together your wardrobe for the trip?

1. See letter 9, n. 2.

67

Vienna, July 4, 1909
IX., Berggasse 19

Dear colleague,

We are not yet doing as well as you assume. We don't leave for Munich until the fourteenth of the month. Our address will then be:

Ammerwald, *Post Reutte* (not Hotel Post)
Tyrol.

I do not dare count on your visiting us this time, since I am assuming that America will consume most of your vacation. We can still decide where we will meet, whether on the way or not until we get to Bremen. Aside from that, there is a *remote* possibility that on Sunday I will be waiting in Budapest between two trains, 1:30–3:20. Couldn't we eat lunch together then? I will telegraph in case the trip should come about. I assume that you are quite lonely now in the summer.

As for wardrobe, besides the travel suits, I will take along a dress coat and a salon jacket. The former can probably be dispensed with. Don't forget a good coat for the ocean voyage. One should buy a top hat there on account of the difficulty in transporting it and then throw it into the ocean before the return trip.

I completed the case of the Rat-Man[1] and am preparing to send it to Jung, but I have reached the end of my capacity for work for now. In the summer only America. I gladly accept your wishes for the vacation. Unfortunately, I can't do anything about the weather. This summer promises little. My daughter[2] has fled the rigors of the Pustertal for Klobenstein auf dem Ritten or Bolzano, which we are also leaning toward for next year.

There will I hope be time on the G. Washington for all scientific conversations, if the sea doesn't bother us. I am very much looking forward to the whole thing.

Your cordially obedient
Freud

1. See letter 64 and n. 2.
2. Mathilde.

68

Budapest, July 22, 1909
VII., Erzsébet-körút 54

Dear Professor,

I hope that no obstacles have come in the way of your vacation plans, and that in the colossal efforts of a psychoanalytic year (about which I also now have a vague idea) you have at last been able to get some rest in the midst of your beloved woods and in the circle of your dear throng of children! Please allow yourself to plunge into your work. [That was a slip of the pen; I intended to write *not* to plunge, and immediately add "although this request struggles against an inner wish to have more and more of you."][1]

I am not so alone as you surmise. A favorable coincidence has made it possible for me to be in pleasant company for the summer months as well.[2]—Still, it was very enticing to me when you spoke of the possibility of my spending a few days in the Tyrolian mountains with you.—Unfortunately, for the time being it won't work!

I have six weeks of leave (from August 16 to October 1). Could you tell me something about the return trip (date of arrival in Europe, port city)? Because if we can't be home on October 1, then I will perhaps stay here somewhat longer and travel directly to Bremen. Otherwise I have four to five days free before boarding, which I am thinking of spending in Berlin or Hamburg. It is not out of the question that I will take a hop over to you in the Tyrol.

I was very sorry that your planned trip to Budapest will not take place. I was very much looking forward to it.—

Only a few more questions. I want to take along 5,000 crowns, 2,000 in my pocket, 3,000 sent ahead in a letter of credit. I calculate 1,200 marks = 1,500 crowns for the trip, 60 crowns per day for the remaining thirty days = 1,800 crowns; that makes a total of 3,300 crowns.—the remainder for unforeseen expenses. Do you think that's enough?

No talk of preparations on my part! An hour of English conversation per day is all that reminds me of America.—Do you have plans for the stay in America, and if so, which places should we visit?

Excuse the many questions.

Kind regards to you and your whole family.

Your obedient
Ferenczi

1. Enclosed in brackets in the original.
2. Possibly the first mention of Ferenczi's love and future wife, Gizella Pálos, née Altschul (1865–1949).

69

Ammerwald, July 25, 1909

Dear Doctor,

It is with pleasure that I attempt to answer your questions, which relate to our planned adventure and can thus arouse only pleasant expectations.

I don't yet know anything about the return trip. Brill has advised against making a reservation now, because one can always get one easily at this time. [The tickets for the G. Washington are sitting in my briefcase; I have paid for half of both of them, so that you have only to pay for the rest in Bremen.][1] I figure, however, that we will go home around September 20, so that a few days will be left to me for Berlin and Hamburg, where, on the one hand, relatives are expecting a visit, and on the other, meetings with people like Marcinowski[2] and Abraham are waiting in the wings. Like you, I want to be home on October 1. We can't know beforehand whether it will come out exactly that way. If you want to use the last days for a visit with us, you will have the joyful assent of all my family. They immediately instructed me to advise you that August 15 is a Sunday, so that you could very easily lengthen your vacation by a departure on the evening of the 14th. We would then leave here early on the 19th and get to Bremen on the 20th, as intended. It would naturally be very nice.

My trip to Budapest would have coincided with a consultation in Salonika, which had already been confirmed but was canceled at the last minute. It was not a case of neurosis but a paralyzed child.

Your financial provisions seem more than ample to me. I figure on getting by with the 3,000 marks from Clark University. But since I won't get it in advance, I will take the same amount along and count on us helping each other out.

I am making fewer preparations than you, although I would have more reason to make them. I have really completely used up my budget of strength for 1909, and I must rest. I will postpone all preparations until the ship. You and Jung should then tell me what I should talk about. I have a few books about America with me, but I'm not looking at them. Yesterday I ordered a few archaeological books; there is still a little spark of interest present for that. I want to be surprised. My only intent is to see Niagara, which is as far from New York or Boston as Abbazia is from Vienna; otherwise I think we should let ourselves be driven by Brill and whatever other influences materialize there.

In expectation of your correspondence during these weeks of vacation, I am

Yours,
Freud

1. Enclosed in brackets in the original.

2. Johannes Jaroslaw Marcinowski (1868–1935), medical director of the sanatorium of Sielbeck am Uklei (Holstein). Freud had come into contact with him shortly before as a result of his article "Zur Frage der infantilen Sexualität," *Berliner klinische Wochenschrift* 46 (1909): 927f. Marcinowski later became a member not of the German but of the Vienna Society (1919–1925).

70

Budapest, August 3, 1909
VII., Erzsébet-körút 54

Dear Professor,

I have not been very well the last few days (I was troubled by an acute intestinal inflammation)—and I didn't want to write you until I was completely recovered. Now I am again quite well and I can look forward to our great journey.—I looked up Ammerwald in Baedeker and on the map, and I noticed how well you have protected yourself this time from the invasion of your acquaintances. I hope you will recover and rest up completely there.—I thank you kindly for the cordial invitation to come there (which I actually provoked myself!). It would, however,—as I had to conclude upon mature reflection—significantly lengthen my railway journey if I made a detour by way of Munich-Ammerwald. I will therefore renounce the great pleasure of reexperiencing the beautiful days of Berchtesgaden and seek a more direct way to Bremen with a few interruptions in Germany. My preliminary decision is to travel by way of Nuremberg (August 15–16) to Frankfurt a. M. (18th) and, in addition to the aforementioned cities, which I don't yet know, perhaps take a short excursion to Rothenburg o. d. T. [ob der Tauber] or to Bayreuth *(Festspiele)*.[1] Would you like to meet in Nuremberg? If so, then I can easily dispense with the Wagner music, which I know doesn't tempt you very much.—All of this is, however, still very much up in the air. The only certainty is that I will get to Bremen in the evening of the 19th or the morning of the 20th and wait for you there.—With your permission, I would like to accompany you on the return by way of Hamburg-Berlin. Relatives[2] are also awaiting me there—and I would also like to get to know our Berlin colleagues.

I am now working less smoothly. The great heat and my unaccustomed condition of bodily illness have crippled my power to work. I am now feeling the way I was before.

I thank the Professor's wife for her kind letter.[3]

Cordial regards from your

Truly obedient
Dr. Ferenczi

1. Ferenczi was a great lover of music with a predilection for the operas of Richard Wagner.

2. Ferenczi's favorite brother, Zsigmond (1862–?), a chemical engineer; his wife, Anne; and their adopted daughter, Rosa.

3. This letter is missing.

71

Ammerwald, August 9, 1909

Dear Doctor,

Your decision has, to be sure, upset the women of the family, but they are not closed to the realization that a few days of complete, i.e., real freedom should probably not be begrudged you. For the same reason I am also not considering curtailing your travel plans through a premature meeting, and will now share mine with you. I am staying here through the 18th, will go to Munich early on the 19th; from there at 4:25 I will take the direct train to Bremen and expect to arrive in Bremen at 5:35 A.M. I therefore need only to know when you will arrive (perhaps by telegram) in order to await you there.

Your indisposition is doubtless a consequence of the exertion of the entire year, which has always manifested itself in symptoms. Let us hope that the ocean voyage will be particularly good for you.

I declare myself definitely unsuited for preparation for America. I haven't read anything but an archaeological work about Cyprus, and the only connection that has with New York is the fact that the largest collection of Cypriot antiquities has made its way to New York, where I also hope to see it. You see, this is virtually an illustration of the words of the Magic Flute: "I can't force you to love."[1] I don't have any illusions at all about America, but I am very much looking forward to our journey together. On the way back, where Jung will probably leave soon after disembarking, we will then finish up in Hamburg and Berlin, which can probably be done together, and then we will separate for the unavoidable duties with respect to relatives.

I am quite well recovered, but intellectually still very lethargic. My family here is doing splendidly. We are all once again united here just now. The eldest daughter, of course, no longer completely belongs to us.

I won't write to you anymore now and await confirmation of your arrival in Bremen. Jung has a complicated itinerary and won't meet us until the ship.

Auf Wiedersehen,
Freud

1. "Zur Liebe *will* ich dich nicht zwingen, doch geb ich dir die Freiheit nicht" (I don't *want* to force you to love, but I won't give you freedom), from Zarastro's aria, act 1; mentioned by Freud in the *Interpretation of Dreams* (1900a, p. 291).

72

Budapest, August 11, 1909
VII., Erzsébet-körút 54

Dear Professor,

It remains as planned: we will meet in Bremen.

My itinerary may undergo some changes in details, but this much stands firm, that I will already be there on the evening of the 19th. I will then await you at the train at 5:35 A.M. and reserve a room for you at the hotel. It says in Baedeker: "Hotels on day before departure of passenger liners for North America often filled. Room reservations recommended." I will therefore reserve the rooms (yours for the 20th) by telegram already on the 17th–18th. I have chosen the first-named *Hotel Hillmann,* not far from the railway station; if there is no room available there I will settle for the *Hotel de l'Europe.* (Both on the *Herdentorsteinweg.*)

It was not easy for me to pass up the visit to Ammerwald. The longing for "real freedom" was not among the motives that brought me to this decision, however. Now I can admit it. I didn't want to disturb your vacation with my visit, which certainly would have degenerated into psychoanalytic conversations.

My intestinal inflammation has disappeared; to be sure, I did everything to achieve that end; I didn't want to be a burdensome traveling companion.

Kindest regards to your dear family. Looking forward to seeing you again soon, I am

Yours,
Dr. Ferenczi

I won't send any more news.[1]

1. Freud, Ferenczi, and Jung met in Bremen on August 20 and departed the next day. After their arrival in the United States on August 29, they first spent a week in New York and then drove to Worcester, Massachusetts, the site of Clark University. During the following week Freud delivered his *Five Lectures on Psycho-Analysis* (1910a [1909]), which he sketched out each morning on walks with Ferenczi. At the closing celebration Freud and Jung received honorary Doctor of Laws degrees. After a visit to Niagara Falls and a stay at James Putnam's camp in the Adirondacks (see letter 85, n. 15), the three men embarked on September 21 and reached Bremen on September 29. Jung immediately went home; Freud and Ferenczi stayed briefly in Hamburg and Berlin (see letter 73, n. 2).

The trip has been described numerous times; see, e.g., Jones II, 53ff; Clark, *Freud*, pp. 264ff, and Nathan G. Hale, *Freud and the Americans* (New York, 1971). A comprehensive account can be found in *Freud/Jung*, pp. 245f.

73

Budapest, October 5, 1909
VII., Erzsébet-körút 54

Dear Professor!

Already on the first day upon my return I was so inundated with work that I can only now finish this letter, which I began on the train.[1]

As a postscript to my story I can add the following:

1. Before she (Frau Seidler)[2] named one of the city names (Vienna, Hamburg), she acted very strained, as though she had far to go. At Vienna the first thing she said was: "The letter (yours) leads me into a city where I already was; first I see the railway station"—"Yes, that is Vienna."

2. At our departure she said to me: "Recommend me, Doctor," even though I didn't introduce myself as "Doctor." She had evidently read the salutation in your letter to me.

When I try to explain what I saw and heard I must admit that I am incapable of doing so.—

Reading through the cloth, i.e., with a blindfold, could be sleight of hand. But guessing the occupation of Prof. Philipps [sic][3] as well as the strange statements about your personality are certainly not. I said nothing that could have helped her do this; I hardly spoke at all—she didn't even let me say a word. The card that she received (and perhaps read, cleverly and unbeknownst to me) says so little that her many pertinent remarks about your interests and intellectual tendencies are certainly striking.

Now, if I assume that she really possesses uncommon abilities, then this could perhaps be explained as a kind of "mind reading," as reading *my* thoughts.

The intensive self-analysis that I undertook immediately after the séance led me to this hypothesis. Most of her statements about you, Prof. Philipp, etc. correspond to trains of thought that I really produced, but partly also those which I could have repressed. Some examples:

1.) "Between you and me stands a scholar" etc.

"Between us both (Frau Seidler and me) there is regret"—

Analysis: I consciously regretted that I—following your advice—made inquiries about a completely strange person and not one who is quite close to me. I also repressed my curiosity about my own future (that is to say, about her oracular prophecies about it).

2.) The remarks about your *maturity*, about your *age* (in the spiritual sense), your overcoming of everything human correspond *exactly* to a long meditation in which I immersed myself on the ship after the somewhat painful acknowledgment of my *infantility* about you and your personality (as an emulative example). First I overcame the spiteful thought: "I would rather be the way I am; that way I am at least happy, a happy child. You (Prof. Freud), however, are obviously intellectually *so old*, explaining everything, resolving all your own passions into thoughts, that you cannot be happy."—I soon recognized, however, that this thought was an attempt at resistance and then undertook to attempt to follow your instructions.

3.) The remark about your dissatisfaction with the Viennese surroundings could perhaps be an allusion to your Viennese colleagues; in all honesty, however, in analyzing your dreams I also had the thought that dissatisfaction and concern about the members of your family must play a great role with you. "Being dissatisfied with one's soul" naturally also always has—in my thoughts—sexual significance.

4.) The not-quite-understanding between both of us (Freud and Ferenczi) has figured prominently in my thoughts in recent weeks. I learned from your dream that with me it is only "11:45" (I interpreted this to mean that you won't find complete understanding in me). The impulses of jealousy with respect to Jung, however, also inspired in me the infantilely strengthened thought that you, too, do not fully appreciate me (my attitude, my good will, my longing for recognition). (I corrected that later.)

5.) That business about the comparison of your knowledge with my faith etc. is complete nonsense. It could correspond to the at most quite ucs. ideas of grandeur in me.

6.) I have almost no idea about how etchings are produced. I believe I read something about it in Goethe's Dichtung und Wahrheit;[4] my conception of it was that one *engraves* or scratches the image with a *needle* on a metal plate and then treats the plate with an etching solution. I have not yet had time to enlighten myself on the matter.

But even if we assumed (which, however, after so little experience would be quite inadmissible) that she really guessed my thoughts, the matter would still be no less obscure. Along with the theory of "psychic induction," one would then also have to think about the possibility of a kind of ecstatic hyperesthesia for minimal expressive movements, i.e., that we all somehow betray our thoughts in our speech, movements, etc. Finally, the time would come for the assumption of a real clairvoyance, telepathy, etc.—There was no talk at all about the future (because of the lack of time).—Perhaps I will send my brother in Berlin[5] to her with a well-thought-out plan. I am also thinking of visiting one of the soothsayeresses in Budapest sometime.

The following is also worth mentioning:

Frau Seidler never seems to know whether she should interpret an idea—an image that appears to her (she is visual)—in a *concrete* or *abstract* sense. So, she talked for a long time quite correctly, but not clearly, about Prof. Philipp's occupation. Then she asked me curiously what he actually was. When I told her Prof. Philipp was an artist—only then did she say "he sticks with a needle."—We also have this uncertainty about concrete or symbolic meaning in the interpretation of dreams.—

In conclusion, I want to assure you (although you are justified in accepting such "assurances" with skepticism) that I am not in danger of lapsing into occultism. The case has certainly aroused my interest, but I also know that it is not my next task to be concerned with these questions.

I would be very grateful to you if you would share your ideas about this case with me—no matter how brief they may be.—

I have received the page proofs of my paper[6] from Deuticke. In reading them I found the first part somewhat superficial but the second part (hypnosis) somewhat better worked through. You must have your paper about technique published soon so that the ambiguities which I have not yet been able to avoid will be eradicated.

America is like a dream. On the whole, it went as I expected—I had much more reward and satisfaction from the company on the voyage than from what I engaged in over there. But I am extraordinarily glad to have made the trip.

Best regards to all.

Your obedient
Dr. Ferenczi

As "supporting material" I am enclosing Frau Seidler's original notes—Prof. Philipp's card and your letter to me.—*Please be so kind as to send me back all this (as well as this letter) when you get the chance.* Perhaps this matter is the beginning of something—then this material would be useful.—[N.B. No asking back in Abraham's sense!][7]

I am also enclosing an excerpt from the *Berliner Tageblatt,* which my brother sent me. Prof. Ostwald's energetic remarks[8] suffer very much from ignorance of psychoanalysis. If he knew something about the mechanism of mania and hysteria, he would find the question of "ecstasies" not so simply, mathematically soluble.

1. The pages of the letter are numbered consecutively with Roman numerals in the upper left-hand corner, written in blue pencil, beginning with II. The first part of the letter, written on the train, is obviously missing.

2. After returning from America, Ferenczi had looked up Frau Seidler, a medium, with the intention of investigating parapsychological phenomena.

3. Possibly the painter John Philipp (1872–1938), a cousin of Martha Freud's, whom Freud had met in 1885 in Paris (see, e.g., Freud's letters to Martha of November 26 and December 3, 1885; *Letters,* pp. 186–188).

4. Goethe, *Aus meinem Leben, Dichtung und Wahrheit,* bk. 8, in *Sophienausgabe* XXVII, 179–181, 213f.

5. Zsigmond Ferenczi.

6. "Introjection and Transference."

7. Enclosed in brackets in the original.

8. Wilhelm Ostwald (1853–1932), a German chemist (won Nobel Prize for chemistry 1909) and philosopher, had formulated an "energetic" theory of happiness: "The feeling of happiness is proportional to the product of the surpluses subject to the will and the total operational supply of energy" see "Zum Fall Wangel," *Berliner Tageblatt,* afternoon edition, February 10, 1909. See also Ferenczi's paper "Ostwald über die Psychoanalyse" (1917, 192).

74

Vienna, October 6, 1909
IX., Berggasse 19

Dear friend,

I can't answer you today nor send back your letter. I want to sleep on it first for a few nights and ruminate over it for a few days. Now, I see only this much: one can go ahead and assume that the person reads with her eyes what has been presented to her—just as you read this letter—by means of some trick. All her declarations and the guarantees proffered by her speak in favor of that. But, apart from that, there seems to be something to the thing. The rest appears to be genuine! Not that the woman [*Frauenzimmer*] possesses particularly great talents. You really don't need to regret that you didn't ask about the future. That always forms itself anew; even the dear Lord doesn't know it in advance. But the transference of *your* thoughts in incomprehensible ways is the strange thing and possibly something new. Keep quiet about it for the time being; we will have to engage in further experiments.

By the end of this week I will have gotten myself together and will be able to express myself.

I have been visited by much work and some hardship here.

Cordially,
Freud

75

Vienna, October 11, 1909
IX., Berggasse 19

Dear friend,

At last I can pull myself together to write to you about your experience with Frau Seidler. I have now overcome the shock and am confronting the matter just like any other, which is not easy.

Let's sort things out:

1.) Setting up experiments to find out whether she knows something about the future would be patent nonsense; we will permit ourselves to keep this prejudice in reserve. It should be kept out of all further experiments.

2.) We seem to be able to presume with certainty that she reads. How she does it is rather uninteresting. But she is quite a stupid person, otherwise she wouldn't reproduce the names so precisely but rather be content with approximations. In the beginning I was very puzzled that she should have guessed Vienna. I had forgotten that the name is printed on the stationery. This point can be decided by a simple experiment that you can commission your brother to perform. Carefully erase the place name from a real letter that you have received and replace it with another, or alter it by adding something if possible. Be sure *not* to explain the forgery to your brother, and you will see that she will name the wrong place and will have no suspicion of the forgery.

3.) I also cannot exclude the probability that she can do something, namely, reproduce your thoughts, whose visual representation in her mind she herself does not understand. All other explanations, like enhanced sensitivity for mimicry and the like, seem to me first of all inadequate, and second, they presuppose a special psychic ability in this woman. The assumption of thought transference alone does not require this but rather the opposite; she may be quite an imbecilic, even inactive person who makes images of what would otherwise be suppressed through her own intellectual activity. In her intention to swindle and to play the magician, she then has the courage and the attentiveness to perceive what has come into being purely physiologically in her. Certain of her behavior traits, like her questions about what is correct in what she says, her (projected) concern about whether one understands her, seem to be genuine.

Thus, as you see, I subscribe to your interpretation that she guesses the thoughts, perhaps the ucs. thoughts of the experimental subject—with the corresponding misunderstandings and convergences of a kind of *distortion* in the transition from one psyche into another. So she seems to have interpreted the images of ships and traveling symbolically in connection with a death, as perhaps she might have done correctly in other cases, because she could not have known that she had a real traveler to America in front of her.

What she says about me, nonsense in and of itself, acquires value if you acknowledge and legitimize it. You then have to take responsibility for it.

I don't understand that business about the ancient books and notes. You would have to analyze that. Are they perhaps dollar bills?

In analyzing the prophecies, the following should be taken into consideration:

1.) Pythia's distortion.

2.) your own resistances.

One may fail any number of times to make an interpretation under such circumstances; if it succeeds, it will do so only under the condition that you adapt what has been said as you do a ψ accomplishment of your own.

Should one now, as a result of this experience, commit oneself to occultism? Certainly not; it is only a matter of thought transference. If this can be proved, then one has to believe it—then it is not a ψ phenomenon, but rather a purely somatic one, certainly a novelty of the first rank. In the meantime, let us keep absolute silence with regard to it. The only one whom I have drawn into the secret is Heller,[1] who also has had experiences with it. We want to initiate Jung at a later date, when we have more to go on; for at the moment it is very little, and by asking clear questions, renouncing the future, and taking into account the little deception, it ought to be easy to get more material. Think out some good plans and have your brother formulate experiments which dispense with analysis in the beginning. We can then take a research trip to Berlin, if you haven't found something as good in Budapest by then.

I am almost afraid that you have begun to recognize something big here, but we will encounter the greatest difficulties in exploiting it.

I am totally immersed in work; nothing new with my daughter[2] (did I already write that she is ailing again?).

Cordially,
Your Freud

Returning enclosures as the beginning of a dossier.

You received Anatole France,[3] I hope.

1. Hugo Heller (1870–1923), Viennese publisher and bookseller, member of the Wednesday Society; first publisher of *Imago* and the *Zeitschrift*. His salon was a center for liberal artists and intellectuals.
2. Mathilde.
3. Anatole France (1844–1924), the French novelist, essayist, and literary critic, was one of Freud's and Ferenczi's favorite authors.

76

Budapest, October 14, 1909
VII., Erzsébet-körút 54

Dear Professor,

I was very gratified that you so quickly and profoundly satisfied my longing for news about your reaction to the Seidler case. For me it was also an experience of the first rank, and I was glad that, despite the effect of a seemingly novel psychic phenomenon, I was able to maintain my total presence of mind and behave like a critical observer. Even so, I was afraid that you would conceive the matter differently, which my intelligence complex struggled against. Then I was all the more pleased by your lines, from which I surmise that you also, for your part, bring to the fore *the* interpretation that I consider the only probable one (I added the others only to cover myself, as it were). Transference of thoughts in heretofore inexplicable ways, arousing visual impressions in a strange psyche through my (cs. or ucs.) thoughts—this was the possibility that also arose in me most distinctly. I can't discover any trace of occult tendency in me; you need have no fear on this account, and I mentioned the story about interpreting ucs. expressive movements only for the sake of completeness. Only I am not *quite* convinced that the woman reads the letters with her own eyes. If we assume the possibility of a transference, then we should not be frightened by the possibility of the transference of images of the sound of words [*Wortklangbildern*], of written images, etc. i.e.: the person, stimulated by *my brain,* could have named, that is, seen the names of persons, localities, etc. That should be ascertainable through further experiments.

Yesterday I wrote to my brother and asked him to visit Frau Seidler and hand over to her three pieces of paper with writing on them.

1.) The first (which he is supposed to give her) is the fragment of a German letter written by a person whom my brother doesn't know; the signature is not a direct one but rather an allusion, almost illegible; the person to whom the letter is addressed knows my brother—but he doesn't know the person. The letter has no date and designation of place; in the contents I have skillfully made illegible the only word that would be revealing ("artist").

2.) The second is a letter that *I* wrote many years ago (1905) to *my younger brother's present mother-in-law*[1] (about whom I have already told you much). The contents are very interesting for my brother, arousing feelings. There is much discussion about the illness of our brother[2] who has since died. I could also learn through Frau Seidler (if she really can do something) whether and what my brother thinks about my relations with the Pálos family. The letter is *written in Hungarian.*

3.) Then I also sent him a closed envelope with the request to open it only at Frau Seidler's and to have her divulge its contents (an apocryphal letter fabricated exclusively for this occasion, written by a young lady of my acquaintance to whom I promised "graphological" information) *without reading it.* This letter is written in German.

I didn't want to complicate this matter any further for the time being, but I did prepare a number of other writings for the future. I also intend to develop an interest in the local "soothsayeresses."

I now have two analyses: my homosexual—and an anxiety hysteria with masturbation (and washing) compulsion. This is a new case—in addition, one or two of my old ones will come back.

The homosexual (who is now in full transference) is going to look you up in Vienna one of these days (as an attempt at flight from me) and ask you "whether homosexuality is curable or not." [Today he had the fantasy that I will allow him to stay overnight in my home, but *not* in the bedroom; if I permit him to do this—he won't go to Freud.][3] He despises all men with whom he is homosexually involved—but this transference to me forces him to acknowledge that he can respect someone and still wish to have intercourse with him [friends, father, mother][4]; but he doesn't want that and represses his feelings toward me. Please, *do not*[5] *mention Dr. Stein's name* in front of him. If he flees to him, it won't do either of them any good.—I must also confirm that *Stein* is turning away from us to a certain extent; he talks in public about the fact that I (and you) "went too far," "want to explain everything in sexual terms," "neglect the self-preservative drive."

My lecture on dreams is being announced for *the day after tomorrow* (Saturday) as this year's first lecture to the Society of Physicians.[6] In the title I emphasized the "pathological" (in consideration of the *practical* interests which predominate here). But I will say mostly purely psychological things and only add the significance of the dream theory for recognizing psychoneurotic and psychotic dream images, as well as the importance of dream analysis for psychoanalysis.—The closer the hour of the lecture comes, the less enthusiasm I have for it. My colleagues are behaving disgustingly; they slander me and psychoanalysis up hill and down dale; they don't deserve to be instructed by my lectures.—But I will only think about the nonspecialists and give the lecture for them.—I think it will come to a discussion which lacks substance, and I fear that I will become very rude. Being together with you and Jung has raised to colossal heights my need for a discussion of these themes; it is *very* hard for me to answer the same objections with the same responses again and again. But if I don't show any signs of life, "They'll throw me to the dead."[7]

I am very sorry that your daughter is ill again! I hope that the thing will once again be cured, and this time radically, for good.

Best regards,
Ferenczi

P.S. 1.) The homosexual patient must naturally not know that I wrote to you about him!

2.) If you should happen to have my last letter "about the Seidler case," then I ask you to send it back for the "dossier," when you get a chance.

1. Ferenczi's friend Gizella Pálos-Altschul. Ferenczi's brother Lajos (1879–?) had married her younger daughter, Magda.
2. Probably Max (Miksa) (1861–?).
3. Enclosed in brackets in the original.
4. Enclosed in brackets in the original.
5. The word "not" is underlined three times.
6. See letter 77 and n. 1.
7. The source of the quotation is unclear.

77

Budapest, October 16, 1909

Dear Professor,

The lecture on dreams is over. The picture of the auditorium as usual. The hall packed, outwardly great success, two insignificant, banal, in fact, stupid "protests" against what was said—which I was easily able to make look ridiculous. I then had the laughers on my side.—

Inwardly I obviously aroused much resistance, which won't be palpable until later.

Cordially,
Dr. Ferenczi

I would like to find a place for the German translation of the dream lecture.[1] Could you help me with this? (Perhaps to get it into a neurological journal?)

1. The lecture, "On the Psychological Analysis of Dreams" (1909, 66; *C.*, p. 94), was published in Hungarian in *Orvosi Hetilap* [Medical Weekly] 44–45 (1909), and in German under the title "Die Psychologische Analyse der Träume" in *Psychiatrisch-Neurologische Wochenschrift* 12 (1910): 102–107, 114–117, 125–127.

78

Vienna, October 22, 1909
IX., Berggasse 19

Dear friend,

I am writing you hurriedly because I couldn't do otherwise. It is an entirely American exploitation; I hardly have time to live, never mind work. And then, to top it all, Stanley Hall, in a really kind letter, has reminded me of my promise about the five lectures.[1] Now, only half a page of them is really finished.

My walk-in practice is still very far behind my regular, so that I still have hardly anything to share. The patients are disgusting and are giving me an opportunity for new studies on technique. Eitingon[2] is here and goes for a walk with me twice a week after dinner, and has himself analyzed at the same time. He is proving to be very intelligent there and in the Wednesday discussions, and he has his feet on the ground. My daughter is doing much better without an operation, but not yet a hundred percent.

I am sending you back your first Seidler letter today. I think you have prepared too many tests at once for the poor thing, so that the later ones might not yield anything clearer. My opinion that she reads with her eyes, like you and me, is based not on theoretical considerations but on what is apparent in the facts. This point will be the easiest to determine experimentally.

I congratulate you on your dream lecture. Just write it down in German; we will endeavor to find a home for it. Do you consider it unsuitable for an English, i.e., American, journal?[3] There it could have a completely new effect. It would be easy to get it translated. Your patient, as you will find out, did not come to see me.

I learned from Jung that Friedländer[4] was with him "sweet as sugar and wagging his tail"! He's a rotten character! I am very eager for further news.

I was more pleased by a little discovery the last few days than twelve articles by Aschaffenburg[5] could have made me. In *1884*, a philologist named Abel[6] published a piece, The Antithetical Sense of Primal Words, which claims no more and no less than that in many languages, Old Egyptian, Sanskrit, Arabic, but also in Latin, opposites are designated by the same word. You will easily guess which piece of our investigations about the ucs. is confirmed by this.[7] I haven't felt so victorious in a long time.

I am also occupying myself with Leonardo da Vinci.[8]

Cordially,
Freud

1. Freud's lectures given in the United States (1910a [1909]) were published in 1910 in the *American Journal of Psychology* 21, nos. 2–3, published by Stanley Hall; in "Lectures and Addresses Delivered before the Departments of Psychology and Pedagogy in Celebration of the Twentieth Anniversary of the Opening of Clark University, Part I"; and in German by Deuticke.

2. Max Eitingon (1881–1943), German physician of Russian extraction. During his practicum as a student at the Burghölzli in 1907 he had visited Freud and the Wednesday Society as its first foreign adherent (*Minutes* I, 92–102); he had also been a guest there two days before Freud wrote this letter (*Minutes* II, 276–281). Eitingon later became a founding member of the Berlin Society (1910), a member of the Committee (1919), and founder of the Berlin Psychoanalytic Polyclinic (1920)—where he introduced the tripartite structure of psychoanalytic training (training analysis, supervision, and theory)—and president of the IPA (1925–1932), as well as of the International Training Commission

(1925–1938). In 1933 he emigrated to Palestine, where he helped found the Psychoanalytic Society of Palestine. His significance lies above all in the organization and financing of the psychoanalytic movement.

3. The paper (1909, 66; *C.*, p. 94; see also letter 77, n. 1) was published under the title "On the Psychological Analysis of Dreams," *American Journal of Psychology* 21 (1910): 309–328, in which Freud's American lectures were also published.

4. Adolf Albrecht Friedländer (1870–1949), German psychiatrist. Although he vehemently criticized psychoanalysis in public, he visited Jung on October 14, 1909 (*Freud/Jung*, pp. 250, 253, 296) and later Freud (see letter 138); see also Jones II, 117.

5. Gustav Aschaffenburg (1866–1944), German psychiatrist. He had worked with Meynert in Vienna and Kraepelin in Heidelberg, where he qualified to teach psychiatry in 1895. In 1900 he became associate professor there, and in 1905 he became full professor at Cologne and director of the psychiatric division at Lindenthal. In 1939 he emigrated to Baltimore. He is the author of numerous polemical articles against psychoanalysis.

6. Carl Abel (1837–1893?), Berlin linguist and social psychologist. Author of *Über den Gegensinn der Urworte* (Leipzig, 1884) see also *Sprachwissenschaftliche Abhandlungen* (Leipzig, 1885), pp. 311–368.

7. For example, the assertion made in the *Interpretation of Dreams* (1900a, p. 318) that the dream thoughts in the manifest content of the dream can be presented positively or negatively through their opposite. Abel's work was especially important to Freud. He reviewed it for the *Jahrbuch* (1910e) and referred to it several times.

8. At the time Freud was reading several books about Leonardo da Vinci and spoke about him a few weeks later in the Vienna Society (see letter 88 and n. 3). He finished writing *Leonardo da Vinci and a Memory of His Childhood* in April 1910.

79

Budapest, October 26, 1909
VII., Erzsébet-körút 54

Dear Professor,

Gratefully confirm the receipt of your letter of the 22nd. I was very pleased to hear about the linguistic discovery. After the fact, one naturally thinks that opposites *must* also flow into one another in speech (as in other psychical structures with great impact from the ucs.). Confirmation of this, however, and from the pre-ψ-α time to boot, is a very valuable supplement to your teachings. Whether this will also impress the uninitiated is extremely doubtful.

I read the report about the Budapest Congress[1] in the *Neurologisches Zentralblatt*—so did you, probably. *Ranschburg*[2] said the stupidest things. He says he does psychoanalyses—but only to the point where he comes to sexuality. Some analyses! And what kind of scientific logic is that, to intentionally (consciously!) leave something factual undiscovered? He criticizes your theory of forgetting, even though I learned more in your first essay about it than from a long-winded book about memory (by Max Offner, Munich),[3] which I unfortunately had to read through; it is written in the boring and at the same time stupid and conceited tone of laboratory psychology. Ranschburg likes that, of course! *Sommer*[4] concedes that psychoanalysis deepens the knowledge of psychoneuroses—but he won't have it as therapy. (In other words, he only wants a therapy that is founded on ignorance of the facts.) Each of your opponents generally admits to a different piece of your theories; one goes wild over Breuer,[5] the other over Jung[6] (like the aforementioned Offner). If one adds up all the critiques, the result is an almost complete recognition of your theories—but each individual opponent's conclusions culminate in a summary condemnation. I would like, sometime, to collect all the critiques which have been published to date and to criticize them without mentioning the authors. You don't like to make advertisements for them.—Friedländer's tail-wagging over at Jung's speaks an eloquent dog's language. I hope Jung gave it to him straight.

News comes from my brother[7] (who is very much interested in the Seidler case) that he found Pythia ill and bedridden; he was, to be sure, admitted, but he was not granted an audience. That speaks to a certain extent in favor of the reality of her indisposition at the time of my visit, which at the time I took to be a fake.

My homo sapiens was in Vienna in the meantime, but was content with the compromise action of a telephone call to you. Upon his return he produced one of his frightful eruptive reactions which always precede an insight on his part.

Another patient, Herr Helvey, who is tied to a sadistic-masochistic love affair, can't get away from it, and is also relatively impotent with his own wife, will probably look you up. He wants to be thoroughly hypnotized; I also tried it a year and a half ago, at his request, but couldn't get through to him. In addition, he suffers from reflex rigidity of the pupils, probably tabes,[8] about which he has no inkling. A very intelligent person; could be cured by analysis. I told him (in accordance with the facts) that I mentioned his case to you last year.

My personal well-being (psychic) was good right up to the last few days as long as it was possible to keep frequent company with Frau Isolde[9] (I will call her that, which was also her name in one of my dreams). The difficult and painful operation of producing complete candor in me and in my relationship with her is proceeding rapidly. Her intelligence and her interest in the psychological side of analysis proved to be strong enough to allow the—not insignificant—resistances to be overcome and the bitterness of the unvarnished truth to be accepted after correspondingly long defense. The matter, of course, makes *much* more rapid progress in me; I dream a great deal, analyze my dreams, and find *lots* of infantilisms. Accordingly, the analyses of patients are also going much more smoothly; I find the solutions better, more quickly.—As far as my feelings toward Frau

Isolde are concerned, I must say that the confession that I made to her, the superiority with which, after some reluctance, she correctly grasped the situation, and the truth which is possible between us makes it seem perhaps less possible for me to tie myself to another woman *in the long run,* even though I admitted to her and to myself having sexual desires toward other women and even reproached her for her age.

Evidently I have *too much* in her: lover, friend, mother, and, in scientific matters, a pupil, i.e., the child—in addition, an extremely intelligent, enthusiastic pupil, who completely grasps the extent of the new knowledge.—

Otherwise, I am scientifically isolated. I have one sole student,[10] but he is just beginning; on top of that he is too poor, and he probably has to go away soon.—So, I have everything that can be distributed by nature between the two sexes combined in a single person.

The young people are beginning to take an interest in you. Today a medical student came to see me under the auspices of the student section of the Galileo Society (Freethinkers' Club),[11] and I once again allowed a lecture to be extorted from me. Next Saturday I will speak there about the psychopathology of everyday life.[12] So I now have five lectures before Christmas![13] That should be very nice, but it makes the really scientific, not pedagogical, work impossible. I won't accede so frivolously to such demands in the future.

In a few days I will send you the *dream lecture* in German, which, I think, should be readily translatable into English. Where is the German supposed to be published?[14]

I had intended today to share with you a few more interesting observations.—In the meantime it is too late, and this letter has become too long, so I will save them for the next time.

Cordial greetings to you all—from your

Truly obedient
Dr. Ferenczi

I intend to publish a collection of my ψ. α. lectures which were previously published in Hungarian.[15] Would you like to write a brief introduction to them? You know most of the lectures; they were also published in German.

1. The first part of the report by Schweiger, "XVI. International Medical Congress in Budapest from August 29 to September 4, 1909," "Section for Psychiatry," *Neurologisches Centralblatt,* October 1, 1909, pp. 1067–72.

2. Pál Ranschburg (1870–1945), neuropsychiatrist; founder of the Budapest Psychophysical Institute (1899); from 1918 professor of psychology at Budapest University. In 1828 he founded the Hungarian Association of Psychologists and became its first president. He is known for works about memory, disturbances in reading and writing, and intelligence in children. At the congress he had claimed that he had "carried through the

Freudian procedure up to the point where he found sexual traces, but didn't press forward any further from there," and he had spoken out "against reducing slips of the tongue and failure of reproduction to sexual complexes" (Schweiger, "Congress").

3. Max Offner (1864–1932), *Das Gedächtnis, Die Ergebnisse der experimentellen Psychologie und ihre Anwendung in Unterricht und Erziehung* (Berlin, 1909). Offner was active as a teacher in Munich, Aschaffenburg, Ingolstadt, and Straubing. In 1919 he became director of the Humanistisches Gymnasium Günzburg a. D. He published in the fields of pedagogy, philosophy, and psychology.

4. Robert Sommer (1864–1937), psychiatrist and researcher in heredity; professor at Giessen (1895); first president of the General Medical Society for Psychotherapy. He had remarked that "the Freudian mode of investigation has brought us further in the knowledge of the mechanism of hysteria, but he points with strong emphasis to damage which arises from its indiscriminate application to all cases of hysteria in practice" (Schweiger, "Congress").

5. That is, for Breuer's and Freud's "cathartic method" and their theory of hysteria, as it was set down by them in *Studies on Hysteria* (1895d). Josef Breuer (1842–1925), Viennese physiologist and internist, qualified in 1875 and was a docent at the University of Vienna until 1895. He was not only a sought-after general practitioner among the upper crust of Vienna but also an influential scientist. (In 1868 he discovered the so-called Hering-Breuer reflex, and in 1873 he investigated the function of the semicircular canals of the inner ear.) Breuer was a fatherly friend and mentor to young Freud. The part he played in the development of psychoanalysis was often emphasized by Freud, even after they had experienced a parting of the scientific and personal ways. See, e.g., Freud (1910a [1909], p. 9; and see the editorial remarks in Freud, *Nachtragsband*, pp. 214ff.

6. Jung's association experiments and his theory of psychic "complexes" (*Diagnostische Assoziationsstudien*, vol. 1 [Leipzig, 1906]; *CW*, vol. 2).

7. Ferenczi's already frequently mentioned brother Zsigmond in Berlin.

8. See letter 56, n. 2.

9. Gizella Pálos.

10. This student remains unidentified.

11. A group of freethinking students, founded in 1908, opposed to clericalism, corruption, economic privilege, and bureaucracy. It later became the cradle of the Hungarian left wing. Several analysts, such as Imre Hermann and Lilly Hajdu, also belonged to the group.

12. See letter 81.

13. In addition to the one mentioned here, he gave another four lectures at the Free School of Social Sciences (see letters 51 and 85).

14. See letter 77, n. 1.

15. See letter 85 and n. 16.

80

Budapest, October 30, 1909
VII., Erzsébet-körút 54

Dear Professor,

I want to share with you a very funny story about symptomatic action. The passages that I have underlined in blue,[1] however, must be made unrecognizable if you want to publish it with the other things. Better yet, eliminate my name altogether.

Frau Isolde, whom I am eagerly at work analyzing, told me recently that she had given her Coffeemaker ("Non-Plus-Ultra," it's called), which, in addition to other features, also announces the end of the brewing process with a kind of bird's chirping, to my brother-in-law (my eldest sister's husband)[2] as a present; he liked the machine so much that she was unable to resist the desire to give it to him. I told her that was a very surprising thing; indeed, she had liked that machine very much herself, and I expressed the supposition that that was a symptomatic action: through the gift of the coffeemaker she had clearly made known her inclination to give her love to the brother-in-law. I reminded her that, just before she told [me] about the gift, she had mentioned the fact that my brother-in-law's and my sister's marriage was not as happy as he deserved it to be. My sister was too strict, too brusque, cold toward him, whereas he, for his part, did everything to please her, etc. Then I told her that she had told me earlier, in fac⁺ several times, that my brother-in-law was a handsome, pleasant man; I reminded her further that we had determined in other analyses that she (Isolde) had great desires to be rich, dominating, e.g., to be the proprietress of a large, comfortable household (my brother-in-law is very well-to-do and the proprietor of an estate). The extreme interest in his hearth and home can be very easily brought into harmony with the gift of a miniature hearth. She is often—I told her further—accustomed to quoting the proverb about coffee (black as night (?), hot as hell, sweet as love). But she usually makes coffee *for me* (I am a great *lover* of coffee); now she wants to do for my brother-in-law what she previously did for me, etc. She denied with conviction, and her doubt about the reliability of psychoanalysis, which comes up now and again, even returned. But the fact that I hit the mark was proved by what came to her mind: "The only thing that speaks for your interpretation is the similarity of the coffeemaker to an organ from which a fluid flows in a thin stream." "This single thought is sufficient to justify my diagnosis," I answered. With that, the matter was settled for a while; afterward, the possibility of a word association with the word *bird-chirping* occurred to me.[3] (Frau Isolde had not previously been acquainted with the corresponding obscene word, but had learned it some time ago in an analysis with me.) I don't know if I can go so far as to consider the "signal," the "chirping" at the end of the brewing process, as analogous to the orgasm at the end of the act.

The day before yesterday my youngest sister,[4] who has now moved to Budapest, her husband, Frau Isolde, and I were sitting at the table. My sister says to me she hopes to see me often at her house; I should come for dinner whenever. Her husband (as chief executive of an insurance company) is often not at home for days, and she would be able to prepare a meal anytime that suits me.—"That depends on whether you can make good <u>coffee</u>," I answered. "By the way, I have a <u>coffee</u>maker that I seldom use; I will lend it to you and drink coffee in the afternoon with you."

Frau <u>Isolde's</u> laughter brings me to the awareness of what I just said and suggested. A brief resistance on my part, then complete insight into the state of affairs. This youngest <u>sister</u> was the one that I liked to "treat" so much when she was sick. (One of the determinants of my *doctor* complex.) I was not completely satisfied with her choice of a mate; I consider her otherwise very good husband, who has gone rather far in his profession, as not intelligent enough (that is *my* intelligence complex); I wanted to find a home for her in the neighborhood (in the house where I live!), in order to see her often; look forward colossally to getting to know her dear, clever four-year-old boy better, etc. etc.! To make the matter even more complicated, it occurs to me that I got this coffeemaker as a gift from your <u>daughter Mathilde</u>, who, for her part, has an idiosyncracy against <u>black coffee</u> (which we, for its part, related to repressions).

After writing this down, it occurs to me that this story loses its value completely when it is communicated in a garbled fashion; the story is more of personal than general value.—So it would best remain unprinted and should find its way to the wastepaper basket!

Best regards,
Ferenczi

1. The underscored words were underlined in blue.
2. Zoltán Jószef, married to Ferenczi's sister Ilona (1865–?).
3. The word for "bird" *(Vogel)* in German is sometimes used as a vulgar equivalent for penis [Trans.].
4. Zsófia (1883–?).

81

Budapest, October 30, 1909
VII., Erzsébet-körút 54

Dear Professor,

Do not be frightened by my talkativeness; I only want to remain true to the tradition of reporting on the progress of my apostolic mission on the basis of fresh impressions. (N.B.: I have already determined that it has to do with the infantile wish to be praised by the father.)

So, today was the lecture about "Everyday Life."[1] I was happy that I could speak before approximately three hundred young and enthusiastic medical students, who listened to my (or, that is to say, your) words with bated breath. I spoke for about an hour and a half but stuck to generalities and could cite only a few examples (among them *a-liquis in extenso*).[2] I didn't spare psychophysics and the experimental psychologists; I was even rather aggressive in regard to them.—After the end of the lecture, the *Privatdozent* in psychology, Dr. Révész,[3] gets up (a rather capable experimental psychologist, who has worked a lot in Göttingen and now has a large following among the students). He must—he said—defend himself against the charge that experimental psychologists are not scientists, that those who are concerned with it are handymen and machinists, as I (Dr. F.) characterized them. He spoke about the accomplishments of their methods, etc. He seems to have been particularly pained by the accusation that everything that they do is sterile, because, instead of first studying the macroscopic anatomy of the mind, psychoanalysis, they work prematurely with their "microscopic" instruments and they don't want to give that up even *now*; I dismissed all their results as worthless because a pure psychology of consciousness can only yield partial, or even false, results. "We can't stand here with open mouths," he replied, "and wait until *Freud* and his adherents have finished everything. For the time being, therefore, I have to continue to bore my audience with the old methods, curves, and calculations." With that, he concluded his talk. (N.B. He only spoke out of false modesty about boredom at his lectures [which he is very proud of].[4]

Having the last word, I held true to my convictions, invited him and the experimental psychologists not to stand there with open mouths but to participate in *Freud's* work. They can also bring their instruments along, for all I care. Or he should try, as *Jung* has done, to extend experimental psychology to the psychology of the unconscious. Then his audience won't be bored by his lectures.

The medical students surrounded me and wanted me to promise them, at any price, to tell them more about these things. I asked for time to think it over.

Budapest seems, after all, not to be such an absolutely bad place. The audience was naturally composed of nine tenths Jews!

Best regards,
Ferenczi

1. Before the Galileo Society (see letter 79 and n. 11).

2. An example of the forgetting of foreign words cited by Freud in *The Psychopathology of Everyday Life* (1901b), pp. 8ff.

3. Géza Révész (1878–1955), professor of experimental psychology at the University of Budapest during the 133 days of the republic (1919). Imre Hermann was among his assistants. After the fall of the republic he emigrated to Holland, where he directed the Institute for Experimental Psychology (1921) and, from 1932 to 1950, was professor of psychology at the University of Amsterdam. He is known for his work on musical talent.

4. Enclosed in brackets in the original.

82

Vienna, October 31, 1909[1]

Dear friend,

Your contribution, very interesting from both a personal and contextual standpoint, will one day be found for the first time among my papers, that is, if you don't ask for it back à la Abraham.[2] The third edition of Everyday Life[3] is already in print.

Best regards,
Freud

1. Postcard.
2. Allusion unclear.
3. *The Psychopathology of Everyday Life* (1901b), 3d ed. (Berlin, 1910).

83

Budapest, November 8, 1909

Dear Professor,

Here I come again with a long epistle and a mass of extras.

I. I am sending enclosed the *dream lecture* in German. I also happened to send it to my brother in Berlin with a request that he improve it stylistically. I am indebted to him for a few useful expressions; he has, however, made some unnecessary changes, partly out of insufficient knowledge of the subject matter, partly out of an exaggerated desire to Germanize everything (as is the custom in Berlin), so that I had to restore these passages and have the whole work retranscribed. On the whole, I am astonished at his relatively very significant insight into the psychoanalytic way of looking at things. Heretofore he has read nothing but my lectures. Only now is he getting your works.—

II. Now to the main thing.

The Seidler case has reached a more serious stage, owing to a second, successful experiment. I want to treat the matter pragmatically, and therefore I am sending you all the pieces of evidence in the original, as before.

In the envelope marked "I"[1] you will find the three pieces of paper with writing on them that were presented to Frau Seidler. To wit:

1.) the fragment of a letter written in blue ink on blueish paper and marked at the end "3 B." It comes from that painter (Schramm),[2] whose name I had such a hard time remembering on board the Washington. My brother doesn't know of its existence, even less about its significance for me and about its role in the life of Frau Isolde, to whom the letter is addressed. (My brother is equally unaware of the last point.) On the next to the last (torn) page *I* transformed the word *artist* [*Künstler*] into the nonsense word *Bärdiar*; above that I changed the word *canvas* [*Leinwand*] into something like *"Kaugründ"* (meaningless). The signature is illegible; the addressee could read it, of course; it says: *Festö bácsi* (= Uncle Painter). Afterwards I reproached myself for not having altered this word, so I asked my brother directly who he thought the writer of the letter was. See his reply later.—

2.) a Hungarian letter that I wrote to *Frau Isolde* in 1905. Content, sender, recipient all known to my brother. Following is the word-for-word translation of the letter:

Tátrafüred, August 20, 1905
Sunday

Permit me to use the time until the departure of the carriage which is supposed to take me to the station of Poprád Felka for my journey home to share with you in a few lines the main impressions of my stay here. My first and most important piece of information is the fact that my brother Max's[3] condition, perhaps under the influence of my intervention, has improved significantly in the last few days. I say "perhaps" because we will not be able to make a final judgment as to the appropriateness of the treatment which has been initiated until more time has passed. In the meantime Max is in good spirits and strengthened physically, easily takes rather long walks, that is, he would like to take them, and I haven't talked him out of it. But I also didn't stand in the way of his trying his favorite diversion, hunting, albeit in moderation. I even accompanied him myself lying in wait*, with a gun on my shoulder. But I didn't have a chance to fire the shotgun; the hunting dogs didn't drive any game toward me. Perhaps it was better that way; at least, I didn't have a chance to shoot a buck**. I also—sitting in hiding—got much more satisfaction from the idyllic peace and quiet of forest solitude than shooting an innocent little deer could have offered me.—I don't know whether the card that I wrote you from the "Silesian shelter" has gotten to you. In the meantime I made the mountain climbs which I had only planned then. In the company of others, I climbed the "Little Viszoka" (2–300 meters higher than the "Polish Crest"). But yesterday, with a guide, I climbed the Lomnitz Peak (2,663 meters). The outing was very interesting from a tourist's standpoint (it cost me a pair of breeches), but at the summit I waited in vain for an hour for the fog to lift. All around the clouds gathered [literally, perhaps more accurately: "clouds whirled around"],[4] and I felt at the summit as if I were standing in the middle of a gigantic kettle breaking out of the magical-fiery vapors. But it was also so beautiful. In order that I might explain the enclosed little flower in the manner of Prof. Constantinus Compactus,***

I will share with you the fact that it is the so-called "Kohlröserl," a flower which is very common in the Austrian Alps but very rare here, with a pleasant aroma. I found it there on the summit and immediately decided to send it to you, the dilettantish botanist. I am afraid its pleasant aroma will fade before you get this letter. I spent the days between the excursions here, in the midst of the spa-crowd of Tátrafüred. I already have so many acquaintances that—in order not to insult anyone—I greet everyone. Getting acquainted snowballs in the manner of an avalanche; every new acquaintance means ten more. Of course, the guests here would be very bored without gossip; but lately they must have been especially starved; not even I have been completely spared from being talked about.—

Last evening on the promenade there was music, confetti-throwing by lamplight. It was a beautiful sight; the weather was also good.

If I am correctly informed, you, gracious lady, will stay in Weisswasser until September. On the one hand, I am sorry; I would have liked to meet you and Elmagda**** upon my return home. On the other hand, I am comforted to a certain extent by the fact that you are feeling well there.—

In the expectation of seeing you again soon, I greet you, gracious lady, and ask you also to extend my greetings to the members of the Propper and Stross families, who are also staying there.

With a kiss on the hand.

Dr. Ferenczi

*A kind of hunt, in which one waits in hiding for game which comes by or is flushed out by beaters. (Dr. Ferenczi.)

**Jocular expression for a miss and for other offenses. (Dr. Ferenczi.)

***Comical figure in a Hungarian humor magazine; a professor of literature who robs the most beautiful poems of their beauty through his analyses.

****Collective name (hybrid word) for both daughters, Elma[5] and Magda.

3.) The envelope within the envelope contains the apocryphal letter which I had fabricated by a young lady. My brother knows nothing about the writer and has *not* read the writing himself; in fact, he kept it sealed inside the envelope until just before he handed it over and didn't read it until *after* the visit.—

In envelope "II" you will find my brother's report about the course of the experiment and, as enclosures to this letter, six pages with stenographic notes in his handwriting.

Envelope "III" contains my response to the report; "IV" his return response, which arrived just today.

These are the documents which I ask you to read through (best in chronological sequence).—

Now, a few concluding remarks.—

It seems to be indisputable that *Frau Seidler* can do things heretofore thought impossible, and, very probably, that she recites the thoughts of others (in the manner that we laid out after the first experiment), mixed with her own thoughts and unaware of the abstract or concrete meaning of the images that she sees (probably also without knowing what belongs to her and what to her partner).

The following part of her oracle, however, remains *totally inexplicable*. My brother does *not* know, as is clear from his letter of today, that the writer of the blue letter is a *painter*; he even thought him to be a poet. How does Frau Seidler, in interpreting this letter, get to speak of "several hands" that "stir in a pot"? If one assumes thought transference, then one must assume that my brother unconsciously knew and knows whom it is about, even though—as far as I know—he could never learn anything about it. (It is, however, not *impossible* that he once heard about him. But it has been about fourteen years since Schramm played a role in Frau Isolde's life!)

I find *the most striking* thing to be the candid confession of not knowing in the case of the converted letter which said nothing and which my brother had never read. My admonition to my brother to *analyze* himself came to naught, of course. He produced only the things that consciously came to mind, and those only sparingly. Nothing else was to be expected. The next experiment with which I entrusted my brother was as follows:

I took two letter fragments (from two different letters) and *encoded* them (both in a different way) in a manner that is very hard to decipher. I sent the one letter with the two encoded writings along to my brother; he knows *nothing* about the other one. I also asked him, for the sake of the experiment, *not* to try to decipher it. (Incidentally, he would hardly be able to do it even if he tried.) Now we will see whether Frau Seidler can do something even if the writing reveals nothing of its contents *even when it is read*. The encoded fragment unfamiliar to my brother is in Hungarian; the other German (likewise encoded).

In the meantime I also found someone here who has herself hypnotized by her husband during soothsaying. I already called on her twice; the first time the woman was not at home, the second time supposedly sick. These people are very distrustful! I'll go back again one of these days.

After the experiences to date our trip to Berlin is coming seriously into question.—

I wrote to Jung last week and received a friendly response from him. I eagerly await your reply.

Cordially,
Dr. Ferenczi

I am full of psychological experiences. Next time you will again simply have to let a long letter wash over you.—

I request that you send back this letter, with enclosures, for the dossier. In the end something will probably come of it.—

1. This Roman numeral is written in red pencil, as are the others used later in this letter.
2. Possibly Victor Schramm (1865–1929), painter and illustrator in Poplet, near Orsova (today in Romania).
3. Max (Miksa) Ferenczi (1861–?).
4. Enclosed in brackets in the original.
5. Elma (1887–1970), Gizella Pálos's elder daughter.

84

Vienna, November 10, 1909
IX., Berggasse 19

Dear friend,

Thank you very much for your interesting reports, which are doubly welcome to me at a somewhat arid time. I will answer you immediately; sending back the material will require a free hour on one of the next few days.

On the whole, I find that these last experiments have yielded little on account of the medium's indisposition. Your organization also seems to me to be somewhat too complicated, a judgment which I would like to expand upon with regard to your attempts at encoding. I believe that, first of all, you don't need any experiments from which the basic fact that is presumed, the mirroring of the other's thoughts, is any more unquestionable than before; rather, you need those that definitively settle the question of whether she reads or not. One should first confront and not inhibit. For example, a letter that evokes certain affects in your brother would be quite appropriate. But even these experiments were not completely unsuccessful, and in some respects very suspicious. I would like once again to review on its own merits the one that you seem to value over and above our assumption. "The several hands that stir in a pot" really doesn't point to new abilities on the part of Frau Seidler. It would also be a strange characteristic for a painter, who doesn't do that with one hand at all. But rather, your brother senses your relation to Frau G., as you correctly assume, and possibly did have knowledge of that painter, albeit very obscure, which influenced him somewhat in expressing his thought, and his thought was that several men there were having to do with a woman; smearing around [herumschmieren], as they say. Frau Seidler is again only guessing his thought. The technique ought to be to eliminate Frau Seidler altogether and to take up the analysis on the object which mirrors itself. Since your brother is introducing a new unknown and refuses analysis, there will be hardly anything left but to go to Berlin with a well-thought-out program, as you indicate.

I very much liked your dream lecture, especially its excellent examples, and I intend to think about putting it to further use. Only one place in the introduction needs revision or correction. Page 2: "But even these authors (the Symbolists) failed to make comprehensible the peculiarities of dreams *or* forcing their explanations into the procrustean bed of an artificial allegoristics." Instead of "or" [*oder*] shouldn't it be "without" [*ohne*]? Allegoristics, by the way, is an impossible word and should be replaced (play with artificial allegory?).[1]

I am scientifically fixated by the American lectures, the last of which has already sailed off. Otherwise I have been lucky with two trivialities, with the antithetical meaning of primal words and with an analysis of— just marvel at the illustrious subject—Leonardo da Vinci.[2] But nothing bigger. The times are otherwise downright arid. I am booked solid and have intentionally cut down on work, but some cases are boring, and the walk-ins are staying out altogether, so I can distribute almost nothing among the "circle." I expect the next thing they'll do is strike and drop out. Jung isn't writing to me at all any more, so I sent him a card today asking why. Eitingon, who picked me up twice a week for an evening walk, where he had himself analyzed, is coming on Friday for the last time and then is going to Berlin for a year. A formidable attack, half demented, half clairvoyant, and dipped in holy venom, has been very deliberately directed against me by Foerster[3] in the *Evangelische Freiheit*. Pfister has been looking forward to responding to him for a long time.

You will certainly be glad to hear that my daughter[4] has become ambulatory without intervention and is again very happy about her life. My health has been severely debilitated by a Viennese cold. I got some pictures from Hamburg that I consider very bad. But if you want one, say so in the long letter that you promised.

Cordially,
Freud

1. Ferenczi followed Freud's suggestion in the published version (1909, 66; *Unbewusstes*, p. 116; *C.*, p. 96).
2. See letter 78.
3. Friedrich Wilhelm Foerster (1869–1966), German philosopher, educator, and pacifist; became a professor in Zurich in 1901 after having had to leave Germany because of lèse-majesté. Foerster was respected as a pedagogical and moral authority. Freud refers to his article "Psychoanalyse und Seelsorge" [Psychoanalysis and Spiritual Welfare], pts. 1 and 2, *Evangelische Freiheit* 31 (1909): 335–346, 374–388. See also letter 96 and n. 2.
4. Mathilde.

85

[Budapest,] November 20, 1909
Dear Professor,

About four weeks ago I visited a Frau *Jelinek* for the first time in the outer Trommelgasse in Budapest in the company of two women, one of whom had once had her fortune told by her.

In a darkened apartment on the ground floor with its entrance under a dark gate, we found an approximately seventy-year-old man, with very energetic features, brewing coffee on the kitchen stove. The place is actually a coffeehouse for very poor people; through the kitchen one gets to the actual guest room, with dirty walls, several round tables, and an icebox containing a large jug of milk. We were not allowed in.—

The second time the husband dismissed me in a rather unfriendly manner, saying his wife was not at home.—I came two more times. First I was turned away with the information that the woman was ill. The third time the man let me in, but he was very mistrustful and asked how I knew her. I heard a conversation in monotone from the next room. But its content escaped me. The man again behaved very morosely and said one should not be impatient here, it was only a question of whether his wife would receive me. After a long wait a very fragile, thin, about fifty-five to sixty-year-old, apparently ill female comes out with a lady, who goes away. She (Frau Jelinek) turns to me with the question, What do I want? When I explained to her that I wanted her to tell my fortune, she told me that if I wanted card reading and the like swindle, I should go away immediately. She was a medium, a somnambulist. I agreed to this and sharply condemned those swindlers and explained that I only believed in extraordinary mental abilities, I already had experience in such matters, etc. That and my intentionally exaggerated politeness, as well as my feigned interest in her well-being (I inquired about her health), favorably disposed her toward me, and she allowed me to come back in two to three weeks. She was now still ill with influenza.

I visited her this afternoon at 2:30. The husband in the kitchen again; he and the little dog received me in an unfriendly manner. She, more amicably.

At the visit before last she explained to me that in her soothsaying she was hypnotized by her husband. [I immediately thought of a "father-hypnosis,"[1] of intimidation by her evidently strict, even violent-looking husband.][2]

Today she received me in *her* room (a room with two windows on the alley and very shabby furniture and an oppressively unpleasant smell). She was sitting by the window, knitting. Her speech is tremulous, her breath short, dyspneic, like that of someone with a heart condition or emphysema. Her husband had me informed by way of the chambermaid that he had no time now; we had to wait a half hour.

In the meantime she talked about herself. She said she likes to "speak" with some, but not at all with others. There are people who come with practical questions (something stolen, etc.): she turns them away and sends them to the police.

She endeavors to get rid of antipathetic people (is happy when they go away).

In response to my question she said: "My husband is very strict. But that doesn't matter." She doesn't suffer under him. "Anyway, there will soon be an end to it; we have been married for forty-three years, and one of us will soon die." The husband is moody, tyrannical.—I wanted to have him summoned. She prevented it: Better not! Let him come himself.

She has been aware of her abilities for forty-two years. *In the first years of her marriage* she was ill for months at a time, had talked crazy; doctors thought it was typhus; "but it was only somnambulism."[*] During a relapse of her illness they took her to a Dr. Gárdas, the oldest magnetist in the city. He magnetized her.

After she awoke from the magnetized sleep, the doctor told her she was a somnambulist (she didn't know the word before; she was a child of poor parents and didn't learn anything). The doctor said further, "If you want to stay healthy, you have to tell the fortunes of people who come to you and let yourself be put to sleep by your husband for this purpose. If you don't do this, you will die."—At first she had been very fearful when people came to her, but she gradually got used to it.—⟨Then the husband came in and interrupted our conversation.⟩

When the man came in, she asked me to take a seat on the chair next to her, to pose the questions to her, and, when I was finished, to wake her up with the *energetic* exclamation—"Wake up." *I must address her as "du."*[3]

The man made a few gestures in the air until she began to tremble and her eyes closed. He went out again. She immediately grasped my right hand and began, without waiting for my question, to speak with a trembling but strikingly fluid voice. Unfortunately I was unable to retain much and couldn't take notes. She talked about the fact that I have much to struggle with, that the ground under my feet often sways, that many people spoil my plans; that I am too good, too unselfish. But I should not waver, should continue as I have begun; there are some who help me, not with money but with words. In the end I will press through, like a hero, "not entirely in my field," "some changes will be necessary." I will only be able to maintain myself, keep myself "in balance," but will not get rich; I won't have to wait long for the satisfaction of recognition, etc. Then all at once she stopped talking.—

These much too general phrases seem, nevertheless, to have awakened in me certain affects (of an infantile nature); I felt a kind of emotion, to which I then, incidentally, intentionally gave in; in so doing, I intended to further the experiment.

1.) Now I asked my first question [about a sister whose relationship to her mother is somewhat disrupted]. She answered with a few very general phrases which I wasn't able to note at all.

2.) Second question: "How and what should I work at?" She again became talkative and repeated the earlier remarks about duration, about my *field*, which I should stay with. "You shouldn't work on [*bearbeiten*] so many things, but only *one thing*, in great depth." She said something about books and suggestion.

3.) Question: *"What do you recommend regarding my relations to Jung?"*

Answer (approximate): "That will work out. He is, to be sure, moody and violent (not quite sure of last word; but she said something like it), but in the end you will find yourselves in mutual work."—

4.) *"What can you tell me about my Viennese friend?"*

You *should remain true to him. A blockage [Sperrung] (sic!) has, to be sure, occurred, owing to the intervention of a third party, but you should not stop sending him the letters, reports. Not only is he useful to you, but also you to him; for that reason never let go of him. Your trust will be very much strengthened until you find recognition.*

This time I didn't want to put her to the test any longer and called: "Wake up." She awoke and was disoriented for a few seconds.

I wanted to give her money (three crowns), but she didn't want to take it under any circumstances; she was angry about it. I (Dr. F.) was not now in a position to give money, she said. Finally, rather annoyed, she sent me away and said I shouldn't be so violent and should not come back until a month later.

Outside, I gave the husband the three crowns.

The experiments with Frau Jelinek seem far and away not so nice as the ones with the Berlin Pythia. Frau Jelinek does not speak with such rich imagery; her phrases are terribly flat and general throughout. She learned that in theosophical societies, where she is much in demand as a medium.

The self-analysis always has to come out positive with such generalities. Even so, some of her phrases correspond *rather precisely* to my trains of thought. That business about "pressing through like a hero" is with me, as it is with almost all people, the crowning of a fantasy of greatness. That I will never get rich is an oft-thought-through and reinforced conviction, obviously the reaction to the wish to get rich. *"Not so many things, one thing in depth"* is an idea that often comes to my mind. I would like to retreat from other, nonanalytic activity (workers' polyclinic, court)[4] The "working on" [*bearbeiten*] sounds somewhat suspicious; but I can't find a corresponding sexual complex in myself.—

The idea with regard to *Jung* is rather transparent.

The strange thing is what she says about *your* relationship to me. Frau Seidler already told me (word for word): *"You draw much from his (?), but he, too, could draw much from you."*

Frau Jelinek says: *"Not only is he useful to you, but also you to him."*

Ideas like that are—*consciously*—quite foreign to me. It is possible that I can have them unconsciously. Consciously I very often have *ideas of smallness;* in the ucs. they can correspond to a colossal desire for greatness and megalomania.—On the whole, the Jelinek case has not been so successful. If we want to pursue these matters further, we will have to go to Berlin.

Best regards from

Your obedient
Ferenczi

Please also send back this report, when you get the chance.—

Continuation, November 26, 1909

I refrained from sending this letter off in order not to disturb you too often. In the meantime, I received your very detailed letter and have learned from it that, even if you can't always answer promptly, you always accept my reports amicably. I am very thankful for your in-depth evaluation of my analytic observations, and your concurrence makes me very proud. I would appreciate being in contact with a neurological journal which appears more frequently, in which such casuistic things could be published. We have too little prospect of being able to work by ourselves on all the various themata on which such observations impinge. By sharing the facts, we would come to the aid of others who are concerned in depth with this or that topic.

I am deeply grateful to you for your efforts on behalf of my dream lecture. *Stanley Hall* answered my letter (in which I asked him for an autograph for the group picture from Worcester) with the enclosed letter.[5] I also received a letter from *Campbell*,[6] which I am also enclosing.[7] I naturally granted him the desired authorization.

Rank is diligently sending me the "Almtanz" lectures from Vienna.[8] I was *extraordinarily* surprised by Wittels's splendid analysis of his anxiety hysteric.[9] I find his analysis exemplary. He (Wittels) has developed colossally in a short time. Apart from Dora and the Rat-Man, no such successful and transparent, and at the same time difficult, analysis has, in my opinion, yet been published. In reading it I got one of my—lately much less frequent—attacks of smallness mania.—I am, to be sure, quite isolated here (that's my excuse), and can't go to you for advice, as Wittels could.

Yesterday I gave the first of the four announced lectures at the "Free School of the Sociological Society."[10] I talked about the ucs. in general (starting with hypnosis, double conscience,[11] etc.), used hysterical anesthesia (Janet's experiments)[12] as a transition to *Breuer's* case,[13] in order to get to psychoanalysis. Then I talked about Everyday Life and gave examples. The audience was *very* interested; a sociologist present immediately wanted to pump me for a paper (Sociological Conclusions from Freudian Theory). I remembered Frau Jelinek's advice and refrained from giving an affirmative answer. The women present were the most attentive (as in Worcester). Next time I intend to tell stories about Everyday Life and begin dreams. The third lecture has to do with dreams and maybe jokes; in the fourth I will treat sexual questions.

Décsy[14] hasn't shown up here yet. But I also haven't—think of that!—looked up *Stein* yet. I will explain in detail in my next public lecture that I came to psychoanalysis by way of *Stein*; that way I will partially pay off my debt. And he won't be able to act insulted anymore.—

Walk-in practice almost zero with me, too. But I have enough to do. Many practicing physicians have a "theoretical" interest in me and my lectures, but here a physician considers it impossible to call in for consultation someone who is not a docent.—I have no prospect of becoming a docent.—Earlier (before analysis) that pained me a great deal, now much less. ΨA. compensates one for the lack of external honors.

I like your portrait very much. I thank you for this gift. Unfortunately, I can't reciprocate. But you have me in the group picture.

I just received the letter from *Putnam*,[15] which I have also enclosed (reply to my letter, in which I wrote to him about his Hungarian friends). I replied to Putnam as well as I can. He is struggling, like every beginner; but he seems to be investigating capably and honestly.—I will write to him that I have to bring the diligent exercise of analysis to bear on his questions.—[I will advise him against any suggestive influencing of patients. The instruction in sublimation must take shape differently in each individual case. If a patient has the capability for it, then he instinctively uses the opportunity which offers itself to that end; there is no need to force it. The cure consists of bringing the patients to the point where they themselves admit to their suppressed libido without pangs of conscience, if possible, abreact a part in a crudely sexual manner, and consciously master what remains. The tension which mounts up from this will find its way to other possible goals; etc.]

Next week I am sending to press a collection of my lectures which have been published to date. The volume will contain six lectures (in Hungarian):

1. The neuroses in *Freud's* sense, etc. (Wiener klinische Rundschau);
2. The lecture on dreams;
3. The paper on impotence;
4. The lecture about psychoneuroses that I gave last semester at the Physicians' Association;
5. A brief article about the significance of *ejaculatio praecox* for women (two pages);
6. A brief excerpt from the Salzburg lecture (Psychoanalysis and Pedagogy).[16]

If you want to write a brief foreword to it, you can do so, since you are acquainted with the content of all these works. But I will *not* be insulted if you are not inclined to do so for one reason or another. If you should, then I will translate it, but also have the original (German) printed.—

I am also sending you an extract from *Pester Lloyd*[17] about reading thoughts. *Kotik*[18] doesn't seem to let much criticism prevail.—In *Löwen-*

feld's collection there is also a volume by a Russian[19] about a clairvoyant who works in a manner strikingly similar to that of our Seidler (visual presentation of thoughts). I read the little volume—hastily—before America; I will read through it again.—

Do you want to come to Budapest to see Jelinek? I would be *very, very* pleased. If you don't come, I will visit you next time in Vienna. Please indicate the Sunday on which I may come without inconvenience. Or—I will wait until Christmas; then I could stay away for two to three days (then perhaps Berlin would be possible).

Best regards,

Your obedient
Ferenczi

Unfortunately, I must get the letter back again with enclosures—because of the occult stories in it.—

*She had a dream at that time (half awake). *A millstone lay on her body.* She "had to see everything that went on in the world," etc.

1. In "Introjection und Transference" (*Schriften* I, 32f; *C.,* pp. 69f) Ferenczi had distinguished between hypnotizing through dread ("paternal hypnosis") and through love ("maternal hypnosis").

2. Enclosed in brackets in the original as are all bracketed remarks in this letter.

3. The familiar form of address in German. Its use between strangers would be considered highly unusual, hence Ferenczi's underscoring it here [Trans.].

4. Ferenczi refers to his activities at the health service and as an expert witness.

5. This enclosure is missing.

6. See letter 13 and n. 4.

7. This enclosure is missing.

8. See letter 18 and n. 5.

9. Fritz Wittels (1880–1950), Viennese physician and writer, since 1907 a member of the Wednesday Society. From 1910 to 1925 he was a physician at the Cottage Sanatorium of Rudolf von Urbantschitsch. His pointed, polemical contributions and publications, e.g., *Die Sexuelle Not* [Sexual Need] (Vienna, 1907), and his coming to terms with Karl Kraus (*Ezechiel der Zugereiste* [Ezekiel the Newcomer] [Berlin, 1910]; see also letter 112 and n. 7) unleashed heated controversy. Wittels left the Vienna Society in 1910, joined Stekel, and wrote a critical biography of Freud, *Sigmund Freud: Der Mann—die Lehre—die Schule* [Sigmund Freud: His Personality, His Teaching, and His School] (Leipzig, 1924). Around 1927 he was readmitted into the Vienna Society with Freud's support; in 1928 he emigrated to New York, where he became a professor at the New School for Social Research. Wittels had spoken on October 27, 1909, at the Wednesday Society in a lecture titled "Analysis of a Hysterical State of Confusion" (*Minutes* II, 282–289).

10. See letter 51 and n. 2.

11. "Double conscience" in English in the original.

12. Pierre Janet (1859–1947), famous French philosopher, psychologist, and psychiatrist; pupil of Jean-Martin Charcot. In 1903 he was made a professor of psychology at the Collège de France, and in 1913 became a member of the Institut de France. Janet had a theory of "unconscious fixed ideas" and had developed a therapy in which traumatic scenes were sought out in hypnosis and replaced through suggestion by a different, nontraumatic version of the event. For hysterical anesthesia, see *L'automatisme psychologique, Essai de psychologie expérimentale sur les formes inférieures de l'activité humaine* (Paris, 1889), pp. 290–299, and "L'anesthésie hystérique," *Archives de Neurologie* 24 (1892): 29–55.

13. The famous case of "Anna O." (Bertha Pappenheim); reprinted in Freud, *Nachtragsband*, pp. 221–243.

14. Probably Imre Décsi (Deutsch) (1881–1944?), a neurologist and psychiatric journalist who was close to psychoanalysis; a directing physician of the neurological section of the outpatient department of the Budapest Health Service. In 1909 he had done a practicum at the Burghölzli. Later he joined the Hungarian section of the Association of Independent Medical Analysts, which was oriented toward Stekel. Paul Harmat, *Freud, Ferenczi und die ungarische Psychoanalyse* (Tübingen, 1988), pp. 47, 157. He became a victim of the Nazis. See also letter 86 and n. 7.

15. James Jackson Putnam (1846–1918), professor of Neurology at Harvard University; co-editor of the *Journal of Abnormal Psychology*. He was a participant in the celebration at Clark University and host to Freud, Ferenczi, and Jung at his camp in the Adirondack Mountains. In 1911 he was founder and first president of the American Psychoanalytic Association. He was interested in combining psychoanalysis and philosophy. Putnam's letter is unpublished. Ferenczi's letters of October 22 and November 27, 1909, are in Hale, *Putnam*, pp. 304–306.

16. The volume of collected papers was published under the title *Lélekelemzés, Értekezések a pszichoanalizis Köréböl* [Papers on Psychoanalysis] (1910, 70), with the works indicated (57, 60, 61, 63, 65, 66; *Fin.*, p. 291; *F.C.*, p. 30; *C.*, p. 11; *Fin.*, p. 280; *F.C.*, p. 15; *C.*, p. 94) and a foreword by Freud (1910b). See also letters 88–92.

17. "Der Flug des Gedankens," *Pester Lloyd*, November 25, 1909, pp. 1–3. *Pester Lloyd* was a German-language newspaper published in Budapest. Leo Veigelsberg (1846–1907), father of the literary figure Hugó Ignotus (see letter 135, n. 4), had been its editor in chief from 1906 to 1907.

18. Probably Naum Kotik (1876–?) from Moscow. See also letter 184.

19. Naum Kotik also wrote *Die Emanation der psychophysischen Energie, Eine experimentelle Untersuchung über unmittelbare Gedankenübertragung in Zusammenhang mit der Frage über die Radioaktivität des Gehirns* [The Emanation of Psychophysical Energy: An Experimental Investigation into Direct Thought Transference in Connection with the Radioactivity of the Brain] (Wiesbaden, 1908). It appeared as volume 61 of *Grenzfragen des Nerven- und Seelenlebens; Einzeldarstellung für Gebildete aller Stände* [Questions at the Frontier of Nervous and Mental Life: Individual Presentations for Educated Persons of all Classes] (Wiesbaden, 1908), edited by Hans Kurella (1858–1916) and Leopold Löwenfeld (1847–1924); see letter 302 and n. 7.

86

Vienna, November 21, 1909
IX., Berggasse 19

Dear friend,

I am a bad correspondent, now that I have to use every free hour, and I don't have many, for writing down the damned American lectures (three have already been sent off). But that should have no repercussions on you, rather the opposite; the less I can give, the more need I have to receive.

After lengthy consideration I have offered your work on dreams to Stanley Hall to be translated and published.[1] I believe that is the best way to make use of it. I made much of it to him, but I have kept the manuscript, because sending it in would have seemed too much like pressuring him. Figuring on the deadlines which are familiar to us, we will now await his decision.

He wrote in his last letter what I am now copying out for you: "I am a very unworthy exponent of your views and of course have too little clinical experience to be an authority in that field. But it seems to me, whereas hitherto many if not most psychopathologists have leaned upon the stock psychologists like Wundt, your own interpretations reversd (sic) the situation and make us normal psychologists look to this work in the abnormal or borderline field for our chief light."[2]

Now, back to Europe and to your interesting communications.[3] I will send them back to you, and my only regret is that in so doing I will gradually lose your entire correspondence; still, this is the best way of exchanging ideas about scientific matters. You don't need to copy out future notices, but send me the originals, which I will then send back after I've looked at them.

(Your notebook has been ordered; I know from experience that these people take their time.)

Ad 1: The analgesic hand as mouse. Excellent. Agrees, by the way, with the conception that I have always maintained of hysterical anesthesia as a sign of possession of the ucs., and it also agrees with the idea, represented by the French, that hysterical paralyses originate by means of a reservation to the ucs. (I. Sammlung).[4] My patient at the time, who played roles with both hands, has been dead for a long time.

[*Ad*] 3: Isaac just as nice. Analogous to my mistake in telling the story of Kronos' castration by Zeus,[5] put forward against mythology, only now explains this mistake to me (Interpretation of Dreams). All of that must be collected and then we can draw from the supply. The same with the analysis of numbers.

[*Ad*] 5: I remonstrate in the case of obsessional neurosis with washing onanism! What you quote me as saying is not a supposition but is so often seen that I have put it down as certain fact.

Your confirmation is again quite flawless. Incidentally, I am treating such a case now. Patient is surprised about her constantly renewed consciousness of guilt and doesn't want to acknowledge its source in her continued washing onanism.

Crazy is quite correct, not responsible for his sexual misdeeds!

[Ad] 6: In the case of the actress, you will run into the problem of how far the identification with the role can go without disturbing the force of the presentation. She suspends complete identification. From that point on access to artistic problems!

[Ad] 8: What is new to me is the relationship of the little penis to the mother's vagina; I only believed in the comparison with the father's penis. In the meantime a mediation results from the fact that the father's penis has filled out the mother's vagina and therefore must be as big as the child (distension at birth is not taken into account because it is unknown).

I will copy out the passage from the military physician's paper for Jung.[6]

My photograph will get to you one of these days. I am so inhibited that I can't take care of anything myself but instead have to draw wife and children to me, especially since my sister-in-law, who normally takes care of all such business, isn't here yet.

In the aforementioned week the third edition of Everyday Life, to which you have contributed so much, will also probably come, and certainly the Jahrbuch. So lots of things are happening.

Decsy (or however you spell him) was here[7] and got little from me. I was too busy to invite him. He looks intelligent—and unreliable.

You will be oriented as to my condition when I tell you that I have the most productive week of my practice behind me, during which I produced one and a half lectures for Worcester. Deuticke has expressed the wish to bring out the lectures in German as well.[8] Only that way they don't contain anything new at all.

I could also be better healthwise; America has cost me much.

My thoughts, insofar as I can still make them perceptible, are with Leonardo da Vinci and Mythology.[9]

I am eagerly looking forward to news from you, factual as well as personal. I am totally without compensation for the pampering of the six weeks of journey.[10]

Cordially,
Freud

1. See letter 78, n. 3.
2. The entire quotation is English in the original [Trans.].

3. This material is missing. Its absence may account in part for the incomprehensibility of some of Freud's comments [Trans.].

4. Possibly a reference of Freud's to his *Sammlung kleiner Schriften zur Neurosenlehre, I. Folge* (Vienna, 1906). See also Freud 1893c.

5. Freud 1900a, p. 256.

6. A Dr. Drenkhahn, staff physician from Detmold, had made a connection between a decrease in cases of alcohol-related illness and an increase in cases of mental illness in the army ("Das verhalten der Alkoholerkränkungen zu den Geistes- und Nervenkrankheiten," *Deutsche militärärztliche Zeitschrift* 38, no. 10 [1909]: 393–396). Freud copied out part of this article for Jung (*Freud/Jung*, November 21, 1909, pp. 588f); Ferenczi referred to it in "Über die Rolle der Homosexualität in der Pathogenese der Paranoia" [On the Part Played by Homosexuality in the Pathogenesis of Paranoia] (1911, 80; *Schriften* I, 78f) and "Alkohol und Neurosen" (1911, 81; *Schriften* I, 92f).

7. On November 17, 1909, Décsi had been a guest at the Wednesday Society (*Minutes* II, 315, and 325).

8. See letter 78, n. 1.

9. Freud was engaged in an active exchange with Jung over questions of mythology (see *Freud/Jung*, November 15 and 21, 1909, pp. 263–266).

10. At the end of November Freud had a "consultation in Budapest, which gave [him] an opportunity to see Ferenczi and share in his work." On this occasion Ferenczi also introduced Gizella Pálos to Freud, who immediately took a liking to her (*Freud/Jung*, December 12, 1909, p. 270).

87

Budapest, December 1, 1909[1]

Dear Professor,

If I am not mistaken, one of these days you should be receiving a small shipment of Hungarian wine. Unfortunately, the consumption tax (which I hope won't be too high) can't be paid from this end.—

Best regards,
Ferenczi

1. Sealed postcard.

88

Vienna, December 3, 1909
IX., Berggasse 19

Dear friend,

Here is the outline of a foreword. I couldn't wait until my writer's cramp, which is supported by all resistances against my activity, has run its course.

Now, give me your opinion of it and tell me whether you want to have a translation made of this or of a modified text.

The Jahrbuch[1] was waiting for me in Vienna; it came out very splendid. Later volumes will, I hope, not be so conspicuously dominated by my name. I am keeping your paper[2] for myself for Sunday, after I send off the Worcester lectures.

The copy of Everyday Life for Frau Gisela, which we talked about, has, I hope, already gotten from you to her.

The lecture on Leonardo on the evening of the day which we began together[3] was not very satisfactory to me. Stein was there. I didn't get to hear any good response; even unusually uninspired and off-the-mark stuff from Adler.

I am now enjoying a bit of leisure, since I am working two hours less. Dirsztay's [a patient] parents were with me and proved themselves quite friendly to the treatment. I am quite eager to see how it turns out with Dr. Pollak.[4]

Putnam has informed us about the photographs from the Adirondacks in a very kind letter.

Cordial greetings to you and Frau G.

Yours,
Freud

[Enclosure:]
Psycho-analytic research into the neuroses (the various forms of nervous illness with a mental causation) has endeavoured to trace their connection with instinctual life and the restrictions imposed on it by the claims of civilization, with the activities of the normal individual in phantasies and dreams, and with the creations of the popular mind in religion, myths and fairy tales. The psycho-analytic treatment of neurotic patients, based on this method of research, makes far higher demands on doctor and patient than the methods hitherto in common use, which operate through medicaments, diet [and] hydropathy . . . But it brings the patients so much more relief and permanent strengthening in the face of life's problems, that there is no cause for surprise at the continual advances made by this therapeutic method in spite of violent opposition.

The author of the following essays, who is a close acquaintance of mine, and who is familiar, to an extent that few others are, with all the difficulties of psycho-analytic problems, is the first Hungarian to undertake the task of creating an interest in psycho-analysis among the . . . men of education in his own country through writings composed in their mother tongue. It is our cordial wish that this attempt of his may succeed and may result in gaining for this new field of work new workers from the body of his compatriots.[5]

Vienna, December 1909   Freud

1. The second half-volume of the *Jahrbuch* (November 1909). Freud was represented in this volume with the analysis of the "Rat-Man."

2. This is evidently a reference to Ferenczi's essay "Introjection and Transference," which was also published in this half-volume.

3. On December 1 Freud had talked about "A Fantasy of Leonardo da Vinci" in the Wednesday Society (*Minutes* II, 338–352), after returning from his visit to Ferenczi in Budapest (see letter 86, n. 10).

4. See letter 89.

5. This text is virtually identical to the published version (Freud 1910b [1909], p. 252). See letters 89 and 97 [Trans.].

89

Budapest, December 7, 1909
VII., Erzsébet-körút 54

Dear Professor,

Thank you very much for the introduction to the Hungarian collection. I am very satisfied with it. Assuming your concurrence after the fact, however, I have added a word; at the place where you note that I am the first Hungarian who etc. . . . wants to initiate "the men of education in his own country," I want to have printed *"the doctors and the men of education* in his own country."[1] I don't want this book to be described as "popular science." Probably no one will notice that in so doing the doctors will be removed from the circle of the educated (even though this ironic conception would not be inappropriate).

Now to Dr. Pollak! he is no longer in treatment with me. The thing went brilliantly. He was quick to learn, confessional, transferred excellently, already began to bring up infantile material. But his wife annoyed him to the quick; she confronted him with the choice: "me or analysis"; talked him into believing I had some kind of base intentions of alienating him from her; declared to him (on the basis of information from Vienna) that the analysis was 1.) dangerous, 2.) immoral, 3.) a swindle. He still didn't let up. Then she made a terrible scene at night: "I will save you, cure you. Come, love me." The poor guy tried it—and couldn't. The wife—very ashamed—implored him not to tell me about it. But he came and told.

Then the wife called in Dr. Lévy,[2] and he,—in an excess of timidity—let the analysis drop. [N.B.: Lévy is in the same situation as Pollak. He married a very rich, ugly girl. He is excessively concerned about his wife.[3] I told him so, and he was—apparently—aware of it.][4] The Pollaks are now in Vienna.—

The matter was instructive. I have the feeling that I could have straight-ened Dr. Pollak out.

The remaining analyses are going very well; I quickly overcame the unpleasantness of the Pollak case.

I wrote Jung a long letter in which I confessed candidly about my "brother complexes" and explained that guerrilla war cannot be the tactic of choice in psychoanalysis; someone must lead, and this one person, besides you, is by nature Jung himself. I also told him (probably in order not to garner any more sympathy) that you have altered your view about the "dead-end" that I have gotten into.[5]

Frau G. thanks you very much for your attention. She sends you the enclosed lines.

What has happened in and with me otherwise you will find in the enclosed "diary pages."[6] I have made an effort to be completely honest, despite the fact that I know that you will read it.

A Russian, Dr. Wrulff (?)[7] from Odessa, wrote me that he wants to review my psychotherapeutic works in an annual report for a newspaper there. Please give me your honest opinion about the work on "introjection." I am well aware of its weaknesses; but one is still always somewhat too lenient with oneself.

Kindest regards.

Your obedient
Ferenczi

1. Freud's foreword was published with this modification (Freud 1910b). See letter 88 and n. 5.

2. Lajos Lévy (1875–1961), renowned Hungarian internist; later became editor of the journal *Gyógyászat* [Art of Healing]; founding member of the Hungarian Psychoanalytic Society (1913). After the First World War he was director of the Jewish Hospital. Lévy was Ferenczi's friend and physician and was also frequently consulted by Freud between 1923 and 1928. Max Schur, *Freud: Living and Dying* (New York, 1972), p. 407.

3. Kata F. Lévy (1883–1969), sister of Anton von Freund; patron of psychoanalysis, and social worker later analyzed by Freud. She became a psychoanalyst and member of the Hungarian Society. In 1954 she and her husband emigrated to London, where they were both supported by Anna Freud.

4. Enclosed in brackets in the original.

5. Jung reported to Freud on December 14, 1909, about Ferenczi's "very nice letter" (*Freud/Jung*, p. 274). Jung's reply of December 6 is in Jung, *Briefe* I, 31.

6. This enclosure is missing.

7. Moshe Wulff (1878–1971), Russian psychiatrist. He had studied in Berlin with Karl Abraham and Otto Juliusburger (see letter 90 and n. 4) and returned to Odessa in 1909. Member of the Vienna Society (1911). In 1927 he emigrated to Berlin and in 1933 to

Palestine, where he became co-founder and, after Eitingon's death, president of the Psychoanalytic Society there.

90

Vienna, December 12, 1909
IX., Berggasse 19

Dear friend,

Many thanks for the enclosures, the nonpersonal part[1] of which will be returned. I only want to say, two more such analyses of paranoia and there will be a splendid contribution to the Jahrbuch. How distinct is the prominence of the homosexual components, namely the re-formation of sublimations. What you yourself fantasize about homosexuality will be saved and at least communicated to Sadger.[2] I will gladly give you my ideas about it when it takes more or less complete shape in you.

Your article in the Jahrbuch is now being read by everyone; instead of giving you my own judgment I am giving you that of a knowledgeable third party. He found the first part quite outstandingly good; the third, about suggestion, less original, since you confined yourself to working out my remark on the theory of sexuality.[3] I have no doubt about the complete success of the whole thing, only I am unsure whether the term introjection will prove to be lasting.

It is small comfort that I was able to predict so well the course of events with Dr. Pollak. Let us be happy that we had so much of him. Meanwhile, these are the things that we have to deaden ourselves against, for which one finds only too ample opportunity. The oversight with the doctors in the foreword occurred to me on the same day that I sent the letter, but not before it was too late to remedy it. I am satisfied with your suggestion, as I would have been with any changes you might have wanted to make.

Dr. Wulff from Odessa also wrote to me recently about a case that he is analyzing. He comes from Juliusburger,[4] and still seems to understand very little.—The fact that you wrote to Jung in that vein once again proves how the trip to America has refreshed and advanced you.

I am still not one hundred percent, but I don't want you to spare me in matters of thought transference. This weakness is about to succumb to being surmounted. The recent experiments with Frau Jelinek seem not to have yielded anything particularly fruitful as far as I am concerned, no matter how well they support our earlier conclusions. I find myself particularly inept in hazarding to recommend to you a scheme for experimentation. So, the matter is still not right with me, deep down. But you will find it alone.

I am now revising the Theory of Sexuality for the second edition[5] and am otherwise recovering slowly as my activity diminishes.

Best regards,
Freud

You should have received the notebook. I will be glad if it reminds you frequently of my inspiration.

1. This material is missing.
2. Isidor Sadger (1867–1942), neurologist and literary critic from Galicia and member of the Wednesday Society since 1906; Fritz Wittels's uncle. He published on matters related to homosexuality, among other subjects. He died in the Theresienstadt concentration camp.
3. See letter 63 and n. 6.
4. Otto Juliusburger (1867–1952), German psychiatrist and psychoanalyst in Berlin. Founding member of the Berlin Society (1908), from which he later resigned. He emigrated to New York in 1941.
5. *Three Essays on the Theory of Sexuality* (1905d), 2d ed. (1910). Freud completed the revision in December; see also letter 92 and Freud's foreword to the second edition in *Studienausgabe* V, 43.

91

Budapest, December 18, 1909
VII., Erzsébet-körút 54

Dear Professor,

Since I am in a great hurry I am writing you only a few lines now. I have a laborious week of self- and patient analysis behind me, the high point of which was my reading of the "Rat-Man," the significance of which is incalculable. (Many thanks for the offprint!)

I will include the report about things that I have thought and seen in my next, detailed letter. This time I would only like to ask you about your decision regarding the use of the Christmas vacation. You may be too tired for Berlin as well as for my visit. If not, then I will come. I hope you will not feel any compulsion on my account and that you will write me without further ado what is preferable to you.

The Hungarian lectures are half corrected—the foreword with the indicated change.

Best regards,
Ferenczi

92

Vienna, December 19, 1909
IX., Berggasse 19

Dear friend,

Thank you for today's offprint. Jung writes that they also especially appreciate your introjection paper in Zurich.[1] Stanley Hall has responded that he has not found your paper[2] among his, but he is looking for it in order to have it translated and published, if it is not too long. He thought he already received it. I enlightened him, sent him the paper, and am now waiting to see how he will react. I hope he won't find it too long. But I didn't neglect to tell him that it is designated for publication in connection with your Hungarian book.

So much for the literary business news. Otherwise I am still hoping that the stationery store has really sent you the notebook. I am recovering quickly as a result of strongly diminishing activity, but I am dissatisfied with the fact that health can only be coupled with poverty. News about your intended coming here is also due.

I am revising the Theory of Sexuality, which, at Deuticke's behest, is being changed so little that it can go to the printer's at the end of January. I now see how flawed and unsatisfactory especially II and III[3] are. But the time has not yet arrived to replace them with something else.

Cordially,
Freud

1. See *Freud/Jung*, December 14, 1909, p. 274, and Jung's letter to Ferenczi of December 25, 1909, in Jung, *Letters* I, 13.
2. See letter 78, n. 3.
3. The essays "Infantile Sexuality" and "Transformations of Puberty" (1905d, pp. 173–230).

93

Vienna, December 21, 1909
IX., Berggasse 19

Dear friend,

A new crossroads! I am responding, therefore, that I am turning down your kind Christmas visit, not out of fatigue but on account of familial unrest and work, and that I am prepared to offer compensation. Work: today the translation of Worcester I arrived, which will soon be followed by the other pieces. They are pressing me from over there to settle the matter quickly, and I have no time for it and for revising the Theory of Sexuality other than the two free days, Saturday and Sunday. *Family:* fortunately, less critical. Yesterday (i.e., early this morning), my brother received his first boy.[1] It was a difficult birth, was completed in the sanatorium, and, because of the size of the child, it would not have turned out all right without help. Now everything is going well, but the family is upset, and the situation is still not certain. My little Anna[2] is supposed to go to the Semmering Monday morning with her married sister[3] as chaperone.

Jung writes to me that we have to firm up the date for Nuremberg.[4] I am very much in favor of Easter, in order to be free in September and to carry out disrupted plans.

In expectation of your announced scientific news,

Yours truly,
Freud

1. Harry, only child of Alexander and Sophie Sabine Freud (1878–1970). He became a lawyer. On February 7, 1948, he married Leli Margaret Horn.
2. Freud's youngest child, Anna (1895–1982). Originally an elementary schoolteacher, she—analyzed by her father—was the only one of Freud's children to become a psychoanalyst. She was a pioneer in child analysis. From 1922 on she was a member of the Vienna Society, and from 1924 a member of the Committee. When her father fell ill with cancer, she became his nurse, secretary, and adviser and remained so until his death. She was co-editor of the *Zeitschrift für psychoanalytische Pädagogik*. In 1934 she took over from Helene Deutsch as director of the Training Institute of the Vienna Society. In London she was head of the Hampstead Nurseries (1940–1945) and the Hampstead Clinic (from 1952 on). In 1945 she founded the journal *Psychoanalytic Study of the Child*. In her works she represented—in contrast to Melanie Klein—the pedagogical trend within child analysis and maintained a clear differentiation between the analysis of children and of adults. Her book *Das Ich und die Abwehrmechanismen* [The Ego and the Mechanisms of Defense] (Vienna, 1936) is considered a classic of psychoanalysis.
3. Mathilde.
4. For the Second Psychoanalytic Congress on March 30 and 31, 1910.

94

Budapest, December 27, 1909
VII., Erzsébet-körút 54

Dear Professor,

In expectation of being able to meet you personally again, I still owe you two letters and many thanks. First, for procuring the pretty notebooks (the price of which the delivery man did not indicate), and then for the effort which you are undertaking on behalf of my work on dreams, and, finally, for the many communications about your activity, which interest me very much.—Instead of the excursion to Vienna, I rested for two whole days, got up late, didn't touch a pen or a book, visited a lot with the family (my mother is staying here). The somewhat worrisome events in your family have in the meantime—I hope—turned out favorably. I would have wished for you to spend the two days without care and work (I also didn't want to go to Vienna for that reason). I am afraid you are overtaxing yourself.—

As far as the Congress is concerned, I have decided on Easter; in that case, to be sure, we will probably have to forgo the presence of the Americans, with the possible exception of Brill, who will certainly come.

It would be appropriate to determine the program in advance and to submit certain important themata for discussion (a reporter would have to be assigned to each theme). Besides the psychological and pathological problems, someone would have to treat the practical experiences to date and the most expedient methods of *propaganda* for our psychological movement. (I don't want to suggest that directly to Jung, in order not to evoke the appearance of unjustified meddling with his authority.)

The criticism of my work on introjection has interested me greatly; Rank has also written to me indicating that the first part is more valuable. I am happy that there is at least something useful in it.—I am now reading the Rat-Man for the second time; Stekel's dream analyses[1] are in part very good, but "botched" in places. I have saved Adler's hard-to-read work[2] for last (as the toughest nut); I am convinced that I will find a lot of good ideas in it. Too bad he judges everything so forcefully from his point of view (aggression, inferiority).

The last of my notes are not actually scientific but purely personal. I will send them to you next time.

Best regards,
Dr. Ferenczi

What do the notebooks cost?

1. Wilhelm Stekel, "Beiträge zur Traumdeutung," *Jahrbuch*, 2d half-volume (1909): 458–512.
2. Alfred Adler, "Über neurotische Dispositionen," *Jahrbuch*, 2d half-volume (1909): 526–545.

95

Vienna, December 28, 1909[1]

Professor Freud and wife[2]

express to you, dear and esteemed Dr., their most cordial thanks for the very splendid holiday cake. You know, of course, how such things are valued and esteemed by us.

Will we see you with us again soon? In any case, I wish you a happy, joyful year and remain your gratefully obedient

Martha Freud[3]

1. Calling card.
2. This line is printed; the remaining text (on both sides) is in Martha Freud's handwriting.
3. In the collection of the Austrian National Library in Vienna there is attached to this card another enclosure which is missing from the photostat folder as well as the Balint folder. Since it is dated February 1909, it has been included with letter 37.

96

Vienna, January 1, 1910
IX., Berggasse 19

Dear friend,

For half an hour I have been able to wish you happiness for the New Year, which I hereby do with all my heart, to you and to those dear to you.

A few hours after I turned you down for Christmas, lectures II and III came back from Worcester, as if to justify me in the face of my most intimate conscience. I was so preoccupied for the holidays, and during the same time I also revised the almost completely unaltered Theory of Sexuality for publication. My practice has picked up again since the holidays, but I am already recovered and cheerful.

Mathilde is on the Semmering with the little one;[1] both are not doing badly, but also not very well. Everything seems to be going smoothly with my brother. The weather, of course, never comes from the quarter that one has been carefully observing.

I am just now awaiting a response from Jung regarding the Congress. I find your suggestions quite useful and don't see why you don't want to write to him about them as soon as the preliminary date has been set, which is not yet the case.

I will gladly entrust to you an insight that I had right around New Year's: the basic reason for religion is man's infantile helplessness. I will spare myself further details.

Jones is now excelling in rueful and contrite letters; his resistance finally seems to be broken. Pfister seems to be looking forward, in a childlike way, to his polemic with Foerster[2] and is as cordial as ever. A few days ago a Moscow assistant, Ossipov,[3] appeared with a few (unfortunately illegible)[4] offprints, which seem to contain very careful reports. He is applying for the Moscow Academy prize, to be awarded in March, which has designated "psychoanalysis" as its theme, and he wants to come to Vienna in May.

Binswanger wants to visit us in January or February. Do you want to come at the same time, or would you rather come alone? I have decided to leave to you when you want to come. Don't make any further inquiries and be here. You are, of course, acquainted with the situation. I am always busy, no matter what day it is.

Incidentally, what do you think of a tighter organization with formal rules and a small fee? Do you consider that advantageous? I also wrote Jung a couple of words about this.

Otherwise I am lazy, gnawing at Leonardo, about whom not a line has been written.

Best regards,
Freud

1. Anna.

2. Oskar Pfister answered Foerster (see letter 84 and n. 3) with "Die Psychoanalyse als wissenschaftliches Prinzip und seelsorgerliche Methode" [Psychoanalysis as a Scientific Principle and Method of Pastoral Care], *Evangelische Freiheit*, N.S., 10, nos. 2–4 (1910).

3. Nikolai Evgrafovich Ossipov (1877–1934), chief physician of the Psychiatric University Clinic in Moscow; co-founder of the Russian Psychoanalytic Society and Freud's translator. In 1920 he emigrated to Istanbul, and in 1921 to Prague, where he became docent for psychoanalysis. As early as 1908 Ossipov had come forward with reports about psychoanalysis (see Moshe Wulff, "Die russische psychoanalytische Literatur bis zum Jahre 1911," *Zentralblatt* 1 [1910–11]: 364f).

4. I.e., printed in Cyrillic script.

97

Budapest, January 2, 1910
VII., Erzsébet-körút 54

Dear Professor,

Many thanks for the New Year's wishes, and the same to you. I don't know whether I have already told you once or several times (in any case, repeating it confirms the truth) how gratefully I think of you every time I get the opportunity to reflect. I know that the many years in which you have been misunderstood have very strongly diminished your receptivity to admiration, recognition, etc. (see in connection to that the passage in the Interpretation of Dreams where you so morosely disdain the effusive admiration of a pupil [in the coffee house][1])—but you must gradually accustom yourself to the fact that times have improved, and that, without the danger of later disappointment, you can rely upon having enhanced the lives and occupations of a very large number of people who were previously striving in vain for recognition. It is my unshakable conviction, however, that these adherents are but the predecessors of all humanity, which, for the time being, is still stuck in infantile resistances, and there is no doubt that your work will leave behind strong traces in world history. I say all of this after appropriate correction, after removing everything that personal adherence, and especially my own father complex, could dictate to me. Without this correction this letter would have come out much more effusive.

I cannot report on events. My mother's presence and my social obligations, which, incidentally, have been reduced to a minimum (and the fulfillment of which I have saved for Holy Week), have impeded me in all scientific work.—I intend to be more diligent in the new year.

As far as the Congress is concerned, I am in favor of Easter; I find your suggestion (tighter organization) extremely useful. The acceptance of members, however, would be just as strictly managed as it is in the Vienna Society;[2] that would be a way of keeping out undesirable elements.

I find the explanation of religiosity by infantile helplessness very plausible; I hope to learn the details of this theory from you at our next meeting.

I will write to Jung about propaganda.

The question whether I should come at the same time as Abraham or alone is a tricky one. If I follow the unpleasure principle, I should come alone, and then I will also do Abraham a favor. But if I consider the advantage that I gained through the trip to America* and think of the necessity of coming closer to Abraham, then that means: "You should go to Vienna when Abraham comes." Neither intention has tipped the scale yet one way or the other—I haven't made a decision yet (I'm behaving like an obsessional neurotic).

I am happy that the storm clouds have receded from the horizon of your family life. In my own there are constantly large and small disturbances, as is not otherwise possible in this difficult situation. More about that later.—(I have not forgotten my promise to send the notes.)

Miss Judith Bernays[3] was so kind as to send me a New Year's card.

Best regards from me and Frau G.—She thanks you for the New Year's wishes.

Cordially,
Ferenczi

I have inserted another word into the foreword to my little book. Where you speak about the earlier therapeutic methods (diet, hydrotherapy), I also added *suggestion*,[4] in order to emphasize the difference between ΨA. and suggestion.

[The following is written on a new page.]

I'm back to my old habits! It drives me to despair! I already put this letter in an envelope, I call for the maid, 1.) to stir up the fire in my room, 2.) to

give her the letter to "mail." At the last minute I read your letter again
(and, to be sure, only the passage where you talk about the expected visit
in February); all of a sudden I notice that up to now I have always been
reading Abraham instead of Binswanger—or maybe I read Binswanger, but
certainly I have been thinking Abraham! That tiresome brother complex
is still playing tricks on me. I was evidently afraid that Abraham would be
the guest; he is the more significant one (perhaps the most significant after
Jung); it is evidently my secret wish to be able to measure myself against
him; not to be capable of it—the motive of anxiety and antipathy!—But if
it is a matter of Binswanger—then the question is much more easily resolved. I would very gladly come at the same time as he; even though I do
hope to have you for myself alone in the meantime.

I am now so terribly ashamed of my mistake, and this affect is for me
the measure of the work that I still have to do on myself. Frau G.'s extensive identification with me is demonstrated in the fact that she also read
the letter and didn't recognize my error. (I shared the content of the letter
earlier with her and in so doing always talked about Abraham.)

* (Jung's presence)

1. Freud 1900a, p. 470; enclosed in brackets in the original.
2. See letter 11, n. 1.
3. Judith Bernays (1885–1977), eldest child of Freud's sister Anna (1858–1955) and
Martha Freud's brother Eli Bernays (1860–1923).
4. See Freud 1910b.

98

Budapest, January 10, 1910

Dear Professor,

Thanks for the letters and shipment.[1] Will answer both in detail.—On
mature reflection I will postpone my trip to Vienna—the egoism of speaking with you alone has won out.

Here is the Hungarian booklet.

Gratefully yours,
Ferenczi

1. The second edition of *Three Essays* (Freud 1905d).

99

Vienna, January 10, 1910
IX., Berggasse 19

Dear friend,

Today I have you to thank for much and little to give you in return. Analyses and writings, as you now do them, are very significant events for one's own person, and the other—if he comes into it at all—has nothing to do but keep a respectful silence.[1] *Favete linguis*.[2] I can hardly admire perspicacity, for I know that it is made up of honesty and firm decision. Certainly you are right in every instance.

Your dream and attempt at clarification in the case of Frau G. naturally belong together. In the analysis you seek to free yourself from the inner drives from which Frau G. has constructed a reproach against you. As to what is real, I have to say that you were by and large undoubtedly correct with your disclosure to the beloved woman. It belongs to the ABC of our worldview that the sexual life of a man can be something different from that of a woman, and it is only a sign of respect when one does not conceal this from a woman. Whether the requirement of absolute truthfulness does not sin against the postulate of expediency and against the intentions of love I would not like to respond to in the negative without qualification, and I urge caution. Truth is only the absolute goal of science, but love is a goal of life which is totally independent of science, and conflicts between both of these major powers are certainly quite conceivable. I see no necessity for principled and regular subordination of one to the other.

I fear that not much new will result from an investigation of what is constitution and what is repression in the sexual character of women. The question will probably be answered with bisexuality and the knowledge that there are women who are capable of everything. A large piece of sexual repression is inextricable from the character of a woman of culture [*Kulturweib*].

The illumination of your medical tendencies in your dream was of great personal interest to me. This need to help is lacking in me, and I now see why, because I did not lose anyone whom I loved in my early years. I found this same personal motivation in Fliess. What is both strong and pathological in him comes from this. The conviction that his father, who died from erysipelas after many years of nasal suppuration,[3] could have been saved made him into a doctor, indeed, even turned his attention to the nose. The sudden death of his only sister two years later, on the second day of a pneumonia, for which he could blame doctors, instilled in him the fatalistic theory of predetermined dates of death—as a consolation. This piece of analysis, unwanted by him, was the inner cause of our break, which he effected in such a pathological (paranoid) manner.

I wonder if you don't also have a secret reason for sharing this analysis of your dream with me, and I think I have actually found it. The dream must also have a relation to me, which has, by the way, also revealed itself to you in a number of places. It is easy for me to find the motive for equating me with your father. On the trip I behaved like someone who is taking his leave, who wants to set his house in order. In camp [Putnam's Adirondacks cabin] I had real appendix pains for the first time, and for at least a day I was quite despondent over the prospect of becoming a burden to Putnam and causing him worry and responsibility. I know that I talked about it later, but I no longer remember whether it was more with Jung or with you. (These pains, incidentally, have come again and again since that time; just today they reminded me finally to write the letter that I had postponed. I am not considering drawing any particular conclusions from them; they are also rather slight, but quite localized, and they increase with every constipation; they also, incidentally, stay away for a week at a time.)

So, that provides a basis for the identification. Again, as then, the death of the father is the signal for a great inner cleansing for you, and for an effort to bind the mother to you.[4] Whether your harping on the year 1909 (twice repeated) is a compliment for the year just past, or whether it is connected with my imminent demise, I have no way of knowing. Let us nevertheless firmly establish that I myself already decided quite a long time ago not to die until 1916 or 17. Of course, I don't exactly insist upon it.

As compensation for this unseemly discussion I want to give you a little piece of theory, which came to me while I was reading your analysis. It seems to me that in influencing the sexual drives, we can bring about nothing more than exchanges, displacements; never renunciation, giving up, the resolution of a complex. (Strictest secret!) When someone delivers up his infantile complexes, then in their place he has salvaged a piece of them (the affect) and put it into a present configuration (transference). He has shed his skin and leaves the stripped-off skin for the analyst; God forbid that he is now naked, skinless! Our therapeutic gain is a substitutive gain, similar to the one that Hans im Glück makes. The last piece doesn't fall into the fountain until death.[5]

The theoretical value of this conception lies in its convergence with the processes in dementia praecox. In practice it is, fortunately, not exactly decisive.

It would be useless to deny that I was happy with the words with which your letter introduced the new year. One is so insensitive only toward reproach, not toward recognition. Only with great difficulty can I, myself, take a position with respect to the question of the value of my works and their influence on the shape of future science. Sometimes I believe in it, sometimes I doubt it. I mean, it can't be predicted. Perhaps the dear Lord doesn't know it yet himself. Still, they may be of some value to us now, and I am glad from the bottom of my heart that I am no longer the only one. If I don't get very old, I will get nothing out of them, and I certainly don't work for the sake of anticipated usefulness or fame, and, cognizant of people's necessary ingratitude, I also don't expect anything for my children later on. All such considerations must play a very small role if we are serious about our belief in the global firm of "Fatum & Ananke."[6]

Very occasionally I sometimes write a few lines about Leonardo, which is still proceeding with great difficulty. At home things are very well, in my practice lively. Your "Abraham" has announced himself for the 15th of the month;[7] I am notifying you immediately of his arrival so that you can choose your time. You will be a great relaxation for the ladies, who have a special kind of liking for this visitor that they don't demonstrate to our other guests.

Your dream analysis will follow tomorrow. Again, I haven't found an appropriate envelope at home.

Cordially,
Freud

1. A letter of Ferenczi's is evidently missing here.

2. "Keep your tongues in check!" (Horace, *Odes* 3.1, 2): the words with which a Roman priest would begin a sacrifice.

3. In fact Fliess's father may well have died by his own hand (communication kindly sent by Peter Swales).

4. Ferenczi's father had died from an intestinal occlusion (according to Ferenczi's sister Zsófia).

5. In the fairy tale "Hans im Glück" (Lucky Hans) by the Brothers Grimm, Hans, as a reward for his work, receives a piece of gold, which becomes a burden to him. He trades it for a horse, trades the horse for a cow, and so on until he is finally in possession of two stones. Because they weigh him down, he puts them on the edge of a fountain, accidentally pushes them, and they fall in. Hans thanks God and, free of all burdens, bounds home to his mother.

6. Latin "fate" plus Greek "compulsion." The concept of *ananke* was first mentioned by Freud in the paper on Leonardo, on which he was in the process of "gnawing" (1910c), p. 125; see letter 96.

7. The Binswangers' visit took place January 15–25.

100

Vienna, January 12, 1910
IX., Berggasse 19

Dear friend,

The Binswangers ("Abraham") are coming to Vienna on Saturday morning, the 15th. The main event will probably be on the following Sunday. I don't need to tell you that you are welcome at any time.

In America everything seems to be excellent and developing rapidly. Putnam acknowledges you very appreciatively in his first paper (Journal of Abnormal Psychology, no. 5).[1] Hall will put your article into the April issue of the American Journal of Psychology; he didn't have it yet at the time of your letter.

Cordially,
Freud

1. James J. Putnam, "Personal Impressions of Sigmund Freud and His Work, with Special Reference to his Recent Lectures at Clark University," *Journal of Abnormal Psychology* 4 (1909–10): 294.

101

Vienna, January 14, 1910[1]

Hearty congratulations on the publication of your first work on ΨA in Hungarian[2] and many thanks for the too modest dedication!

Don't you want to reveal to me what the strange word in the title *(Lélekelemzés)* means? It must be something very beautiful. Your naughtiness in not wanting to come this week has been very much derided in this house. On account of it, things will not go well for Binswanger (Abraham); he will really be taken to the cleaner's.—The organizational plans for the Congress are assuming more definite shape; more about that later. Critique from the British Medical Journal is by Havelock Ellis.[3]

Cordially,
Freud

1. Postcard.
2. See letter 85 and n. 16.
3. Havelock Ellis (1859–1939), versatile English scientist and, above all, sexual researcher; editor of *Studies in the Psychology of Sex* (Watford, 1897–1928). Freud is presumably referring to the anonymously published review of his *Selected Papers on Hysteria and Other Psycho-Neuroses*, Nervous and Mental Disease Monograph Series, no. 4 (New York, 1909), in the *British Medical Journal*, December 18, 1909, p. 1756.

102

Budapest, January 14, 1910

Dear Professor,

This time also no reply to your dear letter—only the inquiry as to whether you will reflect upon one of the two (or both) little figurines which were unearthed near *Nagybecskerek*.[1] The dealer is asking twenty-two crowns for the Hermes and twenty-eight crowns for the primitive Cupid. In case you can't use the figurines, please return them as soon as possible and at this opportunity please indicate whether or not I am burdening you unnecessarily with such requests.

Cordial greetings to the entire family and to colleague Binswanger and his wife.

Your devoted
Ferenczi

The dealer is prepared to take back the figurines in the event that an expert declares them fake.—

1. Grossbetschkerek; now Zrenjanin, in the Vojvodina, about forty miles north of Belgrade.

103

Vienna, January 16, 1910[1]

Dear friend,
Many thanks! Both figurines are good and will be kept. Please tell that to the dealer. More to follow. The Binswangers are very affectionate and will stay here for eight days. I await your news.

Cordially,
Freud

1. Postcard.

104

Budapest, January 18, 1910
VII., Erzsébet-körút 54

Dear Professor,
I have very many things to say about your detailed letter—but again and again things come up that I have to share with you without delay, whereas writing down all the thoughts that reading your letter aroused in me would require an hour totally undisturbed—inwardly and outwardly—which I don't have at the moment.

For the time being, therefore, I will only react to your latest news—confirm receipt of the 50 crowns and both postcards.—

The word *Lélekelemzés* is the word for Ψ-A which I coined and which is a word-for-word translation of it. *Lélek* = psyche (anima), *elemezni* = the

Hungarian word for *to analyze; elemzés* = analysis. [*Elem* = element; to analyze = to reduce to elements.][1] The word *elem* has simply been stolen from the Latin.

The news that the Binswangers are staying so long in Vienna fills me with mixed feelings. You see, I intend to go to Vienna at the end of this week (Friday or Saturday) in order to spend Sunday with you. I know that on Saturday evenings you are at your tarok game;[2] but I could attend your lecture.[3]

I am afraid of two things. First of all that the prolonged presence of the Swiss guests could make a new guest appear undesirable to you—(you can hardly breathe with all the guests). Second (and that would be the less significant one), that finally I would only meet the Binswangers and couldn't speak with you alone.

If I don't receive a letter of refusal from you, then I will come and hope to learn more about the Congress, along with scientific and personal matters.

Your most obedient
Ferenczi

1. Enclosed in brackets in the original.
2. On Saturday evenings Freud customarily played a game of tarok (a popular card game in Austria) at the home of Leopold Königstein (see letter 128, n. 4.). In addition to Königstein, the philosopher Friedrich Eckstein, Oskar Rie (see letter 110, n. 6), and the pediatrician Ludwig Rosenberg were usually his partners.
3. Freud was to lecture at the University of Vienna on Saturday evening between seven and nine.

105

Vienna, January 19, 1910
IX., Berggasse 19

Dear friend,

It is settled that I won't turn you down again. I have no reason to this time. I only want to orient you. The Binswangers are not a strain and not—satisfying. They will still be with us Sunday noon and afternoon. In the evening they are going to+++[1] Obersteiner's.[2] We would be free into the wee hours of the evening. Only, *I* would be grateful for the afternoon; you must choose.

Cordially,
Freud

1. Freud often used the symbol of three crosses before the names of persons toward whom he was ambivalent. According to Jeffrey Masson (*Fliess Letters*, November 5, 1899,

n. 1 p. 382), "This sign was sometimes chalked on the inside of doors in peasant houses to protect against danger."

2. Heinrich Obersteiner (1847–1922), head of the neurological institute and professor of anatomy and the pathology of the nervous system at the University of Vienna. In 1885 Freud had worked in his private clinic for a month. See Freud's letter to Martha Bernays of June 8, 1885 (*Letters*, pp. 150f); Freud 1887d (p. 929) and 1887e (*Nachtragsband*, pp. 105f); and Gerhard Fichtner and Albrecht Hirschmüller, "Sigmund Freud, Heinrich Obersteiner und die Diskussionen über Hypnose und Kokain," *Jahrbuch der Psychoanalyse*, vol. 23 (Stuttgart, 1988), pp. 105–137.

106

Budapest, January 21, 1910
VII., Erzsébet-körút 54

Dear Professor,

I will arrive in Vienna on Saturday (morning or afternoon) and will stay at the Hotel Regina.[1] On Sunday morning I will take the liberty of calling on you right after breakfast in order to abreact something personal as soon as possible. If you have something to do on Sunday morning, I will soon leave you alone and will come only to help amuse the Binswangers (Abraham!). I will be most pleased to go along with the remainder of your program.

See you soon!

Your obedient
Ferenczi

1. Many of Freud's visitors stayed at the Hotel Regina, five minutes' walk from his apartment at what is now called Sigmund Freud Park.

107

Budapest, January 25, 1910
VII., Erzsébet-körút 54

Dear Professor,

At this point I very definitely hope that nothing will stand in the way of my carrying out my travel plans and that I will arrive at the Hotel Regina Saturday noon.

You must have noticed that my letters and replies have lately become too laconic; in order to avoid misunderstandings, I would like to inform you that this was the consequence of a psychic depression which has nothing to do with you, Jung, and science—in fact, it has only a little to do with Frau G. I have undertaken to inform you personally about it, which will be all the easier for me, since I have almost completely overcome this mood swing in the meantime and will certainly have *completely* overcome it by Saturday. Perhaps it is good that Binswanger's presence kept me from visiting you in Vienna—I am now certain that I won't have to spoil your good mood with my sad demeanor.—

If you still have time and the desire to write me a card before my departure, I would ask you to let me know the time and place of your lecture on Saturday.[1] If the theater does not conflict with the lecture, I will be free to invite your wife and sister-in-law to the Burgtheater for a performance of *Hamlet* and request Oli or Ernst[2] to get me three good seats in the parquet. Perhaps we can compromise between lecture and theater (i.e., I could spend an hour at the lecture and then go to the theater).

Kindest regards to all. Looking forward to seeing you again, I am

Yours,
Ferenczi

1. See letter 104, n. 3.
2. Freud's sons Oliver and Ernst.

108

Vienna, January 26, 1910
IX., Berggasse 19

Dear friend,

I really hope that nothing will stand in the way of your visit. If you still bring your depression along, then you won't take it home again. I myself am well and cheerful and have many things to talk about with you. It was quite right for you not to come last week. The Binswangers didn't leave until yesterday. We wouldn't have been able to say a word to each other.

The ladies have asked me to thank you kindly for your invitation, but they are unable to accept it because the children are going out, etc. So we make two suggestions to you. Either give instruction by telegram for a theater ticket (Oli) or come with me to the lecture from seven to nine and then just eat with the rest of the family at our table. The lecture will certainly offer little. Federn[1] will talk about the Bleulerian mechanisms;[2] you see, it is a kind of seminar, but at least you will breathe $\psi \alpha$ air there. I would rather go with you to Hamlet myself, but I have to be there and afterwards also commit the tarok excess. So choose freely, and in any event let us see you Saturday afternoon.

Yours,
Freud

1. Paul Federn (1871–1950), internist and prominent member of the Wednesday Society. He joined the Social Democratic party in 1918. He was Freud's spokesman after the latter's operation for cancer (1923) and was vice president of the Vienna Society from 1924 until its dissolution by the Nazis in 1938. Later that year Federn emigrated to New York, but it was not until 1946 that he became recognized as a physician and consequently as a member of the Psychoanalytic Society there. After his wife died and he contracted cancer, he took his own life. Federn was significant because of his "ego psychology" and his pioneering role in the investigation of psychoses and in popularizing psychoanalysis and its application to related disciplines. He wrote *Ich-Psychologie und die Psychosen* (Bern, 1956) and *Das Psychoanalytische Volksbuch*, ed. H. Meng (Leipzig, 1926).

2. Possibly a reference to Bleuler's essay "Freud'sche Mechanismen in der Symptomatologie von Psychosen," *Psychiatrisch-Neurologische Wochenschrift* 8 (1906–07): 316–318, 323–325, 338–340.

109

Budapest, February 5, 1910
VII., Erzsébet-körút 54

Dear Professor,

The rich—all too rich—"booty" of my latest trip to Vienna is constantly on my mind. A day like that compensates one for months of renunciation and refreshes one's mind and spirit. It is a comforting prospect that in future generations such free and open discourse (without the danger of arousing infantile sensitivities) will not be counted among the exceptions. When you talk about the prospects for psychoanalysis,[1] you should not eliminate this point of view from consideration. Once society has gone beyond the infantile, then hitherto completely unimagined possibilities for social and political life are opened up. Just think what it would mean if one *could tell everyone the truth*, one's father, teacher, neighbor, and even the king. All fabricated, imposed authority would go to the devil—what is *rightful* would remain natural. The eradication of lies from private and public life would necessarily *have to* bring about better conditions; if reason and not dogmas (to which I add the word "morality") prevail, a more purposeful, less costly, and in every respect more economical reconciliation of individual interests with the common good would ensue. (The opposition between the two will not be removed from the world—nor should it be.) I do not think that the $\psi\alpha$ worldview leads to democratic egalitarianism; the *intellectual elite of humanity* should maintain its hegemony; I believe Plato desired something similar.[2] Naturally these must be intelligences that are always conscious of their own weaknesses and do not forget or deny the animalistic-instinctual basis of the human spirit. To put the power of government into the hands of vain, conceited professors would be the most horrible of horrors.—

The scientific usefulness of what Sunday brought me has yet to manifest itself.—The notes that I took about the things that came to your mind were not sufficient to consolidate the clear and virtually self-evident insight into your ideas that I got from them in Vienna. I must wait until experience assists me in discovering, that is, rediscovering these things myself. What completely eluded me in particular was the discovery of the struggle between the individual strivings of the libido, which are supposed to explain neurasthenia![3] I am beating my brains out in a vain attempt to recall this.

Here in Budapest I found everything the way it was; only I myself seem to have changed somewhat: talking things out has eradicated the last traces of neurosis, and I sense—in place of the earlier inclination toward inactivity—a kind of urge to do something. I regained my motivation for work last evening. It came about thus: in light of our discussion, I want to talk about propaganda and organization in Nuremberg.[4] That brought me to the shameful insight that I have certainly created propaganda here but no trace of an organization. So I sent Décsi a patient in order win over his good will, conferred with him over the founding of a $\psi\alpha$ society (modeled on Vienna), and made contact with Stein.

Décsi is a young go-getter, wants to work and publish a lot; he also writes newspaper articles about $\Psi\alpha$ and wants to make a name for himself; at the same time he is very conceited (also, in fact, very intelligent), thinks he is discovering something new everywhere, etc.

I felt somewhat uncomfortable. The analysis gave impetus to the old brother complex: I evidently want to play the little *Freud* here, very eagerly instructing someone quite inexperienced who recognizes me as his master, but to allow myself to be taught by someone younger—that makes me uncomfortable. Despite this insight, it occurred to me today to organize my notes for an article on Everyday Life; I am also preparing the Hungarian translation of the paper on introjection.[5] All that is certainly the consequence of brother envy (perhaps more likely the fear of losing my authority). But in this innocent, indeed, advantageous form, under constant control of reason, one can become aware of one's drives, one's (as *we* know, essentially immutable) uniqueness.

I forgot to tell you that I discovered the pediatrician *Lindner* living here. I recently wanted to read his work on thumb sucking[6] in the original. On this occasion I asked a man who has been employed in the library of the Society of Physicians whether he knew the author. He said, "Yes, he comes to the library now and then." In my first surprise I was seized by the impulse to give him some news about the fate of his work. I wrote to him immediately and called your theory of sexuality to his attention. (I was led by the wish to make amends to the old man, who, I hear, had been ridiculed in his time because of this work.) He replied with the enclosed card. I still don't know him personally.

I believe I have made a not worthless acquisition for our cause in the person of a young doctoral candidate. His name is . . . [The name escapes me for a moment. His name is *Vajda*. That is also the name of my brother-in-law who died at an early age,[7] a lawyer who left my sister with three children and entirely without means. At the same time, an echo of my illness complex.][8] He is clever, grasps things easily, gets into things, and is eager to learn. He is, to be sure, something of a "know-it-all," but he is still young. I will now experiment with him. I picked up a nice case of anxiety hysteria from the Health Service and analyzed him in Vajda's presence, three times a week. He functions as "recording secretary." The thing works! Not uninteresting for *instruction* in psychoanalysis. I want to talk about my experiences in Nuremberg.—I want to train Vajda (naturally also a Jew) up to the level of our *Rank*. The previous student[9] is poor and had to leave Budapest.—

I still can't say anything about the *excavations*. The man hasn't reported to me yet. I hope he will come next week.

Frau G. is now staying in Vienna. She sends you the enclosed lines. She was very pleasantly surprised by your attentiveness.

Best wishes to you all.

Yours,
Ferenczi

1. See letter 126, n. 1.
2. In the eighth book of Plato's *Republic* Socrates says to his pupil Glaukon that in the perfect state "kings are to be philosophers and warriors." See *The Dialogues of Plato*, trans. B. Jowett, vol. 2, 4th ed. (Oxford, 1953), p. 99.
3. Ferenczi may be referring here to Freud's speculation about the existence of two sexual substances, one "male" and one "female," the accumulation or diminution of which may produce neurasthenia in the one instance or anxiety neurosis in the other (January 20, 1909, *Minutes* II, 114). See also letter 110.
4. See letter 126 and n. 1.
5. Published under the title "Indulatáttél és magábavetités," *Gyógyászat*, nos. 19–20 (1910).
6. S. Lindner (1840–1912), "Das Saugen an den Fingern, Lippen etc. bei den Kindern (Ludeln), Eine Studie," *Jahrbuch für Kinderheilkunde und physische Erziehung, Neue Folge* 14 (1879): 68–91, cited by Freud in *Three Essays* (1905d, pp. 179f). See also Ferenczi's note "Ein Vorläufer Freuds in der Sexualtheorie" [Dr. S. Lindner: A Forerunner of Freud's in the Theory of Sex] (1912, 91; *Fin.*, p. 325).
7. Adolf Vajda (?–?), lawyer in Miskolcz, married to Maria Ferenczi (1868–?). The couple had three children: Anna, Laszló, and Ilona.
8. Enclosed in brackets in the original.
9. See letter 63. The French word for student *(éleve)* is used in the original.

110

Vienna, February 8, 1910
IX., Berggasse 19

Dear friend,

Today I can finally forward to you the long-awaited news from Worcester that your article on dreams[1] arrived a long time ago, has been translated by Mr. Chase,[2] the translator of my lectures, and is in press. Stanley Hall adds that he has asked Brill, whom he saw in New York, to write him a paper "which should do for your work on the actions of daily life what Ferenczi attempts to do for the Traumdeutung."[3] The old man is certainly very commendable.

Our talk has also invigorated me greatly.[4] Every day after work I write on Leonardo and am already on page 10. My writer's cramp is in full convalescence. As a consequence of your impressive exhortation to allow myself some rest, I have—taken on a new patient from Odessa, a very rich Russian with compulsive feelings,[5] but I am more capable of accomplishment than ever. My friend Rie,[6] whom I have put in charge of my cecum,[7] explains my malady as a catarrh and considers it highly unlikely that it is life-threatening; he does ask, however, that I go to Karlsbad. The plan now is to undertake the journey for the cure on July 14 with my wife and daughter Sophie and to meet the others three weeks later in an as yet unknown summer residence. The plans for September will not be affected thereby.

You should not be surprised if in my Nuremberg lecture[8] you again hear your thoughts and even some of your formulations. It will be the way it was with the last lecture in Worcester; I have a decidedly obliging intellect and am very much inclined toward plagiarism. I myself, meanwhile, have surely already made the analogy with the Platonic rule of philosophers. I ask you in your own interests to please be careful with organization. Décsi seems to me to be quite an inferior type, and Stein is probably of no use whatsoever. I like your youngster of the Rank series better. Wait until new people come to you. Your book will lead them to you as soon as it has overcome its latency period.

You must, of course, discover my ideas anew; for the time being they have been relegated to the mute processing of your ucs. With your first neurasthenic in ΨA you will again have my idea of conflict *within* the libido. It seems to have sunk in the deepest and to stick the best. Your discovery of old Lindner is lovely. You will certainly see him again. I have not yet met Frau G. in Vienna, which is also not easy unless she goes for a walk on specific streets precisely between two and three.[9] Your little letter is very charming. The absence of news from the antiquities site has disappointed the gang very much. For me as well, that (and the anticipated shipment of samples) is the porcupine[10]—

Kind regards,
Freud

1. See letter 78, n. 3.

2. Harry Woodburn Chase (1883–1955), American educator and psychologist. During Freud's trip to America he was on a scholarship at Clark University, from which he graduated in 1910. From 1910 to 1919 he was a professor of psychology at the University of North Carolina at Chapel Hill, from 1919 to 1930 its president, from 1930 to 1933 president of the University of Illinois, and from 1933 to 1951 chancellor of New York University.

3. The quotation is in English in the original [Trans.].

4. "Ferenczi was a balm to me last Sunday; at last a chance to talk about the things closest to my heart; there is another man I am really sure of," Freud wrote to Jung on February 2, 1910 (*Letters*, p. 291).

5. Sergei Konstantinovich Pankejeff (1887–1979), the patient known as the "Wolf-Man," whose treatment Freud had begun in January. See Freud 1918b; also Muriel Gardiner, ed., *The Wolf-Man by the Wolf-Man* (New York, 1971).

6. Oskar Rie (1863–1931), pediatrician, a close friend and tarok partner of Freud, and Freud's family physician; brother-in-law of Wilhelm Fliess. Rie is the "friend Otto" in Freud's dream of Irma's injection (1900a, esp. pp. 106–121) and coauthor of Freud 1891a. He and Ferenczi were accepted for membership in the Vienna Society in the session of October 7, 1908. One daughter, Margarete, married Hermann Nunberg, a psychoanalyst and coeditor of the *Minutes*. The other, Marianne Kris, became a renowned psychoanalyst in her own right.

7. Appendix. During his stay in America, Freud had been stricken with a mild appendicitis.

8. "The Future Prospects of Psycho-Analytic Therapy" (1910d).

9. The time of Freud's daily walk on the Vienna Ringstrasse.

10. During his trip to America, Freud had seen a dead porcupine, "on which incident hangs a tale. He had made the interesting observation that, when faced with an anxious task, such as the present one of describing his startling conclusions to a foreign audience, it was helpful to provide a lightning conductor for one's emotions by deflecting one's attentions onto a subsidiary goal. So before leaving Europe he maintained that he was going to America in the hope of catching sight of a wild porcupine *and* to give some lectures. The phrase 'to find one's porcupine' became a recognized saying in our circle" (Jones II, 59).

111

Budapest, February 8[1]
VII., Erzsébet-körút 54

Dear Professor,
Here is the archaeological postscript to my last letter.
The excavator was here and brought a few rather nice clay pots, a spear-

head, a string of glass beads, and a bronze bowl, all of which I bought from him for twenty crowns and am sending you herewith.

He supposedly unearthed these things two weeks ago. He hopes to accomplish more in better weather. He showed me a lot of very nice silver coins; he also has a number of the familiar little lamps in different shapes. Do you want some of them?

The man is very poor. He made the suggestion that I give him an advance of fifty or sixty gulden within two to three weeks (about ten florins a week), with which he wants to pay the day's wages. They will certainly find things—so he says. (There is a Roman cemetery there.) What they find is then appraised cheaply, and he demands half of what remains after subtracting expenses.

He lives in Duna Pentele;[2] all the farmers bring him what they find. Unfortunately, Duna Pentele is very hard to reach; four hours on the Vicinal Railway from Budapest! Under those circumstances and with the impossibility of any supervision (he can pocket the nicest things!), I can't advise you to take him up on his suggestion to buy half of a supposedly certain discovery site, 1,000 square fathoms, for 600 gulden. He is supposedly a respectable man (although he has already been tried and acquitted for a criminal act committed in the heat of the moment).

The best thing would be to give him very small advances (twenty to thirty crowns) and to buy from him cheaply—what he brings. All other approaches are, in my opinion, impracticable, in view of the impossibility of supervision.

Kind regards,
Ferenczi

I am also including a rusted piece of bronze with the blurred head of a man. Site of discovery likewise Duna Pentele.

February 10

Just received your letter with thanks; pleased about your "plagiarism," about the news from Stanley Hall (archipater psychoanalyseos), about Rie's diagnosis, about the improvement in the writer's cramp as a sign in you of a more active desire to write. Your view of Décsi gives me pause. The work is going smoothly. The booklet (for which I thanked you by letter, albeit not personally) is filling up. In order to force myself to write things down more exactly, I promise next time to report to you scientifically in more detail. [This *forcing oneself* belongs to micropsychosis; not very strongly present in me.][3]

Frau G. is coming back tomorrow, already.

I finally turned down my friend Schächter[4] for *Corfu;* don't want to be "ill."—

I received the invitation for Nuremberg from *Jung*. A few more Congresses and we (as experienced Americans) will be jubilant.

How was the seminar on Saturday? Did Dr. Sachs review the paper correctly?[5]

Please write to me soon; the need for me to be apprised about the matter of the excavations can serve as a motivation.

Kind regards,
Ferenczi

1. No year given. The sequence was determined from the content and from the date of the postscript.

2. A former Roman military camp, Intercisa, from the first to the fourth centuries A.D. (communication from Thomas Pekary), situated on the Danube approximately seventy kilometers south of Budapest; now called Dunaujváros. Subsequent variations in the spelling of the name are true to the original [Trans.].

3. Enclosed in brackets in the original.

4. Miksa (Max) Schächter (1859–1917), physician and fatherly friend of Ferenczi, who gave him the nickname "little Schächter." Chief editor of the journal *Gyógyászat* [Art of Healing], a liberal forum in which many of Ferenczi's articles appeared and which was continued after Schächter's death by Ferenczi's friend and physician Lajos Lévy. See Ferenczi's obituary tribute "Barátságom Schächter Miksával" [My Friendship with Max Schächter] (1917, 199). Schächter went on vacation every year to Corfu; Ferenczi accompanied him in 1913.

5. Hanns Sachs (1881–1947), Doctor of Laws; from October 1910 member of the Vienna Society. In 1912 he, along with Rank, became editor of the newly founded *Imago*. He was a founding member of the Committee and a training analyst at the Berlin Institute (1920–1932). In 1932 Sachs emigrated to Boston, where he was a prominent but isolated exponent of lay analysis. Sachs was one of the first to become interested in the application of psychoanalysis to the humanities. His essay on Ferenczi's "Introjection and Transference" (see also letter 112) was the starting point for a correspondence between the two. See letter 122 and Sachs, *Freud, Master and Friend* (Cambridge, Mass., 1944), pp. 49f.

112

Vienna, February 13, 1910
IX., Berggasse 19

Dear friend,

I would like to push myself to answer your letter quickly, since the matter itself amuses me, and I now have little to do with other correspondence, which is something halfway between intellectual work and rest.

So, first the business. In view of the unfavorable location of Duna Pentele there is really no other possible alternative but your suggestion, even though the beautiful, fantastic hopes have to be given up in the process. I will thus give you a few hundred crowns, which you should see that the excavator gets little by little as an advance, but from which you should also deduct the costs of packing and mailing. There is no compensation for your interest and effort. The man has to earn something in the process, and for that we can let him take care of himself. The objects which arrived yesterday are certainly quite modest, but in any case very cheap, and as samples of forepleasure they are not to be disdained. If the peasants bring him whatever they find in the way of better objects (glass, rings, statues), then he must be able to promise them that we will take them. In any case we don't want to give up the mine of Duna Pentele.

Now to more serious things. Yesterday Sachs reviewed the first part of of your paper[1] with much understanding, but more autoerotically, without proper consideration of the———[2] As for his statement that libido is withdrawn from pleasurably toned complexes, from which you derive the "passion" [Süchtigkeit] of hysterics,[3] it created very interesting and difficult discussions about the correctness, i.e., efficacy, of this description, and we all saw that our language of imagery is still very imprecise and inconsistent. I myself am not clear about it, that is, am now too stupid to be able to think about it. But in this we seem to be in agreement about the fact that in hysteria the libido remains in possession of primal complexes and is not detached from them, which contradicts your presentation to a certain extent. There will be further negotiations about this next time. Those are the most beautiful and most difficult questions, the ones about the manifold mechanisms of repression, and we will have to deal seriously with such metapsychological mechanics at some time or other.

Now, on to further news, not all pleasant. Yesterday I received a manuscript from Riklin[4] about the "Bekenntnisse der schönen Seele,"[5] a study in the psychology of religion, but it is so flat, colorless, and boring that I dislike it very much. It is actually only a translation into ψα jargon, the way Sadger likes it. Now, it isn't pleasant to write him this, but it will have to be done. It is storming and raging again in some corner of Jung, erotically and religiously, and he is writing me with visible displeasure, and when he does that, as today, it sounds as though it is coming from afar. He is working for the Congress, and today he enclosed the list of those to be invited. He expresses great misgiving about the medal for ethics and culture; he thinks I want to be the promoter of religion, whereas my intention was based on purely practical considerations, and I have already renounced it in conversation with you.[6]

ΨA is being threatened by a vicious attack from the "Fackel" because of Wittels's lecture about the "Fackel-neurosis." You know the boundless vanity and insubordination of this talented beast, Karl Kraus.[7] I have given the word to withhold all reaction. We will certainly survive it, but the popularity that the Fackel gives one is almost as unpleasant in the negative as in the positive. So today, on the whole, I am in a bad mood, and I would very much like to flee to Leonardo, if only I can today.

The Worcester lectures are also already typeset and are supposed to have been corrected. Stanley Hall has accepted the dedication.[8]

A few discoveries and ideas have moved me in the last few days, but they are not yet the treasures that we are trying to raise in Duna Pentele. I have suddenly found unsuspected old coprophilic drives in an erythrophobia, and I think that they are similarly significant for this form as osphresiophilia is for the fetishisms. Science and brooding mania come closer to each other, and the like.

On the whole I am only a machine for making money and have been working up a sweat in the last few weeks. A rich young Russian,[9] whom I took on because of compulsive tendencies, admitted the following transferences to me after the first session: Jewish swindler, he would like to use me from behind and shit on my head. At the age of six years he experienced as his first symptom cursing against God: pig, dog, etc. When he saw three piles of feces on the street he became uncomfortable because of the Holy Trinity and anxiously sought a fourth in order to destroy the association.

Clay lamps are very appropriate as gifts. When the man comes again, please take from him only those things that you like yourself.

Frau G. called me on the telephone. I forgot (choice of mood!) that your simile of the catalytic effect of the physician has found general approval. You will also find it in the text of the Worcester lectures.[10]

Don't hold today's crookedly folded letter against me, but accept it as resistant. Sometimes it can't be any other way, and tomorrow maybe it'll be better.

Kindest regards,
Freud

1. "Introjection in the Neuroses," the first part of "Introjection and Transference" (1909, 67).

2. The end of the sentence is missing.

3. Ferenczi explained the general "*passion for tranference* of neurotics" from their "*flight from their complexes* . . . that is to say they withdraw the 'sexual hunger' from certain ideational complexes that were formerly charged with pleasantness" (*Schriften* I, 18; *C.*, p. 45).

4. Franz Riklin (1878–1938), Swiss psychiatrist; collaborator on Jung's association studies. After the Nuremberg Congress he became secretary of the IPA and, with Jung, editor of the *Korrespondenzblatt*, which was founded there. Riklin followed Jung in the latter's break with Freud. His manuscript, which was submitted for the series *Schriften zur angewandten Seelenkunde*, was based on a lecture in the Swiss Society (1907). It was not published.

5. A reference to *Confessions of a Beautiful Soul*, book 6 of Goethe's novel *Wilhelm Meisters Lehrjahre* [Trans.].

6. Freud had originally had the idea that the Psychoanalytic Association should be-

come affiliated with the International Order for Ethics and Culture, founded by the apothecary Alfred Knapp (Zurich), and whose president was Auguste Forel. Jung responded: "Religion can be replaced only by religion. . . . I imagine a far finer and more comprehensive task for ΨA than alliance with an ethical fraternity. I think we must give it time to . . . absorb those ecstatic instinctual forces of Christianity" (Freud/Jung, February 2, 1910, p. 294).

7. Fritz Wittels, a former co-worker of Kraus's, had spoken in the Wednesday Society on January 12, 1910, about the "Fackel" neurosis (Minutes II, 382–393; see also letter 85, n. 9). At the age of twenty-five Karl Kraus (1874–1936), Viennese satirist, writer, and actor, had founded the journal Die Fackel [The Torch], which he published singlehandedly up to his death and which achieved enormous significance among intellectual circles in Austria. Originally Freud held Kraus in high esteem and used Die Fackel as a podium for taking a position on the Fliess-Swoboda-Weininger plagiarism affair (see letter 163, n. 2). In 1906 he even wrote to Kraus: "The few of us should . . . stick together." Quoted from E. Hartl, "Karl Kraus und die Psychoanalyse," Merkur 31 (February 1977): 162. As early as 1908 Kraus had begun to criticize psychoanalysis in Die Fackel, but he stepped up his polemic after Wittels's lecture. Later Kraus assumed a place "at the very bottom of [Freud's] ladder of esteem" (Freud/Arnold Zweig, Correspondence, February 12, 1927, p. 3).

8. The dedication reads: "To DR. G. STANLEY HALL, Ph.D., L.L.D. / President of Clark University, Professor of Psychology and Pedagogics / This Work is Gratefully Dedicated" (Freud 1910a [1909], p. 8).

9. See letter 110 and n. 5.

10. Ferenczi, "Introjection and Transference," Schriften I, p. 14f; C., pp. 39f; and Freud 1910a (1909), p. 55.

113

[Vienna,] February 13, 1910[1]
(Postscript)

Dear friend,

With your consent (?) I will direct to you a medical student in his tenth semester, Joseph Neumann, who, inspired by Lélekelemzés,[2] has turned to me and asked me to let him have some books; perhaps he can enlarge your circle. If *you* advise me to do so, I will send him what I still have a few copies of, the Studies and Everyday Life.[3] One should be distrustful, although his letter makes a *good* impression.

Cordially,
Freud

P.S. I can send you a few copies for propaganda purposes in any case.

1. Postcard.
2. Psychoanalysis; see letter 85, n. 16, and letters 101 and 104.
3. The Studies on Hysteria (with Breuer, 1895d) and The Psychopathlogy of Everyday Life (1901b).

114

Budapest, February 16, 1910
VII., Erzsébet-körút 54

Dear Professor,

I will prove myself worthy of your very quick and detailed answer by at least replying promptly; in terms of content, my letters must turn out much more meager for numerous reasons.

The crooked folding of the letter is revealed right at the end of the first page, where you say that Sachs's criticism was more autoerotic, "without [proper] consideration of the . . ."—the rest is missing; you forgot this "transference" onto the next page; resistances must have prevailed there. I must tell you that I am and have always been in complete agreement with the insight that the libido in neurotics remains fixated on the nuclear complexes. This fixation, however, holds true primarily for the unconscious. In the conscious, the neurotic *flees* from these primal conflicts, that is, from their too strong libidinal cathexis; so, in lieu of that, he is forced to encounter all inwardly or outwardly associable objects with exaggerated interest. *In the ucs. all this interest naturally applies to the original objects.* In all situations that make possible the pure sublimation of the libido [reverence for father, mother, attending the sickbed of parents, etc.][1] they also remain consciously fixated on their parents; they remain dependent children for their whole lives. But as such, they cannot live out their sexuality; the childlike-parental relations do not suffice for that. *The quantity of libido not brought to bear in this manner* is appended as a complex-fleeing affect to the introjectable things of the outside world. In this way I understand my statement about the broadening of the circle of interest, under which I also naturally mean the exaggeratedness of the negative affects.—If that can't be read out of my paper, then it is solely a matter of the inadequacy of the presentation. Please also share this with Dr. Sachs when you get the chance, so that this contradiction, which is only apparent, may disappear.

The man from Duna-Pentele was here today. I gave him a small advance and conveyed your wishes to him. I bought five clay lamps (at one gulden) and a small bronze receptacle (supposedly from the Bronze Age) also for one florin.—Our treasure hunter definitely works very cheaply.

Tomorrow evening I am very probably going to the winter spa of Tátra-Lomnic, where I am supposed to spend Friday, Saturday, and Sunday with a a hysterical baroness. The family doctor wants a neurologist to observe an attack; they "hope" that an opportunity will present itself within three days. For my part, I believe that the patient won't produce any attacks on those specific days, but I'm going anyway, 1.) because they are paying me and the three days of Tátra air will do me good. 2.) because I would like to make an analytical case (the first aristocratic one) out of it. They are not Jewish barons;[2] I can count on the physician (an old friend). Still, it is doubtful if anything will come of the affair.

Nuremberg will do Jung good. I will do everything in my power to contribute to the solution of his crisis. I wrote him yesterday and showed him the title of the paper which I'm delivering about the motives and methods of an organization of Freudian adherents.[3] I don't have anything more than the title at the moment.

What do you think about the possibility of combining the Nuremberg trip with an excursion to Berlin? (Seidler.) It would certainly be a discord in the psychoanalytic harmony of the Congress days; but you told me yourself, I shouldn't spare you.—

If Riklin is boring, that proves that he hasn't changed since the "fairy tale."[4] At the same time, he is a diligent, respectable worker; only he should concern himself with medical matters that can better withstand his dry tone.

It is with difficulty that I venture to take up a literary theme, although a case just recently totally illuminated Ibsen's *"Peer Gynt."*[5] It is the patient to whom I owe our connection with the treasure hunter. The identity with the liar-hero Peer Gynt is astonishing—it coincides with minute details of his fantastic plans.

All these wish fantasies are rooted in the wish to appear great in the eyes of the mother (i.e.: to make a child for her). But what Ibsen and my patient were able to make out of this terrible complex is worthy of admiration. After the breakdown (in Peer Gynt as well as in the patient), comes the fear of death and the flight to the old mother [with P. Gynt to the old lover, who is only a new edition of the old Aase].

So there I have the second Ibsen theme; the first, already partially set down in notes is the "Lady from the Sea."[6]—

Since his twelfth year *my* Peer Gynt has lived on a high (he is now fifty-three), not an alcohol high but a self-imposed grandiose optimism. The impetus to it was, strangely, caused by the circumstance that his little brother, who had been infected by him, died of diphtheria, while he re-mained alive. That gave him—who had previously been very fearful—"toughness," courage. He wanted to achieve the highest aim, *in all areas of human achievement and knowledge.* He could not stand compulsion, authority. He reacted to the breakdown (which he still doesn't want to comprehend) with—agoraphobia and a number of other anxieties.—All warnings, reprimands, curses that he encountered for twenty years and that he laughingly repressed are now unconsciously coming due. The burning wish for greatness has really made a colossally many-sidedly talented person out of him, who, however, never did anything right.—

Now I will stop "talking shop."

Kindest regards,
Ferenczi

The colossal optimism in this patient reminds me of the manic production of pleasure along the lines of Gross.[7]

Budapest
VII., Erzsébet-körút 54

Postscript

Dear Professor!

The young *rigorosant* (Neumann) reported to me. A very poor, neurotic boy with a stutter. Not a suitable individual. After completing his studies he will immediately have to seek a position as a district physician. Otherwise respectable and modest. I promised him nothing and told him that at the moment, as far as I knew, you had only a very few copies of your work at your disposal. He will, however, buy the studies, in any case. If you want to honor his interest, send him a copy of Everyday Life. He lives in Budapest V., Nádor-utca 74. IV. 21., and his name is Joseph Neumann.

I am enclosing a communication from Putnam with this letter.[8]

Your obedient
Ferenczi

1. Enclosed in brackets in the original, as is the similarly enclosed phrase later in the letter.

2. Certain Jewish families received titles of nobility in recognition of their accomplishments in the economic sector, but there was a distinction between those who had been recently ennobled and those who belonged to old noble families. Ferenczi refers to this distinction.

3. See letter 126 and n. 1.

4. Franz Riklin, *Wunscherfüllung und Symbolik im Märchen; Schriften zur angewandten Seelenkunde,* vol 2 (Vienna, 1908).

5. In the play *Peer Gynt* (1867) by Henrik Ibsen (1828–1906), Peer Gynt, who has been accused of being a liar by his mother, the widow of the farmer Aase, seduces Solvejg, whom he then leaves. He becomes rich in Africa, but returns home a poor old man to find Solvejg still waiting for him.

6. See letter 15 and nn. 1 and 2.

7. Otto Gross (1877–1920), author of *Das Freudsche Ideogenitätsmoment und seine Bedeutung im manisch-depressiven Irresein Kraepelins* [The Freudian Factor of Ideogenity and Its Significance in Kraepelin's Manic-Depressive Illness] (Leipzig, 1907), was the son of Hans Gross, renowned professor of criminology at the University of Graz. In 1902 Gross, who was addicted to cocaine and morphine, was at the Burghölzli for the first of many drug cures. In 1908, at Freud's request, he was analyzed—unsuccessfully— by Jung ("Whenever I got stuck," wrote Jung, "he analyzed me"; *Freud/Jung,* May 25,

1908, p. 153). In 1914 he went back into therapy with Stekel. In the meantime, Gross practiced and published as a talented and controversial analyst; he was also known for his anarchistic sympathies.
    8. The enclosure is missing.

115

[Tátralomnic,]
February 17, 1910[1]

Dear Professor!
Heartfelt greetings from the Tátra [Mountains] in winter. This would be something for Martin.[2] One does nothing here but sledding, bobsled riding, skiing.

Yours,
Dr. Ferenczi

    1. Picture postcard from Tátralomnic. The caption reads: "A Magas-Tátra (the High Tátras)."
    2. Freud's son Martin was an enthusiastic mountain climber and cross-country skier.

116

Vienna, February 21, 1910
IX., Berggasse 19

Dear colleague,
I recommend to you this countryman of yours, who doesn't know German, with a rather old disorder of the right peroneus[1] (paralysis, contraction, and hyperesthesia) for further diagnostic clarification and, one hopes, the introduction of a successful local therapy.

Collegially yours,
Freud

    1. A disorder of the fibula.

117

Budapest, February 25, 1910
VII., Erzsébet-körút 54

Dear Professor,
The consultation in Tátralomnic went as follows:
The patient is the young, unmarried Countess Vay; her mother is the sister of our present prime minister, Count Khuen-Hédervary.[1] The patient broke her leg while riding a bobsled, then lapsed into unconsciousness,

talked gibberish, cursed, raged, and "defended herself" when she was attacked (attacked in the sense of touched). After the usual "absolutely
negative" information about sexual antecedents, I learned from her
mother, who was, incidentally, comprehensible (whose favor I won, whereupon the patient immediately adopted a resistant stance), that, although
always cool with respect to men, she still (or therefore?) had terrible experiences last year. She became ill in the middle of the highway [journey], in
the carriage. When she came to, the coachman bent over her and asked,
"How are you, Countess?" "I don't know what happened to me," she said
to herself, and then complained, in tears, to her mother. She then remembered Cagliostro,[2] who abused a girl in a hypnotic sleep [wish to be used
by the coachman].[3] The present accident (not caused by her, by the way),
with the ensuing unconsciousness, evidently motivated the reigniting of
these fantasies.—She now has strange spells of *half-consciousness with
"rapturous sucking" of the back of her hand or the corner of the pillow*. It
naturally hasn't come to analysis. The leg is not yet healed.—Tomorrow
the family is coming to Budapest and—so I hear—will keep the patient in
treatment with me. The following data as illustration: The young countess
was already treated for menstrual complaints with 1.) irrigations, 2.) *massage of the uterus per rectum*, 3.) general massage. 4.) To reassure her that
"nothing had happened" to her, they had her examined locally several
times.

The three days in the Tátra were a good rest for me. Even the last traces
of depression have vanished. I am analyzing diligently; I am less diligent
in working over my really nice material. I have the feeling that one should
work just as many hours daily on one's cases as one analyzes. The ground
is so virginal, and even if one doesn't always find significant things—one
should note and consolidate even the small novelties!

I am having luck with homosexuals. Now my sample card has been
enriched with a third type: namely, a *passive* homosexual; *even before he
saw me*, he transferred his fantasies onto me (something similar has also
happened to me with women). Chance is evidently urging me to concern
myself with the problems of homosexuality.

I again bought some little things from the treasure hunter for twenty
crowns, among them a string of glass beads, supposedly from a Sarmatian[4]
grave in Duna Pentele, with interesting, peculiarly inlaid ornamentation;
the one (blue) piece of glass is magnificently iridescent! Furthermore: a

small bronze receptacle, five lamps (some with trademark); a small rusted ring, silver, I think. A peculiar bone platter in the shape of a fish (which was dug up in Duna Pentele but whose significance is problematic); and a piece of glass.

The string of beads is in the bronze receptacle; the ring is in an envelope; please unpack the things carefully.

My antique dealer now wants to fix me up with a few freshly unearthed—incidentally quite interesting-looking—*belts* (Roman ones, with some gold ornamentation). Reflect on such warlike things. He is asking 60–100–150 crowns per item.

Received the enclosed letter[5] from Jung; the tone is very gratifying. At the same time I am sending a few notes—and an observation[6] which I have started, about which I have already made many notes and which I intend to finish before long.

Best regards,
Ferenczi

1. Count Károly Khuen-Héderváry (1849–1918), major landowner in Croatia, confidant of Emperor Franz Joseph, and prime minister of Hungary from January 11, 1910, to April 22, 1912; co-founder of the National Workers' party in February 1910 and its president from 1913 to 1918.

2. Alessandro Graf von Cagliostro (pseudonym of Giuseppe Balsamo) (1743–1795), Italian adventurer, healer, hypnotist, alchemist, and freethinker. He achieved the highest social recognition in Paris and in England, but in 1791 in Rome he was condemned, first to death, then to life imprisonment, for heresy.

3. Enclosed in brackets in the original.

4. An ancient tribe of nomads who inhabited the steppes of Sarmatia, in southern Russia [Trans.].

5. The letter is missing.

6. The enclosure is missing.

118

Vienna, February 25, 1910
IX., Berggasse 19

Dear friend,

I am returning Putnam's letter, which is enclosed. I don't know why he makes such great demands on ψα influencing, especially after three months' work. Has he been spoiled by the successes of earlier treatments?

Jung is writing more freely again, and the Congress is gradually taking shape. So far he has had twenty-two applications; ten to fifteen will be added from Vienna. I don't think we will be numerous, and we don't need to be. But we should do good organizational work. About lectures: *Abraham* on fetishism, *Marcinowski* on sejunctive processes in the genesis of neuroses (which emphasizes its special position already in the title), *Adler* on ψ hermaphroditism (on Wednesday he gave us the lecture,[1] which is full of *anagrammatic* misunderstandings and is packed with will-o'-the-wisps; the genesis of neuroses is supposedly as follows: the child suffers from its inferiority, which it takes to be feminine; from that there develops an uncertainty about its gender role, which is the original basis for all later doubt; it attempts a masculine defense, and when that fails, neurosis results—a bad speculation!). I want to ask *Stekel* to give a lecture on initiating research in collecting symbols and typical dreams. He should then become head of the committee elected to do that, put to good use and at the same time held in check by the others. In addition to that, there will be our three lectures (Jung, you, I). There will probably be others.[2]

I think that we can go to the Congress together, that you will pick me up, and the like. It's still up in the air whether Jung's contribution will take place a day before or a day after; it depends on his call-up for military service, which still hasn't been firmed up.

Today Jones had two very good letters come in. Today the first introduction by letter from Häberlin.[3] So much for external news.

Your book on Ibsen should come into being one day. The student got his copy of Everyday Life. You should have received 200 crowns for antiquities from Duna Pentele.

I will no longer avoid the fortuneteller. But it is very questionable how things will go timewise in Berlin, especially since my time there is not my own.

I was saved just short of the point of exhaustion by the departure of my main client[4] for Frankfurt yesterday and will now be able to write Leonardo.

Cordially,
Freud

1. On February 23, 1910, Adler gave a lecture titled "Psychical Hermaphroditism" (*Minutes* II, 423–434), the theme of his Congress lecture. Freud had originally proposed that he speak in Nuremberg addressing the question: Is psychoanalysis compatible with every worldview, or does it force adherence to a particular faction? (undated letter of Freud to Adler, Library of Congress).

2. See letter 126 and n. 1.

3. Paul Häberlin (1878–1960), a native of Jung's birthplace, Kesswil; Swiss philosopher and professor of philosophy at Bern (1914–1922) and Basel (1922–1944). For Freud's response to Häberlin, see Freud 1987h, pp. 283f.

4. Elfriede Hirschfeld, who, with a few interruptions, was in analysis with Freud from the end of 1908 until 1914, but was also treated by Muthmann, Janet, Jung, Pfister, and Ludwig Binswanger. She played a significant role in the conflict between Freud and Jung.

Her case was briefly described by Freud in "An Evidential Dream" (Freud 1913a) and
formed the basis for his work "The Disposition to Obsessional Neurosis: A Contribution
to the Problem of Choice of Neurosis" (Freud 1913i), in which Freud introduced the
concept of pregenital libido organization.

119

Vienna, March 3, 1910
IX., Berggasse 19

Dear friend,

In consequence of an attack of writing frenzy which has advanced
Leonardo to page thirty, I have postponed thanking you for the interesting
mailings. I am now freer, work and earn less, and would like to be finished
with Leonardo by the time of the Congress.

The antiquities are meager but still worth the price. The bronze receptacle was not included, the glass beads are beautiful, the lamps, to be sure,
overpriced at 1 crown each, but it doesn't matter if it gives the old guy
pleasure. I naturally can't take the belts without seeing them; he would
have to send them along for examination.

Excuse me if I give second place to the more valuable scientific mailings.
I am happy to see that you are now doing things exactly the way I did at
the time, only I wasn't able to show my notes, with their intimations and
confusions, to anyone. You seem only to have found the same things with
your homosexuals as Sadger and I did with ours. It would be funny if that
were already the rule. The theories of the Scientific-Humanitarian Committee[1] are naturally tendentious deliria.—I didn't have a moment's doubt
that Silberer's observations[2] permit the same continuation as every dream.
If I say little about your communications, partly on purpose in order not
to disturb you, that shouldn't keep you from sending me more.

The American mail has again brought pleasant things: a complete commitment to our teachings from Putnam in his second article[3]: in it he gives
the three of us the following beautiful characterization from the heart of a
Puritan: . . . but I see the volume has already been lent out, and I can't
write out the quote for you! Then a magnificently turned-out paper on
Hamlet by Jones,[4] who has now happily overcome his obstacles and, it
seems to me, will soon win precedence over Brill thanks to his multifacet-
edness and dexterity. It was good that we didn't sacrifice him back then.[5]

Jung has again emerged from his personal perplexities, and I was quickly
reconciled with him, for I was not angry, only concerned. I am now awaiting his suggestions about the details of the Congress. I am continuing to
scuffle with my ill-mannered boys in Vienna and am expending much
educational work on them, probably in vain.

Have I shared with you yet my solution about the nature of the ucs.? I am completely without perspective because of the interruption. If not, it will come next time, if you ask for it.

With kind regards and in expectation of much news still before Nuremberg, I am

Yours,
Freud

1. The Scientific-Humanitarian Committee was brought to life by the Berlin sex researcher Magnus Hirschfeld (1868–1935) in the struggle for the legalization of homosexuality. Homosexuality was seen by Hirschfeld as neither curable nor punishable but a quirk of nature.

2. Herbert Silberer (1882–1923), sports journalist, balloonist, and private scholar; member of the Wednesday Society from October 1910. He was interested in the investigation of dreams and symbols, alchemy, and occultism. Freud is referring to his "Bericht über eine Methode, gewisse symbolische Halluzinationserscheinungen hervorzurufen und zu beobachten" [Report on a Method of Eliciting and Observing Certain Symbolic Hallucination Phenomena], *Jahrbuch* 1, 2d half-volume (1909): 513–525.

3. James Putnam, "Personal Impressions of Sigmund Freud and His Work, with Special Reference to His Recent Lectures at Clark University," pt. 2, *Journal of Abnormal Psychology* 4 (February/March 1910): 372–379.

4. Ernest Jones, "The Oedipus Complex as an Explanation of Hamlet's Mystery: A Study in Motive," *American Journal of Psychology* 21 (1910): 72–113 (published in German as vol. 10 of the *Schriften zur angewandten Seelenkunde* [1911]).

5. At Freud's American lectures, at which Jones had been present. Freud later wrote to Jones: "I remember the first time when I got aware of this my attitude towards you, it was a bad one; when you left Worcester after a time of dark inconsistencies from your side and I had to face the idea that you were going away to become a stranger to us. Then I felt it ought not to be so and I could not show it otherwise than by accompanying you to the train and shaking hands before you went away." Letter of February 24, 1912, in R. Andrew Paskauskas, ed., *The Complete Correspondence of Sigmund Freud and Ernest Jones, 1908–1939* (Cambridge, Mass., 1993).

120

Budapest, March 4, 1910
VII., Erzsébet-körút 54

Dear Professor,

In order that the last crossing of our letters will not result in an interruption, I am writing this time without having anything special to communicate, other than the postscript that I have received the 200 crowns for antiquities in good order.—

Our man has not shown up for ten days; let us hope he will surprise us with something better.

I bought—relatively cheaply—six very ornamental little porcelain figures in an antique store. [Trademark: Capo di Monte.]¹ Should the occasion arise, may I also buy these kinds of semi-antiquities for you?—Certainly it is good if, to a certain extent, one reins in one's desire to buy—otherwise one's home very soon becomes a junk shop.

I am doing very well—except for a low-grade influenza from which I have already almost recovered. I am doing analysis without getting overtired, evidently with more psychic economy than before. My patients and the court have also brought me materially favorable successes in the past half year. Within six months I was able to set aside 4,000 crowns (the cost of the trip to America). I will be able to increase the honorarium that I am now asking (ten crowns) next year, perhaps by half, if the demand becomes stronger. The book "Lélekelemzés"[2] appears to be going well. Forty copies of it have already been bought in a provincial city alone (Debreczin).

I have grounds for dissatisfaction only with myself—the resistances to (scientific) work are still there. Instead of the hard work of writing and stylizing I use every occasion to lecture Frau G. or to read Anatole France or Mereschkowski.[3] I know the precise motives for this resistance, but I am too weak to fight them. ("Laziness is a Hungarian disease," according to a local proverb.)

Cordially,
Ferenczi

1. Enclosed in brackets in the original.
2. See letter 85, n. 16, and letters 101 and 104.
3. Dmitri Sergeyevich Merezhkovski (1865–1941), Russian symbolist writer, poet, and critic. Freud cites his book *Leonardo da Vinci* (Leipzig, 1903) from the novel trilogy *Christ und Antichrist* several times in his own work on Leonardo (1910c) and ranks it among his favorite books in a letter of November 1, 1906, to his publisher, Hugo Heller (*Briefe*, p. 268). Ferenczi read *Tolstoy und Dostojewski als Menschen und Künstler* [Tolstoy and Dostoyevski as Men and Artists] (Leipzig, 1903). See letter 133.

121

Vienna, March 10, 1910
IX., Berggasse 19

Dear friend,

I hear from someone supposedly close to you that you are a Hungarian lazybones. Don't believe it, it's slander. I congratulate you heartily on the success of Lélekelemzés. I am sure that hardly forty copies of any of my books can be dug up in Linz or Klagenfurt.[1]

And now for the big news! Jung suddenly left for Chicago, called by McCormick, who has fallen very ill, and has his wife assure us that he will be back for the Congress.[2] Nice, eh? The [ship] Crown Princess Caecilie is arriving in New York on the 15th, is leaving again on the 22nd, and lands in Cherbourg on the 28th, so he can be in Nuremberg on the evening of the 29th or at 5 o'clock in the morning of the 30th. Since Jung doesn't come into consideration for the Easter holidays, I can ask you perhaps to spend a day at Easter with us in Vienna, in any case to travel with me and to devote the day before the Congress to me. I was thinking of leaving Vienna on Monday evening.

Yesterday morning my poor Mathilde was again subjected to a follow-up operation, which has removed a number of bad growths and cystic scars. The doctors are very satisfied, but her subjective condition is still very bad.

My sister-in-law Minna, alarmed by a telegram, went to Hamburg to see our 80-year-old mother (I just came from the North Station). My wife was, of course, detained [from going] by the operation.

The old dog[3] is especially strong and in good health and is vacillating as to whether he shouldn't rather pass up Karlsbad. I (I want to lift the incognito) am writing every free hour, i.e., every third day, on Leonardo and have brought it up to p. 40. My secret hope is to be finished by the time of the Congress, especially if I can take a day at Easter to do it. The Theory of Sexuality is here;[4] I will send it to you if you don't have it; it has been enriched only by a few notes. Pfister's reply to Foerster is also here.[5] I recently acquired some antiquities of outstanding quality. Dunapentele will have difficulty reaching that standard.

Lueger died yesterday.[6] You see, all kinds of things are happening. Let me hear something good in response now.

Cordially,
Freud

1. Now the capitals of the Austrian states of Upper Austria and Carinthia.

2. See *Freud/Jung*, March 8, 9, and 16, 1910, pp. 301–303. The Chicago industrialist Harold Fowler McCormick (1872–1941), later a patron of analytical psychology, had consulted Jung in Zurich in 1908 and 1909.

3. Written in English in the original [Trans.].

4. The second edition of the *Three Essays on the Theory of Sexuality* (1905d).

5. See letters 84 and n. 3, 96 and n. 2.

6. Karl Lueger (1844–1910), Doctor of Laws; founder of the Christian Socialist party (1890); populist and anti-Semitic mayor of Vienna from 1897 until his death. Cited by Hitler as his political model.

122

Budapest, March 15, 1910
VII., Erzsébet-körút 54

Dear Professor,

I cannot serve up such interesting news as you, and certainly cannot report on such a depressing event as Mathilde's recent operation. I confidently hope that your strong constitution will also easily overcome this shock.

Dunapentele is not proving its worth. The man is too poor—hence, unreliable. You can't trust him with money—otherwise he won't show up for weeks on end. I gave him forty-four gulden as an advance—since then he reports only sporadically. With the exception of two so-so glass receptacles, he has brought nothing. The supposed "bronze" receptacle mentioned in my letter should be understood as the little *clay* receptacle in which the beads arrived.

Jung's mobility deserves much recognition. Let us hope he won't arrive too late!

I am in complete agreement with your plans. I am considering arriving in Vienna on the evening of Easter Sunday—but I won't disturb you that evening if you are still writing on Leonardo—but rather I will appear at your home on Monday morning.

I have been corresponding with Dr. Sachs since his paper; it is astonishing that someone who doesn't himself analyze can penetrate so deeply.

My laziness is on the wane. I have already written down the Nuremberg lecture, i.e., the motivation for rallying,[1] as well as the preliminary draft of statutes. The latter still has to be talked through precisely. I am now writing a lecture on "Everyday Life," which will be given at the Physicians' Association in April and will also appear in print.[2] The paper on introjection is also awaiting translation into Hungarian. These two works have been designated for a second volume of my "Lélekelemzés."[3] The enclosed review of the latter from the pen of Arthur Schwartz appeared in Pester Lloyd.[4] The local organ for medical professors is also writing similar but more trenchant things about it.[5] Everything is explained in favor of the mutual suggestion of doctor and patient, and at the same time the associative exploration of the "subconscious" is recognized as possible. The results of suggestion cures (which are directed at forgetting the psychotraumas) are at least as successful; psychoanalysis is often harmful. It hasn't been proved that "sexual psychotraumas" are the cause of neuroses, etc.— As a consolation, as usual, intellectual richness and style are praised.

Pfister wrote me a very cordial letter and sent in his paper (the polemic against Foerster). He could still become one of the most capable men.

Stanley Hall responded in a very friendly manner to my request to send back the German manuscript of the dream paper and permitted its translation "in any language you like."[6] After the English original comes out, I want to publish the dream lecture in German (or French).[7]

I naturally have the Theory of Sexuality, but I can't pass up the new notes and will gladly buy the book if you have only a few copies.

Kind regards,
Ferenczi

Please send back the excerpt when you get the chance!

1. Reassembling scattered troops.

2. This lecture was never published, to the best of our knowledge.

3. Published in December 1911 under the title *Lelki problémák a pszichoanalizis megvilátásában* by Manó Dick in Budapest (1912, 98); see letter 262 and n. 2.

4. See *Pester Lloyd*, March 13, 1910 p. 24.

5. Review by Jenö Kollarits (see letter 173, n. 4) in *Orvosi Hetilap* 54, no. 11 (1910): 195.

6. Written in English in the original [Trans.].

7. See letters 77, n. 1 and 78, n. 3.

123

Vienna, March 17, 1910
IX., Berggasse 19

Dear friend,

Understood. I will be finished with Leonardo before Easter, will therefore await you at our house on *Sunday* evening, and on Monday evening at 8:30 we will travel through the night to Nuremberg. Colleague Steiner[1] is reserving a sleeping compartment, at least for two people.

The Theory of Sexuality ought to have reached you already. I am enclosing the excerpt again. Schwarz is still bearable, a tasteful person at least.

My daughter is doing so well that she can come home the day after tomorrow. Let us hope this operation has been of lasting benefit to her, but *quien sabe?*

Dunapentele is vexing. During the last few days I acquired some very beautiful things, essentially to keep me in a good mood, which I will show you in Vienna. You have yet to learn antiquities and mushrooms from me.

There are dark rumors going around here about a big strike that the clinicians are going to launch against those of us from ΨA.[2] Sinister things, which one has to confront with equanimity.

I am being so brief because I want to write on Leonardo.

Kind regards,
Freud

1. See letter 12, n. 3.

2. Prominent neurologists in Germany were speaking out in favor of boycotting clinics in which psychoanalysis was being practiced (*Minutes* II, 478, April 14, 1910). See also letter 130 and n. 4 and letter 186, n. 3.

124

Budapest, March 22, 1910
VII., Erzsébet-körút 54

Dear Professor,

This will, I think, be my last letter before Nuremberg.—I gratefully acknowledge your arrangements for the trip and will appear on Sunday evening. It is not clear to me from your letter whether I should reserve a sleeping berth for the night trip from Vienna to Nuremberg for myself, or whether one of the places reserved by colleague Steiner has been designated for me. I therefore request a very brief communication in this regard via correspondence card.—Pfister wrote to me in great detail; a very nice person, full of enthusiasm for the cause. Strangely, he believes that "our Freud has endowed *theology* with a methodology that is of no less significance for it than spectral analysis is for physics." He doesn't yet suspect that the analytical conception *carried through to its conclusion* does away with theology. He has yet to come to that.

The news of the clinicians' conspiracy has indeed made me uncomfortable. This could be the beginning of a crusade against us, in which clerics and "liberals," united, turn against us. I am certain only of the fact that we can count on the understanding of *one* sector of the population—neurotics themselves. That is evident, for instance, in the interest that these people bring to my "Lélekelemzés." Will you also mention the possibility of such a holy war in your lecture on the *prospects* of psychoanalysis?[1]—

I would like to recommend to you another point for consideration (in case you haven't come upon it yourself). That is the *sociological* significance of our analyses in the sense that in our analyses we investigate the *real* conditions in the various levels of society, cleansed of all hypocrisy and conventionalism, just as they are mirrored in the individual. The analysis of a typesetter, for instance, gave me the opportunity to see clearly the terrorism that so horribly oppresses the individual worker from the side of the party, and the action toward him that mocks all "brotherliness." At the same time, I analyzed the owner of a print shop, who had to expose all his swindles, with which he knew how to get around the rules of the "Association of Print Shop Owners." The brief analysis of a young countess showed me the inner hollowness which characterizes the life of her social class, from which her fantasies involuntarily flew to the kind and natural—coachman. A talk with this countess's maid revealed to me the infantile source of the peculiar circumstance that she prefers to work for aristocrats for lower wages than for bourgeois for better pay. (Masochistic component of the sexual drive, stemming from the parent complex.)

These and similar observations should further sociology more than all

statistics and speculations. Next to the "Iron Law of Wages," the psychological determinants are sadly neglected in today's sociology.[2]

I am now reading Gross's book about inferiority[3] and am delighted by it.
There is no doubt that, among those who have followed you up to now, he
is the most significant. Too bad he had to go to pot.

———————

I thank you kindly for the Theory of Sexuality. You are gradually giving
me an entire library!

Congratulations on your daughter's successful operation and best regards
to the patient.

Auf Wiedersehen!

Yours,
Ferenczi

1. In ' is lecture at the Nuremberg Congress, Freud touched on society's resistance to
psychoanalysis in only a general way (1910d, p. 147).

2. In his later writings Ferenczi returned numerous times to the issues discussed here
(see, e.g., 1913, 103 [*F.C.*, p. 424]; 1922, 241; and 1928, 283a). He described the case of the
young countess in "Soziale Gesichtspunkte bei Psychoanalysen" [Social Considerations
in Some Analyses] (1922, 245; *F.C.*, pp. 413ff; *Schriften* II, 127–130).

3. Otto Gross, *Über psychopathische Minderwertigkeiten* (Vienna, 1909).

125

[Vienna,] March 22, 1910[1]

Steiner is reserving the place in the sleeping car for you.
Auf Wiedersehen.

Freud

1. Postcard.

126

Vienna, April 3, 1910
IX., Berggasse 19

Dear friend,

I went home with Steiner yesterday noon, arrived here in the evening,
and today I still feel very tired after recovering from Easter, and need to
chat with you, in the manner of an epilogue, about the Congress.[1] There is
no doubt that it was an extraordinary success, yet the two of us, personally,

had the least luck. My lecture evidently fell flat, and I don't know why; it contained much that was worthy of interest. Perhaps it betrayed my inner tiredness too much. Your impassioned pleading had the misfortune of unleashing so much opposition that they forgot to thank you for your significant inspiration. Every society is thankless; that doesn't matter. But we are both a little at fault, since we didn't sufficiently take into account the effect this would have on the Viennese; it would have been easy to omit entirely the critical allusions and to take up the direct promise of scientific freedom, and we could have made resistance on their part rather difficult. I believe that my aversion toward the Viennese circle, which has been accumulating for a long time, and your brother complex have had the combined effect of making us shortsighted.

But that is not the essential thing. It is more important that we have accomplished a big piece of work that will have a far-reaching influence on the shape of the future. I am happy to state that we have both found ourselves in clear agreement, and I thank you very much for your decidedly successful support.

Events will now continue. It has become clear to me that the moment has now come to carry out a decision which has been long in the making. I will resign the leadership of the Vienna group and in so doing withdraw from all official influence. I will transfer the leadership to Adler, not out of inclination or satisfaction but because he is the only [prominent] personality and because in this position it will perhaps be necessary for him to share the defense of the common ground. I have already communicated this to him; I will tell the others officially on Wednesday. I don't even think they will regret it very much; I was already close to the point of falling into the role of the dissatisfied and superfluous old man. I don't want that, and for that reason I would rather go early, but voluntarily. The leaders will then all be of equal age and position and will be able to develop freely and settle their differences among themselves.

Scientifically I will certainly participate to the last breath, but I will be able to spare myself all the effort of directing and holding myself in check, and enjoy my *otium cum dignitate*.[2] With my stepping down, all kinds of changes will certainly come about in the Society; the meeting place will not be kept the same, etc.

I very much hope that you will find suitable persons for the Budapest group. You have not come as far in overcoming your brother complex as you had hoped. Unfortunately the two, Stein and Décsi, do not seem to me to be quite the right co-founders. Don't you perhaps want to advertise a course for doctors and students, as Abraham has done?[3] I had a good day with Jung in Rothenburg.[4] He is right at his peak and will, I hope, keep himself that way. He is now attacking the paranoia of mythology,[5] as we have seen, and has made a brilliant catch in Honegger.[6] I vehemently talked him into not letting the young man out of his sight, but to engage him long-term as his assistant, which his circumstances permit, and I hope to have gained some influence over his reserve. The personal relationships among the Zurichers is altogether much more repectable than it is in Vienna, where one often wonders where the ennobling influence of ΨA on its adherents actually is.

The infancy of our movement has ended with the Nuremberg *Reichstag*; that is my impression. I hope that a rich and beautiful youth is now coming.—

I found the Worcester lectures at home in the yellow box; I am not actually supposed to send them to you until the volume of the American Journal of Psychology[7] has arrived here. Leonardo goes to press tomorrow; I will then soon write down the little matter about the "maternal etiology,"[8] and perhaps also publish the work about technique. Sending me your "precipitates" will, as always, please me very much. Best regards to Frau G.

See you soon!

Yours,
Freud

1. The Second International Psychoanalytic Congress took place on March 30 and 31 in Nuremberg. Freud opened it with a lecture, "The Future Prospects of Psycho-Analytic Therapy" (1910d). Ferenczi gave his "Report on the Necessity of a Closer Amalgamation of the Adherents to Freudian Doctrine and Suggestions for Founding a Permanent International Organization" (1910, 69; published under the title "Zur Organisation der Psychoanalytischen Bewegung," in *Bausteine* I, 275–289). Freud's and Ferenczi's plan to move the seat of the IPA to Zurich and to vest in Jung exceptional powers as president for life (every lecture or article was to be presented to him for approval) produced resistance, especially from Adler and Stekel. The power of the president was thereupon lessened and his term of office limited to two years. As a countermove Freud offered Adler the chairmanship of the Vienna Society and, with Stekel, the editorship of the new *Zentralblatt für Psychoanalyse: Medizinische Monatsschrift für Seelenkunde*. The *Korrespondenzblatt* [Bulletin], edited by Jung as president and by Riklin as secretary of the IPA, was founded as the official organ of the association.

2. "Leisure with dignity," i.e., an honorable retirement, an expression often used by Cicero (106–43 B.C.).

3. On eight evenings in March Karl Abraham had taught a course in his home on Freud's theory of neuroses.

4. Following the Nuremberg Congress.

5. Jung was indulging in his "mythological dreams with almost autoerotic pleasure" (*Freud/Jung*, April 17, 1910, p. 308). These efforts led to the publication of "Wandlungen und Symbole der Libido," *Jahrbuch* 3 (1911): 120–227, and 4 (1912): 162–464, the work that precipitated his scientific break with Freud.

6. Johann Jakob Honegger (1885–1911), Zurich psychiatrist, student, and close collaborator of Jung's. Barely a year later he committed suicide (see letter 207). Freud held him in high esteem, saying of him, "He has made a splendid impression on me too by an attempt to analyze me" (*Freud/Jung*, February 2, 1910, p. 291).

7. Volume 21, nos. 2–3, in which Freud's American lectures were published.

8. Freud's essay "A Special Type of Choice of Object Made by Men" (1910h), which appeared in the next issue of the *Jahrbuch* and in which he traced the type of choice described there to an "infantile fixation of tender feelings on the mother" (pp. 168f).

127

Budapest, April 5, 1910
VII., Erzsébet-körút 54

Dear Professor,

Your letters always give me extraordinary satisfaction in my intellectual and emotional isolation. This time your letter had this effect to an increased degree; being together for days with people of like mind spoiled me—and this evening I caught myself singing a Hungarian song with the following text: "On the great ball of earth no one so orphaned as I."[1]—You told me once in Berchtesgaden: "Man *must* love something." That could also be craft and science. But obviously not exclusively. One must also love *people* if one wants to be happy.—Now, I'm not quite lacking in that respect, either. I have such a person, as you know. But external circumstances, enviousness of people (who appear to have conspired downright maliciously to persecute every happiness that doesn't have the authorities' official stamp of approval), make our encounters as difficult and infrequent for us as possible. The few hours that I spend in this company, which brings me intellectual and emotional satisfaction, are practically everything that life offers (apart from the satisfactions of work). Obviously that is not enough for me, and I have to say that *Jung* is right when he urges me to gather young men around me whom I can teach and perhaps also love somewhat. For the time being, you must—for better or for worse—allow me to attach such a large portion of libido to you. Possibly, no, undoubtedly, you are right in your supposition that brother envy has not yet been overcome within me. As an antidote to this it will also be good to take younger brothers under my tutelage; the teacher (father) role will satisfy my ambition, and I will be able to walk up to my older brothers (Jung, Adler) *sine ira et studio*.[2]

The other solution (getting serious about Frau G.) has often been discussed between us. There are actually no material difficulties, except for those that concern for her unnmarried daughter[3] and for the two-sided (partly communal) relationship[4] entails. Add to that the uncertainty about nephritis![5]

It is tactless of me to weigh you down with such purely personal matters; I could work those out by myself. But you will find that understandable and forgivable, considering my unsatisfied need for support.

As a transition to the business side of my letter, I would like to write down a supposition, namely, that my continuing analytic practice brings with it an *increase* in this need for support. Already, before the establishment of your requirement of "suppression of countertransference,"[6] we all did this instinctively, and this continual suppression *has to* add up to something disturbing when one such as I, after ten to twelve hours of work, is so completely isolated and does without every love object. In fact, it is in the evenings when I feel this isolation particularly painfully.

I deliberately put the personal part of this letter first. So, now that I have taken care of that, I can come back to your very important and correct remarks about the Congress.

Its success is unquestionable. I scarcely believe that Strohmayer, for example, ever participated in a congress where, as in Nuremberg, one could really learn from *everyone*. Also, the general impression of being able to do much, which psychoanalysis helped us to achieve, must amaze someone on the outside—certainly no one's conscience will be able to remain completely at rest in the face of this. *Abraham* was, as always, clear and clever. *Jung's* lecture was deep and beautiful; everyone was delighted by it. *Honegger's* ideas (the mythological in paranoia) were deep, his style and presentation congenial. *Maeder* was somewhat too dry—but to the point. *Stekel* was in his element; *very much* good is contained in *Adler's* all too generalized explanations. The beginners (Marcinowski, Stegmann) are very promising.[7]

I don't find that your lecture had no deep effect, but I can only judge from my own perspective, since everything you said was already known to me. But even with this in mind, I followed your lecture with *great* pleasure.— Anybody who didn't like it (and I know of no one) didn't understand the great significance of your ideas.

I was somewhat depressed by the disappointment of encountering the *personally* motivated resistance of the Viennese to my suggestions. My brother complex was *certainly* operative in me (e.g., I didn't want to sacrifice the critical passages that they complained about!). But I wasn't prepared for such an unanalyzed brother complex as the one of Adler and Stekel with Jung. It distressed me considerably to have to observe that in people who have lived in your vicinity for almost a decade. Jung is right: every community grows wild without a "complex community" [*Komplexgemeinschaft*]. But the father and brother complex is raging among the Viennese. I called their attention to it on the trip back (very carefully; I said: "You have to analyze one another"). "We don't have time; the Zurichers have time for that," was the mocking reply.

On the other hand, I was struck by the deep sadness which the transfer of the Central Office to Zurich produced in *Adler,* and I felt myself freed, as if from a pressure, when I learned of your plan to make him the head of the Vienna group. You have also created the corresponding substitute for *Stekel's* other ambitions. You have have kept in reserve for me the expression of your trust (in your last letter). I can maintain with psychoanalytic honesty that that is worth more to me than honors from outside (although I do not disdain the latter).—

So now you have "fed" your people and now you want to withdraw from directing the menagerie. If, in so doing, you gain some more time for *recuperation* and for *scientific work*, then I am not dissatisfied with this change, but I hardly believe that much more than formal change has taken place. As gratified as I was by the robust and pugnacious attitude of the Zurichers, some supervision on your part is still in order. The trace of *mysticism*, which is revealed in their utterances, must still be corrected with time. That would be the Christian reaction to ΨA. Still, it is more welcome than the Jewish (in Stekel)—which has to be monitored no less closely.

You will therefore, for better or for worse, still have to scrap and fight with your trusted ones, and there is not much hope for the *"otium cum dignitate."*

Now, again something from me. The local Budapest group will perhaps be a reality once and for all. A Dr. Hevesy (chief director of the National Theater),[8] whom I initiated two years ago, has uninterruptedly taken up the ΨA. of the theater and the actors in the interim. In a long discussion he acquainted me with the *very good*, partly surprising things that he found. Perhaps a paper for the *Jahrbuch* will come out of it. I have another writer (Dr. Szilágyi);[9] very well oriented and enthusiastic for the cause.

We are still missing *doctors.* Last week a doctor from the provinces came to me for literature.—I had already decided in Nuremberg to teach the course. Your letter strengthened me in my resolve.—I will postpone organizing it until doctors are in the majority.

One of your patients whom you sent to me has been here for two days. The other (young Zayda from Pressburg) canceled.[10]

Once again many thanks for your kind letter, and obedient greetings.

Yours,
Ferenczi

1. "Az ég alatt, a föld szinén nincsen olyon árva mit én." Seventeenth-century song (personal communication from Béla Stoll).
2. "Without anger and without affect," i.e, partiality (Tacitus, *Annals*, 1.1).
3. Elma.
4. Magda, Gizella's younger daughter, was married to Ferenczi's brother Lajos.
5. Ferenczi was afraid that he was suffering from a kidney infection, but it was not confirmed; see letters 344 and 352.
6. Freud had used the expression *countertransference* for the first time publicly in his Nuremberg lecture and had expressed the opinion that "we . . . are almost inclined to insist that [the physician] shall recognize this countertransference in himself and overcome it" (1910d, pp. 144f).
7. The lecturers and titles of the lectures were: Abraham, "Psychoanalyse des Fetis-

chismus" [Psychoanalysis of Fetishism]; Jung, "Bericht über Amerika" [Report on America]; Honegger, "Über paranoide Wahnbildung" [On Paranoid Delusions]; Maeder, "Zur Psychologie der Paranoiden" [On the Psychology of Paranoids]; Stekel, "Vorschläge zur Sammelforschung im Gebiete der Symbolik und der typischen Träume" [Proposals for Group Research in the Domain of Symbolism and of Typical Dreams]; Adler, "Über psychischen Hermaphroditismus" [On Psychic Hermaphroditism]; and Marcinowski, "Sejunktive Prozesse als Grundlage der Psychoneurosen und andere Behandlungsarten in der nervenärztlichen Praxis" [Sejunctive Processes as the Foundation of Psychoneuroses and Other Types of Treatment in Neurological Practice].

8. Sándor Hevesi (1873–1939), director, theatrical producer, and writer; pioneer of modern theater direction in Hungary. "Hevesy" is Ferenczi's spelling.

9. Géza Szilágyi (1875–1958), poet, journalist, and theatrical producer; member of the Hungarian Society.

10. Zayda did go into treatment with Ferenczi. See letters 128 and 129.

128

Vienna, April 12, 1910
IX., Berggasse 19

Dear friend,

Professor Modena from Ancona[1] just left, a pleasant Judeo-Italian who has translated half of the Theory of Sexuality and is still looking for a publisher for it. We will perhaps be able to visit him on the trip to Sicily.

Your discussion in the last letter got me busy in certain directions. I see much that can't be changed and that I have always regretted. But the next thing that can happen is obvious: that you advertise a course in ΨA for physicians and others. That seems to be the way to make yourself the center of a circle and to constitute the Budapest group soon. As far as the rest is concerned, accept it with ψα resignation and write to me as often and as much as you want. I think I understand all that.

The Viennese here were very friendly in the reaction after Nuremberg and definitely wanted to found the Republic with the Grand Duke at the top. I at least had to keep leading the discussion in scientific sessions, but I will be able to withdraw gradually. A committee—Adler, Stekel, Steiner, Federn, Hitschmann,[2] Sadger—is occupied with the necessary new arrangements. I don't believe that my resignation will turn out to be only a formal change. Oversight may be necessary, then as now, but I can't provide it, and the matter will probably not continue quite in the way we mean it to, since the others are not so united among themselves as the two of us. The newest Dioscuri, Adler-Stekel, are considering publishing a ψα Zentralblatt [Central Organ], which is supposed to perform search-and-destroy missions alongside the heavy artillery of the Jahrbuch.[3] I think that will be a good place for some of the notes that you sent me for review.

In the week since the Reichstag in Nuremberg I had to do a little paper on psychogenic disturbances of vision as a contribution to a *Festschrift* for Königstein's sixtieth birthday on the 24th of the month.[4] It doesn't amount to much, like everything done on request, but precisely because of that it has eaten up every evening of the week.

The last shipment from Dunapentele contained a glass which produces a magical play of colors after being scratched in the appropriate spot. I wish you could have seen it. The little bronze things are not worth anything; still, the man does produce something. Isserlin's critique[5] already sounds much more polite; the case is perhaps not completely hopeless. The best technique here seems to be no treatment at all.

The Worcester lectures are ready. You will receive them as soon as the issue has arrived from America, which should be tomorrow. Jones writes quite charmingly; every letter from him shows more value and content. Brill, on the other hand, declares himself to be tired and nervous and is longing for a friend who can analyze him. We are all weak people.

Fackel-Kraus has unleashed a few stupid rockets of his wit against ΨA.[6] It is interesting, in any event, to learn what a "culture-fighter" [*Kulturkämpfer*] in Vienna allows himself to do. The secret is—don't let this get out—he is a crazy half-wit with great theatrical talent. He can, for example, also present himself as intelligent and outraged.

When I have overcome the present tired bad spell, I will probably write the first contribution to human love life: the characteristics of "maternal etiology."[7] That is not the permanent title, but you know what I mean.

Your young man from Pressburg [Zayda] is also dissatisfied here with Sadger; he likes you better as a person, and he wants to go back to you—if his acquaintances in Budapest don't bother him. He also had something against Rekawinkel.[8] He thus doesn't want to do anything at all. I had a few rude things to say to him by way of his mother. I will take this opportunity to point out to you how wrong it is for you to charge ten crowns per session when Sadger demands twenty. You see, the ten didn't keep him with you and the twenty didn't keep him from going to Sadger. Promise me you will improve!

We are freezing now; it is a harsh early spring, and I am longing for spring proper.—Havelock Ellis sent me the new, last volume of his studies (sex in relation to society).[9] Seems very much worth reading. Your motto "Hold your tongue and serve on" often goes through my mind.

Kindest regards,
Freud

1. Gustavo Modena (1876–1958), neuropsychiatrist and acting director of the asylum at Ancona. In 1907–8 he had met Ernest Jones in Kraepelin's clinic in Munich, and the former had interested him in psychoanalysis—which Modena later sharply criticized,

however. The first Italian translation of *Three Essays* (by Marco Levi Bianchini) was not published until 1921.

2. Eduard Hitschmann (1871–1957), internist; member of the Wednesday Society since 1905. He was head of the psychoanalytic outpatient clinic in Vienna from 1922 until the Society was disbanded by the Nazis. In 1938 he emigrated to London and in 1940 moved to Boston, where he was active as a training analyst. See also letter 130 and n. 6.

3. In the session of April 6, 1910, the Vienna Psychoanalytic Society was founded, with Adler as president and Freud as scientific chairman. It was also decided to publish the *Zentralblatt* (*Minutes* II, 463–471); bylaws and organizational questions were discussed a week later (ibid., pp. 472–478). See also letter 130.

4. *The Psycho-Analytic View of Psychogenic Disturbance of Vision* (1910i). Leopold Königstein (1850–1924), professor of ophthalmology in Vienna, was a close friend (and tarok partner) of Freud's. The topic chosen by Freud is also interesting because in 1884 Königstein, at Freud's urging, had also examined the anesthetizing effect of cocaine on the eye. The experiment had failed because Königstein had used an inappropriate solution. As is well known, another friend of Freud's, Karl Koller, became famous because of this discovery (see, for example, Freud's letter of August 15, 1924, to Wittels, in *Letters*, pp. 350–351). In 1885 Königstein had operated on Freud's father's eye while Freud and Koller themselves prepared the local anesthetic with cocaine.

5. Max Isserlin (1879–1941), neurologist and, at that time, Kraepelin's assistant in Munich, had sharply criticized Freud and Jung in an article titled "Über Jungs 'Psychologie der Dementia Praecox' und die Anwendung Freudscher Forschungsmaximen in der Psychopathologie," *Zentralblatt für Nervenheilkunde und Psychiatrie* 30 (1907): 18. On April 12, 1910, Freud wrote to Jung about the work mentioned here, "Die psychoanalytische Methode Freuds," *Zeitschrift für die gesamte Neurologie und Psychiatrie* 1 (1910): "Isserlin seems to be almost having lucid moments" (*Letters*, p. 306).

6. In the issue of *Fackel* published at the end of March 1910 (no. 300, pp. 26f), Kraus polemicized about, among other things, "a certain psychoanalysis [which] is the activity of lascivious rationalists who reduce everything in the world to sexual causes with the exception of their activity . . . Children of psychoanalytic parents wilt early . . . One can talk about happiness when such a one reaches the age where the youngster can confess a dream in which he has violated his mother . . . The new psychology has dared to spit into the mystery of genius . . . But we will withdraw Kleist and Lenau from ordination! . . . Neither doctors nor lawyers know this: that in eros there is neither a demonstrable truth nor an objective finding . . . In short, that it is high time to drive lawyers and doctors out of a world that belongs to thinkers and poets." See also letter 112, n. 7.

7. See letter 126 and n. 8.

8. A sanatorium for nervous diseases in Rekawinkel, a summer resort near Vienna. Its director, a Dr. Weiss, was recommended for acceptance in the Vienna Society the next day (*Minutes* II, 477f), but there is no further mention of his candidacy in subsequent minutes.

9. Havelock Ellis, *Studies in the Psychology of Sex*, vol. 6, *Sex in Relation to Society* (Philadelphia, 1910).

129

Budapest, April 17, 1910
VII., Erzsébet-körút 54

Dear Professor,

I must extend the validity of your statement, according to which physicians are in ψα treatment, *to the adherents* of your doctrines as well. The difference is only that we are treated not with "nonobservance" but rather according to all the rules of the art. I scarcely believe that the treatment of your patients ever caused you as many headaches as ours. Your newest principle (which, by the way, is becoming more and more clear to me)—that technique has to direct itself according to the uniqueness of each case—is becoming completely valid with us. The personal sensitivities, childish ideas of jealousy and grandeur, personal destinies: all this becomes a burden to you, so that you also have to bear the concerns of all your pupils in addition to your own. I am aware of the fact that only the capacity for *total* self-analysis, the bringing out of one's inner conflicts without outside aid, signifies the final *cure* of a person, and I am firmly resolved to make use of your offer to write to you as much and as often as I want only in the sense that I will communicate to you the results of previous self-analysis; you will probably also find something in this that doesn't appear to be perfectly clear to you. In this way I hope to be able to spare you a lot of care and work. You certainly have enough of both. If it were in my power, I would recommend similar procedures to all our colleagues. In addition to consideration for you, there also comes into play the egoistic wish on my part to spare you superfluous matters so that you can work with fewer distractions.

The experiences in Nuremberg have certainly not encouraged me very much, to the extent that I had dared to hope that in the not too distant future psychoanalysts would get serious about the *energy expended against themselves.*

I will gladly send smaller pieces for the Zentralblatt; we are up to our ears in those things. I just revised my little notebook and will (now that I have finished the Hungarian translation of the first part of the "Introjection" paper) begin to put the material, which has been piling up for a long time, on paper. I will then send you the "loose leaves" [*fliegende Blätter*][1] which result from this.

Kraus's expectorations come out as very feeble. They don't differ in any way from the humoristic fancies of the Berlin harlequin (Neurologisches Zentralblatt).[2]

I want to offer the course. I will put a notice to that effect into the two more significant medical journals right away.—The question as to whether

I should also take on students has already led, by the way, to a rather acrimonious dispute between my friend Dr. Schächter and me. He is afraid that I am corrupting the youth and that the youthful stormers will corrupt us. I, for my part, am afraid that this friendship will not last in the long run, which, by the way, I am sorry about.

Isserlin's critique has made a big impression here. Our ignorant opponents are again happy that they have done away with us. Yet the critique contains absolutely nothing new and significant; he wants to have "proof"—but he doesn't look in the only place where it can be found, in analytic practice. These people always forget that Ψα. is not a *hypothesis* but a sum of empirical experiences that are brought into an intellectual context.

The case of the young Pressburger is a wonderful case of *paranoia*. The case was originally a neurosis—at a very specific point in time, two years ago, the patient projected everything troublesome onto the outside. I was successful (probably with the help of remnants of neurosis) in winning him over to a certain extent by taking the standpoint of his delusional ideas. Naturally, I don't know if I can effect the retransformation of his projections into neurosis with this "hypomochlion."[3] The case is not suited to Sadger's somewhat coarse manner. The extraordinary role of projected homosexuality in paranoia is also confirmed here. So, probably a new contribution to the planned work on paranoia. In future I will heed your advice to charge more than ten crowns. I haven't done it yet in Zayda's case, in order not to be inconsistent.

Frau G. sends you kind regards and thanks you for your repeated inquiry.

Kind regards,
Ferenczi

1. A reference to a satirical German periodical of the same name [Trans.].

2. Attacks on psychoanalysis appeared frequently in the *Neurologisches Centralblatt*; this could be an allusion to the report mentioned in letter 130, n. 4.

3. Fulcrum of a lever; in obstetrics, the part of the infant's body that forms the starting point for its bending around the pubic arch.

130

Vienna, April 24, 1910
IX., Berggasse 19

Dear friend,

I am not entirely happy with the tone of resignation and melancholy in your letter. I consider it to be a residue of the Nuremberg experience, for which I share the blame, and I hope that it will soon ease. Your standing among the "hostile brothers" will again increase, and the future will have to prove you right.

For the time being the treatment has done them good; since they have the work in their own hands, they are much friendlier toward me and, for the moment, still in agreement among themselves. We are now meeting in the Doktorenkollegium[1] in Steiner's house, 2 Rotenturmstrasse 19, where the library will also be moved. We have covered the cost through a long-term subscription. Outwardly the matter has not yet progressed very far; Zurich has also not been formally constituted because Bleuler is still in the hospital—or at least he was at the time of Jung's letter.

Deuticke is making things difficult for the new Zentralblatt because Stekel doesn't seem to him to be trustworthy. Stekel made all kinds of superfluous comments to him, from which Deuticke concluded that the purely scientific character of the periodical is not assured. I appeased Deuticke, and I think he will still do it.[2] I will certainly not commit myself much further, but rather let them test out the measure of their capabilities. The Zentralblatt is a sword that cuts both ways, certainly very powerful when it is used correctly.

You must also have been very pleased about the issue of the American Journal of Psychology.[3] That is thus the first fruit of our expedition. Immediately afterward I sent out the copies of the German edition. Now we will hear that there is nothing new in it. Among the latest attacks, the letter about the session in Hamburg is noteworthy (correspondence of Hamburg Physicians, April 4, 1910).[4] There they make the argument I had wanted to deflect by moving to Zurich, namely, that Viennese sensuality can't be found elsewhere! You can still read between the lines that we Viennese are not only pigs but also Jews. But that wasn't printed.

I recently received a paper from Strohmayer (Moll II.2), "Zur Analyse und Prognose psychoneurotischer Symptome,"[5] which is quite genuine in its conviction. An enclosed letter gives one to understand why he can't befriend the Interpretation of Dreams and the therapeutic benefit, and it will give me cause for a sharp attempt at analysis (in the sense of your treatment).

Jung writes that he is deeply immersed in mythology, from which something significant will come. I am correcting Leonardo and otherwise doing nothing. Today Rank and Hitschmann read to me out loud a few chapters of the "synthetic presentation" of my Theory of Neuroses,[6] which they wrote. It will be quite usable, especially when it undergoes revision in later editions. The first textbook of ΨA, so to speak, at the moment still somewhat too much of a chronicle and compilation.

I hope you are asserting all your rights as a member of the Vienna ψα

Society;[7] I will occasionally remind you about them here. I am very curious about the first success of your advertisement. You may sooner be able to put your group together with laymen than with doctors.

My daughter[8] does indeed seem to be recovering now. She is more active, and this week she was with us for the first time in months.—By the way, I count eighty-one days until the beginning of vacation.

A small contribution to the psychology of love life for the next Jahrbuch (II.2)[9] will probably yet be written before vacation. Otherwise I consider it good to pause. Let's go to Sicily together then, and in conversation something will certainly break out of its latency. By the way, what do you think about asking Brill to take this trip or a part of it with us? He complained in his last letter that he was exhausted and neurotic, and asked in the next sentence where I want to spend the summer. I had to attach a hint of an invitation to it, the serious repetition of which naturally depends on you. It would mean a loss of intimacy, but otherwise a gain in comfort and something of the fulfillment of an obligation. I am, of course, not convinced that he wants or is able to come along.

Kind regards in expectation of your reports.

Yours,
Freud

1. The Vienna Doctors' College, where Freud had given his three-part lecture "On Hysteria" (Freud 1895g) in 1895.

2. The *Zentralblatt* was finally published in the Bergmann Verlag in Wiesbaden.

3. The issue, already mentioned several times, in which Freud's American lectures and Ferenczi's article on the dream were published (see letter 78, nn. 1 and 3).

4. The meeting of the Medical Society of Hamburg on March 29, 1910, at which several neurologists proposed to boycott agencies where psychoanalysis was practiced. A further report appeared in the *Neurologisches Centralblatt* 29, no. 12 (1910): 659–662; see also Jones II, 116.

5. *Zeitschrift für Psychotherapie und medizinische Psychologie,* ed. Albert Moll, 2, no. 2 (1910).

6. Hitschmann's book *Freuds Neurosenlehre: Nach ihrem gegenwärtigen Stande zusammenfassend dargestellt* (Vienna, 1911) was the first systematic presentation of psychoanalysis. Rank did not sign on as coauthor. On May 26, 1910, Freud characterized the work to Jung as "a kind of manual for elementary schools" (*Letters,* p. 321).

7. See letter 12, n. 1.

8. Mathilde.

9. See letter 126 and n. 8.

131

Budapest, April 27, 1910
VII., Erzsébet-körút 54

Dear Professor,

I have rather gotten out of the habit of saying "no"; still, I think that the somewhat resigned mood of my last letter has *less* to do with the impressions of Nuremberg than with the personal events to which I recently alluded. In your reply *you* advised somewhat more resignation; as an obedient pupil I seem to have obeyed you immediately. But there is no question that in all this, the events at Nuremberg may have *increased* my sensitivity at the opposite pole (private life). One constantly vacillates back and forth between homosexual (public-communal) and heterosexual (exclusive, private) interests. If one deceives oneself here, one then seeks solace there and suddenly perceives the personal situation which one has perhaps already previously accepted with resignation as unbearable. I repeat, however, that this time actual events (a paranoid would say: a concentrated attack against all of us) also helped to bring about the depression.

The mood swing, however, had already been analytically dissolved at the time of my last letter; I feel well, am working very hard, and find much satisfaction in work. My sleep, the indicator of my mental condition, is restful and undisturbed by anxiety dreams.—The plan to invite Brill immediately aroused my slumbering brother complex. [I want to tell you how I came upon it. I received your letter during an analytic hour and didn't have time to read it; but in my impatience I skimmed through the letter and immediately discovered the place where you talk about the invitation to Brill. Then I put the letter in my pocket—but it was not until an hour after the end of the analysis that I remembered that I hadn't yet read the letter.][1] The analysis of this symptomatic omission helped me to recognize that I have something against this invitation; a further deepening of this train of thought convinced me, however, that I can't raise any objection to the invitation other than the unjustified infantile desire to be the first and only one with the "father." I like Brill very much and am *in complete agreement* that you should invite him. But between the two suggested modalities I would still like to choose the one that states that the three of us make only *a part* of the journey. That is not only a small concession to my complexes (which I usually handle as badly as Spitteler does his "Poor Konrad"),[2] but it also has its logical foundation. There are questions (of both a personal and scientific nature) which we can settle much more economically alone than in Brill's presence; these should also get their due.[3]

I am very much looking forward to the trip. Sometimes September seems infinitely far away to me. America was not a real recuperation: physical effort and bad diet were paired at that time with the self-analytic crisis of the brother complex. I can therefore say that I have actually not allowed myself any recuperation at all for two years. I haven't looked forward to a vacation this much since my Matura.[4] (In Berchtesgaden I was still full of unexplained inhibitions, which have only been explained and resolved since then.)

I thank you very much for putting in a good word for my rights at the Vienna Society. As long as I live I will also always belong to the Vienna Society, along with the Budapest Society, which may yet be founded.

My founding is not yet progressing. Here people are talking much about Ψα—colleagues are beginning to consult me, etc., but not a single application has come from the advertisement that came out on Sunday.

I thank you for the Worcester lectures; you have certainly prophesied the critiques correctly. I was just thumbing through a brochure by *Frank,* which impudently calls itself *"the* Psychoanalysis,"[5] although it contains only *his* impoverished analysis, discarded by the authorities.

I am now often immersing myself in the psychology of paranoia; chance is helping me in this. The reciprocal relationships of homosexuality and paranoia are becoming more numerous. I now have three homosexuals and in the next few days I will be getting a second case of paranoia. The mechanism of projection can be traced back in spots to generally present infantilisms (of childhood). But this time I don't want to preempt my detailed report on scientific observations and ideas.

Kindest regards to the entire family.

Yours truly,
Ferenczi

1. Enclosed in brackets in the original.

2. Carl Spitteler (1845–1924); Swiss writer who won the Nobel Prize for literature in 1919. The character Viktor in his novel *Imago* (1906) "was accustomed . . . to calling his body Konrad in a comradely way, because he got along so well with it" ([Frankfurt, 1979], p. 21). Freud borrowed the expression, which became standard in psychoanalytic circles, and often spoke of "poor" Konrad (see, e.g., letter 325).

3. Brill turned down the invitation (Jones II, 81).

4. The qualifying examination for admission to German universities [Trans.].

5. Ludwig Frank, *Die Psychanalyse, ihre Bedeutung für die Auffassung und Behandlung psychoneurotischer Zustände* (Munich, 1910). Frank (1863–1935), an adherent of Forel's, was a neurologist in Zurich and practiced a variation of the original Breuer-Freud cathartic method.

132

Vienna, May 1, 1910
IX., Berggasse 19

Dear friend,

You would be gratified to see how mild the Viennese "brothers" have become since that great revolt at the Nuremberg Reichstag; they are downright affectionate and respectful with me. Above all, it has to do with the new monthly,[1] which Deuticke doesn't quite want to bite into, and about which we are therefore in the process of negotiating with Bergmann. I think it will indeed come into being and will appear in October. I hear little from Jung; the latest, a telegram: advice on what to do because Bleuler doesn't want to go along. No explanatory text since.[2]

The vacation this time is very important to me as well. The last two summers I, too, did not have the fairy-tale feeling of living in freedom and beauty. I am very much in agreement with your decision about Brill, for the same reasons. Write to him yourself in this vein. It is quite doubtful whether he can come with us anyway.

Our plans for the summer are beginning to take shape. I have been forced into a decision in favor of the sea by the need to be no further than a day's journey from Hamburg,[3] and my Dutch patients here have been the decisive factor in choosing a beach in Holland. We have been looking at a place near Leyden that is spelled something like Nortwyige, and we will probably make a decision soon. From there I can probably best travel to our meeting place by ship if Holland is too far for you to go. That will give us nice material for plans and decisions in the next few months.

Your work on paranoia should come into being. It doesn't make sense to stay away from it because Jung is working in the area, and our understandings about the attempt at cure,[4] about the hypocrisy of paranoia and the like that we reached in the woods,[5] should be taken up there. I recommend to you as well the case of Hofrichter[6] as exquisitely typical, especially now after the establishment of his love for his wife, which, as the amorous adventure in the hotel shows, was evidently very tenuous.

I must ask you if anything remains of the funds for Dunapentele and what we can expect from the man. The Worcester lectures have brought with them an honorarium, which should be spent.

My wife and Sophie are going to Karlsbad for a week.

I send kind regards and will probably soon have something scientific to share with you.

Yours,
Freud

1. The *Zentralblatt.*

2. Bleuler wanted to be neither the head nor a simple member of the Zurich Society. See *Freud/Jung*, letters of April 26, and 30, May 2 and 5, 1910, pp. 311ff; and letter 18, n. 2.

3. Because of the illness of Freud's mother-in-law, Emmeline Bernays.

4. "The delusional formation, which we take to be the pathological product, is in reality an attempt at recovery, a process of reconstruction," wrote Freud in his analysis of Schreber (1911c [1910], p. 71).

5. During their vacation together in Berchtesgaden in 1908.

6. First Lieutenant Adolf Hofrichter was then being tried for murder and attempted murder. The allusion could not be explained further.

133

Budapest, May 6, 1910
VII., Erzsébet-körút 54

Dear Professor,

I seem to myself to be like an old railway engineer I know, who (retired after fifty years of service) stops in front of a locomotive standing on the tracks and cries out with naive admiration: "That's really a beautiful invention!"[1]:—For years I have been occupied with psychoanalysis from dawn until dusk, I am a wage earner of this method, it is my craft and my daily bread. But hardly a day goes by when I don't—sometimes in the midst of work—have to stop to admire the uncommon progress in the understanding of sick and healthy humanity. "It is indeed a beautiful invention!"

The occasion for this remark was provided by the impression I received this evening from a woman to whom I had been called who had fallen ill with overwhelming puerperal mania. I hadn't seen a mania for several years. And what did the same clinical picture that I perceived earlier as a strange conglomeration of inexplicable "symptoms" tell me now? At that time I was already preaching that there were no such things as "fools," only mentally ill people. Only now do I see that I, like all preachers and paranoids, inwardly believed the opposite. Without Ψ-A, one *must* consider mentally ill people to be fools—people with "nonsensical" ideas and actions.

Instead of the "euphoria" from that time I saw erotic allusions, demands, gestures. Instead of "madness" I saw the elemental outbreak of violence, instead of "verbigeration,"[2] unconcealed truths that the patient flung in the face of her surroundings.

They brought me the "puerperium"[3] only in the way of an anamnesis. But in five minutes I got out of the family doctor the fact that it was a *mariage de raison*[4] (she had a photography studio, he was her competitor and asked for her hand in order to unite the firms); that the husband did not bring about defloration (the introitus was "too tight," she had to be operated on]; that he was altogether a cool man and she was passionate; etc.

How simple-minded, how poor we were, as if struck blind, as long as we let these things pass by unnoticed.

One naturally thinks, after the fact, that one should have intimated all that. But I become more and more convinced that a monstrous distance, a chasm, separates intimating from knowing.

I just finished reading *Mereschkowski's* excellent work "Tolstoi und Dostojewski als Menschen und Künstler."[5] I already read through two thirds of the book with increasing admiration in the firm belief that the man knows everything we know—maybe even more! And in the last third I learn that all these things were only *intimations* of the writer's—which he uses as the building blocks of a *completely erroneous* metaphysical-religious "knowledge." He knows everything—but he doesn't know the true meaning of the unconscious—and his entire worldview ends up on the rocks from this not-knowing. You must read this book! The attitude of this intimating writer reminds me of your meaningful remark according to which there are *two kinds* of preconscious.

Imagine! My appeal remained completely unsuccessful. Only one person applied, and he is unusable. Of course, I don't think anything of it; the poor people should be pitied. Still, it was interesting to set up this experiment! The doves will one day return with the olive branch. For the time being I feel very pleasant and comfortable in Noah's ark and have no particular longing for the more boring times of the becalmed, quiet period of ΨA.—

Should I give the course for Stein, Décsi, and two to three nonphysicians?

The vacation plans interest me very much. I will study the map and measure off the temporal and spatial distance between Holland and Sicily. My first concern is to spend as few vacation days as possible alone, i.e., not in your company. I will cook up something: maybe a meeting on the way.—

Up to now I have expended 215 crowns for Dunapentele. Tomorrow I will send Steiner thirty-five crowns as a contribution to the Society's fund; please give the fifteen crowns that I paid for you likewise to Steiner in order to increase the amount to fifty crowns.

As regards Dunapentele, the man from D[una] P[entele] is unproductive and unreliable. He brings lots of trash, so I chased him away. I will write to the mayor of D[una] P[entele] that the peasants can come to me directly with their finds.

In the meantime you don't need to send me any money; if something turns up, I'll buy it.

Kind regards,
Ferenczi

1. This anecdote was repeated by Ferenczi much later, in his lecture in honor of Freud's seventy-fifth birthday, "Kinderanalysen mit Erwachsenen" [Child Analysis in the Analysis of Adults] (1931, 292; *Fin.*, p. 142; *Schriften* II, 288).
2. Constant repetition of seemingly nonsensical words and sentences
3. Childbed.
4. Marriage of convenience.
5. See letter 120 n. 3.

134

Vienna, May 17, 1910
IX., Berggasse 19

Dear friend,

You will witness the fact that I have seldom neglected to talk to you, if possible, and you should now learn that since the 5th of the month (your delightful letter arrived just after my 54th! birthday) I have been laboring under an influenza which first caused me to lose my voice, and now my strength. I was in Karlsbad over Whitsun, where I met my blossoming wife and daughter and where I brought back with me not convalescence but rather a nice nephrite.[1] The week before the holidays was the busiest of the entire year, and I braced myself for the necessity of not sacrificing any earnings to the illness. Now I have, I hope, apologized to you, and your thinking will not seek any other motives. Today I can write again, if not eat properly.

I think you should announce the course again after a while and wait at your post as a general, until the army returns. For Duna Pentele, my thanks for all your efforts. Your contribution has been in Steiner's hands since Wednesday.

We are working very assiduously in Vienna. The contract for the Zentralblatt has been signed with Bergmann, and the first issue is set for October. I will sign on as the editor, in accordance with Bergmann's wishes, and will open with the lecture in Nuremberg.

Jones is writing magnificent reports about battles and victories in America.

Our summer has been set to the extent that we will arrive in Noortwiyk near Leyden (Hotel Nordsee) on August 1. The previous two weeks have not been determined. I will occupy myself vigorously with plans for the possible trip through the Mediterranean. Think about it, the same trip that we had to give up on account of Worcester!

I won't write you any more today because I am very inactive, and I also haven't slept for two nights on the train, which is quite contrary to my constitution, and I hope now to hear from you very soon.

Most cordially,
Freud

1. A type of jade, regarded as a remedy for diseases of the kidney.

135

Budapest, May 18, 1910
VII., Erzsébet-körút 54

Dear Professor,

A woman patient whom I had to throw out some time ago in the state of transference used the catastrophe threatened by the comet as a moving farewell to me.[1] I myself belong to those optimists—more correctly skeptics—who don't want to believe that such a great cataclysm will happen precisely during my lifetime, and I will go ahead and go to sleep. That is, I was about to do so, when the idea "freely came to mind" that I haven't written to you for a long time.—Naturally, it soon came out that I do have something to share with you—and if one wants something, then such a far-fetched association (Halley's comet) suffices to bring the idea to mind.

For yesterday I was invited into a private circle of sociologists to give a lecture about your theories.[2] It was the most intelligent and understanding audience that I have heretofore had the opportunity to address. *That* must have animated me to the extent that, without any preparation, I put together such a good, concise summary of what distinguishes psychoanalysis from every earlier psychology as I could certainly not put on paper now. When I think about what I had to say in conclusion about the anticipated social effects of your ideas, the association with the comet becomes clear to me. In fact, I can't go to sleep so easily, because—you see, such a great revolution in psychology and in everything connected with it could arrive in my lifetime, and, in defiance of every reckoning of probability, with my co-workers, no matter how modest they may be. As a schooled obsessional thinker, I do have to consider: "If one came, then the other must come as well"—namely, the comet. On the other hand, of course, skepticism stirs in me and says: if one has come, then the other will probably not arrive.—

But this time skepticism has been somewhat delayed: the letter is already finished—in fact, it sounds a little bit like an imitation of the moving farewell that my patient gave me!—That, too, has its reason: like the patient, I wanted to extort something—namely, news from you. You have been pampering me very much lately—that was incautious of you; you know, of course, how easily one gets used to good things.

The course could also come into being, if not in the form originally planned. A total of two doctors applied, both unusable: I succeeded in frightening them away by demanding an honorarium of 200 crowns each. Instead, I will give the course for free to a small group of young doctoral candidates (seven or eight). I will finally give up wanting to get involved with older, practicing physicians. There is no longer any doubt, youth is our only hope. These young people are full of enthusiasm for the idea; perhaps two or three of them will remain with the cause. I will bring into the course three nonphysicians (an educator,[3] a literary man,[4] and the chief director of the National Theater[5]), and I intend to lecture them for four weeks three times a week from nine to eleven P.M. (Yesterday I spoke for two hours without getting tired; psychoanalytic training is certainly not useless.)

I am now reading a charming book by *Anatole France* with much enjoyment, "Le livre de mon ami."[6] One of the best books about the souls of children, and at the same time one of delightful sensitivity and depth of feeling. Please read it!

Were you perhaps in Karlsbad over the holidays? I hope you and your family are well.

Best regards from Frau G. and from your obedient

Ferenczi

Postscript:
Just received your letter, whereby mine actually became superfluous. Please let me know, if only by correspondence card, how you are. I will answer next time in detail.

F.

1. At that time the newspapers were full of reports about the approach of Halley's comet. It had been calculated beforehand that on May 19 the Earth would be brushed by the comet's tail, and some people were afraid that the gases might poison the atmosphere.

2. This lecture may have been based on the text "Zur Erkenntnis des Unbewussten" [Exploring the Unconscious] (1911, 81a).

3. Perhaps Sándor Varjas (1885–1939 or 1940), a high school teacher at the time; collaborator on the periodical *Huszadik Század* [Twentieth Century], in which he published several articles about psychoanalysis.

4. Hugó Ignotus (pseudonym for Hugó Veigelsberg) (1859–1949), editor in chief of the periodical *Nyugat* [Occident], founded in 1908; it played a major role in Hungarian cultural life as a radical organ of modernity and renewal, and many articles about psychoanalysis were published in it. Ignotus was a founding member of the Hungarian Society and a translator of Freud, with whom he also carried on a correspondence. In 1919, after the fall of the Hungarian republic, Ignotus went to Vienna, but he was again active in Budapest during the 1930s. In 1938 he emigrated to New York, then returned once again to Budapest in 1948.

5. Sándor Hevesi; see letter 127 and n. 8.

6. Anatole France, *Le livre de mon ami* (Paris, 1885).

136

Vienna, May 20, 1910
IX., Berggasse 19

Dear friend,

The world has not ended here, either. I, too, still exist to alleviate your concerns; only I am still miserable in a bourgeois sort of way and am counting the days until July 14. There are still fifty-five. I hope to be compensated by a very nice vacation. Just study the timetables in your free time.

I am sorry that you are so lonely. It is soothing not to have so much interaction and communication; still it is something that one shouldn't give up. The lecture with the socialists[1] must have been very interesting.

Otherwise, not much is happening. Hirschfeld sent his book about transvestites.[2] He is finally becoming clear about the distinction between inversion of object and of person, i.e., homosexuality and feminine mixing.

I will order Anatole France today. I miss that sort of thing, since I can't produce anything now.

I request that you give me a word of confirmation of my having sent you Kleinpaul, the Essence of Witches,[3] if it's true. Not for the sake of the book itself!

Many thanks.

Yours,
Freud

1. As in the original; cf. letter 135 [Trans.].

2. Magnus Hirschfeld, *Die Transvestiten, Eine Untersuchung über den erotischen Verkleidungstrieb* (Berlin, 1910). Ferenczi took up the distinction in his concepts of subject-object homoerotism in "Zur Nosologie der Männlichen Homosexualität (Homoerotik)" [On the Nosology of Male Homosexuality] (1914, 136; *C.*, p. 300; *Schriften* I, 186).

3. Rudolf Kleinpaul, *Modernes Hexenwesen, Spiritistische und antispiritistische Plaudereien* (Leipzig, 1900).

137

Budapest, May 27, [1910][1]
VII., Erzsébet-körút 54

Dear Professor,

Left completely in the lurch by my professional colleagues and the older doctors, I organized the course for young, enthusiastic students, who are overjoyed finally to hear something new and beautiful after their arid university lectures. I lecture three times a week from nine to eleven in the evening. I chose ten auditors from the large number that applied: two doctors (very young ones), a pedagogue, four medical students, two law students, and a specialist in music.[2] The last (a Ph.D.) is a valuable acquisition. After a brief introduction, I immediately began with the analysis of a case of hysteria and explained hysteria in light of this case; naturally, also the interpretation of dreams and the ancillary questions (myth, joke, everyday life, etc.). The lectures late at night and after the exertions of the day take up a great deal of my energy, but the great interest of the audience makes me forget all fatigue. In the fall I will found the branch society with the better elements of the course and then, of course, also bring in Stein and Décsi.

The eagerness of the Vienna circle is precious; we hear too little from Zurich. The Zentralblatt will surely prosper; I, too, will eagerly take part in it. I can find places for only a few articles in Hungarian.

I am writing this letter late at night and am rather exhausted, which accounts for its laconic brevity and incoherent content. I only wanted to give a sign of life on my part and thank you for your kind letter.

Kind regards,
Dr. Ferenczi

The Essence of Witches is here.

1. The letter has been put in sequence on the basis of its content.
2. Possibly Sándor Kovács (1886–1918), musicologist and educator. He was the first in Hungary to introduce psychological principles into music education.

138

Vienna, June 5, 1910
IX., Berggasse 19

Dear friend,

I just received the enclosed very interesting letter from Brill.[1] So I hope to see you now in June in Vienna, and I leave it to you to sound out Brill regarding the trip. His participation will certainly not be very probable by virtue of this visit. I acknowledge your intensive efforts to create the Budapest group, but I think you have made things too difficult for yourself with the lectures three times a week from nine to eleven. Think about the fact that you don't intend to go on vacation until September, and a hot summer lies ahead.

Jung is still having difficulties in Zurich that he has not mastered. The group is rudimentary, and the Korrespondenzblatt[2] is being delayed. But these are now essentially his problems. How necessary the founding of the Zentralblatt was is being proved by the practice of Alzheimer's[3] of dismissing as unscientific works that are scientific in our sense.

Two interesting visitors recently. On May 28 Friedländer[4] (!), who was with me from nine in the evening until one o'clock in the morning, and yesterday Ossipow[5] from Moscow. I will put off the description of Friedländer until I can give one orally; it was a pleasure for me to see what a liar, rogue, and ignoramus he is (no discretion necessary). I treated him very badly. The Russian is a magnificent chap, clear head, an adherent of honest conviction; he will be a good acquisition. He will translate the Worcester ΨA into Russian.

After two bad weeks I decided to seek medical treament, and since then I also feel much better. It is surely only a colitis without involvement of the appendix. I am on a diet, use a hot water bottle, etc. You see, I don't want to lay on you the burden of having to spend your vacation with an invalid.

This morning my wife and Sophie returned from Karlsbad. In June, part of the family is going to Bistrai to see Jekels,[6] where I will follow on July 14. We won't go to Noordwijk until August 1.

I send kind regards and hope soon to hear personally what you have to say about Leonardo.

Yours,
Freud

1. The enclosure is missing.

2. The *Korrespondenzblatt*, founded at the Nuremberg Congress as the official organ of the association, was supposed to appear monthly. The first issue came out in July.

3. Alois Alzheimer (1864–1915), German neurologist and psychiatrist, who described the disease that was named after him, edited the *Zeitschrift für die gesamte Neurologie und Psychiatrie*, of which he was co-founder.

4. See letter 78, n. 4.

5. See letter 96, n. 3.

6. Ludwig Jekels (1867–1954), neurologist and psychiatrist, member of the Wednesday Society since 1909, analyst, and tarok partner of Freud's, had invited the family to Bistrai in Austrian Silesia (now Poland), where he was director of a sanatorium. Jekels introduced psychoanalysis to Poland.

139

Budapest, [ca. June 5, 1910][1]
VII., Erzsébet-körút 54

Dear Professor,

Many thanks for *Leonardo*. I have already heard everything essential about it from you personally, and yet it is only now that I have gotten the complete impression of your idea. Since our trip from Budapest to Komorn[2] at night, where you first explained the idea to me, I have learned a great deal from my homosexual, and what appeared to me then as a possibility became the only possible thing.—The vulture fantasy *can* find no other explanation than the one that you give in your Leonardo.[3]

You are certainly not mistaken about the impression that the book will make. Nothing more shocking has appeared since "Little Hans"[4]—shocking this time not so much in a moral as in a *logical* sense. People don't suspect that in mental life other than logical rules exist, and they will again make you out to be a dreamer and draw the most unfavorable conclusions about your other works.

What will happen with you will be something like what has happened with me, namely, that I—as has been confirmed to me by various sources—have been decried as a homosexual, evidently because I am concerned with homosexuality. You are interpreting a fantasy—ergo, you are a dreamer [*Phantast*].—And the funniest thing in all of this is that this error in thinking is made by none other than the logicians!

I found a passage in your Leonardo[5] that also characterizes me: I evidently also belong to those who, gripped by the grandeur of the phenomena unfolding before their eyes, feel that they are too small and not capable of actively meshing in with the machinery of the world. I see, learn, find new things, but immediately spin everything into a great context which scares me away from coming to grips with it. So the things remain undescribed.—

In the last few months I have been occupied with a series of hypochondriacal anxiety hysterias, more often than not complicated by obsessional thinking. With great regularity I found in them the exceptional significance of a repressed miser complex. These are people who, in reaction to the miserly father, are *consciously* cavaliers, but unconsciously they are forced to sympathize with the father's miserliness. Every expenditure of money (especially family expenses) makes them ill; in place of "impoverishment" the hypochondriacal idea of "going to ruin" through illness and death steps in. *Money* is the valuable thing that belongs to the father, onto which the struggle for the mother is displaced—at the same time it is a substitute for renounced coprophilia. Money is a terribly important nodal point—it also takes upon itself the worries about masturbation, about "loss of semen"—

(the husband, for instance, has carefree intercourse with his wife and becomes afraid of death from small expenditures of money).[6]

Have you made similar observations? It goes without saying that the interpretation of the fear of death is not exhausted with this. It also signifies the identification with the beloved person (father, wife) whose death one wishes (out of covetousness, envy)—and the divine and earthly punishment for such wishful fantasies of death.

Brill writes to me today that he is coming to Europe with a patient and will also visit me. But he wants us to make no mention of this patient in front of the Americans and Jung. I am looking forward to seeing him again.—

The course is going well. The young people are diligent and interested. The day before yesterday it was so hot that I had to give the course on the upper deck of an omnibus and in the city park. Very peripatetic!

I would very much like to hear something about your ideas on the vacation trip. Let us hope nothing distracting will get in the way.

How is your health?

Kind regards,
Dr. Ferenczi

1. The letter has been put in sequence on the basis of letter 140 from Freud.

2. Komorn (Komárom, Komárno) is approximately halfway between Vienna and Budapest (now in Slovakia). Ferenczi may have accompanied Freud up to that point on the latter's return from a visit to Budapest in November 1909 (see letter 86, n. 10).

3. "I recall as one of my very earliest memories that while I was in my cradle a vulture came down to me, and opened my mouth with its tail, and struck me many times with its tail against my lips." (Leonardo da Vinci, quoted in Freud 1910c, p. 82). The vulture is interpreted by Freud as a symbol of the mother, and the fantasy is translated as meaning: "It was through this erotic relation with my mother that I became a homosexual" (ibid., p. 106). Freud's interpretation breaks down because of an error in translation, which rendered *nibbio* (kite) as "vulture."

4. Freud 1909b.

5. "Investigating has taken the place of acting and creating as well. A man who has begun to have an inkling of the grandeur of the universe with all its complexities and its laws readily forgets his own insignificant self. Lost in admiration and filled with true humility, he all too easily forgets that he himself is a part of those active forces and that in accordance with his personal strength the way is open for him to try to alter a small portion of the destined course of the world—a world in which the small is still no less wonderful than the great" (1910c, pp. 75f).

6. See Ferenczi, "Zur Ontogenie des Geldinteresses" [The Ontogenesis of the Interest in Money] (1914, 146; *C.*, p. 319), in which—according to Freud in letter 140—he characterized hypochondria as a "fermentation product of anal erotism" (*C.*, p. 323; *Schriften* I, 200).

140

Vienna, June 7, 1910
IX., Berggasse 19

Dear friend,

Our letters have crossed each other. Don't worry about Leonardo. For a long time now I have been writing only for the small circle that enlarges daily, and if the others didn't get angry over Leonardo, I would have gone astray in my judgment about him. It is also a matter of indifference what these others are now saying. We will all get more thanks and posthumous fame from ΨA than is good for us at present, while we are at work.

Our colleagues seem to like Leonardo. Pfister has become a visionary through him and sees the outline of a vulture in the white cloth around the body of Mary[1] (test: Where is the cat?)[2] and gets stuck with the correspondence of γυψ *(Geier)* [vulture] and *Gyps* [gypsum]. The latter is, unfortunately, superfluous; the former seems possible to me. Pfister has become perspicacious through his homologous mother complex.

So you have direct news from Brill. I expect you in Vienna when he is there; we can talk about the trip then. My mood is good in spite of the heat; I hope to have made my large intestine travelworthy by that time.

You now seem to be on the way to a great discovery if you can show that *hypochondria* is a fermentation product of *anal erotism*; in other words, that it relates to hypochondria in a similar way as does sadism to obsessional neurosis. If you yourself seem to be paralyzed in your energy by admiration, I will see to it that you feel yourself to be part of a power[3] again.

Kindest regards,
Freud

1. See Oskar Pfister, "Kryptolalie, Kryptographie und unbewusstes Vexierbild bei Normalen" [Cryptophasia, Cryptography, and the Unconscious Puzzle Picture], *Jahrbuch* 5, 1st half-volume (1913): 117–156; cited by Freud in *Leonardo* in a footnote added in 1919 (1910c, pp. 115f). Freud's impression of the color is based on a black and white reproduction. The cloth is actually blue in the original.

2. The reference is to a picture puzzle; see the unpublished letter of Freud to Pfister of June 9, 1910, Library of Congress.

3. See letter 35, n. 2 [Trans.].

141

Dear Professor,

The exotic stationery[1] can be explained by the fact that today, Sunday, I am visiting Frau G.—She sends warm regards.

I found Pfister's vulture at first glance—it is really amazing.

One is astonished not to have found the bird oneself—although one has this feeling with all discoveries. Your Leonardo makes a deep impression even on those who already essentially knew its content.—There are so many ideas distributed among the few pages that they give one something to think about for weeks.—This first psychoanalytic pathography (Sadger's Lenau[2] is too oversimplified) will serve as a model for all time. The explanation of your philosophy of life made the deepest impression on me: willful subordination under the rule of "Ἀνάγκη."[3]

Something occurred to me yesterday: the myth of Deucalion and Pyrrha about the story of the origin of man[4] is the mythological explanation of the infantile "Lumpf" theory (humans originate from bones (garbage)[5] which *are thrown backward between the legs*).

The question of hypochondria is occupying me constantly. It really appears as though anal erotism and sadism are at the base of *hypochondria + obsession*—; I encounter this etiological mixture again and again in a case where these two states are combined.—

I still have the Pressburg case in treatment (Zayda); his paranoia has become more transparent to me—not to him!

I will bring along a very interesting case of *circular alternation of sadism and masochism* for the trip.

I find Adler's expression "masculine protest"[6] prejudicial.

I am discharging the first cured case of severe obsessional neurosis in the next few days.

As you can see, I am completely busy—but as you guessed correctly, the courses have taken too much out of me; there are only eight days left of them. I am not completely satisfied with the "material" provided by the auditors.

If Brill comes, I will go to Vienna for a Sunday. I am looking forward to seeing you again.—

Perhaps Jung has been upset by the founding of the Zentralblatt.[7]—In any case, it is good to keep two irons in the fire, and the competition between Vienna and Zurich can do the cause good. Vienna now has the advantage!

Kind regards,
Ferenczi

1. The letter is written on very small folded sheets of pale green paper with a watermark. Ferenczi had used the same stationery once before (letter 40).
2. Isidor Sadger, *Aus dem Liebesleben Nicolaus Lenaus* [From the Love Life of Nicolas Lenau], *Schriften zur angewandten Seelenkunde* 6 (1909).
3. "Fate." Freud 1910c, p. 125; see also letter 99 and n. 6.
4. According to this Greek myth Deucalion, son of Prometheus, and his wife, Pyrrha, were the only two survivors of the Flood. The new human race consisted of the stones that were thrown behind them, the "bones of the great mother" Earth.
5. Parentheses in the original.
6. On June 8, at the conclusion of a debate in the Wednesday Society on the harmfulness of masturbation, Adler had termed it a form of "masculine protest" (*Minutes* II, 569ff). The concept of masculine protest was destined to play a central role in Adler's individual psychology.
7. See letter 126, n. 1.

142

Vienna, June 20, 1910
IX., Berggasse 19

Dear friend,

I naturally cannot examine this Hungarian girl and am sending her to you. She was sent to me for hysteria, but in the meantime I notice facial paresis[1] of the right side and biting of the tongue, and I am not sure of the diagnosis.

Cordially,
Freud

1. Paralysis.

143

Budapest, June 27, 1910
VII., Erzsébet-körút 54

Dear Professor,

The stomach pains that I began to feel last year at this time are making their presence known again. But I was warned—and two days' diet has put everything back in order. Unfortunately, they happened to be the days that I wanted to use for the trip to Vienna; I would like to hope that the brother complex had nothing to do with this stomach trouble.

You have learned from Brill details about the sudden end of the American adventure[1]—which was certainly hopeless from the beginning. I am actually glad; the man would have given me too much to do. Incidentally, he behaved quite nicely.

The Hungarian-Jewish patient whom you sent me is a Jacksonian epilepsy;[2] the ophthalmologist to whom I sent her saw the attack (cramps on the right side—localized to that of the facial paralysis). I sent her home, prescribed mercury, then iodine, and told her to come back in six weeks.

The trip in the fall is the main object of my daydreams, which I catch myself at during some of the more monotonous analyses. I, too, am beginning—to count the days. Unfortunately, I have too many of them!

Brill's presence[3] hindered the otherwise very refreshing scientific and personal talk with you. I must console myself with the fall.

You were right when you advised me not to limit the idea of the pathological significance of the "latency period" to the "small penis" and "big mama" complex.[4] I find almost daily new points of departure for maintaining that this significance is a much more general one.—

Please write me how you are and how the evening on the Hill of Constantine[5] went.

Kindest regards,
Dr. Ferenczi

A Hungarian artist donated 159 *very beautiful* Roman glass pieces to the local "Industrial Arts Museum." I must show them to you next time you come to Budapest.

1. Possibly a reference to an American female patient on whom Brill had reported; see letters 139 and 141.
2. Focal-motor attacks, named after the English neurologist and epilepsy researcher John H. Jackson (1834–1911), the founder of modern neurophysiological theories.
3. See letter 144.
4. Ferenczi had evidently talked with Freud about his work "Über obszöne Worte, Beitrag zur Psychologie der Latenzzeit" [On Obscene Words] (1911, 75; *C.*, p. 132), in which he cited these complexes as examples for the assertion that "the latency period actually brings about an isolated inhibition in the development of individual repressed complexes" (*Schriften* I, 68; *C.*, p. 148).
5. The traditional celebration at the end of the work year; see letter 64, n. 4.

144

Vienna, July 3, 1910
IX., Berggasse 19

Dear friend,

The brother complex ought not to have upset your stomach. The evening did not come into being because Brill wished to be free of his burden as quickly as possible and therefore wanted to leave Monday morning. It is useless, however, to bring people together on Sunday, for everyone is then uncomfortable staying over. So I didn't do it. I will gladly satisfy your curiosity as to how things are here. We are quite exhausted and in considerable perplexity about the summer. We sent an advance guard, consisting of an aunt and two trifles,[1] to Dr. Jekels in Bistrai, and the two elders then wanted to follow on August 1 and send the boys off to adventures in the meantime. But we found out that Bistrai doesn't have enough room, and nothing else is going right, either. The boys, including Martin, were unable to find lodging, and so I called it off with Jekels and am at a loss as to what to do. The both of us will probably go to a Dutch boardinghouse in the Hague with two boys and will do a bit of sightseeing in the cities until there is room by the sea, and the other party is still looking for shelter in Germany somewhere along the way. As for myself, I am already quite exhausted, and I even refrained from work for a day because of a fever. But it was an attack of sinus infection. My intestine is doing much better, but this is not the time for a restoration. All hopes are concentrating themselves on the September trip, which should be the subject for warm reflections later.—Work has been reduced by only one hour and naturally ends with a bang on the 14th.

Hoche's lecture in the Berlin clinic was amusing and has received the greatest recognition to date.[2]

A few days ago the first editorial session[3] took place, and everything was still very disorganized. Perhaps people can't be changed. A critique of Stekel's about Neutra's book had to be confiscated on account of florid indignation.[4] The Jahrbuch[5] is still not here. Jung is writing much about a work of his which I found some fault with.[6] Everything is getting a bit stuck.

I will write to you as soon as I know more about our plans, then about three other works, the germ of which I am carrying around in me. Best regards to Frau G.

Cordially,
Freud

1. Minna Bernays and Sophie and Anna Freud.

2. Alfred Hoche, "Eine psychische Epidemie unter Ärzten" (Vortrag auf der Wanderversammlung der Südwestdeutschen Neurologen und Irrenärzte), address delivered in Baden-Baden, May 28, 1910; see *Medizinische Klinik*, June 26, 1910, pp. 1007–10. Hoche, (1865–1943), professor of psychiatry at Freiburg in Breisgau and one of the bitterest opponents of psychoanalysis among the German psychiatrists, had railed in his lecture against the "strange medical frenzy movement" of psychoanalysis and its "dragging out the sexual" [*Hinzerren auf das Sexuelle*], and had also termed it a "medically prohibited" method from which one should "dissociate oneself most emphatically."

3. Of the newly founded *Zentralblatt.*

4. The review of William Neutra's *Briefe an nervöse Frauen* [Letters to Neurotic Women], 2d ed. (Dresden, 1909), was finally written up by Freud himself (1910m) and published in the *Zentralblatt* 1 (1910–11): 49f (*Nachtragsband*, p. 500). An agreement was reached between Freud as editor and Adler and Stekel as associate editors that each would have veto power over the publication of a text. Stekel believed, incidentally, that Freud's first veto had been exercised not against this review but against his paper "Die Verpflichtung des Namens" [The Obligation of a Name], *Zeitschrift für Psychotherapie und medizinische Psychologie* 3 (1911); see *The Autobiography of Wilhelm Stekel* (New York, 1950), p. 131.

5. Volume 2, first half.

6. See letter 126, n. 5. Freud's critique and Jung's response are in *Freud/Jung*, ca. June 22 and June 26, 1910, pp. 332–337.

145

Budapest, July 9, 1910
VII., Erzsébet-körút 54

Dear Professor,

My birthday the day before yesterday—my 37th—released a few thoughts in me that I don't want to keep secret from you, first of all because I know that you are interested in my personal fate, and second, because they are—I believe—of general interest. The thoughts are a continuation of your pessimistic line of reasoning about the immutability and unchanging nature of men.—I must contradict it.—I have already often thanked you for beautifying my profession, in fact, my whole life, through the ψ-analytic way of looking at things. But if I compare my inner psychic existence before and after ψ. α. insight, I must regard the most valuable thing to be precisely that inner change that you deny. It was only through Ψα. that I became a man from a child, only since its mastery in me can I better subordinate the "pleasure principle" to the "reality principle" and better inhibit the senseless waste of affect. Infantile sensitivity plays a much smaller role in me than before; I have more or less reconciled myself to the thought of dying and being ill. I learned to treat and regard human beings as sick people, and I bear them no ill will because of their malice: they can't help it. I inhibit ambitious daydreams by tracing them back to their infantile roots.

I am also more optimistic than you in another respect. I believe that ψα. honesty can be effected, not only among friends but also among life's companions of various genders. The analytic association with Frau G. is making decided progress, after at times overcoming very great resistances.—As the "ménage à trois" on the George Washington[1] became a signficant experience for me and provided the occasion for unshackling my infantile complexes, so did the visit of a sister from Italy[2] prove to be a ferment for Frau G., which activated her heretofore inadmissible impulses of jealousy, hate, etc. *Two people* get along easily. It is not until one gets to *three* that one constitutes a small society, with all of its positive and negative passions. The family: father, mother, child or father and two brothers—is the primal type of a society, a "mikrodemos," and at the same time the school of later social life.—It will take a while before Frau G. has overcome the turmoil; but her love is stronger than the unpleasure that the analysis arouses in her, and she will pass the test of endurance.

The persecution of blacks in America reminds me of the case that Jung so sagely presented, according to which the blacks represent the "unconscious" of the Americans.[3] Thus, the hate, the reaction formation against one's own vices. Along with the circumcision/castration complex, this mechanism could also be the basis for *anti-Semitism*. The free, "fresh" behavior of the Jew, his "shameless" flaunting of his interest in money, evokes hatred as a reaction formation in Christians, who are ethical not for logical reasons but out of repression. It is only since my analysis that I have understood the widespread Hungarian saying: *"I hate him like my sins."*

I always find renewal and confirmation in our Anatole France. Today I found the following great passage in "L'Anneau d'Améthyste"[4]:

"Pecus" (that's what he calls the masses)—"Pecus est nourri de mensonges antiques. Son aptitude à l'erreur est considérable. Se sentant peu propre à dissiper par la raison les préjugés héréditaires, il conserve prudemment l'héritage de fables que lui viennent des aïeux. Cette espèce de sagesse le garde des erreurs qui lui seraient trop nuisibles. Il s'en tient aux erreurs éprouvées. Il est imitateur; il le paraîtrait davantage, s'il ne déformait involontairement ce qu'il copie. Ces déformations produisant ce qu'on appelle le progrès. Pecus ne réfléchit pas. Aussi est-il injuste de dire qu'il se trompe. Mais tout le trompe et il est misérable. Il ne doute jamais, puisque le doute est l'effet de la réflexion. Pourtant ses idées changent sans cesse. Et parfois il passe de la stupidité à la violence. Il n'a nulle excellence, car tout ce qui excelle se détache immédiatement de lui et cesse de lui appartenir. Mais il erre, il languit, il souffre. Et il faut lui garder une profonde et douloureuse sympathie. Il convient même de le vénérer, parce que c'est de lui que sortent tout vertu, toute beauté, toute gloire humaine. Pauvre Pecus."[5]

If psychoanalysis is a paranoia, then I have already been successful in overcoming the stage of persecution mania and replacing it with megalomania. You see, I find our opponents in no way different from Anatole France's *pecus*.

The odyssey of your scattered family will, I hope, end pleasantly, and everyone will soon see the Dutch sea resort, happily reunited. I also have more peaceful times from Monday on: two patients are going on vacation. Every day I think frequently about our approaching vacation; please entrust dear Oli with the task of studying the timetables.

Cordial regards to all.

Obediently yours,
Ferenczi

Frau G. thanks you for remembering her.

1. During walks on the deck of the *George Washington* on their trip to America, Freud, Ferenczi, and Jung had analyzed one another.

2. Sarolta Morando, née Altschul (see Ferenczi/Groddeck, July 8, 1922, *Briefwechsel*, p. 44).

3. In his "Report on America" at the Nuremberg Congress, Jung had spoken about the American "Negro complex." According to Rank's record in the *Zentralblatt* I (1910–11): 130, Jung was of the opinion that "living together with the Negro . . . [had a] suggestive [effect] on the laboriously subdued instincts of the white race" which made it necessary for whites to take "defensive measures."

4. Novel written in 1899. The quotation has been edited in accordance with the Calmann-Lévy edition (Paris 1899), pp. 261f.

5. *Pecus* [Latin for "sheep" or "cattle"] "is nourished by lies brought from long ago. Its ability to err is considerable. Since it feels itself little suited to destroy its inherited prejudices through reason, it carefully preserves the inheritance in fairy tales that have come over to it from its ancestors. This kind of wisdom protects it from errors that could harm it. It clings to the preserved errors. It is an imitator; one would be better aware of that fact if it did not involuntarily distort what it copies. These distortions then produce what one calls progress. *Pecus* does not reflect. Thus, it is also unjust to claim that it deceives itself. But it is deceived by everything and it feels miserable. It never doubts, because doubt is, after all, a consequence of reflection. Its ideas change constantly, however. And sometimes it goes from stupidity to violence. It has nothing outstanding, for everything that is outstanding is immediately detached from it and then no longer belongs to it. But it wanders around, it yearns, it suffers. And one must maintain a deep, painful sympathy with it. It is even appropriate that one honors it, for all virtue, all beauty, and all human fame emanate from it. Poor *Pecus*."

146

Vienna, July 10, 1910
IX., Berggasse 19

Dear friend,

Did I really ever doubt that persons like you could develop themselves? I think my pessimism had more to do with the weak people whom we are supposed to change through our influence, not those who can bring about something from themselves, with the support of external influences.

I am glad that you are already as far along as I am in relation to our opponents. Isn't it best that way? Paranoia certainly contradicts inner contentment. The paranoid is dissatisfied and must continually restructure. To change the subject, your work on paranoia must go forward once and for all; it will be material for the time when we are together.

My address from the 17th until the end of July is Hotel Wittebrug, The Hague. I am going with Oli and Ernst; my wife will stay here and then go to Hamburg. On August 1 there will be a big reunion in Noordwijk. Only four more days of work; I am very pleased about that, but I still have some things to work out.

I am straining hard to restore my health to the point where our plans for the fall won't be disrupted. I, too, am not doing badly. Great progress was certainly not possible during the time of intense work. As soon as we are settled by the sea, I will begin to approach you with suggestions.

You have doubtless read Hoche?

I, too, gratefully acknowledge the elevation of life through ΨA. A more complete view of life should certainly be based on it. Now is not the time, in the fatigue of year's end.

I send kindest regards and hope to hear from you soon.

Yours,
Freud

147

Dear Professor,

According to the information I received, a ship of the *North German Lloyd* is leaving from Antwerp with the following route:

from	Antwerp	Aug. 29
"	Southhampton	Aug. 30
"	Gibraltar	Sept. 3
"	Algiers	Sept. 4
"	Genoa	Sept. 8
arr.	Naples	Sept. 9

As soon as you are in a position to decide, we will have to make reservations.

More next time.

Kind regards.

Yours,
Ferenczi

1. In the original, the date is at the end of the letter; no address is given.

148

[Postmark: 'sGravenhage,]
July 17, 1910[1]

Just arrived. Received your suggestion, agreed in principle, please give more information.

Cordially,
Freud
Hotel Wittebrug

[In different handwriting]
Best regards,
Ernst

1. Picture postcard. The caption reads: "'sGravenhage [The Hague], Binnenhof met Ridderzaal."

149

Budapest, July 22, 1910
VII., Erzsébet-körút 54

Dear Professor,

It is terribly hot in Budapest now. I have to bathe twice a day in cold water in order to stay halfway capable of working.

At Adler's request I put together a paper about the Hungarian psychiatric literature of the last few years.[1] I soon noticed (despite the greatest restraint) that I will not be able to avoid making those colleagues who have heretofore only been opponents into enemies through my critiques. They just write too much stupid stuff!—The Zentralblatt will serve us well; it will hold up well as a defensive, and especially as an offensive, weapon, in addition, of course, to having the advantage of being able to publish works of smaller caliber more quickly.

The medical periodicals are now going absolutely wild in opposition to you and the whole movement. Hoche's article had a liberating effect on the spirits who, out of prudence, have not dared to rebel against us up to now. My friend Dr. Schächter, for instance, whom Ψα. has heretofore "given something to think about"—all of a sudden sees clear as day that we are the victims of a colossal self-deception.

On the other hand, I get much joy from a young scholar, a physicist and a first-rate thinker whom I acquainted with your works and who subsequently, with the aid of autoanalysis, recovered from a severe neurosis to the extent that he became capable of work.—It's too bad that he lives in Klausenburg; he would be a pillar of our branch society.

In the meantime I have been unable to learn any more about our travel plans. You are closer to reliable sources there in The Hague; perhaps Oli or Ernst (whom I thank kindly for the greeting) will take the trouble to inquire at a North German Lloyd travel agency.

Near the end of August we are having a *Hungarian* "hiker's meeting of physicians and natural scientists" right in Miskolcz, my hometown; my friend Docent Schächter is one of the organizers of this congress. I couldn't absent myself, and I also agreed to give a lecture, with the title *Psychoanalysis and Homosexuality*.[2] But the audience at this congress is not the right forum for this lecture. I will therefore probably cancel or talk about a less difficult topic.

I hope that you are already very well—and I do so not only for egoistic reasons. As much as I yearn to wander through Sicily in your company, I must nevertheless ask you to be guided in your decision only by considerations of your health. Should you suggest something else instead of Sicily, I will also gladly go along. It would be very, very painful to have to give up the trip altogether—of course, I would have to reconcile myself with this eventuality if your condition or other personal circumstances demanded it.

For the time being I live in the certain hope of having the pleasure of seeing you soon and, with cordial greetings to your family, I remain

Yours,
Ferenczi

1. Ferenczi, "Aus der ungarischen neurologischen-psychiatrischen Literatur," *Zentralblatt* 1 (1910–11): 74–78.
2. See letter 164. The Hungarian physicians and natural scientists had been meeting for thirty years in such gatherings, which took place every year at a different location (*Orvosi Hetilap* 35 [1912]: 657).

150

Hotel Wittebrug, July 25, 1910

Dear friend,

Immediately after the receipt of your letter I got the information from the agency in The Hague and can report to you the following about the trip.

On August 29 the Yorck leaves from Antwerp (not Rotterdam) for East Asia and takes on passengers as far as Genoa or Naples. It stops in Southampton, Gibraltar, Algiers, and arrives at Genoa on the 8th and at

Naples on the 9th. The price is 396 marks first class, perhaps somewhat more or less (certain details). From Genoa we could also go with an Italian or other ship directly to Palermo, just as you wish. I would be totally involved, my health would not suffer, I am already very much recovered, my colitis much better; I would not pass anything up on account of a little constipation. There remains a certain risk in making reservations weeks ahead of time and risking 200 marks each, but that can hardly be avoided. The only thing that could disrupt our travel plans is what happens in Hamburg, where the old woman is wretchedly decrepit. I am certainly not directly affected by this to the extent that, for example, I would have to go to Hamburg, but if the end came right during those days—it could still drag on for months—it would naturally be painful for me to leave the women alone just then. So if you want to risk it, give me permission to reserve two cabins here. I have no way of judging if the demand for these trips is great or small. My brother, who is also here, thinks it is not great, since those who actually travel to Asia make the trip by rail.

I have sensed even more interest in your scientific innovations. Hoche has amused me very much and shaken me very little. Deuticke asks that I write a preface to the second edition of the Collection, First Series,[1] which has now become necessary; maybe I will make a funny essay about opponents and resistance out of it, but very gently, because I am in a good mood.

At present I can't easily imagine heat. It is cold here, it rains several times a day, a mean wind is blowing from the sea, but we bathe every day and are very comfortable in The Hague. My boys are behaving very respectably and are already good company.

Antwerp is only three hours from The Hague, i.e., Leyden. Perhaps you will thus pick me up a day earlier in Noordwijk, or we won't meet until Antwerp.

With kind regards and in expectation of hearing from you soon,

Yours truly,
Freud

P.S. Here until Sunday the 31st, then Noordwijk, Hotel Noordzee.

1. *Sammlung kleiner Schriften zur Neurosenlehre*, 1st ser., 2d ed. (1911). Freud never published any such preface.

151

Budapest, July 25, [1910][1]
VII., Erzsébet-körút 54

Dear Professor,

A gentleman who recently made the trip Bremen–Antwerp–Gibraltar–Genoa gave me the enclosed brochure.

From the also enclosed official schedule of North German Lloyd you see (from the line underlined in blue) the timetable of the ship that is right for us. The ship is supposed to be large and comfortable (it goes to Yokohama), the service excellent.

We can perhaps get a ticket only as far as Gibraltar, where we would arrive on September 3. There we could wait for the North German Lloyd steamer "Berlin," which goes to America and arrives punctually on September 4, and then we could go *directly to Naples*, where we would arrive on September 7. That would mean gaining two days for Sicily and sparing us the superfluous trip to Genoa and back. There is always enough room on the "Berlin." On the other hand, many Englishmen travel to the Orient (Egypt, India) with the German postal service steamer, so one has to make timely reservations. The best are (naturally) the upper-deck cabins; the middle-deck cabins are good—but the ones on the lower deck are bad. One should (according to my reliable source) ask for cabins with windows opening directly on the sea.

That is what I wanted to bring to your attention and will be able to share with you in all haste.

Best regards,
Ferenczi

1. In the original the date is given at the end of the letter, without the year. The letter has been placed in sequence based on its content.

152

Budapest, July 27, 1910
VII., Erzsébet-körút 54

Dear Professor,

Our—quite identical—letters crossed each other. I am hurrying so that my reply will still get to you in The Hague.

I am happy that you have recovered to such an extent in such a short time, in and for itself, as well as with regard to our travel plans. It goes without saying that I can in no way influence your decision and declare myself in agreement with your arrangements at the outset. I.e., I request that you also make arrangements in my name with regard to the cabin at whatever time and in whatever manner you deem appropriate. I ask you—if you make the decision in the affirmative—to pay the 200 marks for me.—

If the trip does materialize, I will pick you up in Noordwijk, if at all possible.

I hope I'm not disturbing you too much in your vacation mood by also "talking shop" in my letters.—

In a collection of litarary critiques by our Anatole France (La Vie Litteraire. *4 volumes*) I found a short newspaper article titled "Les fous—dans la littérature" [The Insane in Literature] (from the year 1887). He speaks so clearly and understandably, and at the same time so beautifully and sagely there about the functional psychoses that I asked Adler to translate the little essay for the Zentralblatt.[1]

I want to put on paper a few strange experiences about things that correspond to one another that came to my mind and that of a patient (belonging to the *Seidler* documents) and send them to you.

The analysis of the young man from Pressburg (paranoia) shows that the draft accords of Berchtsgaden were *completely* correct. Projection, negative sign, failed withdrawal of interest—everything makes sense and can be genetically traced. Homosexuality has been inserted between the nuclear complex and paranoia. What is interesting in this patient is the reciprocal representation of obsession and mania.

The triad: hypochondria–miserliness–anal erotism is becoming increasingly clear and understandable.

I have a case that will perhaps aid in explaining *masochism*.
I greet all your dear ones and await news.

Yours,
Ferenczi

1. Anatole France, *Les fous dans la littérature*, in *La vie littéraire* (Paris, 1888–1892). Ferenczi translated parts of this work for his article "Anatole France als Psychoanalytiker" (1911, 76) in the *Zentralblatt* 1 (1910–11): 461–467.

153

Noordwijk, August 2, 1910

Dear friend,

I am writing you just after a glowing red sunset from the breezy balcony of our apartment in the Pension Noordzee, where we arrived yesterday morning after we three[1] had drawn the other members of the family to us. My sister-in-law stayed in Hamburg, where our old mother is slowly expiring from marasmus, behind which an intestinal carcinoma is also concealed.[2] Despite all our recognition of the inevitability of dying, this brings about a serious mood and disturbs the contentment which would normally accompany a sojourn such as this. For years I have been following a certain pattern in a vacation: in the first days after stopping work very cheerful and well, then after about two weeks I get into the real misery of exhaustion that understandably goes along with the end of the work year, and I also behaved this way recently and am writing you today in this very mood. It is an unedifying condition, something like when one can't fall asleep and is still too tired to wake up. I feel as though the remnants of work leave me no peace; what I would need is to collect myself in order seriously to get to work, but I am completely incapable of accomplishment. I think, certainly, that walks in the beautiful, dense woods would allow me to collect myself, but that is probably a deception, for I have sea and dunes in front of me and can blame my laziness on their influence. In reality I can't do anything now, not even enjoy the rest which the situation really requires, and I have to wait and see.

So I haven't done a thing to confirm our trip on the Yorck. Excuse: if Grandmother's death coincides precisely with our departure, my wife would have to go to Hamburg and the children would be alone when we would have to move out of our lodgings. There could even be something in this; the main thing, in any case, is my reluctance to do anything, to decide, for instance, whether to continue this letter now, for which the increasing darkness again offers good excuses.

More in the morning.

Aug. 3

In reality, it is beginning to get terribly pleasant here, a kind of primitive luxuriousness in the house, and nature, which holds everything that one expects from her. Matters with our trip should also stay the way we decided. I agree that you should leave all the arrangements to me, and I will now see if I can decide to make an early commitment. This week I will go to an office of North German Lloyd and will confirm our requirements. I heard that one can always find room from Antwerp to Genoa, since serious passengers don't get on until then. In Genoa we will easily find another ship to Palermo. Leaving out Genoa would also, I think, entail the same for Algiers, and one really would like to have been in Africa. If I can't decide to commit myself, then, when the time comes, you could come to Noordwijk; we will try the same route or another, whatever the situation permits, and we will keep our objective.

I almost forgot to tell you that the most unexpected company awaits me for the middle of the month. Jones is participating in the congress in Brussels[3] and on August 8 is arriving here, where his sister-in-law[4] owns a villa. It's a small world.

The little ones arrived here in mint condition; they will all be happy to see you, and we will all talk much with one another.

Best regards,
Freud

My best to Frau G.

1. Freud and his two younger sons, Oliver and Ernst.
2. Freud's mother-in-law, Emmeline Bernays, died October 27.
3. The first congress of the International Society for Medical Psychology and Psychotherapy, founded in 1909 by Auguste Forel, Oskar Vogt (see letter 221, n. 8), and Ludwig Frank, which took place in Brussels on August 7–8, 1910. Freud had been invited by Vogt to give a lecture, but he turned down the invitation (*Freud/Jung*, March 2, 1910, p. 300).
4. A sister of Loe Kann, possibly named Hortense, had a house in Noordwijk (personal communication from Andrew Paskauskas). Kann and Jones were not married but presented themselves as a married couple.

154

Noordwijk, August 9, 1910

Dear friend,

Only a few words to keep you current. I have reserved two cabins to Genoa from the North German Lloyd agency in The Hague of the quality which you emphasized, and I am now waiting to hear if we can get them. The deposit is, fortunately, small and not yet made. If it works out that way, it would be nice if you could come here early enough so that we have one more day for Antwerp and Bruges; the latter is supposed to be incomparably worth seeing. You remember that the ship leaves from Anvers on the 29th. Don't forget to bring along a Baedeker for southern Italy, latest edition, when the trip is confirmed.

There is no change in Hamburg; very pleasant here, but I am completely incapable of accomplishment. I am very well physically. I am very annoyed about the Jahrbuch; it is invisible; Stekel and Hitschmann seem to be working enthusiastically. Jones is supposed to come day after tomorrow, and he will probably awaken me from my summer sleep.

Kind regards,
Freud

155

Budapest, August 10, 1910
VII., Erzsébet-körút 54

Freudtòl
visszakèrtem ès kaptam
910. november[1]

Dear Professor,

Both halves of your last—very detailed and kind—letter gave me not only precise explanations of the chances for our vacation trip and about your internal and external situation but also renewed confirmation of an observation that can very freqently be made. The letter that you wrote late in the evening of August 2 is pervaded by distinct depression as well as by a feeling of indecision, of "laziness," as you express it. You look for pretexts to avoid all kinds of decisions.—The postscript sounds quite different: you find the dunes "terribly pleasant," whereas the day before you were still sorely missing the forests of the Alps. You make up your mind to go to Leyden in order to commit yourself early to the trip; on the day before you were—according to what you said in the letter—worlds away from even thinking about this active intervention into the course of events.

I know that this observation is banal. But it is still not explained, no more than are the normal periodic swings of emotional life that return with astronomical punctuality. I am thinking here not at all of Fliess's periods, but rather of the well-known fact that there is such a thing as a morning, afternoon, evening, and night mood.

I have often reflected on this matter and have gathered observations in me and in my patients, and I have come to the conclusion that this question cannot be settled by light (sun) and by physiology alone. It could have to do with the daily buildup and destruction of a complicated psychological edifice whose foundations may certainly be purely physiological. I find the physiological basis in sexuality and think about the matter somewhat like this: every movement, every bodily sensation and every sense arousal, indeed, every phase of metabolism has a pleasurable component (one could say that the entire external and internal body is *one* erogenous zone, only that there is a different emphasis at different locations). These accumulate from morning till evening and bring the complexes of the ucs. associated with them to constantly increasing arousal. The biological aim of this process seems to be preparation for the sexual act, which is, by nature, carried out at night.[2] But the arousal can also be sublimated; it can be lived out in work, in fantasies, in artistic enjoyment, etc. In the evening the fantasy is incomparably more lively and more productive; every kind of intellectual production goes much more smoothly in the evening (worse, by contrast, is purely mechanical, mindless work, e.g., calculation).

Sleeping (along with its psychic parallel process, the dream) makes all these states of arousal disappear (under normal conditions). That, and not rest, is the main function of sleep and of the dream. The physiologists say: in sleep, processes of reorganization take place in elements of tissue which are decomposed by activity. We, however, see that the best-protected rest cannot replace sleep and dreaming. I believe that there occurs in the course of the night a kind of *decomposition* of those chemical compounds that cause the pleasurable components of the day's existence to be stored up. Sleep is thus a gradual sexual leveling-off, prolonged for several hours, a kind of coitus equivalent, and *for that reason* every dream is a wish fulfillment, i.e., the ψ. parallel process of this slackened sexual leveling-off. The *content* of dreams is naturally influenced by the complexes and experiences of people.

At night the path of the sublimations (as in neuroses and psychoses) seems to be difficult to travel: the erogenous zones achieve direct connection with the organ of consciousness (censorship-sleep) by regressively reviving the remnants of childhood.

The diminished need for sleep in old people would speak in favor of the connection of depth of sleep (and duration) on the one hand and sexual arousability on the other. But how do we explain, in light of this assumption, the extraordinary need for sleep in infants? Or can there perhaps be a further consequence of this that infantile (and embryonic) development (growth) occurs with the aid of the same chemical agents that are later designated to procreate the race?[3]

This time I want to give free rein to my fantasy and speculate further.—

I refer to the analogy of a theory (certainly rejected by many) of *heredity* with my assumption of the summation of pleasurable components from all organs. This is the hypothetical process (called *pangenesis*, if I remember correctly) whereby every cell of the body provides a material (or dynamic) contribution to the construction of every germ cell. In that way it then becomes a matter of "growth over and above the individual," in other words, of the reproduction of individual characteristics.

Of course, I am not confusing the gradual development of sperm and egg cells with the periodic need for discharge and fertilization, respectively. These two processes must, however, be intimately connected somewhere, probably in chemism.

Pathology shows that sleep and sexuality belong inwardly together. Strangely enough, however, satisfaction brings on sleep, and dissatisfaction sleeplessness. But I believe that one can find without difficulty an explanation for this that does not contradict the sexual-chemical theory of sleep and dreaming.

A personal observation:
I never have sexual intercourse at *night*—always only in the morning. But one is "sober" in the morning; the compulsionlike urge (i.e., a part of the libido) is missing in the act. But if one still lets oneself be enraptured to moderate excesses, one becomes almost incapable of work during the day because of neurasthenic parasthesias, headache, heaviness in the legs, etc. I.e., the act had the character of masturbation. The satisfaction, as well as potency, was *incomparably greater,* and, in fact, devoid of the slightest pathological reaction if the act was carried out without exception in the late afternoon.

The argument that castrates (eunuchs, oxen) also sleep, and that the former also dream, does not prove anything to the contrary; the "erogenous zones" would still be in their possession, and they would remain sources of sexual arousal. [It would be interesting to learn something about the dreams of castrates.][4]

If, after these fantasies (for whose adventuresomeness I am fully accountable) I return to the point of departure of my letter, then I think to myself that the tragic mood that one often falls into toward evening and that makes everything appear in a more elegiac light is essentially identical with the infantile fear and anxiety during the night hours; both are reactions to the insufficiently usable libido which has accumulated from all sense zones in the course of the day. At night the unusable surplus is reduced—and so in the morning one becomes fresh and sober again, difficulties appear to one to be easily surmountable, one is in a good mood for all work (except that which requires fantasy).

A neurotic who can bear less libido would have to show all these things on an enlarged scale.

———————

Now, enough chatter. I want to talk about more sensible things again.

I can't tell you how sorry I am that your mother-in-law's illness so acutely disturbs the tranquillity of your vacation. Last year, America was bought at a high enough price; I hope this time you will be able to travel without external and internal hindrances.

I don't want to give up hope that it will be that way. But if it turns out otherwise, I ask you then to dispose of me as you see fit. I don't believe I have to tell you in particular that—as much as I would like to see Italy—I place a much smaller value on this trip than on being together with you, and that I would gladly be prepared to visit you anywhere at all. I would only dispense with the latter if you wished to be alone in consideration of your rest, health, or family.

Give my regards to all the dear members of your family. The distance does not permit me to appear with the usual supply of melons. Too bad, for we are having a superb year for melons.—We are now having cool, rainy fall weather. Italy certainly would be nice!

Regards also on behalf of Frau G.

Yours,
Ferenczi

Jahrbuch published! Very good!

Regards to colleague Jones (by whom a good paper on American literature was published in it, but without mention of Putnam's latest works and Stanley Hall's volume.)[5] But please don't tell him about my somewhat immature fantasies.

1. "Requested return by Freud, and received November 1910" (these three lines are written diagonally across the top of the page beneath Ferenczi's preprinted letterhead); see also letters 181 (next-to-last sentence before the closing) and 182.

2. A short time earlier Freud had presented a similar view, namely, that "the sexual and ego instincts alike have in general the same organs and systems of organs at their disposal" ("The Psycho-Analytic View of Psychogenic Disturbance of Vision," 1910i, pp. 215f). Ferenczi extended his thoughts further with the concept of "amphimixis of erotisms" in the act of ejaculation in *Thalassa: A Theory of Genitality* (1924, 268, p. 369; *Schriften* II, 321–334) and in "Organneurosen und ihre Behandlung" [Organ Neuroses and Their Treatment] (1926, 272; *Fin.*, p. 22).

3. See *Thalassa: A Theory of Genitality,* chap. 9, "Coitus and Sleep," pp. 200–207.

4. Enclosed in brackets in the original.

5. Ernest Jones, "Bericht über die neuere englische und amerikanische Literatur zur klinischen Psychologie und Psychopathologie," *Jahrbuch* 2, 1st half-volume (1910): 316–346. "Hall's volume" is *American Journal of Psychology* 21, no. 4 (1909–10), published by Stanley Hall, which was dedicated to psychoanalysis and in which Ferenczi's paper "Psychoanalyse der Träume" [On the Psychological Analysis of Dreams] (1909, 66; C., p. 94) appeared.

156

Budapest, August 11, 1910
VII., Erzsébet-körút 54

Dear Professor,

I gratefully confirm your latest news about the travel plan, which is now beginning to take more definite shape. Up to now the all-too great uncertainty was an obstacle in my ability to succumb uninhibitedly to a mood of expectation. Now I am beginning to concern myself more seriously with Baedeker and the timetable.

The Jahrbuch is very rich in content. Abraham's work is outstanding: clear, moderate, convincing. I find points of contact between my fantasies of yesterday about sleeping and dreaming and his explanation (read today) of "dream states."

Skipping over Jung, Maeder, and Pfister, I read for the time being only Jung's astute critique of Wittels's book and then the foreign reports from Italy and Russia. The latter are incomplete (mention of the Russian translation of Everyday Life[1] is missing). The Antithetical Sense of Primal Words (about which I was already informed in principle) never ceased to astound me in your paper.[2] We are still missing a competent philologist.

All in all, the Jahrbuch is very impressive; our opponents will certainly get thoroughly annoyed again.

As for myself, I am still stuck in contemplation; but I am full of good intentions, which now, of course, I can't actualize until fall.

I definitely hope to be in Antwerp one day before embarkation, and I am looking forward to the honorable city of Bruges.

I ask you for occasional (if brief) reports.

Yours,
Ferenczi

1. Published in 1910 in the translation by V. Medem.

2. The works he mentions are Abraham, "Über hysterische Traumzustände" [Hysterical Dream States]; Jung, "Über Konflikte der kindlichen Seele" [Psychic Conflicts in a Child]; Maeder, "Psychologische Untersuchungen an Dementia praecox-Kranken" [Psy-

chological Investigations in Dementia Praecox Cases]; Pfister, "Analytische Untersuchungen über die Psychologie des Hasses und der Versöhnung" [Analytic Investigation
of the Psychology of Hate and Reconciliation]; Jung, "Randbemerkungen zu dem Buch
von Wittels: Die sexuelle Not" [Marginal Notes on Wittels's Book *Die Sexuelle Not*];
Assagioli, "Die Freudschen Lehren in Italien" [Freud's Theories in Italy]; Neiditsch,
"Über den gegenwärtigen Stand der Freudschen Psychologie in Russland" [The Present
State of Freudian Psychology in Russia]; and Freud, "Über den Gegensinn der Urworte"
[The Antithetical Meaning of Primal Words].

157

Noordwijk, August 14, 1910

Dear friend,

It is not my fault, nor that of my hesitation, if I still can't tell you whether
we are passengers on the Yorck through Gibraltar. I was in The Hague and
reserved from a Lloyd agent there two cabins, upper deck, outside window,
confirmation of which would be sent to Noordwijk, whereupon payment
would follow; but after a few days I received a foolish, actually incomprehensible notification from him, so I went directly to Lloyd in Bremen. I am
enclosing the notification; I still have no answer from Bremen and don't
want to postpone any longer thanking you for your latest letters, which are
rich in content.

I think that the outcome of these negotiations will alter little in our
plans. You should come here as soon as possible, go with me to Antwerp
and Bruges, if time permits, and there either we will look for another ship
or we will decide on a trip over land, while we keep Sicily the objective of
our journey, and, as you say, our being together will be the main thing. I
hope you will find a happy solution to the mental dullness which is holding
me prisoner in my present state of great well-being.

Jones was here and laid intensive claim to me for two and a half days,
but he was kind and interesting. He left before your great letter. I was still
hoping to be able to show him the Jahrbuch, which Deuticke promised to
send me, but it's not here yet today. I am happy that you like it. Our
responses to all attacks should be of that sort.

Your fantasy didn't seem to me to be so unfounded according to the
present constellation; it certainly deserves more attention than I have
devoted to it up to now. We will talk about it, and I am looking forward to
a friend and traveling companion between whom and myself not a hint of
discord is possible. I also received yesterday an epistle from Jung[1] which
again shows him to be at his peak and in full possession of those qualities
which justified his election.

According to your wish I will communicate frequently about the situ-

ation here and ask you to make your trip as early as possible so that you
will still see something of Holland and my family.

Yours truly,
Freud

1. *Freud/Jung*, August 11, 1910, pp. 344–346.

158

Dear friend,

I am enclosing the letter that I received today from North German Lloyd
in Bremen. Leaving aside whether my hesitation or the ineptitude of the
agent in The Hague spoiled our chances with the Yorck, the fact of the
matter now is that we wouldn't be in Genoa before September 14 nor in
Palermo before the 10th, and we would therefore have too little time for
Sicily. Actually, with this objective in mind we would have been cutting
it close even five days earlier—with the Yorck. To pick out other ships
where accommodations and service are certainly not as good as with Lloyd
is perhaps not so enticing. In view of this it seems apparent that both
aims—Mediterranean cruise through Gibraltar and comfortable stay in
Sicily—are not easily compatible in the short time left at our disposal, and
it behooves us to give one of them up. I suggest to you that we give up the
Mediterranean and keep Sicily.

Many things speak against the cruise. We were on one not long ago and
are able to form an opinion. The trip from Antwerp to Genoa corresponds
to a ten-day-long imprisonment in a confined space. According to the letter
from Lloyd we can again get only two bad cabins, or we would have to
share a single better one. I know we would both feel confined. Think about
the fact that no ship would have such large rooms for the passengers as our
Washington, and that even there we didn't know what to do in the space
of a cabin. But inside cabins would probably be very uncomfortable in the
Mediterranean at the height of the summer. I also long to chat with you
and to do some work, and I know that one is quite cramped on a ship,
something like here by the sea. The freedom of innervation by one's surroundings seems to me to be a condition for intellectual activity.

Something else speaks in favor of giving up the cruise. If you come here
in the last week of August, you could still go swimming with us and then
at your leisure see Ghent, Bruges, and Brussels with us (for which we have
the Baedeker). Then a fast train would take us, e.g., from The Hague at 4:20
P.M. to Milan, 3 A.M. with sleeping car, and from there on to Rome, where
we would pause for one day in order to see the new excavations on the

Palatine[1] and the new monument on the Capitoline.[2] Then I would hold open the possibility that you might see Vesuvius and perhaps Pompeii for a day, and then we would soon be in Palermo and would in any case have a full three weeks for the beautiful island. We are free in any case to insert a shorter cruise on the Mediterranean if we wish, perhaps on the way back. I think we will gain time and freedom if we do without the voyage.

Should you come here at all if the itinerary is altered in this way? It is quite a bit of railway travel for you, but I think the two to three days in Holland and Brabant would be worth it, and the expenses don't come into consideration when compared with those of the voyage (330 marks). At the same time I haven't taken into account how happy we would all be about your coming. I calculate about a week for the entire first leg as far as Palermo.

So I put this itinerary before you. In a certain sense I have made the decision in the manner in which you transferred it to me; for if I had waited for your response, the opportuniity on the Seydlitz would probably have been lost, as was the earlier one on the Yorck. But if you prefer it that much, we could still try to get another booking from Antwerp at a time that suits us. My sympathies are strongly in favor of the land journey, not being tied down, with accommodations sprinkled in.

It would be very nice if you came here soon. Every day earlier means a possibility to see more and to move about freely.

Now on to other things: I got a letter from Putnam; he promises to bring the American society to life.[3] The Jahrbuch is still not here. I am already quite impatient to write something, but I have to be content with reading my very first works in corrected proof, which, however, please me with their naive freshness (the second edition of the Theory of the Neuroses).[4] We are all basically well; no change in Hamburg. Climate and bathing here are charming; I could almost say, along with Tannhäuser: I pine for adversity.[5] The very pleasant smoking also doesn't permit any real urge for activity to emerge.

I greet you cordially and count on your not staying away long after your reply.

Yours truly,
Freud

1. Presumably the excavations of the Italian archaeologist Rodolfo Lanciani (1847–1929).

2. Presumably the Roma Fountain.

3. See Putnam's letter of the end of July 1910 in Hale, *Putnam*, pp. 102–104. The American Psychoanalytic Association was founded on May 9, 1911.

4. See letter 150, n. 1.

5. Richard Wagner, *Tannhäuser*, act 1, sc. 2.

159

Noordwijk, August 17, 1910

Dear friend,

Postscript to yesterday's treatise. Today I spoke with the agent in The Hague on the telephone and learned that he had in fact reserved a double cabin for us on the Yorck (August 29) on the main deck, and thus fulfilled none of our stipulations. Travelers to Italy on these ships are given no choice, they don't get to know their number until they are on board; they are, so to speak, stopgaps. For this reason we will regret all the less having changed our minds.

Finally received the Jahrbuch. Very nice. Jung shows himself much to his advantage in his critiques and remarks about Wittels. He is too discreet and inhibited in his paper about his Agathli; the analyst has not yet overcome the father.[1] On the whole this volume is again a brilliant piece of countercriticism against Friedländer, Hoche, etc. If I knew, by the way, that the critiques in the Zentralblatt would show the same cheerful superiority as those by Jung here I would gladly remove its muzzle, but it seems more secure to me not to do that.

Cordially,
Freud

Enclosure: letter from Bremen.

1. In his essay (see letter 156, n. 2), Jung had described the case of his daughter.

160

Budapest, August 17, 1910
VII., Erzsébet-körút 54

Dear Professor,

This is not supposed to be a reply to your kind letter of today, only a notification that I will reply to you tomorrow.

I am sending you extracts from the Wiener klinische Rundschau[1] and a few "self-observations," which I request that you preserve.

Kind regards,
Ferenczi

[Enclosure]

August 17

A few recent observations
(on the theme of thought transference)

It has already frequently occurred to me that a patient, a homosexual with strong resistances and equally strong ucs. transference to me, sometimes includes things in his associations that occupy me with particular intensity. But I remained for a long time with this uncertain impression (which I also, incidentally, once communicated to Prof. Freud). Lately (in the face of resistance and transference which was becoming more and more intense) these correspondences were accumulating, so I decided to pursue the matter and note down precisely the individual occurrences.

1.) Note of July 25, 1910

The patient lies down as usual. But he immediately jumps up excitedly. "I smell a strong odor of phosphorus matches." "What kind of worms do you have on the couch?" "Shoemaker and laughing gas" [allusion to a Hungarian joke].[2] "Solom alechem. Salem Aleikum."

Observations [free association]:

I had sexual intercourse on the same day. The thought occurred to me that it is not right to use the same couch for one's occupation and for making love. The woman with whom I had intercourse calls spermatozoa "little worms" [a special Hungarian word "kukac"]. On the same day I thought of the possibility that a person with a fine sense of smell could sense that something took place there. [It is improbable that material traces had remained on the couch. That had been seen to. But such a thing cannot be dismissed.]

On the day before (in the company of the same woman) I spoke with a gentleman who was giving his opinion about Jewish jargon; I mentioned, among other things, the words *Salem Aleikum,* which *he* corrected as Scholem alechem.—On the night before the analytic hour I dreamed, among other things, about the words *"Mein Volk";* in the morning (in analyzing the dream) I associated the conversation about the jargon and also the words *Salem Aleikum* etc. to these words.

Subsequent to these thoughts the patient made further associations that have a direct bearing on his illness, or, more precisely, his person.

2.) July 26. The following comes to mind:

A fantasy: "I am lying. My clothes are empty, as if there were no body in them at all."

Self-analysis: In the early evening before falling asleep, I (Dr. F.) was reading a newspaper article by Anatole France, "Les fous dans la littérature,"[3] in which a lunatic is described putting clothes on an armchair, sticking in a pole as a backbone, slapping a hat on the pole, and looking at this phantom as an old, sick friend. The article made a big impression on me; I found in it confirmation of our views on the content of psychoses.—

3.) In the same analytic hour (immediately after the previous association):
"I am sweating. I am lying in salt, acid, potash, sodium, or what are those things in chemistry called? I seem to be like a woman, I throw off the covers. I am lying in childbed."

Analysis:
I slept poorly the night before. I perspired, threw off the covers. Couldn't fall asleep for hours, was depressed. Thought often about my kidney ailment and thought about whether the sweating wasn't perhaps compensation for the insufficiency of my kidneys. *I smelled the sweat to see if it didn't have the odor of urine.*
[N.B. a very transient and not severe attack of hypochondria.]
I note that the patient's "thought-reading" associations always come at the beginning of the analysis.

4.) August 3.
First things that come to mind: Get off at "Abrudbánya" (name of a city). Nagy-Káta. Kis-Káta.⁴ A man with a large beard directs. His wife directs. The wife in velvet pants."

Analysis: In the morning I was riding with the wife of a colleague. I see her often and was ashamed that I didn't notice until now that she is very pregnant. I helped her get on the tram with a certain tenderness (which I analyzed immediately). She told me that she was *going away* (I understood this to mean that she was going away today). I ask her: "Naturally again to *Nagy-Káta?*" "To Paks!" she corrected me. [Through this error I revealed the other (suppressed) error about her pregnancy.—N.B.: After four-five days I met her, still in Budapest; at the time it came out that she had recently given the mistaken impression that she wanted to go away on the same day. This whole chain of errors has to do with my blindness at the time toward my mother's pregnancies.]
I note that countertransference is mostly derived from the content of present or ucs.-aroused complexes (dreams, errors, unresolved matters).

5.) August 11. Patient sees (in fantasy) a girl lying on the dissecting table [as if in a caricature of "Le Rire,"⁵ where a naked woman who is about to be operated on is surrounded by doctors]. A doctor holds her from below, binds her with a *cambric bandage as wide as a hand;* another doctor operates on her. "My Rosmarin, my Georgine" [Hungarian song]. She wriggles her legs (feet?). Her upper body is separated from her lower body. As if screwed in.

Self-analysis [I won't repeat the patient's analysis]:
On the same day I was assisting my friend Schächter with a surgical intervention on Frau G.'s elder daughter.[6] The poor girl became infected about three months ago during the extraction of a wisdom tooth, and the pus had to be surgically emptied four to five times. She causes us much worry. Cosmetically not affected for the time being, but the danger is always there. During the last-mentioned operation she was sitting on a chair; Dr. Schächter in front of her; her legs between those of Dr. Schächter. I was standing behind her and was holding her head. After the surgery I made her a gigantic bandage; the cambric bandage was very wide (wider than the breadth of a hand), they were laughing about my excess of zeal. During the surgery she was wriggling her legs.—

6.) August 16. What comes to mind: "The sun lay on the moon, the moon on the stars. They carry out the movements of coitus."

Analysis:
In the morning another patient, the proprietor of a print shop, was telling me that in his print shop a book on natural philosophy was being printed, in which the author, a certain *Aszlányi*,[7] talks about the *love of the world* and gravitation, the earth's magnetism, etc., identified with sexual attraction. "Sun and Earth are having coitus with each other," said my confidant. This talk reminded me at the time of Möbius, Fechner,[8] as well as a conversation with a young music aesthete and philosopher, Dr. Kovács,[9] who is about to write a metaphysics based on psychoanalysis. Actually one should say, "The sun loves the Earth," he said further.
I couldn't stay long with these ideas in the printer's analysis; I turned my attention to his complexes.

These things have no influence at all on the progress of the analysis. The patient immediately associates to them things that concern him. If something in this transference is true, then the transferred words have no different effect from that of *Jung's* stimulus words.[10] Everyone "introjects" them according to his own needs.

My homosexual is a first-rate masochist (his cruelty, naturally, is lodged behind it). This masochism (possibly) enables him to apperceive impulses toward which others are unreceptive. I *project* the stimulus words ucs., he *introjects* them. [I act like a man, he like a woman; he is, of course, a homosexual.] N.B.: My young philosopher considers every artistic production to be a *projection* and every artistic reception to be *introjection* [something like empathy]. Naturally *this physical projection and introjection* should be sharply distinguished from the psychic,————[11]

1. Karl Camillo Schneider, "Wiener Psychologie," pts. 1–4, *Wiener klinische Rundschau*, July 24, 1910, pp. 467–469; July 31, 1910, pp. 483–486; August 7, 1910, pp. 498–500; and August 14, 1910, pp. 516–518. The fifth installment was not published until after Ferenczi's letter, in the issue of August 21, pp. 530–532. See letter 163 and n. 1.

2. Enclosed in brackets in the original, as are similar remarks throughout this letter.

3. See letter 152 and n. 1.

4. "Large Káta," "Small Káta" (Káta is also the Hungarian diminutive of Katherine).

5. Contemporary French satirical periodical.

6. Elma.

7. Deszö Aszlányi (1869–1947), a writer and philosopher of minor significance.

8. Gustav Theodor Fechner (1801–1887), noted physicist, psychologist, and philosopher; founder of experimental sensory physiology (psychophysics). Fechner's theories exerted a great influence on Freud, which the latter expressly acknowledged: "I was always open to the ideas of G. T. Fechner and have followed that thinker upon many important points" (1925d, p. 59). Thus, Freud saw the pleasure principle as a special case of the Fechnerian principle of the tendency toward stability (Freud 1920g, p. 9).

9. See letter 137, n. 2.

10. In Jung's association experiments the time between the utterance of a "stimulus word" [*Reizwort*] and the subject's response (the first word that came to mind) was measured.

11. The remainder of the letter is missing. The notes are written on long double sheets; half of the last sheet is torn off.

161

Budapest, August 19, 1910
VII., Erzsébet-körút 54

Dear Professor,

With the telegram I sent today[1] I only wanted to inform you that I am in complete agreement with your arrangements. I believe that chance has only helped us.—The rich program that is offered as a substitute for the ocean voyage makes it easy to forget the lost joys of the voyage. I am looking forward to it very much—but because of a mountain of work I can't for a moment give in to the anticipations of the trip.—On Sunday I am going to *Miskolcz* for a day to the Hungarian "Hikers' Meeting of Physicians and Natural Scientists," where I will give a lecture Monday on *Psychoanalysis and Hypnosis.*[2] Miskolcz is my hometown; I couldn't stay away, in consideration of Dr. Schächter, the organizer of these meetings.

I will bring along Baedeker's   1.) Italy in one Volume
                               2.) Southern Italy
                               3.) Holland

The spring course seems to have worked out well after all. A small circle of disciples, thirsty for knowledge, is crowding around me, and I am devoting myself to them whenever I can.—

So I have to be active up to the moment of departure and don't even have time to go into your kind and extensive letters in detail.

Enough of that: I am *very* satisfied with all your suggestions and am looking forward to seeing you again and to the beautiful days in Italy.

I will give you the time of my arrival in Noordwijk, but I would be very grateful if you would recommend a good hotel in The Hague.

Best regards to everyone!

Yours,
Ferenczi

1. This telegram is missing.
2. See letter 164.

162

[Budapest,] August 19, 1910[1]

Dear Professor,

Postscript to today's letter: I just saw on the map that *Leyden*, not The Hague, is the nearest major station. I therefore request that you correct my telegram of today to you to the effect that I will arrive in *Leyden* on the evening (Saturday) of the 27th (via Nuremberg). Please tell me also if you are taking along a smoking jacket or a tailcoat, so that I can organize myself accordingly.

Best regards,
Ferenczi

1. Postcard. The date, but not the address, is given at the end.

163

Noordwijk, August 20, 1910

Dear friend,

Many thanks for letter and affirmative dispatch. I ask you now to give me timely information as to when you are arriving in The Hague. Since I have to go there myself to withdraw money from my letter of credit, I could wait for your train at the same time.

Your—carefully preserved—observations on your masochist seem to me finally to shatter the doubts about the existence of thought transference. Now it is a matter of getting used to it in your thoughts and losing respect for its novelty, and also preserving the secret long enough in the maternal womb, but that is where the doubt ends.

Your newspaper extracts were very amusing. That philosophical animal skinner, who naively distributes immortalities, has evidently misunderstood the main thing in the interpretation of dreams, namely, interpretation, if he can doubt the necessity of "dream distortion."[1] He is probably a personal friend of Swoboda's[2] and substitutes liking for understanding.

Very nice here, but occasionally so windy that one's existence becomes difficult. I will not be averse to opening up a new chapter on geography.

Kind regards,
Freud

1. Karl Schneider, the author of the "Wiener Psychologie" (see letter 160 and n. 1), was lecturer in zoology at the University of Vienna and a proponent of vitalism; see *Ursprung und Wesen des Menschen* (Vienna, 1908) and *Vorlesungen über Tierpsychologie* (Leipzig, 1909). In his newspaper articles he had designated Otto Weininger, after Freud and Hermann Swoboda, as the "third Viennese psychologist who is certain of immortality" (p. 517) and criticized Freud's theory of the dream as wish fulfillment, since some dreams can be understood as the satisfaction of a "spiritual need" *(geistiges Bedürfnis)*.

2. In his article Schneider praises Swoboda's theory of psychic periods and his views on the dream. Hermann Swoboda (1873–1963), Doctor of Law and Philosophy; since 1905 *Privatdozent* in psychology and the history of psychology at the University of Vienna. He had played a role in a plagiarism controversy in which Freud, Fliess, and Weininger were also embroiled: Fliess had claimed that Freud's analysand Swoboda and, through Swoboda, his friend Weininger had learned from Freud about Fliess's thoughts on the periodicity of human life and on bisexuality, and that they had subsequently plagiarized them. Hermann Swoboda, *Die Perioden des menschlichen Organismus in ihrer psychologischen und biologischen Bedeutung* (Vienna, 1904); and Otto Weininger, *Geschlecht und Charakter* (Vienna, 1903); see also Freud, *Fliess Letters,* pp. 461–468.

164

Miskolcz, August 22, 1910[1]

I found here an audience raving about Ehrlich's discovery[2] and none disposed to listening to ψ.α. subtleties. For that reason I didn't give the lecture. Traveling today to Budapest and hope to be with you according to plan.

Regards!
Ferenczi

1. Picture postcard. Written in pen is the notation "Miskolcz—Széchenyi utca."
2. Paul Ehrlich (1854–1915), German medical doctor and serum researcher; won the Nobel Prize for medicine (1908) for work on immunology. In 1909 he developed Salvarsan (arsphenamine) as a treatment for syphilis. At the turn of the century an estimated 70 percent of the men in Vienna suffered from syphilis; see Harry Stroeken, *Freud und seine Patienten* (Frankfurt, 1992), p. 47.

165

Noordwijk, August 22, 1910

Dear friend,

These are the final arrangements: if you travel in such a way as to arrive in Leyden (or The Hague) in the evening, then I can't meet you there, for we wouldn't get back to Noordwijk until half past 12 in the morning. So stay overnight in Leyden, *Hotel Lion d'or,* and come over on Sunday on one of the early trains (steam train 52 mins.).

I consider smoking jacket and tailcoat to be out of the question and take them to be an American reminiscence of yours.

You will find Baedeker's Holland here, but better yet, you bring it along. You can contact us first by telephone from Leyden.

So, *auf Wiedersehen,*
Freud

166

Budapest, August 23, 1910
VII., Erzsébet-körút 54

Dear Professor,

Upon my return from the Miskolcz diversion I received your letter of August 20, in which you indicate that you have something to do in The

Hague and want to meet my train. As a consequence of this I will keep to my original, then altered, travel plan and herewith confirm finally that I will arrive in The Hague on August 27 (Saturday) at 9:22 in the evening. The trip from Budapest to The Hague will take thirty-three hours without interruption; I fear that I will be useless for anything on the evening of my arrival.

If you should decide not to go to The Hague, I ask you to inform me of your intention by telegram.

I am a little frightened by the fact that you view my observations on thought transference as proven. All kinds of doubts, or, better said, a feeling of uncertainty, a desire for further, for many, confirmations have been aroused in me. I can certainly warm up to these things theoretically; I also know that they don't shake up psychoanalysis, they only make it more complicated. Perhaps one struggles against such discoveries, however, precisely because of the unexpected complications. But I know that it is a Danaan gift[1] when one gets such ideas, that is to say, has such experiences.—We have time, though, to think about the thing's fate.

Best regards,
Ferenczi

1. Ominous gift; originally the Trojan Horse, according to Virgil: "Quidquid id est, timeo Danaos, et dona ferentes" (Whatever it may be, I fear the Danaans [Greeks], even when they bring gifts); *Aeneid* 2.49, in Allen Mandelbaum, trans., *Norton Anthology of World Masterpieces*, vol. 1, 4th ed. (New York, 1979), p. 590.

167

[Postmark: Budapest,
August 25, 1910][1]

Dear Professor,

I thus confirm that I will stay in the "Lion d'or" in Leyden on the evening of the 28th and will arrive Sunday morning at the Hotel Noordzee (where I ask you to reserve a room for me).

Regards,
Ferenczi

Thursday evening. (Departure tomorrow A.M.)

1. Undated postcard.

168

Budapest, September 28, 1910
VII., Erzsébet-körút 54

Dear Professor,

Following your wise counsel, I am still enjoying the *dolce far niente*. Aside from the fact that today I have again assumed my duties at the Health Service and am at home in the afternoon between three and four, I am living here as if I were my own guest—I indulge myself with hour-long walks with Frau G., shop for large and small items, deal with the appropriate framing of the Sicilian photographs with a serious expression on my face, etc.—Still, the absence of overpowering expressions of art and nature is already having an effect: I am beginning to feel a desire for work and notice that in the course of the month of rest there has indeed been a buildup of reserve strength that requires activation. But I still have no inkling whatsoever of how I will work, and what on. The beautiful days that I spent in your company, the ideas that were stimulated in me at the time will, I hope, have a favorable influence on my activity. My general psychic and intellectual development and self-education must also benefit from this trip (as was the case with America). Still, I am sorry that you had in me a travel companion who is still so much in need of education.

You will probably think that I have begun to subject the events of our living together, the manner in which I reacted to them, to extensive self-criticism.[1] And if I hope, in spite of this, that our personal and scientific relations will not have diminished in intensity as a result of closer acquaintance, then that is based on the one hand on the conviction of my own good intentions (which stand up to the most far-reaching analysis)—and on the other on the justified hope that you can forgive the unavoidable "chimpanzee,"[2] who so often thwarted good intentions. Perhaps in our correspondence I will have the opportunity to return now and then to particulars regarding these things. For the time being, I only wanted to show the first signs of life from me and to thank you most kindly for the trouble that you took as tour leader. Please give my regards to all the members of your family and send me favorable news about your state of health as soon as possible.

Yours,
Ferenczi

1. There was an incident during their trip together to which we have access only by way of Ferenczi's version, written eleven years later: "[Freud] was too big for me, too much of a father. The result was that in Palermo, where he wanted to do the famous work on paranoia (Schreber) in collaboration with me, right on the first evening of work, when he wanted to dictate something to me, I rose up in a sudden burst of rebellion and

explained that it was not at all a collaboration if he simply dictated to me. 'So that's the way you are?'—he said, astonished. 'You perhaps wanted to take the whole thing?' Having said that, he worked alone every evening from then on" (*Ferenczi/Groddeck*, December 24, 1921, pp. 36f).

2. Allusion to a remark by Anatole France, according to which human beings are actually chimpanzees (see Freud's unpublished letter to Pfister of November 6, 1910, Library of Congress).

169

Vienna, October 2, 1910
IX., Berggasse 19

Dear friend,

Your letter has reminded me of the fact that I am the same person who picked papyrus in Syracuse, fought with the railway personnel in Naples, and bought antiquities in Rome. My identity has been restored. It is strange how easily one succumbs to an inclination to isolate the formations of personality.

You will believe me when I say that I think back about your company on the trip only with warm and pleasant feelings, although I often felt sorry for you because of your disappointment, and I would like to have had you different in some respects. Disappointment because you certainly expected to wallow in constant intellectual stimulation, whereas nothing is more repugnant to me than posing, and I then often let myself go in the opposite direction. So I was probably mostly quite an ordinary old gentleman, and you, in astonishment, realized the distance from your fantasy ideal. On the other hand, I would have wished for you to tear yourself away from the infantile role and take your place next to me as a companion with equal rights, which you did not succeed in doing; and further, in practical perspective, I would have wished that you had carried out more reliably your part of the task, the orientation in space and temporality. But you were inhibited and dreamy. So much for my educational efforts.

The following has happened here: everything well at home. Martin, since yesterday, a trim soldier.[1] After putting my letters, books, mailings, etc. in order, I came across a lecture by Putnam of July 21 in the Boston Medical and Surgical Journal which seemed to me so excellent and well suited to be an apology for ΨA that I wrote him that I wanted to translate it for the Zentralblatt, with his permission. The translation has been completed in the meantime and took up my vacation days.[2] My reading of Schreber[3] was interrupted in so doing but will resume today.

Hitschmann is out,[4] Pfister done.[5] A manuscript by Graf, Richard Wagner in the Flying Dutchman, is ready and waiting to form the next volume.[6]

Deuticke is reminding me of the third edition of the Interpretation of Dreams, which I promised him for January-February. Wittels has *resigned* as a result of the publication of his novel.[7] The first session will take place on Wednesday the 5th. The Zentralblatt is supposed to be the first thing on the agenda. The Suicide of Students[8] was published a long time ago.— That's what's been happening in the land of literature.

I myself wrote Bleuler a letter requesting clarification.[9] Maeder left Constance and is going to England.

The most beautiful and interesting female patient of my first office hour wants to undergo a thorough cure with you. I don't need to recommend Dr. Stricker [*sic*][10] to you.

Best regards for today to you and Frau G. Your idyll will also soon be at an end.

Yours truly,
Freud

1. As a student Martin became a so-called one-year volunteer with the artillery. Nonstudents had to serve in the military for three years. See Martin Freud, *Sigmund Freud: Man and Father* (New York, 1983), pp. 168ff.

2. Freud's translation of Putnam's essay "On the Etiology and Treatment of the Psychoneuroses," *Boston Medical and Surgical Journal* 163 (1910): 75–82, was published, with a supplementary footnote by Freud, in *Zentralblatt* 1 (1910–11): 137–154 (Freud 1911j).

3. Daniel Paul Schreber, *Denkwürdigkeiten eines Nervenkranken* (Leipzig, 1903). Freud used this book for his "Psycho-Analytic Notes on an Autobiographical Account of a Case of Paranoia (Dementia Paranoides)" (1911c [1910]), on which he had worked in Sicily.

4. See letter 130 and n. 6.

5. Oskar Pfister, *Die Frömmigkeit des Grafen Ludwig von Zinzendorf* (*Schriften zur angewandten Seelenkunde,* vol. 9 (Leipzig, 1911), was based on a lecture for the Wednesday Society.

6. Max Graf (1873–1958), a noted Austrian musicologist, writer, theater critic, musician, and professor at the Vienna Conservatory, was a member of the Wednesday Society and a friend of Freud's. He was the father of "little Hans" (Freud 1909b). His work *Richard Wagner im "Fliegenen Holländer," ein Beitrag zur Psychologie künstlerischen Schaffens* (*Schriften zur angewandten Seelenkunde,* vol. 9 (Leipzig, 1911), was based on a lecture for the Wednesday Society.

7. Wittels had written a roman à clef about Karl Kraus, *Ezechiel der Zugereiste* (Berlin, 1910). See letter 85, n. 9, and letter 112, n. 7.

8. *Über den Selbstmord, insbesondere den Schülerselbstmord* (*Diskussionen des Wiener psychoanalytischen Vereins* (Wiesbaden, 1910), edited by the leadership of the Society; Freud was represented in it by an introduction and an afterword (1910g). See also *Minutes* II, 479–506.

9. In his letter of September 28, 1910, published in F. Alexander and S. T. Selesnick, "Freud-Bleuler Correspondence," *Archives of General Psychology* 12 (1965): 2f, Freud tried to persuade Bleuler to reverse his decision not to join the IPA, newly founded in Nuremberg.

10. Laura Striker, neé Pollacsek (Pólanyi) (1882–1959), had received a doctorate in

English and history in 1904. She was married to the businessman Sándor Striker and commuted between Budapest and Vienna. She founded an experimental private school (see letter 281) and participated in the activities of the Galileo Society, the Free School for Social Sciences, and feminist associations. She emigrated to the United States in 1938. See also letter 184, n. 4.

170

Budapest, [October 3, 1910][1]
VII., Erzsébet-körút 54

Dear Professor,

I was anticipating your letter with no slight tension—I almost wrote "anxiety." I have already tried to familiarize myself—in fantasy—with *all* eventualities and even prepared myself for the situation in which, with respect to the disappointment that I caused you, you would no longer find it worthwhile to be interested in me, etc. My "heroic" plan was to remain loyal to you without consideration for our personal relations, that is to say, for *your* change of heart. It is well that heroism remained dispensable and that in the tone of your letter I found the same warmth and friendliness, and in its content the same honesty, for which I was always so grateful to you. Already during the trip, but even more so since my return home, I have analyzed what I did and did not do and have found the cause of the inhibitions—just as you did—in my infantile attitude. On this occasion I have also rather ruthlessly brought to light the resistance against my own homosexual drive components (and the uncommon sexual overestimation of women which goes along with it), and I believe I have gained much personal and some scientific advantage from this.

To this extent we are also in agreement about me. But I must contradict you on some essential points and—with reference to ψα. candor—clarify the issue as follows:

It is *not correct* that I have always sought only the great scholar in you—and was disappointed by the realization of human weaknesses, etc. The letters that I wrote to Frau G. from Italy could prove the opposite to you. To the extent that you concerned yourself with scientific matters altogether (and you were kind enough to share with me everything that you were occupied with at the time), I had to be astonished and pleased about the wealth of scientific novelties—and so I was. It didn't occur to me to ask for more.

What made me inhibited and taciturn—and at the same time somewhat stupid was *the same thing that you are complaining about.* I was longing for personal, uninhibited, cheerful companionship with you (and I *can* be cheerful, indeed, boisterously cheerful), and I felt—perhaps unjustifiably— forced back into the infantile role. To be sure, I did, perhaps, have an exaggerated idea of companionship between two men who tell each other the truth *unrelentingly*, sacrificing all consideration. Just as in my relationship with Frau G. I strive for *absolute* mutual openness, in the same manner—and with even more justification—I believed that this, apparently cruel but in the end only useful, clear-as-day openness, which conceals nothing, could be possible in the relations between two ψα.-minded people who can really understand everything and, instead of making value judgments, can seek the determinants of their ψ. impulses.

That was the ideal I was looking for: I wanted to enjoy the man, not the scholar, in close friendship.

But what I forgot—in my egocentric blindness—was that these things didn't move *you* at all: you wanted nothing but to spend four weeks after a strenuous year of work in very well-earned rest and in beautiful surroundings in the company of a compatible traveling companion; and that it was so terribly inconsiderate of me to want to spoil your vacation time by allowing myself to be educated by you, allowing my errors to be shown to me—al o, to be sure, with the entitlement on my part of being permitted always to speak the most unpleasant truth.—

I know very well that this passage sounds pompous and histrionic. I also now know that the entire (unconsciously strengthened) homosexual drive component is behind it. But I am making use of the opportunity and am writing—in free association—what comes to my mind so that you see me as I really am.

My dream in which I saw you standing naked before me (naturally without feeling the slightest conscious [indeed, also in the dream still unconscious][2] sexual arousal) was the transparent symbolization of 1.) the ucs. homosexual tendency and 2.) the longing for absolute mutual openness.

This wish for openness was not one of pure curiosity! In it I understand primarily our right to say everything *unpleasant* to each other. I would, for example, have been very grateful if you had said what you wrote in your letter while we were under way. It would have had a liberating effect.—But that *I* should begin: for that I lacked the strength. Despite constant broodings I didn't bring out more than a few weak allusions. But how happy I would have been if you had accommodated me in that!

Do you know which hours of our trip retain the most pleasant memories for me? The ones in which you divulged to me something of your personality and your life. It was then, and not during the scientific conversations, that I felt free of inhibitions, like a "companion with equal rights," as you always wished me to be and as I so much would like to have been.

You will ask yourself—and me: Where does this tragic mood in me come from? How do I come to demand still more—indeed everything—from someone who treated me with such extraordinary kindness and so much undeserved interest! Where do I claim the right to expect that you will make such a "distinguished" foreigner your confidant? How might I be permitted to learn from you things that you have perhaps not yet uttered to any mortal? (N.B.: Do not think that I presume any grandiose secrets in you.)

The longing for such a friend and the instinctual impulses that underlie it were not the sole causes of this perhaps irrational fantasy formation. I usually tend more toward modesty and self-deprecation—at least I always see my actual smallness.—But don't forget that for years I have been occupied with nothing but the products of your intellect, and I have also always felt the man behind every sentence of your works and made him my confidant. Whether you want to be or not, you are one of the great master teachers of mankind, and you must allow your readers to approach you, at least intellectually, in a personal relationship as well. My ideal of truth that strikes down all consideration is certainly nothing less than the most self-evident consequence of your teachings. I am convinced that I am not the only one who, in important decisions, in self-criticism, etc., always asks and has asked himself the question: How would *Freud* relate to this? Under "Freud" I understood his teachings and his personality, fused together in a harmonic unity.

So I am and have been much, much more intimately acquainted and conversant with you than you could have imagined. Strangely—and that is the point of my case history that appears neurotic, even demented—I forgot to take into account the fact that you could not have known all that—and even if you did know it, it would on no account have obliged you to dispense completely with your justified distrust of people (even of friends—after the *Fliess* case) and give yourself over to someone, e.g., an enthusiastic, impertinent youngster. But I have only just now, here at home, arrived at this insight (which I ask you to take literally; I am now talking without a trace of irony or self-irony). During the trip I played the ridiculous and certainly very repugnant role of one who is misunderstood (like the Sicilian asses, perhaps)—and I was waiting for your accommodation in order to be able to tell you all this. My behavior again only ignited resistance in you, and so it came to a vicious circle that I would now like to hack apart in the same way as my great namesake[3] did to that knot, only with these strokes of my pen, to be sure, but with a measure of personal courage that should not be disdained, and at the risk of jeopardizing interests that are dear to me.

You once told me that ΨA. was only a science of facts, of indicatives that should not be translated into imperatives—the latter are paranoid. According to this conception there is no ψ.α. worldview, no ψ α ethics, no ψ α. rules of conduct. I also know of no ethics other than those of pure reason; but the extension and expansion of reason into hitherto unconscious areas has also had a very significant influence on the worldview and behavior of nonparanoids. The final consequence of such insight—when it is present in two people—is that they *are not ashamed in front of each other, keep nothing secret, tell each other the truth without risk of insult or in the certain hope that within the truth there can be no lasting insult.* If you had scolded me thoroughly instead of being eloquently silent! I would perhaps have felt grievously wounded in the first instant, but, just as now—if I had also very, very soon admitted the truth to myself—in fact, I would have owed you a very large debt of gratitude for it.

I must come back again and again to the fact that I am aware of the excessiveness of my demands. But I believe that you underestimate much too much the ennobling power of psychoanalysis if you don't believe that it makes people who have completely grasped its meaning absolutely worthy of trust. Each time I visited you in Vienna for a few days I was colossally strengthened by the fact that you communicate to me so much, indeed, so much more than to anyone else, of yourself and of your nascent ideas. It was not until we were together for a longer time (America doesn't count, since there were three of us) that I was shown that *much* is no compensation for the *whole*—and, according to my ψ α. ideal, there are no halfway standards; all consideration for people and conditions disappears beside my ideal of truth. Please don't misunderstand me. I really don't want to "reform" society, I am not a paranoiac. I would only like to see *thoughts* and *speech* liberated from the compulsion of unnecessary inhibitions in the relations of ψ α.-minded men.—

Unfortunately—I can't begin, you have to! After all, you are Ψα. in person!

I wouldn't believe that, after all this, you are thinking back about my company "with pleasant feelings" even if you hadn't gone out of your way to invite me to believe it. But I believe many other things. I believe that you will in no way misunderstand the tone and content of this letter; I believe that our trip means not the end of an intimacy but rather the beginning of a real understanding.

Be that as it may, I have introduced myself to you once again unadorned—with all infantile weaknesses and exaggerations. And if this terribly long epistle were otherwise uninteresting to you: it will perhaps interest you as the confession of a man who exists in psychoanalytic ferment.

Yours, thirsty for honesty
Ferenczi

Addendum to 170

Budapest, October 4, 1910
VII., Erzsébet-körút 54

Dear Professor,

I already put on paper yesterday the letter that I am forwarding to you here. But as I was about to mail it today, it suddenly occurred to me to wonder whether there would be any use at all in occupying you in this way with my personal matters, whether I am risking too much by letting it get to you? etc.

I have successfully overcome this feeling of faintheartedness, but as a reward for this I am expecting that you will not leave me for long in uncertainty as to how you judge the content of the letter. You yourself will gather from the letter that I am counting not on unqualified agreement but only on unembellished expression of opinion, and that I would very, very much like to have myself instructed by my better.

1. The date of the letter is suggested by the first sentence of the appended letter.
2. Enclosed in brackets in the original.
2. Alexander the Great (Sándor = Alexander).

171

Vienna, October 6, 1910
IX., Berggasse 19

Dear friend,

It is remarkable how much better you can present yourself in writing than in speech. Of course, I knew very much or most of what you are writing about and now need to give you only a few clarifications pertaining to it. Why didn't I scold you and in so doing open the way to an understanding? Quite right, it was a weakness on my part; I am also not that ψα superman whom we have constructed, and I also haven't overcome the countertransference. I couldn't do it, just as I can't do it with my three sons, because I like them and I feel sorry for them in the process.

Not only have you noticed that I no *longer* have any need for that full opening of my personality, but you have also understood it and correctly returned to its traumatic cause. Why did you thus make a point of it? This need has been extinguished in me since Fliess's case, with the overcoming of which you just saw me occupied. A piece of homosexual investment has been withdrawn and utilized for the enlargement of my own ego. I have succeeded where the paranoiac fails.—Add to this the fact that I was for the most part not very well; I suffered more from my intestinal troubles than I cared to admit. And I often said to myself: he who is not master of his Konrad[1] should not travel. The honesty should have begun there, and you didn't seem stable enough not to become overconcerned.

As far as the unpleasantness that you caused me is concerned—including a certain passive resistance—, that will go the way of memories of travel in general; small disturbances vanish through a process of self-purification, and what is beautiful is left over for intellectual use.

It was plain to see but also easily recognizable as infantile that you presumed great secrets in me and were very curious about them. Just as I shared with you *all* the scientific matters, I also concealed from you very little of a personal nature, and the matter with the national gift [*National-geschenk*][2] was, I think, indiscreet enough. My dreams at the time were, as I indicated to you, entirely concerned with the Fliess matter, with which, owing to the nature of the thing, it was difficult to get you to sympathize.

So, on closer inspection you will find that our coming to terms doesn't need to be as momentous as you perhaps thought at first.

I would rather direct you to the present and tell you that your name is missing from the list of members of the Vienna Society in the first issue of the Korrespondenzblatt, which you should complain about; and that the first evening yesterday went very well and brought six new recommendations for members.[3] Now that Jung has stirred as president and has circulated bylaws, the Korrespondenzblatt, and a recruitment pamphlet, one gets the impression that the organization has been a success. One will then remember what a great part you played in this work.

Did I already write to you that I finally went to Bleuler myself with a request for clarification of his action and with a detailed explanation of my motivation in founding the Association? Response still forthcoming.

And that I translated Putnam's paper for the Zentralblatt, which I have to have published without my name as a courtesy?

But I have certainly not yet written that I worked through Schreber, found confirmation for the kernel of our assumptions about paranoia, and have taken from this all kinds of opportunities for serious interpretations. I have asked Stegmann[4] to find out all kinds of personal things about old Schreber.[5] How much I can say about this publicly depends on these reports.

What would you think if old Dr. Schreber had worked "miracles" as a physician? But was otherwise a tyrant at home who "shouted" at his son and understood him as little as the "lower God" understood our paranoiac?[6] Contributions to the interpretation of Schreber will be eagerly acknowledged.

Cordially,
Freud

1. See letter 131, n. 2.

2. According to Jones (II, 83, n. 1, and pp. 389–390), Freud meant income from consultations, which he used for the acquisition of antiquities.

3. At the session of October 5 applications for membership were received from Guido Holzknecht (1872–1931), a roentgenologist and friend of Paul Federn; Hanns Sachs; Herbert Silberer; Paul Klemperer (1887–1964), cousin of Paul Federn, at that time still a student, later a professor at Columbia University and noted pathologist; Federn's friend Gustav Grüner (1884–1941), Karl Koller's nephew; the pediatrician Richard Wagner (1887–1974); and the economist Leopold Rechnitzer (1851–1916). They were all unanimously accepted at the next session (*Minutes* III, 2, 8).

4. See letter 64, n. 5.

5. Dr. Daniel Gottlob Moritz Schreber (1808–1861), father of the renowned paranoiac and the man who gave his name to the Schrebergärten and Schreber Societies, which promoted the cultivation of private gardens and are still popular today in Germany and Austria, was at that time a well-known author of popular books on health and gymnastics. He favored methods of education that aimed at establishing complete control over the child, and he played a decisive role in the psychotic world of his son. See, e.g., William G. Niederland, *Der Fall Schreber* (Frankfurt, 1978); Morton Schatzmann, *Die Angst vor dem Vater, Langzeitwirkungen einer Erziehungssmethode* (Reinbek, 1974); Han Israels, *Schreber: Vater und Sohn. Eine Biographie* (Munich, 1989); and the introduction and appendix to Daniel Paul Schreber, *Denkwürdigkeiten eines Nervenkranken* (rpt. Frankfurt, 1973).

6. See letter 173, n. 10.

172

Vienna, October 10, 1910
IX., Berggasse 19

Dear friend,

I just read Maeder,[1] whom I find quite far advanced. His first case bears some similarity to Schreber. His comment about the paranoiac's understanding of symbols stimulates me to ask you to get serious about exploiting your patient as a symbol sleuth and then venture to make that public. Perhaps you should test Stekel's expected new symbols[2] in this manner. Or my "rescue" and the "necktie."[3]

Today Mr. Holmos was here with his deaf-mute wife. I naturally sent him back to you energetically. I ask you not to give credence to his stupid objection that ten crowns is too much for him; that is, if he comes again, which one can never know, of course.

From tomorrow on I will be fully booked up, but with patients who don't want to stay very long. I will lecture on the "two principles" at the Society on one of the next evenings.[4] Strangely, I am not very productive, as is normally always the case after a trip.

Kind regards,
Freud

1. "Psychologische Untersuchungen an Dementia praecox-Kranken" [Psychological Investigations in Dementia Praecox Cases], Maeder's article in the recently published *Jahrbuch* 2, 1st half-volume (1910): 185–245.

2. At the Nuremberg Congress Stekel had stimulated interest with his "Proposals for Group Research in the Domain of Symbolism and of Typical Dreams" (see letter 127, n. 7) and was engaged in writing *Die Sprache des Traumes* (Wiesbaden, 1911).

3. Regarding the symbol of rescue, see Freud 1910d, p. 143; Freud 1910h, esp. pp. 172–173; and the supplement in the *Interpretation of Dreams* (1900a, p. 403). On the symbol of the necktie, see *Interpretation of Dreams*, p. 356 (1911 supplement). See also letter 446 and nn. 3 and 4.

4. Freud, "Formulations on the Two Principles of Mental Functioning," Lecture in the Vienna Society, October 26, 1910 (*Minutes* III, 27–34); see also Freud 1911b.

173

Budapest, October 12, 1910
VII., Erzsébet-körút 54

Dear Professor,

Before I—in acceding to your request—turn my attention to the present, I must still return—albeit briefly—to personal matters. They have been temporarily resolved through my reply and your response to it; each of us has defined his point of view, and determined the motives of his actions to the fullest extent possible. I call this resolution *temporary* because I do not want to give up hope that you will let a part of your withdrawn homosexual libido be refloated and bring more sympathy to bear toward my "ideal of honesty." You know: I am an unimpeachable therapist. I don't even want to give up the paranoiac as a *total* loss. So how could I warm up to the fact that you extend your—in part, justified—distrust to the entire male sex! There is certainly much that is infantile in my yearning for honesty—but it certainly also has a healthy core.—Not everything that is infantile should be abhorred; for example, the child's urge for truth, which is only dammed up by false educational influences. (See Freud, Leonardo da Vinci; see also Freud's views on the enlightenment of children[1]—etc.) I still hold firm to the conviction that it is not honesty but superfluous secrecy that is abnormal, although I do admit that the former can be overly emphasized by infantile influences. I am grateful to you for every word that you say or write about my behavior, no matter how unpleasant it may be.

Now, to return to the present, I must at the outset actually come back to your first letter. I am very pleased about the many new literary publications (Pfister, Graf, Putnam,[2] Stekel[3]), and, in my consciousness of the future, I am beginning to dismiss the silly and malicious pranks of our opponents. I even overcame the urge to respond to a local lecturer in neurology (Kollarits),[4] who, in a paper on Isserlin,[5] talks about the "regrettable victims of psychoanalysis," whom the remaining neurologists later have to restore. But I have a great desire to have my Nuremberg lecture published in the Zentralblatt—only I am afraid that the editors won't accept it for personal reasons. It doesn't hurt if one of us writes in a more trenchant tone for once.—What do you think?[6]

I thank you for making me aware of the fact that my name was left off the membership list in the Korrespondenzblatt. I immediately wrote to both Jung and Adler and am vehemently insisting on my rights.

I am conducting a seminar this year with the better students from my earlier course. We meet once a week in my home. Actually, the Budapest group is already meeting there, but I want to notify Stein and Décsi (that is to say, formally establish the branch society) only when the members have had a chance to work themselves into our spirit and can independently represent their points of view vis-à-vis Stein and Décsi.

My time is completely taken up with professional affairs. I am actually working too much. An hour at the Health Service, an hour at the office, a house call now and then, paperwork and court sessions, five–six–seven hours of analysis a day. So I have too little time left for working out the impressions gained, for meditation and for literary activity. But I can't give up the court, because it would entail too much of a material loss (5–6,000 crowns); the hours at the Health Service also amount to 3,000 crowns, with some prestige to boot. I can also show the young medical students there something. So, literature must remain the victim.

In twelve days I am giving a lecture about your "Jokes"[7] in the sociological "Free School." So I have to read it now and don't have time for *Schreber*. I especially want to study the case of my paranoid compulsive (Zayda, Pressburg).

In addition to this I have an interesting case of neurotic stool incontinence in a certain Schlesinger, an engineer, who is a close friend of *Dr. Fliess*. He wants to find out about psychoanalysis from Fliess. I am curious as to how he will respond.

In addition to that, I have a brilliant young patient, a prospective medical student, of whom I expect a great deal (if he is capable of working).[8]

Otherwise, there are a lot of old cases.

Frau Stricker [*sic*] didn't come, probably because she is the sister-in-law of Prof. Sarbó,[9] who is the author of that pretty interruption about the "analyzed-out ten gulden."

Strangely enough, I have no recollection of the name Holmos, nor, for that matter, of a patient who has a deaf-mute wife. That must be a rather old story. I will charge her not ten but fifteen crowns; I made a beginning with Schlesinger—and see, it went all right.

A patient told me that he spoke with Magnus Hirschfeld, who is supposedly not in complete agreement with your Leonardo. Magnus Hirschfeld is supposed to come to Budapest at *Stein's* request in order to lecture here on homosexuality. In any event, I want to intervene in *this* discussion.—

Next time I want to write you more about scientific themata, if I find time to collect my thoughts in the meantime.

Yours truly,
Ferenczi

Your explanation of the "bellowing miracle" is very plausible to me![10]

1. "The Sexual Enlightenment of Children" (1907c).

2. See letter 169, nn. 2, 5, and 6.

3. It is not clear which works of the uncommonly productive Stekel Ferenczi is referring to, for "his panegyrics [to psychoanalysis] were continually appearing in the daily press"; Fritz Wittels, *Sigmund Freud: His Personality, His Teachings, and His School* (London, 1924), p. 132.

4. Jenö Kollarits (1870–1940), author of the book *Charakter und Nervosität* (lectures on the essence of character and nervousness given at the Medical Faculty of Budapest in the first semester of 1910–11 academic year), published shortly thereafter (Berlin, 1912), in which he sharply criticized psychoanalysis. See also letter 295.

5. See letter 128 and n. 5.

6. In the *Zentralblatt* 1 (1910–11): 131, there appeared only a summary of Ferenczi's lecture (1911, 79; *Fin.*, p. 299) by Otto Rank, which was first published in Hungarian in *Gyógyászat*, no. 31 (1911), and was not published in German until 1927.

7. See letter 85. The lecture was published under the title "Die Psychoanalyse des Witzes und des Komischen" [The Psychoanalysis of Wit and the Comical] (1911, 78; *Unbewusstes*, pp. 164–177; *F.C.*, p. 332).

8. Possibly Sándor Radó; see letter 222 and n. 4.

9. See letter 7 and n. 2.

10. As soon as Schreber succumbed to "thinking nothing" [*Nichtsdenken*], the "bellowing miracle" [*Brüllwunder*] appeared, "when my muscles serving the process of respiration are set in motion by the lower God (Ariman) in such a way that I am forced to emit bellowing noises"; Schreber, *Memoirs*, p. 165.

174

Vienna, October 17, 1910
IX., Berggasse 19

Dear friend,

I hadn't intended to write to you until the Zentralblatt was out, but I have had a tiring day today and am disposed only to write letters. So you are the victim.

So, you are still asserting your point of view, and, I concede, ardently and with good arguments. But there is nothing obligatory in that. Perhaps you are imagining completely different secrets than [those] I have reserved for myself, or you think there is a special suffering connected with that, whereas I feel myself to be a match for anything and approve of the overcoming of my homosexuality, with the result being greater independence.

It occurs to me that a paralyzing influence emanated from you to the extent that you were always prepared to admire me. Since I am very jealous of my self-criticism, especially in scientific matters, I naturally gave no cause for admiration. Self-criticism is not a pleasant gift, but it is, next to my courage, the best thing in me, and it has caused me to be extremely selective in publishing my works. Without it I would have been able to publish three times as much. It is more valuable to me than anyone suspects.

I am now completely booked up, from eight to eight and a half hours, and I already find the activity somewhat monotonous. But there are always small harvests. I have nothing as multifaceted to compare with the report of your activities. At the moment correspondence is costing me much time. Bleuler has replied to me with a letter eight pages long, and I responded with one ten pages long.[1] His arguments are remarkably dim. If he gives me possibilities for sewing up the rift, perhaps I will go to Zurich over Christmas.

Jones's Hamlet[2] is before me in German translation. I will have it published as the tenth volume of the *Schriften,* as Deuticke has suggested.

If you want to give your colleague a hefty rebuff, I certainly have no objection to it. You won't require censorship. I just don't want the energy of my Viennese directed into the channels of polemics, and so I am keeping them like dogs on a leash. The public at large is probably not yet ready to listen to your Nuremberg lecture. It was totally in-house.

I send kind regards and hope for good news.

Yours,
Freud

1. See letter 169 and n. 9.
2. See letter 119 and n. 4.

175

Budapest, October 18, 1910
VII., Erzsébet-körút 54

Dear Professor,

I thought I heard from you that you had along in your travel bag the letter in which I ventured to make a few very hypothetical attempts at explaining the problem of the pleasurable character of dreams; I therefore presume that you still have it. In the meantime, what I said there has been somewhat consolidated for me after reading "Jokes," only I can no longer reproduce the content of the letter precisely enough. I would therefore like to ask you to send it back for me to use temporarily (if it's not too much effort for you to look for it).

Altogether, I have not had such pleasure in a long time as I now have in studying your book on jokes. I am reading it again from an entirely different perspective, and I find great correspondences, intimations of things that came much later or are only now in process.—I was even tempted, in reading the section on smut,[1] to write a small article on the psychology of the obscene for the Zentralblatt. Perhaps I will do it.[2]

Otherwise I am not doing badly. I wasn't able to keep the engineer (Fliess's friend); he is over fifty, and perhaps I didn't approach him in an appropriate manner. Even the paranoid is striking—he is frightened by the neurotic anxiety that is surfacing in him through analysis. So now I have more time and am happy about it.

The seminar is going along. Last week Dr. Hevesi, the director of the Hungarian National Theater, gave a lecture about $\psi\alpha$. observations in the theater.

I have amicably come to terms with the Vienna Society. *Jung* left out my name (perhaps out of excessive consideration for Hungarian particularism).[3]

Kindest regards to all your dear ones and to you.

Yours truly,
Ferenczi

1. *Jokes and Their Relation to the Unconscious* (1905c, pp. 97ff). A more precise rendering of the German *die Zote* than James Strachey's "smut" would be "the dirty joke" [Trans.].

2. Ferenczi, "Über obszöne Worte, Beitrag zur Psychologie der Latenzzeit" [On Obscene Words] (1911, 75; C., p. 132), *Zentralblatt* 1 (1910–11): 390–399.

3. Ferenczi is referring to the omission of his name from the membership list of the *Korrespondenzblatt* (see letter 173).

176

Vienna, October 27, 1910
IX., Berggasse 19

Dear friend,

I am now so intensively involved with all kinds of work (not to mention an extensive correspondence with Bleuler) that it has taken days for me to find the letter you wanted. So here it is. Meanwhile, the Zentralblatt has come out; although not yet technically complete, it is still a significant moment in the development of the cause. Yesterday I spoke in the Society about the "two principles of ψ functioning."[1] Unsatisfying. Even I didn't like it anymore at the end. It's getting more and more difficult to get along with these people. A mixture of shy admiration and stupid contradiction *quand même,* not in the same persons. Adler is becoming disagreeable with his new theories, the inappropriateness of which I am becoming more convinced of every day. I should have begun with the purely factual, with the analysis of Schreber, which has flourished considerably.

For the second volume of the Zentralblatt Jung has delivered the facade, and I a little didactic paper, "'Wild' ΨA."[2] We already have an excess of material and a shortage of space, but one must have an inventory, and you shouldn't curtail any of your plans.

Grandmother died today in Hamburg,[3] and my wife left for the funeral. The poor woman had to hold out until the last gasp. Ernst, who has become rheumatic since we were at the sea and looks bad, will be sent to Merano for a few weeks after Mama's return. I always consider editions like that [2nd ed. Sammlung][4] productive. My memories of Rome have recently been awakened by the almost nightly visits of my friend Loewy,[5] who talked about his association with the royal couple[6] and found the acquisitions from the "national gift"[7] very nice. The little Mercury is recognized by all parties, but no one wants to take responsibility for the Tanagra figure.

Strange that I am writing to you about this right at this hectic time; like the woman who rescues the bird cage during the fire.

I send kind regards and beg your consideration for this scribbling.

Yours truly,
Freud

1. See letter 172 and n. 4.

2. "'Wild' Psychoanalysis" (1910k), published in the third issue of the *Zentralblatt* 1 (1910–11): 91–95.

3. Freud's mother-in-law, Emmeline Bernays.

4. Enclosed in brackets in the original. Freud is evidently referring here to the royalties from his *Sammlung kleiner Schriften zur Neurosenlehre* (see letter 150 and n. 1).

5. Emanuel Löwy (1857–1938), professor of archaeology in Rome until 1915, then from 1918 on in Vienna. A lifelong friend of Freud's "who pays me a visit every year and

usually keeps me up until three in the morning" (November 5, 1987, *Fliess Letters*, pp. 277f).

6. Victor Emanuel III (1869–1947), king of Italy, and Elena di Montenegro Petrovich-Njegos (1873–1952).

7. See letter 171 and n. 2.

177

Budapest, October 29, 1910
VII., Erzsébet-körút 54

Dear Professor,

In your letter of October 17 there was another retort directed at my last remarks about our trip to Italy. But for the time being I think it would be better to let this subject mature in me and become clarified. If I come to Vienna sometime, then "everything, everything will turn out all right."[1]

I pity you about your difficult correspondence with Bleuler, even though I see that one should not give up on such a personality so soon. I mean this in particular regard to his reputation as a full professor, for otherwise I find him petty and vain.

The difficulties with the Viennese are also regrettable. How rare objectivity is in the world! One could speak with more justification about the maliciousness of the subject than about that of the object.

I wish you much humor in all of these difficulties. After all, you invented the theory of humor yourself; you should also be able to apply it.

As you see, I am still living half in the memory of my study of your joke book. My announced lecture about jokes took place the day before yesterday in the Sociological Society. I was very successful, and I think I have gained a few adherents (nonphysicians). The lecture will be published in a Hungarian review. Should I translate it for the Zentralblatt?[2]

I am happy about the noble contest between Vienna and Zurich. The Korrespondenzblatt is courageous and pugnacious. I haven't seen the Zentralblatt yet—only your contribution,[3] and I thank you kindly for sending it to me.

I will write a little paper on the psychology of the obscene as soon as I have time.[4] Do you want to read it before I send it to the Zentralblatt?

I fear that I have disturbed you unnecessarily about the "sleep and dream letter." The things that occurred to me in connection with it are not of the first quality, and I am beginning to see that my request was a symptomatic action. In Italy I silenced, along with many other things, the wish to talk this matter out with you. So perhaps it was a "retrospective reaction" [*Nachträglichkeit*].[5]

Why didn't you mention the "shy admiration and mute contradiction"[6] in Italy? Everything could have turned out differently.

Kind regards,
Ferenczi

I ask you to forward my letter of condolence to your wife.

I think I have found in a case the connecting bridge between certain neuroses that we are familiar with and "thought transference." I will write about it next time.

1. Possibly an allusion to the refrain in the poem "Frühlingsglaube" [Spring Faith] (1812) by the popular German romantic Ludwig Uhland (1787–1862): "Nun, armes Herz, vergiss der Qual! Nun muss sich alles, alles wenden" (Now, poor heart, forget the pain! Now everything, everything must change).
    2. The article was published in *Gyógyászat*, no. 5 (1911): 76–77, and no. 6 (1911): 92–94, but not in the *Zentralblatt*.
    3. "'Wild' Psychoanalysis"; see letter 176 and n. 2.
    4. See letter 175 and n. 2.
    5. James Strachey's translation of this term as "deferred action" in the *Standard Edition* has been the subject of recent criticism [Trans.].
    6. Ferenczi misquotes Freud here.

178

Vienna, November 8, 1910
IX., Berggasse 19

Dear friend,
    I am replying immediately on account of the enclosure. I have corresponded with Jung about the same small themata and don't share his views this time. Limiting membership to academicians would have no prospects at all of getting through in Vienna.[1] In contrast to you, I also don't share the opinion that the Korrespondenzblatt is being harmed by the Zentralblatt. The Korrespondenzblatt is not a scientific organ at all, and is meant only for personal communication from the Central Office to the members, which is of no interest to the public. Unfortunately, I must concede that Adler-Stekel's tactlessness and lack of consideration make understanding very difficult. I am chronically annoyed with both of them. But even Jung, as president, could cast aside his sensitivities about earlier events. It is difficult to have to educate so much.
    Your case[2] is very nice and should be studied closely. I just didn't want to postpone the work. I have even immersed myself in the work on Schre-

ber, and in so doing I flee all personal bitterness. It will occupy me until Christmas. Five pages are already extant.

Wife and sister-in-law have been back since Saturday[3] and thank you sincerely for your words of condolence.

Regards, for the present.

Cordially,
Freud

1. The enclosure is missing. On October 29 Jung had written to Freud: "Further, in Zürich we have the rule that *only holders of academic degrees* can be accepted as members . . . I say this because I fear that Ferenczi is starting something with that stage director," meaning Hevesi (see letter 127, n. 8); *Freud/Jung*, p. 363.

2. A communication from Ferenczi is evidently missing here. See also letter 180 and n. 3.

3. From the funeral of Emmeline Bernays.

179

Vienna, November 15, 1910
IX., Berggasse 19

Dear friend,

Quickly, a piece of news for you to fix (in your possession), which brings strong evidence for thought transference. That will certainly be *your* great discovery. So listen.

In Munich there is a court astrologer, a woman, who foretells the future with the aid of astronomical tables. One of my patients (Dr. Weil, a serious person not to be suspected of lying) had his future foretold by her. He gave her the birthday of his brother-in-law (his only sister's husband), and she thereupon produced not a bad description of him! What struck him most was the fact that she prophesied that the brother-in-law would undergo a poisoning from oysters or crayfish in July which would give his intestines trouble for quite a long time. The prophecy was made in January; it *didn't* come true in July, to be sure, but the commendable thing about it remains that the brother-in-law actually had experienced a poisoning from a lobster in July of the previous year. She thus simply prophesied the past again!!! My objection that this is the worst disgrace imaginable for a prophet made no impression on the storyteller, evidently because he *so* very much liked the prospect.

Another session in April of this year. He presented her with his own birthday and learned that there would be a death in this person's family in October; at the very latest, it would drag out until mid-November. It made a particular impression on him that she said *the same thing* upon hearing of his sister's birthday, even though she didn't know that it was his sister. He consciously related it to his father or uncle. Of course, again, only his brother-in-law could have been meant. Now, the timing fits the following context. A short time earlier he had set a date for his treatment with me for which *exactly the same thing* was arranged. He then came on October 10. Then he made the prophecy come true in this guise on November 15 by confessing to me that he was expecting his brother-in-law's death!!!!¹

If you want to publish Παranoia, hurry up, because my Schreber is being readied for the third volume. After that, you will lose the effect. But that way I can still refer to your communications.

I am up to my ears in hard work. Many thanks for the other things you have written.

Yours,
Freud

1. This case is described and discussed by Freud in "Psycho-Analysis and Telepathy" (1941d [1921], pp. 182–185) and in *New Introductory Lectures on Psycho-Analysis* (1933a, pp. 43–45).

180

Budapest, November 16, 1910
VII., Erzsébet-körút 54

Dear Professor,

Many thanks for the interesting "cases of transference." They will go into the collection! In the meantime I experienced something of this sort from my homosexual patient. E.g., the day before yesterday I was talking with Frau G. about my vanity complex and was citing to her your views about the childishness and nonsense that lie in fantasies of immortality (immortality in the sense of fame after death). I was also talking about my own desire for notoriety and money. That took place in the morning.

At six o' clock in the evening, in analysis, the following occurs to my homosexual:

1.) A poem that begins with the (Hungarian) words: "When I run through my bumpy path and find peace in the grave," etc. Thereupon, 2.) *"Prof. Freud* is an egoist if he counts on being famous after his death. It is egoistic to seek money or fame; it serves the person and not humanity."—

Another case:

Yesterday afternoon I was reading a novel written by a homosexual, in which there is talk about Capri.

A patient (impotent) gives these associations in the evening: Vàradi (a local inkeeper)–Capri–goat–Krupp. [Patient was, indeed, himself in Capri, was interested in the case of Krupp,[1] and as a child he had fantasies of bestiality (with cows, horses).][2] But that may have had only a *salutary* effect.—

After mature consideration, and proceeding from the view that a reaction formation against vanity would be just as nonsensical as vanity itself, I have decided to publish our hypothetical ideas from Berchtesgaden along with their subsequent confirmation as *bare facts*, without much alteration and explanation. But I don't want to meddle with your ideas about paranoia since then.—Since I had given up the paranoia plans, I did *not* note down the case (of the teacher) that I recently communicated to you. Would you please send back to me the letter that contains it, as well as the letter with the *case of draftiness* (of the lady who could feel things from a distance).[3] I promise from now on to spare you such requests, which are surely burdensome.

Best regards,
Ferenczi

In the month of December I am probably going to Vienna in the matter of Frau G.'s daughter.[4]

The manner in which my homosexual guesses my thoughts speaks in favor of the notion that *quite abstract* ideas (i.e., those already clothed in verbal images), and not only visual representations, can also be transferred. My patient is, to be sure, a very intelligent person.

The paper on *obscene words* is ¾ finished.

Maybe I will combine my trip to Vienna with an excursion to the soothsayer in Munich. Could you get me her address?

1. Friedrich Alfred Krupp (1854–1902), weapons manufacturer and founder of the industrial empire that bears his name, was the head of a family and a homosexual. He committed suicide when his secret was revealed in the newspapers.

2. Enclosed in brackets in the original.

3. These cases were evidently described in letters or enclosures that have not been preserved.

4. See letter 192 and n. 1.

181

Budapest, November 22, 1910
VII., Erzsébet-körút 54

Dear Professor,

Thank you for sending back the letters! As regards the planned work on paranoia, I don't know what I should reply to *Jung*, who just asked me whether I have something to submit for the *January* or the *August* issue of the Jahrbuch. In which one is *your* work on Schreber coming out?

Please send brief reply (correspondence card will suffice). I know how busy you are.

Kind regards,
Ferenczi

182

Budapest, November 22, 1910
Grand Hotel Royal

Dear Professor,

Interesting news in the transference story. Imagine, *I am a great sooth-sayer, that is to say, a reader of thoughts!* I am reading my patients' thoughts (in my free associations). The future methodology of ΨA must make use of this.

After a few rehearsals with Frau G.—which were downright stimulating—today I ventured toward my homosexual patient. Resounding success. I did four experiments. He had to think about people whom I don't know.

1st experiment. [He thinks of *Taral*, the English jockey who went to America.][1] I begin with the idea of an *English material* (of course, down deep I am thinking about Frau G.'s dress!), then (after a few other associations), come *spats, hunt, map, cheater, counterfeiter, swindler* [all things closely associated with sports in America].

2nd experiment. [He thinks of his boss, the managing director of a bank.] I begin with a *paper scissors, desk,* then (among other associations) *editing.* The *director of a newspaper office.* I said "director."

3d experiment. [He thinks of a deceased uncle.] I constantly associate reminiscences of the foul-smelling Negro chambermaid at *Brill's.* [Explanation: my patient has decidely *necrophagous* thoughts in the ucs.—so in the cs. he is idiosyncratic with regard to all odors.]

4th experiment. [Patient thinks of the millennium monument by the sculptor *Zala.*][2] I (among fifteen to sixteen associations): Elisabeth Bridge, bookstore, the hysterical wife of an engineer. *Lévay* (a name derived from the name of the city *Léva*). *Zala* is the name of a county.

This method will be suitable to catch the patient's *most active* complexes at work.—It can be refined even more!

When I come to Vienna, I will introduce myself as "court astrologer of the psychoanalysts."

Best regards,
Ferenczi

1. Enclosed in brackets in the original, as are similar remarks throughout this letter.

2. István György Zala (1858–1937), with Albert Schickedanz creator of the monument commemorating the millennial celebration (1896) of the Kingdom of Hungary, located in Heroes' Square (Hösök Tere) in Budapest.

183

Vienna, November 23, 1910
IX., Berggasse 19

Dear friend,

Here is the address in Munich:

Frau Arnold, Klenzestrasse 15.

As regards paranoia, it would be better for you to make yourself independent of me. Up to now I have completed the first chapter of the work on Schreber (twenty-four pages) and would like to be finished by January, but I don't think it will work because I am struggling with time and energy, and, in addition, I am getting terribly angry with Adler and Stekel. I had been hoping that it would come to some kind of clean separation, but things are getting reconciled again, so I have to go on slaving away with them despite my belief that nothing can be done with them. The others are also not gratifying. Bleuler's reply is still not forthcoming, as is also the decision as to whether I will go to Zurich over Christmas.

I tell you, it was often nicer when I was alone. Excuse my poor and meager letters under these circumstances.

Kind regards,
Freud

184

Budapest, December 2, 1910
VII., Erzsébet-körút 54

Dear Professor,

The "independence" that you have granted me in the question of paranoia evidently doesn't agree with me. I have postponed beginning work again and again with the most meager excuses—not a line of it has been written yet. But I consider it a favorable symptom that I worked myself up to writing this letter; I believe that I will now improve.—No doubt the bad mood that characterized your last letter has infected me. Perhaps, as in the case of the Russian, *Naum Kotik*,[1] the "psychophysical emanation" has fixed onto the paper and infected me. I hope (*also* [!][2] with consideration for you) that in future your reports will originate from an improved frame of mind.

I frittered away the time that remained to me from analytical work on experiments with transference. For the time being nothing new to report about it—except perhaps the following supposition (already touched on with *Kotik*): if one is somehow upset and not quite with it (in regard to the experiment)—then one may be a good subject for emanation, but one is not suitable for perceiving. A calm mood is more favorable. The most sensitive are those in love (with the aid of their masochistic components). It is not beyond the realm of possibility that this "difference in voltage" and the thought transference conditioned by it also plays a certain role in ordinary life by influencing associations, and through them also mood, action, etc. Greater significance would accrue to it only in pathological cases.

The perceiving person reacts to the transference with his own ucs. complexes, but he chooses among these only those closest to the ucs. complexes of the one posing the task.

Here is such a case:

I am thinking of a woman whose visit I am expecting.

The homosexual patient is given the task of guessing what I am thinking about, and he produces the following associations:

1.) A woman; she gives her child a lollipop.

2.) *Nurses [Wärterinnen] come and go.*

2.) What is the doctor's name in Zurich? Yes! Now I know. *Forel's* book about hypnosis;[3] there Forel relates the dream of a nurse, in which a horse appears. You, Doctor, interpreted the dream in such a way that *Forel* himself portrays the horse without knowing anything about it.—

The woman whom I was expecting is a Frau Pollatschek,[4] the mother of that patient with the beautiful eyes whom you sent to me (in the first office hours after the trip to Italy), but who didn't come.—This lady (the mother) is herself neurotic, you see, and was just in analysis for four months with *Bircher-Benner*[5] in *Zurich*. At the time she was making a lot of nasty remarks about my "obscene" lectures; now she has been completely converted, is full of enthusiasm for the cause, and wants to go back to *Bircher* in order to dedicate herself there to ΨA., as a *nurse*. She told me recently she was concerned whether I might not have problems with my *mother complex* (vis-à-vis her).

During the experiment I was *not* thinking about these things; I was thinking quite vaguely about Frau Pollatschek—The ucs. association to the thought *mother,* which was *preconscious* to me, aroused the patient's ucs. mother complex.

My pcs. thoughts, Zurich, nurse, etc. aroused in the patient the *only* idea that he could have about psychiatry in Zurich: his recollection of my interpretation of Forel's dream.

In this case the complexes aroused in the patient are those that I also possess.—In other cases, where he doesn't have such *mutual* complexes at his disposal, he says something of his own, but something similar.—

I notice that, inwardly, I judged Bircher's analysis somewhat contemptuously. That corresponds to the ridiculous role of Forel when he talks about dreams that he doesn't understand.—

By the way, I learned something interesting from this lady about the way in which Bircher conducts his analyses. The ladies go around all day with the thought that they have to prepare for the next analysis. There are many *Dutch women* among them, who want to make a *theosophical* science out of ΨA., and they talk about the ucs. only as the *race-mneme.* The symptoms are "taken up" in order. "I have been cured of three symptoms; the fourth has not yet been 'taken up,'" said the patient, etc.

Frau Pollatschek is, incidentally, a very intellectual, very well educated lady, who has an excellent grasp of the sense of psychoanalysis.—

On the twelfth I am going to Miskolcz to visit my mother, who is celebrating her 70th birthday. It will be a regular "family day"—ten living siblings and the many grandchildren!

In expectation of good news and with kind regards, I am

Yours truly,
Ferenczi

I almost forgot to tell you the most important—and, naturally, the most unpleasant—thing.—I finally saw that the time had come to work energetically on founding the group. But first I had to come to terms with *Stein* and *Décsi.* I therefore wrote to both of them and communicated to them that I would like to transform the former *course evenings* into *discussion evenings,* and I invited them to the last session (which took place on

Tuesday). I expressly asked for a reply. *But I didn't receive any.* Just today I received a letter, from *Décsi* alone. He apologizes for not having come, he is now a bridegroom, etc. At the time he had written that he couldn't come, but unfortunately he forgot to mail the letter (as proof, he enclosed a sealed, stamped letter dated last Monday).

I am now perplexed about *Stein.* His hurtful behavior is—in view of his sensitivity—understandable; I am also not angry with him. But, for reasons of expediency, I must somehow react to his rudeness! When we met by chance he has treated me downright despicably a few times; he avoided the opportunity to extend his hand to me, etc.—I will probably respond to his last great rudeness, the failure to reply to my invitation, by neglecting to address him with the familiar *"Du."* The whole thing is an embarrassment. I really feel sorry for Stein.

1. See letter 85 and nn. 18 and 19.
2. Enclosed in brackets in the original.
3. Auguste Henri Forel (1848–1931), noted Swiss psychiatrist and psychologist, who also made a name for himself with his research on ants. In 1879 he became a professor of psychiatry in Zurich and, until 1898, was Bleuler's predecessor at the Burghölzli, for whose fame as a progressive institution he was responsible. He was, like Bleuler, a leader in the antialcohol movement. His portrait appears today on Swiss 1,000 franc notes. The book mentioned here (*Der Hypnotismus, seine Bedeutung und seine Handhabung in kurzgefasster Darstellung* [Stuttgart, 1899]) was reviewed by Freud in 1889 (1889a).
4. Cecilia Pollacsek/Polányi (1862–1939), née Wohl, mother of Laura Striker (see letter 169 and n. 10 and letter 231, n. 4). Widowed since 1905, she conducted a renowned literary salon in Budapest. Four of her six children—Laura, Adolf, Karl, and Michael—became well known through their work in education, law, economics, and chemistry and scientific theory. Karl (1886–1964) was, in addition, the founder of the Galilei Society.
5. Maximilian Oskar Bircher-Benner (1867–1939), Zurich dietitian and physiotherapist; founded a clinic for internal diseases and psychoneuroses in 1897; inventor of Bircher-Müesli. In 1909 he opened a psychoanalytic practice (see *Freud/Jung,* October 1 and December 25, 1909, pp. 247–248, 280) and was a member of the Zurich Psychoanalytic Branch Society until 1914.

185

Vienna, December 3, 1910
IX., Berggasse 19

Dear friend,

You will certainly be astounded that I didn't react earlier to your earth-shaking communication to the effect that you were yourself a medium. I wouldn't even be able to write yet today if I weren't rather miserable with influenza and hadn't canceled the lecture (as well as the tarok game). You see, otherwise I am Schreber, nothing but Schreber, of course not until after

10 P.M., and there is a struggle for liberation connected with this work, the literary fruits of which still don't satisfy me.

I could not, of course, prevent your news from occupying me greatly. I see destiny approaching, inexorably, and I note that it has designated you to bring to light mysticism and the like, and that it would be just as futile as it is hard-hearted to keep you from it. Still, I think we ought to venture to slow it down. I would like to request that you continue to research in secrecy for two full years and don't come out until 1913; then, certainly, in the Jahrbuch, openly and aboveboard. You know my practical reasons against it and my secret painful sensitivities.

Now, I would like to know when you are coming to Vienna, since you have indicated you would come in December. Eitingon has announced his arrival here from Damascus on the 5th to the 8th.

The matter with Bleuler seems to be working out more favorably; he will stay with us in some form or other, although perhaps not in the Association. I am about to rendezvous with him in Munich (during Christmas), and Jung has promised to follow from the rear when he leaves.

It is constantly raining insults from Germany; Putnam has submitted his second paper for ΨA, just as chivalrous and decisive as the first but more practical. (Journal of Nervous and Mental Diseases, Nov. 10). The first one will be published in the January issue of the Zentralblatt.[1] The journal is, I think, awaiting original contributions from you. I will keep a close watch on the editorial board now. The matter with Adler and Stekel seems to be on the way to a peaceful solution, but my position in Vienna is difficult.

I hope you will now give up your gracious consideration for me and that you will write again soon.

Kind regards,
Freud

P.S. Do you know the "Man Weary of America" by Kürnberger?[2] Emmes![3]

1. For Putnam's first essay, see letter 169 and n. 2. The second, "Personal Experience with Freud's Psychoanalytic Method," Journal of Nervous and Mental Disease 37 (1910): 630–639, was published somewhat later in translation by Otto Rank in the Zentralblatt 1 (1910–11): 533–548.

2. Ferdinand Kürnberger (1821–1879), Der Amerikamüde, Amerikanisches Kulturbild (Leipzig, 1855; rpt. Frankfurt, 1986). A liberal Austrian writer, raconteur, and essayist, Kürnberger wrote this book in response to the "European weariness" of the reactionary Metternich era, which had found its expression in the novel Die Europamüden (1838) by Ernst Willkomm. The novel's hero, a noble physician and poet of Hungarian origin, finds the American ideal of freedom to be an illusion in a land where the law of the jungle, deceit, and the desire for profit prevail, and a human being becomes "an automaton that produces a dollar" (p. 267).

3. Yiddish for "True!" A joke of Freud's was: "What is the opposite of Emmes? S. M." (Seine Majestät = His Majesty).

186

Vienna, December 6, 1910
IX., Berggasse 19

Dear friend,

Imagine that we are still in Palermo in the Hotel de France in the morning and I gave you the following contribution to the notes on paranoia. You see, I have just overcome an error that was holding me up at that time, and I can produce the following simple formulation.

Let us break down *repression* into
a) *fixation*, b) *actual repression*, c) *return*.

(*Breakthrough*)
[The significance of these terms is, of course, familiar to you],[1] so a main statement goes:

I. *Breakthrough occurs at the point of fixation.*

This is already known to you [but unclear]. The obscurity lay in the relationship between repression and breakthrough; I assumed the same mechanism for both. That was misleading.

II. *The mechanism of breakthrough is independent of that of repression.*
and now, the third:

III. *The mechanism of breakthrough depends on the phase of development of the ego, that of repression depends on the phase of the libido.*[2]

If this is true, then you can have a hundred oxen slaughtered for us, despite the shortage of meat. It would be too beautiful: Hoche, Friedländer, Oppenheim,[3] et al., on the *Ara* of Hiero,[4] which we saw.

Eitingon arrived from Palestine.

I great you cordially and send regards to Frau G.

Yours,
Freud

1. Enclosed in brackets in the original, as is the bracketed remark in the next paragraph.

2. See Freud's analysis of Schreber (1911c [1910], pp. 66ff) and his "Formulations on the Two Principles of Mental Functioning" (1911b, pp. 244–245), where he says it "is plausible to suppose that the form taken by the subsequent illness (the *choice of neurosis*) will depend on the particular phase of the development of the ego and of the libido in which the dispositional inhibition of development has occurred."

3. Hermann Oppenheim (1858–1919), Berlin neurologist and head of a private clinic which he founded in 1891. He was related to Karl Abraham by marriage. Two months earlier, at the fourth annual meeting of the Society of German Neurologists in Berlin (October 6–8, 1910), he had called for a boycott of clinics that used psychoanalysis.

4. Altar of Hiero in Syracuse. Hiero II (306?-215? B.C.), king of Syracuse, had a 200-meter-long sacrificial altar erected, on which 450 bulls (not oxen) were sacrificed annually in memory of the fall of the tyrant Thrasybulos in 463 B.C.

187

Budapest, December 9, 1910
VII., Erzsébet-körút 54

Dear Professor,

I think I can also jubilate about your "Eureka." Now, all of a sudden, much has become clear to me! (Much that I darkly intimated but couldn't make clear.) Among my many plans for work there is a note about "types of onset of hysterical illness," where I seem to have been aware of the fact that *repression* as such is *symptomless,* and that its return only then signifies the beginning of the illness. But it is only the determination that it is *always* this way that makes this idea significant.

But all this is nugatory and insignificant in comparison with the progress that your theory signifies for our understanding of the *choice of neurosis.*[1] "Constitution" has again fallen a notch—and what remains of it has become more comprehensible. Its great simplicity speaks decidedly in favor of the truth of your theory.

I can deliver a few oxen to you from Budapest for Hiero's altar, but I think you will find enough in Germany!

I won't go to Vienna until next year—probably in January. I am very much looking forward to seeing you again. The trip has not left behind anything unpleasurable *in me* (that I haven't tamed through insight).

Here is a little piece for the Zentralblatt.[2] Please read it through and write to me about it; I would like to hear your opinion before I send it to the editors.

Tomorrow I am going to Miskolcz.

Again, I congratulate you on your beautiful solution to the question of the choice of neurosis.

Cordially,
Ferenczi

1. See letter 186, n. 2, and Ferenczi's essay "Über die Rolle der Homosexualität in der Pathogenese der Paranoia" [On the Part Played by Homosexuality in the Pathogenesis of Paranoia] (1911, 80; C., p. 184; Schriften I, 91).

2. "Über obszöne Worte" [On Obscene Words] (1911, 75; C., p. 132); see also letter 175 and n. 2.

188

Vienna, December 16, 1910
IX., Berggasse 19

Dear friend,

Your work was naturally submitted to the editorial board without censorship. Issue no. 3 of the Zentralblatt came out today. Schreber is finished, except for a few notes. Tough work. Mocking laughter or immortality or both;[1] this step in psychiatry is probably the boldest that we have taken so far. The essay recently came into being, "fleeting improvised" [flüchtig hingemacht][2] during ten to eleven hours of analytic work, which has been especially unpleasant recently, but it does exhibit the nice parts known to you. On Sunday I will write down the brief formulations about the reality and pleasure ego.[3] I will bring both to Jung in Munich. I still haven't received anything definite from Bleuler about our meeting. He will certainly cause problems at the eleventh hour.

Christmas will not be celebrated here on account of mourning.[4]

The next, the fourth, issue of the Zentralblatt will contain Putnam's nice lecture in Toronto.[5] Things are going generally well in the literature. I have three volumes prepared for the Schriften zur angewandten Seelenkunde: Jones's Oedipus essay,[6] a juridical work on patricide by a completely unknown writer from Zurich,[7] and Abraham's study on Segantini,[8] which was, of course, just announced.

My health and mood are not quite keeping pace with the pleasantness of these things. Not surprising. If only one didn't have to get rich!

I have now overcome Fliess, which you were so curious about. Adler is a little Fliess redivivus, just as paranoid. Stekel, his appendage, is at least called Wilhelm.

I send cordial regards and await your response to my suggestion concerning the publication of thought induction.

Yours,
Freud

Maybe I really will go to the court astrologer in Munich.

1. "Or both" is written in English in the original.

2. An allusion to an expression used by Daniel Paul Schreber (Memoirs, p. 74).

3. "Formulations on the Two Principles of Mental Functioning" (1911b); see also letter 172 and n. 4.

4. On account of the death of Freud's mother-in-law.

5. The text translated by Freud (see letter 169 and n. 2).

6. See letter 119, n. 4.

7. Adolf Josef Storfer, *Zur Sonderstellung des Vatermordes* (published in 1911 as vol. 12 of the *Schriften*). Adolf (after 1938, Albert) Storfer (1888–1944), journalist and writer of Romanian origin, studied philosophy, psychology, and linguistics at Klausenberg and Zurich, where he also began the study of law. He went to Vienna in spring of 1913 and later became the business manager of the *Internationaler Psychoanalytischer Verlag* (1925–1932). He was co-editor of Freud's *Gesammelte Schriften* (1924–1934) until the next-to-last volume and, until 1932, editor of the journals *Die psychoanalytische Bewegung* (1929–1933) and *Almanach der Psychoanalyse* (1926–1938). After the Anschluss he fled to Shanghai and from there to Melbourne, Australia, where he died in poverty.

8. Karl Abraham, *Giovanni Segantini, Ein psychoanalytischer Versuch* (published in 1911 as vol. 12 of the *Schriften zur angewandten Seelenkunde*).

189

Budapest, December 19, 1910
VII., Erzsébet-körút 54

Dear Professor,

I didn't respond to your wish expressed in regard to thought induction because, in view of our earlier discussions, I thought we had decided to treat this matter with extreme caution. It goes without saying that I am in complete agreement with the date 1913; perhaps I will want to extend it even further.

In the meantime I have been collecting some material. It is interesting and valuable to know that we will be able—so it seems—to do without professional mediums. But I would need a few hints as to determining the *limits* of this possibility.

I, too, am doing well now and then. E.g., Frau G. is thinking about a trip we took together by car to a sanatorium for pulmonary diseases where I was discharging my duties as a court physician.

I associate: *knee, blood*, "blood and blood everywhere, the son murders the father, the brother the brother."—"That was said (I continue) by *Széchenyi* about the Revolution of '48; then he died, in the sanatorium at Döbling."[1]

[It is worth mentioning that the patient whom I went to visit had died the day before of pulmonary bleeding—which we didn't learn until we were outside. *Knee* = a sexual reminiscence of the excursion.][2]

If the experiment succeeds, the percipient must be in a mood that is as calm and cheerful as possible, but still not too lively. If he is excited, then he is not suited for projecting the psychic rays. Impatience disturbs.—The game reminds one of children's games of hiding; while associating, the questioner monitors what is good or inappropriate in what comes to his mind and seems constantly to give direction to the receiver. One sometimes sees outright how the receiver begins very distantly with his own complexes and is gradually led to the proximity of what is supposed to be guessed. A mute "warm" or "cold" is constantly being called out to him. Wonderful compromises come about between one's own complexes and the preconscious ideas of the questioner.

A second example.

[Frau G. is thinking about the Hungarian king Ludwig II,[3] who died in the battle of Mohács,[4] where he fell from his horse and drowned in a stream.]

I associate: "I am thinking of the letter L . . . Kleinpaul says that L imitates flowing, the flowing of a stream; I now see a flowing stream . . . I am thinking of an old pistol . . . the figure of a warrior (a Chinese barbarian) that I gave you; he is sitting on his horse and slashing with his saber. Now I am thinking about my miser complex." [In these thoughts all elements of what Frau G. has imagined are presented with my complexes. Miser complex = the miserliness of my brother *Ludwig*,[5] whom we were talking about on the same day.]

I am *very* curious about Schreber. I am astonished by your capacity for work; but I can't approve of *this* overexertion.

The solution: Adler = Fliess is *certainly* correct. Now I also understand Adler's hate theories; he doesn't want to love, and therefore he has to hate and thinks he is being hated; in so doing he projects all this into his theories.

It is strange, and certainly no coincidence, that both Fliess and Adler emphasize *bisexuality* in this way; the homosexual origin of their character is expressed therein.

I wish you a pleasant recuperation and enjoyment for Munich; give my regards to Jung.

Yours truly,
Ferenczi

1. Count István Széchenyi (1791–1860), an important figure in the history of Hungary; founder of the Hungarian Academy of Sciences. He sought to persuade the Hungarian nobility to institute reforms, but his efforts were preempted by the more radical ideas of Lajos Kossuth. He felt responsible for having caused the outbreak of the Revolution of 1848 and the war of independence. He was committed, with a diagnosis of melancholia, to the sanatorium at Döbling, where he took his life after having written his memoirs.

2. Enclosed in brackets in the original, as are similar remarks throughout the letter.

3. Lajos II (1506–1526), king of Hungary and Bohemia.

4. Decisive defeat of Hungary by Turkey (1526), after which Hungary lost its independence, and large portions of the country were occupied by the Turks for a century and a half.

5. Lajos Ferenczi; see letter 76, n. 1.

190

Vienna, December 29, 1910
IX., Berggasse 19

Dear friend,

I returned from Munich yesterday morning.[1] Since I had left in a very poor frame of mind, I had given myself a vacation day as a bonus during the two holidays. Bleuler arrived a quarter of an hour before me, and then we went for a walk and debated until evening, with interruptions, to be sure, from the marvelous meals at the Park Hotel. I arrived at a complete understanding and good personal relations with him; he, too, is only a poor devil like us and wants people to love him a little, which has perhaps been neglected from a decisive quarter. It is almost beyond doubt that he will join the Society in Zurich. With that, any schism there might be is rectified.

He left at 12:50, and Jung came at 5:15. In the meantime I slept, very exhausted by a bad night. Jung was again magnificent and did me a lot of good. I poured out my heart about many things, about the Adlerian movement, my own difficulties, and finally about my distress about thought transference. You should know that I had intended to write to the court astrologer, and had forgotten to take down her address, and in Munich I remembered only the street. I gave in to such signs of inner weakness and initiated Jung into the matter, told him about your findings, my confirmation through that prophecy, and my proposal of a latency period until 1913. He laughed and admitted that he had been convinced for a long time and had himself initiated very substantive experiments, praised my caution, and declared himself ready for an agreement with you, if it should come to that. He sees all the dangers just as we do, but he still wants to risk it with ΨA. I am glad he has such broad shoulders. I found this burden almost too heavy for me. Now, don't be jealous, but take Jung into your calculations. I am convinced more than ever that he is the man of the future.

His own work has gone deep into mythology, which he wants to open with the key of libido theory. As gratifying as all that was, I still asked him to return to the neuroses at the proper time. That is the motherland where we first have to secure our mastery against everything and everyone.

I brought along my work on Schreber for him, merely read aloud the smaller one about the two principles, and took it home for revision. In the evening Seif[2] happened by, enthusiastic and flourishing as always. I took my leave of them at 10:40 P.M. at the station.

The *entrevue*[3] did a lot of good for my sinking life spirits. I now intend to exert myself somewhat less, and a decline in my practice unprovoked by me seems to be ready to support me in this. I brought along a splendid Japanese toad made of nephrite as a souvenir.

I expect to see you here in January, and, since our correspondence has been a bit wanting of late, to discuss many things with you.

Kindest regards,
Freud

1. Freud had originally planned to visit Bleuler in Zurich in order to persuade him to join the Zurich Society of the IPA. He also hoped to use this occasion to see Jung. In order for Freud not to have to meet Bleuler and Jung simultaneously, since there was some disagreement between them, Jung had proposed that Bleuler and Freud meet in Munich, where he would arrive after Bleuler's departure. In Munich Bleuler appeared "won over," as Freud reported in the Vienna Society (January 4, 1911, *Minutes* III, 101f) and wrote to Abraham (January 20, 1911, *Letters*, p. 98).

2. Leonhard Seif (1866–1949), Munich neurologist, and founder (1911) and head of the Psychoanalytic Society there. In 1913 he separated from Freud and joined Adler.

3. Meeting or discussion, especially among monarchs.

191

Budapest, December 31, 1910
VII., Erzsébet-körút 54

Dear Professor,

I don't want to wait with my New Year's wishes until I have time to respond to your interesting and gratifying report on the trip to Munich (which, I hope, can happen tomorrow).

May the new year, which begins under good auspices—in an esoteric regard—be a year of peace and also lead to a Viennese peace.

I wish you few but very well paid analyses, and health. The rest will come.

Myself—less practice and more literary diligence.

I greet you all most cordially.

Dr. Ferenczi

192

Budapest, January 3, 1911
VII., Erzsébet-körút 54

Dear Professor,

You are right. One must from time to time interrupt communication by letter with a personal one, otherwise one all too easily loses contact with reality and corresponds not with a really living person but with one that one makes up in fantasy at one's pleasure. I also don't want to postpone my trip for long, but am waiting for the impending trip to Vienna of Frau G., who is going there with her daughter[1] toward the end of this month to correct the scar which resulted from a tooth periostitis (in the daughter). I want to be of help to her in this matter.

If you offer us an opportunity to do so, we will also make use of our presence to ask your advice in a rather difficult matter (marriage and love affair of this same daughter). This business is causing poor Frau G. a lot of worry, and I am much too interested in it to be able to judge and act quite calmly.

As mentioned, I am very pleased about the peacemaking with Bleuler. Jung will have to strive to bind him to himself and to the cause with more tender treatment.

After mature reflection I must also unreservedly share your opinion about *Jung's* future role in psychoanalysis. His two great deeds: his courageous and independent stand in recognizing your ideas—as well as the first experiments in psychiatry assure him this role, even if he didn't accomplish any more. Where the Viennese have a head start over him is in the psychoanalytic *routine* acquired with you. But I see in my own case that only some practice and a little sense for solving psychological riddles is required to acquire *this.* But what eludes the Viennese and what Jung possesses in ever increasing measure is the recognition that psychoanalysis must begin with self-criticism, without which every analysis can acquire a paranoid wrapper (see *Adler*).

On the other hand, Jung easily succumbs to theological speculations, and he is also inclined to work too soon with metaphysical thought processes before what is inductively accessible has been exhausted. Your instruction that he should return to "mother earth" will be very useful to him.

When I think of the resistances that Jung has to deal with as a faithful Christian, before he became such a total adherent of yours, I must also praise his insight and tractability. As a full-blooded human being he obviously also has to struggle a great deal with his temperament, especially with his lust for power and his ambition. That will probably be the last thing he overcomes.

But these affects fit in very well with the activity that we expect from him—assuming that he doesn't let himself be dominated too much by them.

I am now thinking about the role that you once reserved *for me*, that of the "wise adviser" at Jung's side.

It would be childishly inveighing against fate for me to want to rebel against this. But I do see more and more that, by virtue of constitution and experience, I am much more disposed to contemplation than to activity. Perhaps I will still have the opportunity to come personally closer to Jung and bring the influence that you wish to bear.

I am not jealous of Jung, i.e. I have *completely* mastered this instinct. But I am sorry that we didn't strike the same tone in Italy that refreshed and gratified you in Munich.

Kindest regards,
Ferenczi

P.S. I will soon approach Jung with the "thought transference" business.

1. Elma Pálos, Gizella's elder daughter.

193

Vienna, January 3, 1911
IX., Berggasse 19

Dear friend,

As a New Year's present, the following prophecy for your collection, perhaps the nicest piece that you have to date, as far as I am familiar with the material.

Woman, 37 years old, fallen ill with an obsessional neurosis since being informed by her husband that the cause of her childlessness lay in his azoospermia.[1] Beginning with symptoms of anxiety in her 27th year. A year later (28th yr.) It was prophesied by a soothsayer in Paris from the lines in her hand that she would go through great struggles and have two children by her 32nd year. She consoled herself with that for a time; so now the prophecy is five years late.

Analysis. The struggles are clear from the situation. She had always wanted children; she, herself, was the eldest of five siblings. She vacillated at that time about whether she shouldn't leave her husband. Still, it is strange that the soothsayer told her this and revealed her wish to have a child directly, without questioning her further. But where do the time limit and the number two for the children come in?

My question: How old was your mother when you were born?

Answer: She was 30 when she was married. (Immediate correction:) she was thirty when I came into the world.

Question: How large is the age interval between you and your nearest sister?

Answer: One and a half years.

I: So, your mother didn't have any children at the age of 28. You consoled yourself by thinking, "I will be like *my* mother and already have two children at the age of 32."

Your struggles don't come into consideration as far as your mother is concerned?

She: No.

I: What does this fantasy further presume? That you separate from your husband or that he dies, so that you still have time, despite the year of mourning, not to stay behind your mother.

She: I always have the great fear that something will happen to him. When he wanted to leave yesterday evening, I had difficulties talking him into taking this morning's train. What if an accident happened with the train that I recommended![2]

Cordially,
Freud

1. Lack of sperm in the seminal fluid.
2. Freud describes and explains this case in 1941d [1921], pp. 185ff, and 1933a. pp. 40ff.

194

Budapest, January 8, 1911

Dear Professor,

Next Sunday afternoon I intend to go to Vienna with a patient whom I have been treating for impotence for some time with considerable success (and whom *Stekel* sent me at the time), and I would like (if at all possible) to consult with you and Stekel on Sunday morning about the matter of his marriage.

I am considering arriving in Vienna at 9 o'clock.

If you happen to be at your tarok game, please let me know. If not, I will come to see you on Saturday evening. But don't let me disturb your game!

It is probable that I will come again on the following Saturday in the matter of the *Pálos* operation, so that I will have the prospect in the next few days of being together with you frequently and discussing many things.

Thank you very much for your contribution to the induction business. The example is, in fact, *very good.*

Kind regards,
Ferenczi

195

Vienna, January 10, 1911
IX., Berggasse 19

Dear friend,

I am very happy about the opportunity which you told me about of seeing you several times this month. I have, however, a lecture on Saturday evening and then a game of tarok afterwards, and if I don't let myself be disturbed, I won't be able to see you until Sunday. You will certainly come for lunch.

I will also ask you why your last letters, insofar as they were not about factual matters, revealed an elegiac character. I am awaiting the connection to our trip, but I will not let that stand.

Unfortunately, I must also tell you that Martin suffered a fall on a ski trip on the Schneeberg[1] on Sunday and was left lying with a fractured thigh. He wasn't brought in until this evening and is now with Fürth[2] and will be examined by Schnitzler[3] tomorrow. His general condition is good, the injury perhaps not too severe. Let us hope it will still turn out all right with a few months in sickbed and superarbitrium.[4]

Kind regards,
Freud

1. Popular recreational mountain for the Viennese near the Rax, where Freud had his conference with "Katharina" (Freud 1895d, pp. 125–134).

2. Otto von Fürth (1867–1938), associate professor of medicinal chemistry and, from 1923 on, full professor and director of the Medicinal Chemistry Institute of the University of Vienna.

3. Julius Schnitzler (1865–1939), brother of Arthur, a well-known surgeon; since 1902 chief surgeon at the Wieden Hospital and since 1905 titular and, from 1928 on, associate professor of surgery. Julius Schnitzler was a friend and occasional tarok partner of Freud's.

4. Determination of irrevocable unfitness for military service. Martin Freud described this incident in his book *Sigmund Freud: Man and Father* (New York, 1983), pp. 175ff. Through Freud's intervention, Martin entered a private rather than a military hospital, which probably saved him from having his leg amputated.

196

Budapest, January 24, 1911
VII., Erzsébet-körút 54

Dear Professor,

I don't need to linger over my impressions of the latest Viennese excursion, for I am in the pleasant position of informing you that I will again be in Vienna next Sunday, the 29th. The Pálos family will probably be occupying me in the morning and certainly at noon as well. But I would like to meet you in the afternoon, if at all possible. I am arriving Saturday evening at the Hotel Regina, where you can perhaps leave a message for me.

I hope your Martin is already doing much better. Give him my regards.

I am analyzing diligently, but in the last few days I was somewhat more "mundane" (two tea evenings and a reprise of the opera). It was quite a pleasant change for me.

Recently a more successful thought transference:

(A lady is thinking of a gentleman named *Postás* (= postmaster).—The first things that come to my mind: "A flute. A *horn*, as is printed on a certain brand of Egyptian cigarettes. *Tra-ra! Tra-ra!*"

The lady interrupts me: "You have guessed it. His name is Postás. He always smokes Egyptian cigarettes.")—I am reading the Jahrbuch[1] in my free time. Very good!

Kind regards,
Ferenczi

1. The second half of the second volume had been published in December.

197

[Vienna,] February 5, 1911[1]

Dear friend,

If I ever imposed a book by Kleinpaul on spiritualism[2] on you, would you be so kind as to write out the Σατυροζ[3] dream in it for me so I can use it as a citation.

I was very pleased today by a visit from Frau G.

Cordially,
Freud

1. Postcard.
2. Probably Rudolf Kleinpaul, *Die Lebendigen und die Toten in Volksglauben, Religion, und Sage* (1898), cited by Freud in *Totem and Taboo* (1912–13a, pp. 58f).
3. *Satyros* (satyr).

198

Budapest, February 7, 1911
VII., Erzsébet-körút 54

Dear Professor,

My last stay in Vienna has left behind particularly pleasant memory traces in me. I found you mentally and physically fresh and active, the most burning scientific controversies on the way to a solution; I found myself objective, free from complex inhibitions. The diagnosis that you made—in the way of a supposition—about Elma Pálos, did, to be sure, have a rather depressing effect. But afterwards I was able to determine that two things were especially to blame for this depression. First, the unjustified effect that the *words* "dementia praecox" had on me as a result of its associative connection with *severe* cases of this kind. Second, I allowed myself to be surprised by your diagnosis, which should have warned me of the fact that I—attuned part and parcel to neuroses as I am—must have overlooked something in the psychiatric sphere. I think that that can only be helped by an—at least temporary—visit to a psychiatric ward.

"*L'autre danger*" that the psychoanalyst is subject to (at least I found myself inclined to it) is that, in lovingly going into the determinants of a neurosis, one finds them, so to speak *justified*. One is actually right in doing so: everything that exists is *eo ipso*—from a philosophical point of view—justified in existing. The only thing is that this all too forgiving understanding can make one too inclined to take a position in favor of the patient (i.e., in favor of fantasy) and against those close to him (i.e., reality).

Besides monitoring the countertransference, one must therefore also pay heed to this "being induced" by the patients. (Perhaps it is only a question here of a form of countertransference.)

Jung confirmed his receipt of my———[1]

1. The rest of the letter is missing.

199

Vienna, February 8, 1911
IX., Berggasse 19

Dear friend,

I am writing to you during a hiatus that an unpunctual patient has left me. Your letter just arrived, and in the morning Kleinpaul's book, in which

I unfortunately didn't find the Σατυροζ dream. Martin came home in a cast and is making attempts at walking. Frau G.'s visit was very nice; her conversation is particularly charming. Her daughter is made of coarser material, participated little, and for the most part had a blank expression on her face. Otherwise, of course, there was not the slightest abnormality noticeable in her. The scar is really inconspicuous and gives good opportunities for her undeniable vanity.

You are quite right about the danger that you have unearthed; it really branches out from the transference. Now, the fear of the name of the illness is another such danger. Hysteria is already familiar to us as small change, dementia praecox not yet. The diagnosis says nothing about its practical significance. So let's hope for the best.

My well-being, which I owe to your communication, is continuing undisturbed. So, it was certainly that. Putnam ordered 400 copies of his paper in the Zentralblatt[1] by wire, so he evidently wants to make big propaganda with it. Today he agrees to come to Europe to the Congress in September if we guarantee to him that he can board ship in Genoa on the 28th.[2] I will report this to Jung, and it can be very nice. I again enclose Jung's card (which my address immediately influenced). I don't want to have the Crown Prince on foreign journeys so long.[3]

On Wednesday I spoke, at first in a measured tone but decidedly in opposition to the Adlerian heresies. Today there will be a continuation of the debate, in which the others will probably show their reaction to my speech. He himself had responded weakly, almost pettifoggingly.[4]

Rank is now very helpful to me with the third edition of the Interpretation of Dreams.

Kind Regards,
Freud

1. See letter 169, n. 2.
2. The Third International Psychoanalytic Congress, which Jung first wanted to hold in Lugano, then in Nuremberg, finally took place in Weimar on September 21 and 22.
3. Possibly Freud is referring to Jung's "excursions" into the land of mythology, away from the "medical motherland" (Freud to Jung, January 22, 1911, in *Freud/Jung*, p. 388). The Freud-Jung correspondence gives no reason to assume that Jung had been in America, as Jones (II, 140) asserts on the basis of this passage.
4. On November 16, 1910, Hitschmann had proposed a detailed discussion about Adler's views and their relation to those of Freud. Freud agreed, with the stipulation that Adler himself should talk about the relation of masculine protest to the theory of repression (*Minutes* III, 59). Adler accepted. In the session mentioned in the letter, Freud's criticism culminated in the remark that the "oneness of the neuroses" was actually a "uniformity" [*Einerleiheit*] (p. 146). The discussions, which finally ended with Adler's resignation, were continued on February 8 and 22.

200

Budapest, [February 11, 1911][1]
VI.,———[2]

Dear Professor,

First, I want to join Frau G. in thanking you from the bottom of my heart.—Then, I ask you to excuse the fact that I didn't answer your kind letter appropriately until later. Today I am busy with a lecture that I want to give tomorrow at the "Physicians' Association" about *"Suggestion and Psychoanalysis."* Do you want to print this lecture (intended for a general audience) in the Zentralblatt? If so, then I will translate it.[3]—

I wrote the enclosed little article for the Zentralblatt. Please return it next time; I want to send it, along with a number of other trivia, direct to Adler or Stekel.[4]—

After the lecture I will write to tell you how it went. Probably no one will dare to stand up to us.

Kind regards,
Ferenczi

1. The letter has been dated on the basis of Ferenczi's reference to his lecture in the Physicians' Association, which he gave on February 12, 1911 (see the brief report about it in the *Zentralblatt für Psychoanalyse* 1 [1911]: 372).

2. The remainder of the preprinted letterhead, with the obviously no longer valid address "Ndrassy-ut 25. (Drechsler-Palotr)," has been crossed out.

3. Ferenczi, "Suggestion und Psychoanalyse" [Suggestion and Psychoanalysis] (1912, 94; *F.C.*, p. 55; *Unbewusstes*, pp. 194–206), lecture at the Budapest Physicians' Association on February 12, 1911. The lecture was published in Hungarian in *Gyógyászat*, no. 51 (1911): 242–246, but not in the *Zentralblatt*, where only a brief note by Ferenczi, "Aus ungarischen Vereinen" [From Hungarian Societies], 1 (1910–11): 372, appeared.

4. In addition to Ferenczi's brief essay "Aus ungarischen Vereinen" the *Zentralblatt* also published his "Reizung der analen erogenen Zone als auslösende Ursache der Paranoia, Beitrag zum Thema: Homosexualität und Paranoia" [Stimulation of the Anal Erotogenic Zone as a Precipitating Factor in Paranoia] (1911, 77; *Fin.*, p. 295; *Zentralblatt* 1 [1910–11]: 557–559) and a report, "Aus der neurol.-psychiatr. Sektion der königl. Gesellschaft der Ärzte in Budapest," (*Zentralblatt* 1 [1910–11]: 372–374.

201

Budapest, February 16, 1911
VII., Erzsébet-körút 54

Dear Professor,

In the lecture that I gave at the Physicians' Association I used the tactic of limiting myself to the explanation of the methodological difference between suggestion and Ψ.A., but this time I refrained from treating the content of what is uncovered by means of analysis (sexuality). I wanted thereby to take into account the audience's resistances. And everything went smoothly; the people listened attentively. But I had barely concluded when a speaker (an insignificant hydrotherapist whose name you don't need to note) rose in opposition and read aloud a long prepared lecture against ΨA. He was not prepared for the fact that a Ψ-analyst would give a lecture without "hanky-panky" [*Schweinereien*] and made a real fool of himself when he (quoting from Stekel's book) referred to the outrageousness of the method. Even so, he was successful in evoking some indignation. His main points were as follows: 1.) The ucs. is *"non existens"* for the psyche. 2.) Analysis is a wayward doctrine which creates illness and destroys culture. (He was lying through his teeth when he said that Freud wants to let loose the untamed drives onto society.)

Encouraged by this, a dermatologist, who is competent in his field but known as a jokester, stood up and said (jokingly) something like this: 1.) Analysis is pornography; so analysts belong in jail. 2.) Analysis is, at the very least, a dangerous poison; one would first have to prove its curative power before one applies it.

Finally there spoke up (quite unnecessarily) a young, inexperienced doctor, who wanted to flatter me—since I am his boss in the workers' clinic—and rose to my defense.

In my response I first protested against my defender by proving to him that his opinion was absolutely worthless, inasmuch as he had no experience.

Well, then I energetically repudiated the lies and stupid jokes of the previous speakers.

The only thing that is of interest in this whole affair is that the most scholarly German neurologists and the most unsuspecting Hungarian non-specialists react to ΨA. almost word-for-word with the same remarks. An absolutely democratic uniformity of stupidity prevails in this matter.

I intend to translate the lecture into German—perhaps for Bresler's journal[1] (or for the Zentralblatt?).

Kind regards,
Ferenczi

1. The *Psychiatrisch-neurologische Wochenschrift*, a journal edited by Johannes Bresler; see also letter 12 and n. 4.

202

Vienna, February 19, 1911
IX., Berggasse 19

Dear friend,

I pity you, that you tussled with such a pack of swine, and I admire your patience, since you are, in fact, doing right by them. I am hardly in the mood for a polemic with Adler, whose neurotic character is revealing itself more and more clearly as a secondary disturbance.

The news these days has to do with America. Putnam has confirmed his presence in September at the Congress in Lugano.[1] Before that he will spend some time in Zurich, and since I, too, want to be with Jung for a while in September (with my wife), the nicest thing would be if you also came. We will discuss details later.

I will send back your interesting little observation,[2] as you wished, and hope to find you again soon with increasing regularity in the Zentralblatt's file. There is already an overabundance there. The *gaffes* in no. 4[3] will not have escaped you, no less than their connection with the Adlerian complexes.

Owing to an absolute lack of time, I am not progressing, despite good health and Rank's willingness to help with the Interpretation of Dreams (3d ed.). My brother[4] has now fallen ill with severe influenza, which looked very serious (pneumonia) at first but is running its course all right. And so there is one disturbance after another. What I am calling "the great synthesis"[5] is lying dormant and waiting for freer hours, which I probably won't find until July–August in Karlsbad.

Regards to you and Frau G.

Cordially,
Freud

1. See letter 199, n. 2.
2. See letter 200 and n. 4.
3. A lecture by Adler of January 4 in the Vienna Society was mistakenly reviewed under the title "Herbert Silberer: Magie und Anderes" (January 18, 1911). In it Adler had termed the libido of the neurotic "not genuine" (*Zentralblatt* 1 [1910–11]: 186); a paper by Pierre Janet was called "Le subconscions" (ibid., p. 181), and in the title "Nervous and Mentral [sic] Disease Monograph," the word "Series" was left out. In a letter to Adler of February 13, 1911 (Library of Congress), Freud remarked that the readership could get the idea from these errors that the libido used in editing the *Zentralblatt* was "not genuine."
4. Alexander Freud.
5. This could be the first indication of Freud's plan for a comprehensive metapsychological presentation of psychoanalysis.

203

[Budapest,] March 9, 1911

Dear Professor,

Nothing significant has been happening here in the last few weeks; that is why I have been silent for so long.

It must have been very stormy in Vienna in the meantime, as I gather from the latest minutes of the "Society." I am uncommonly pleased that you seem to have observed that ΨA.—both in Vienna and "internationally"—will still require leadership from you, lest it become the victim of neurotic or infantile tendencies. At the same time I observe with satisfaction that you can be active without interruption, well in both body and mind.—

As for polemicizing against opponents, I am entirely of your opinion. This kind of polemic is also boring and painful to me. And yet I also want to force myself to do it in the future.

The sad thing is only that I don't have any *doctors* as collaborators. The young medical students are immature, and the talented artists and lawyers can't acquire any real analytic practice. [In the meantime, analysis is being practiced clandestinely at all the clinics; at Moravcsik's,[1] the "*Veraguth*"ian (sic!) psychogalvanic reaction[2] is even being tested, and *Jung's* results are being recognized.][3]

I am very much looking forward to seeing Putnam again. It is astonishing what that old man was capable of accomplishing. Your plan, that we meet in Switzerland before Lugano, is very agreeable to me. That would be a kind of "pre-Congress" of psychoanalysts of strict observance.

I would like to come to Vienna once again, especially in order to inform myself about the latest events in the Society. But I have to go to my sister's in Nyiregyháza on Saturday regarding family matters.[4] On Monday I will be back here, where an uninterrupted schedule awaits me. I am conducting seven analyses daily, among them one at 20 crowns, two to three at 15 crowns, one at *6 crowns* (!), one at 8 crowns, one on credit, and the other at 10 crowns. Despite these discounts I am able to save something (especially with the aid of other income). The total income could represent an increase of 2–3,000 crowns over last year.

It might interest you to know that *Dr. Rosti*, a lawyer in *Baja*[5] (a Jew), gave a lecture on psychoanalysis at the "Free Lyceum" there. He recently made contact with me, is enthusiastic about your works, but can't warm up to Stekel's style of writing.—

The man from Dunapentele finally did offer us the earrings for 40 crowns. I bought them in order to make him happy. I'll send them to you next time.

Kind regards,
Ferenczi

1. Ernö Moravcsik (1858–1924), professor of psychiatry and director of the Budapest Neurological and Psychiatric Clinic. He was tolerantly disposed toward psychoanalysis.

2. Otto Veraguth (1870–1944), neurologist and university professor in Zurich. He was the first to use the galvanometer to measure psychic tendencies. Ferenczi's "sic!" may be a reaction to the priority of Veraguth's work over Jung's own galvanometric investigations (1907; see *Freud/Jung*, April 11, 1907, and February 20, 1910, pp. 31, 297).

3. Enclosed in brackets in the original.

4. In Nyiregyháza, about 200 kilometers east of Budapest, there was a branch of the Ferenczis' bookstore, which was run by Sándor's brother Miksa. It could not be determined which of Ferenczi's four sisters (Ilona, Maria, Gizella, and Zsofia) he is referring to here.

5. A small city on the Danube about 160 kilometers south of Budapest.

204

Vienna, March 12, 1911
IX., Berggasse 19

Dear friend,

I no longer know how it came to be that you could be surprised by the latest events. I had much foreign correspondence and was finishing the Interpretation of Dreams. I will now fill you in on the essentials. The Adler debates have left behind a very unfavorable impression of him, and occasionally I had to put him down with a decisive word. The unconscious signs—forgetting, misspeaking—were against him, so he took the consequences and resigned. Stekel, who is now quite wild and is stirring up strong personal opposition to himself, took advantage of the opportunity to affirm his friendship with Adler.[1] The rest took place very quietly. The fallen are pouting, are now sitting at the "foot" of the table and refusing to take part in the debates, etc. To be sure, I have that same impression that you were talking about, that it was not the right time to resign and that much damage has been done in the process; but I also have another one, namely, that there is only one of all the Viennese who has a scientific future, and that is little Rank, who has held on very valiantly alongside me.

Now, I admit that I would also like to get rid of both of them in the Zentralblatt, in order thereby to consummate the revenge for their behavior toward you and me at the Congress and also to place the organ entirely in my hands. But they know that and are careful, i.e., polite and accommodating. I would throw them overboard here at the slightest difficulty over principle; I am completely fed up with them. But since I don't actually want to be malicious, I have to continue to work with them as long as possible, i.e., as long as they show themselves to be obedient.

I am toying with the idea of making the Zentralblatt the official organ of the IΨA from the Congress on, so that every member would then be a subscriber by paying the Association dues, which would then be raised a little. The Korrespondenzblatt would cease to exist, and the Central Office would keep a column open in the Zentralblatt for its communications. Jung thinks the plan is very good. Bergmann[2] has not yet been won over to it, but we will continue to work on him.

I am really completely capable of accomplishment, but I have had less to do for two weeks and have the prospect of new interruptions accompanied by small inflow, so I can't get very rich this year. That hasn't prevented me from presenting myself with various treasures in honor of the twenty-fifth anniversary of my practice (Easter Sunday),[3] which you will be obliged to admire the next time you are here. Your earrings arrived right on the day of the purchase and suffered in comparison. I thank you now for having put up the money for me when the prices went down.

Last Sunday I had a visit from our far-flung adherent Sutherland[4] from Sagar in India, who is a magnificent person; he is translating the Interpretation of Dreams. Behind him stands another, younger man, Barkley (?) Hill,[5] who is practicing ΨA on the Hindus and confirming everything with them, and will also publish his results. Two days ago another part of the world showed up, Australia. The Secretary of the Neurological Section of the Australasian Congress is declaring himself a subscriber to the Jahrbuch and requests a brief report on my theories, which is supposed to be printed in the Congress publication, since these theories are still completely unknown in Australia.[6] Still no sign of life from Africa.

You are privileged to hear two comparisons which just happened to come to my mind. When we uncover the perverse bases for our moral reaction formations and bring the patient into renewed conflict which he thinks has been settled, then that is comparable to the *recrystallization* of the mineralogist, who in so doing hopes to get more beautiful and purer crystals.—The transference is the still soft and productive *cambium* layer of neurosis, while the symptoms are comparable to being in anorganic ossification.[7]

I hope soon to be able to firm up a few of the basic configurations of the nuclear complex, by which the Adlerian heresy will be theoretically done away with. Perhaps the summer in Karlsbad will bring inspiration along with it.

Martin is already doing well, although his knee is stiff. He is allowed a year's leave and will take up his law studies again in the meantime. I would

like to go to Bolzano for Easter to look for a summer home on the Ritten.—
What is Frau G.'s daughter doing?

Kind regards,
Freud

The paper on Anatole France will go into the double issue 7/8 of the
Zentralblatt.[8]

1. On February 22, 1911, Adler resigned as president and Stekel as vice president of
the Vienna Psychoanalytic Society. In an extraordinary general meeting on March 1 Freud
was thereupon elected the new president by acclamation. It was further unanimously
resolved to thank Adler and Stekel and to inform them that the greatest value was being
placed on their continued collaboration, and it was resolved by a majority that the Society
would refrain from recognizing the incompatibility between his scientific position and
his function, which was cited by Adler as grounds for his resignation (*Minutes* III, 178ff).
2. J. F. Bergmann, the publisher of the *Zentralblatt*.
3. In 1886 Freud had opened his practice in the Rathausgasse on Easter Sunday, a public
holiday.
4. W. D. Sutherland (1866–1920), military physician in what is today Madhya Pradesh.
He later became a member of the American Psychoanalytic Association and a founding
member of the London Psychoanalytic Society (1913).
5. Owen A. R. Berkeley-Hill (1879–1944), staff physician in Bengal, then Bombay. Like
Sutherland, he was first a member of the American Association and then a founding
member of the London Society.
6. Andrew Davidson (1869–1938), born in Scotland, a psychiatrist in Sydney, was
secretary of the psychological medicine and neurology section of the Australasian Medical Congress.
7. Freud did not publish the comparison with recrystallization in this form (but see
Freud 1916–17a, p. 390, and 1933a, p. 59); he did mention the comparison with the
cambium layer (the layer of plant tissue capable of dividing) in the *Lectures* (1916–17a,
p. 444).
8. Ferenczi, "Anatole France als Analytiker" (1911, 76; *Zentralblatt* 1 [1910–11]: 461–
467).

205

Budapest, March 17, 1911
VII., Erzsébet-körút 54

Dear Professor,
Many thanks for your detailed communications. I admire your stamina
and punctuality in your correspondence, and I sometimes also have pangs
of conscience about helping to waste your valuable time with our correspondence. But I am much too selfish to take the appropriate step in that
regard. There has certainly never been any *intellectual* movement in which
the *personality* of the discoverer has played such a great and indispensable

role as yours has in psychoanalysis.—You see, it is *literally* true: you are not only the discoverer of new psychological facts but also the *physician* who treats us physicians. As such you have to bear all the burdens of transference and resistance. It is, of course, unpleasant when you have to deal with incurable or not easily accessible physicians (e.g., an infantile-perverse Stekel and a paranoid Adler). In comparison to them, even I must qualify as quite a simple "case"; I am in approximately the same stage as the patient who came to see me after *a year's hiatus* in order to free herself from the last remnant of her illness, her transference to me. I think I have pretty well freed this patient—as well as myself—from this neurotic character trait (which you got to see in Sicily last summer).

I am very happy that the sowers of discord (Adler + Stekel) can no longer protect themselves with your name. It would be good if, in your next publications, you also publicly took a position with regard to Adler, so that his special position becomes clear to those not so firmly initiated.—I just analyzed a typical case of "ψ. hermaphroditism + masculine protest"[1] in a woman. What Adler says, the patient told me completely consciously. It was only analysis that uncovered the *repressed urethral- + anal-erotism* as the main root of her suffering. She became terribly accustomed to retaining stool and urine; she also accepted this compulsion but avenged herself by *otherwise* tolerating no compulsion whatsoever. She is actually still "protesting" against the restriction of her anal-erotic freedoms. Most of her *compulsive manifestations* can be explained in this manner, e.g., the obsessive fear of saying something unpleasant to people. That means the same as uninhibitedly farting in front of everybody, without concern for the opinions of others. She used the presumed (in part, real) preference for *boys* in her family as a pretext for displacing her unpleasure which stems from her anal erotism onto man-woman relations. (Men are freer; they can "let themselves go," etc.; they can do what they want, when they want, etc.) In this way hermaphroditism and masculine protest came from anal erotism. A childhood screen memory ("God makes pee-pee" = wee-wee) and a dream, in which the patient allowed herself to be admired by officers while defecating, put me on the trail of this. The fact that she finally (before the beginning of treatment) wanted to poison herself with mercuric chloride in order not to take second place to her brother, who committed suicide, and in order to break her father's pride, these are all secondary things.

Could this case be published in abbreviated form?

March 21

I am continuing this letter after several days' hiatus; I interrupted it in expectation that something worth communicating to you would happen in the meantime—which, however is not the case.

I have very often been occupied lately with the social and sociological consequences of psychoanalysis. I think that a lecture for the Congress will come out of this.[2]—

In conclusion, another confession:

The equinoctial storms have fanned the flames of unsublimated erotism in me in the form of very youthful impetuosity. After rather lengthy fantasizing about *youthful* sexual objects, I satisfied myself with a (not completely uninhibited) attempt on a—30-year-old divorced woman (not a patient). The result was the firm conviction that I am unshakably fixated on Frau G. and that I should avoid such experiments in the future. All this played itself out without exaggerated anxiety of conscience, however, certainly a sign of relative normality of mood.

But since I had to unburden myself by means of this confession, my conscience does not, in fact, seem to be completely clear.

Excuse these unreasonable demands on your personal interest.

Yours truly,
Ferenczi

1. Adler's concept of psychic hermaphroditism is not derived, as is Freud's, from biologically predetermined bisexuality; instead it "supposes only the antithesis in the valuation of male and female as it actually exists." Alfred Adler, *The Neurotic Constitution* (New York, 1917), pp. 105f. The devaluation of the feminine role would then lead to the reaction of "masculine protest." See also Alfred Adler, "Der psychische Hermaphroditismus im Leben und in der Neurose" (1910), in *Heilen und Bilden* (Frankfurt, 1973).

2. See Ferenczi, "Die Bedeutung der Psychoanalyse für Rechtswesen und Gesellschaft" [On Psycho-Analysis and its Judicial and Sociological Significance: A Lecture for Judges and Barristers], delivered October 29, 1913, before the Imperial Society of Judges and Prosecutors in Budapest (1913, 103; *F.C.*, p. 424; *Nyugat* 11 [1913]: 704–711; *Gyógyászat* 6 [1914]: 88–90; *Unbewusstes*, pp. 207–216).

206

Budapest, March 31, 1911
VII., Erzsébet-körút 54

Dear Professor.

I received Jung's circular, in which he proposes Nuremberg as the site for the Congress.—I replied to him that, as a member of the Vienna Society, I have no right to a separate vote, but that I would personally like to voice my opinion in favor of keeping *Lugano*.—The situation in the Vienna group, about which the minutes have kept me quite well informed, must be causing you much inconvenience. An exodus of the two disturbers of the peace would perhaps be the best solution.

I am reading Stekel's book[1] with strong feelings of displeasure. I am ashamed that an analyst could have something like that printed. Whatever there is of value in it could be put into a small pamphlet; the rest is useless for the initiate—harmful for outsiders. Much makes a direct impression of being fabricated. One of us has to decide to take a position against this type of publication. If you want, I will write a paper about it for the Jahrbuch.[2] [It would be even better to give this task to a more distant and generally respected person such as *Putnam*].[3]

I have nothing personal to report.

Kind regards,
Ferenczi

1. Wilhelm Stekel, *Die Sprache des Traumes, Eine Darstellung der Symbolik und Deutung des Traumes in ihren Beziehungen zur kranken und gesunden Seele, für Ärzte und Psychologen* (Wiesbaden, 1911).
2. There is no record of any such essay by Ferenczi; a critique of Stekel's book was published by Bleuler in *Münchener medizinische Wochenschrift* 58 (1911): 1142f).
3. Enclosed in brackets in the original.

207

Vienna, April 2, 1911
IX., Berggasse 19

Dear friend,

Yesterday evening I thought to myself, it is strange that you write to me so seldom, as if we had nothing more to say to each other. Then I remembered that I owed you another reply and decided to do it today. Then came your letter.

Your first letter would have made a personal communication more desirable than a written reply. Nevertheless, I will venture a small suggestion on condition that only essential concerns and not secondary considerations guide you in assessing it. I want to utilize the Easter holiday for a little trip, perhaps leave here on Thursday evening and return Tuesday morning. Destination: the Ritten near Bolzano and the Val Sugana (near Trent), where I have my eye on a few possibilities for housing. If you want to come along—I will otherwise be alone—then you are quite welcome, but don't force yourself. Of course, I can't preclude a change of destination yet.

My wish with regard to the Congress is entirely in accord with yours, but Jung is right in taking the wishes of the others into account. It ought to be not Nuremberg but Munich, as long as the accommodations don't present any difficulties. Vienna is rather disgusting. I come out as somewhat more domineering and can still lean on a number of the faithful. Rank is going to Greece for two weeks on a university excursion.[1] I wrote to

Stekel that Jung is requesting a critique of his dream book from me, and that this critique would have to turn out "bipolar,"[2] and whether he had anything against it, in which case I would drop it. If he doesn't boastfully request me to write the critique, then we will certainly be in a big dilemma, which your offer could get us out of. So, I thank you for your willingness to help. We make so many demands on Putnam that we can't possibly expect him to wash our own dirty linen.

I am quite well, physically, am making good progress with my appendix, and for that reason I am not working. I have known for a long time that I can't be diligent when I am in very good health, but I need a bit of discomfort from which I have to extract myself. I am almost finished with correcting the work on paranoia,[3] and it gradually pleases me more.

Jones seems to be wobbling in Toronto;[4] his unsteadiness is again finding excuses. We will very much miss his presence there. Jung was recently in Berlin at Kraus's clinic[5] and reports that everyone there is infected. He had a splendid reception there. Honegger,[6] for whom I had great hopes, has poisoned himself with morphine. A missed opportunity; too bad! Maeder is with Bircher-Benner (Institution "Living Force"); I was able to send him two patients last week. I sometimes write to Bleuler, only he is frozen stiff again. He has promised in the meantime to report on the "Berlin Congress,"[7] altogether to take on the more serious opponents as "Minister of Defense."

Yesterday Oli went to London with the money that he has been saving for a long time. I, too, took my first trip to England when I was about his age.[8] Martin has been set back a year. Sophie is sadly awaiting Karlsbad; she will leave right after Easter. That is our private news. I send cordial regards and look forward to your reply.

Yours,
Freud

1. Freud had "given him money for it [the excursion] in return for the work he had done on the third edition of *The Interpretation of Dreams*" (*Freud/Jung*, April 27, 1911, p. 418).

2. An allusion to Stekel's concept of the bipolarity of affects and symptoms, comparable to Bleuler's concept of ambivalence (*Minutes* II, 397f, 434, 450; and *Minutes* III, 80). Freud subsequently read aloud the draft of his review of Stekel's work (see letter 209) at the Vienna Society on April 26 (see *Minutes* III, 236, and letter 214) but didn't publish it.

3. The analysis of Schreber (Freud 1911c [1910]).

4. Jones was at that time associate professor at the Medical Faculty in Toronto. In January a former patient of his had complained to the president of the university that Jones had abused her sexually, and she had threatened to shoot him. Thereupon Jones had paid her $500 (Hale, *Putnam*, pp. 252–256). Although a scandal was avoided, the affair strengthened Jones's resolve to leave Toronto. In June 1912 he returned to Europe, at first for a few months, then permanently in 1913.

5. Friedrich Kraus (1858–1936), professor of medicine in Berlin and head of the medical clinic at the hôpital de la Charité there.

6. Johann Jakob Honegger (see letter 126, n. 6) had taken his life on March 28 in the Rheinau Clinic, where he had been assistant physician for two months.

7. Eugen Bleuler, "Freud'sche Theorien in der IV. Jahresversammlung der Gesellschaft deutscher Nervenärzte, Berlin, 6.–8 Oktober 1910," *Zentralblatt* 1 (1910–11): 424–427.

8. In the summer of 1875 Freud, then nineteen years old, had visited his half-brothers Emanuel (1833–1914) and Philipp (1836–1911) in Manchester. In letters to his boyhood friend Eduard Silberstein, Freud described his positive impression of England and declared that he "would sooner live there than" in Vienna (September 9, 1875, *Letters of Sigmund Freud to Eduard Silberstein, 1871–1881*, ed. Walter Boehlich [Cambridge, Mass., 1990], p. 127).

208

Budapest, April 4, 1911
VII., Erzsébet-körút 54

Dear Professor,

I joyfully accept and am already in fantasy more in sunny South Tyrol than in this Nordic city, now so chilly, where, after a few beautiful spring days it is snowing again and an icy wind is blowing.—I have not yet studied the itinerary. (Since Oli is absent I have to do it myself.) I don't think we'll meet until we are down there. When and where is naturally reserved for you to decide. I am looking forward to this vacation very much the way a child does, and I gauge from this joy how much I actually slaved away this winter.

The local "Galileo" Society (Society of Freethinking Students)[1] has come to me with a request that I should ask you to give them a lecture sometime. If you consent, they will send you a formal invitation. The best thing would be for us to talk this matter out in person. Incidentally, I didn't hold out much hope to the boys; I know what a day and a trip mean to you.

I would be very pleased if Stekel did *not* reject your critique; what I want to write about his book will be interpreted by Stekel and Adler as an echo of your opinions, which won't prevent me from writing the critique, however.

Jones writes to me from Toronto with much conviction, so that I can only interpret his "wobbling" in such a way that he can't get along with the prudish Scots (about whom he complains a great deal).[2]

Tomorrow I will send you a paper—which is kept somewhat speculative and leans too heavily on the side of consciousness but is not devoid of intellect—by a local initiate, *Dr. Kovács*[3] (former patient; music aesthete). He would like to have the work published as a volume of the "Schriften zur angewandten Seelenkunde." Would you make an entirely objective judgment about this and then let me know what you think?

I will write to you very soon, but I am also awaiting details about our trip.

Kindest regards,
Ferenczi

1. See letter 79, n. 11.

2. Jones writes in his autobiography that a large number of influential people in Toronto were of Scottish extraction (*Associations*, p. 177).

3. On Kovács, see letter 137, n. 2, and letter 160. His essay "Introjektion, Projektion und Einfühlung" [Introjection, Projection, and Empathy] was later published in *Zentralblatt* 2 (1911–12): 253–263 and 316–327 (see letter 211).

209

Vienna, April 6, 1911
IX., Berggasse 19

Dear friend,

Many thanks for your preparedness. I hope this trip will come into being, even though I am now not yet sure about our arrangements for the summer. Today I am sending you the intended critique of Stekel; he has declared himself willing to have me write it. I ask you to return it soon and will be very grateful for comments about it. I will then show it to him before it goes off to Jung, who is presently taking his Easter trip. I am constantly annoyed about the two—Max and Moritz[1]—, who are also developing with great rapidity in a backward direction and will soon have arrived at a denial of the unconscious. But I am quite powerless against them, especially as long as I can't throw them out of the Zentralblatt. Enemies are much more comfortable; you can at least ignore them. I would also like to discuss this situation with you.

Best regards,
Freud

1. This is a humorous reference to Alfred Adler and Wilhelm Stekel, the editors of the Zentralblatt. "Max und Moritz," a popular cartoon (1865) by the German artist and humorist Wilhelm Busch (1832–1908), depicts the pranks and the bad end of these two boys. Freud kept a Busch cartoon album in his waiting room.

210

Budapest, April 8, 1911
VII., Erzsébet-körút 54

Dear Professor,

I find your critique *very good*, only a bit too *tame*. I think you ought to take a position here, if only a very general one, against the Adlerian prin-

ciples (hermaphroditism, masculine protest). I consider another consultation with Stekel or submitting the paper to him before sending it off
superfluous. That is also not in the direction in which you are justifiably
heading (throwing them out of the Zentralblatt).

I have not yet read the book[1] from cover to cover. In reading the first half
I made a few marginal notations, which I am enclosing here. It is a painful
task for a clear-thinking person to read through this hodgepodge. Your
analogy of "a pig wallowing in a flower bed" is totally applicable. You
shouldn't hold that back in your critique, even if it isn't quite proper.

But even if you don't change anything in the paper, it will seem like being
freed from a nightmare when at last censure is being voiced from one's own
camp against such "sloppiness" [*Schlampereien*].

There are only four more days separating us from Thursday.[2] Please write
to me very soon when you decide so I can catch up with you at the proper
time. Perhaps we can meet on the way and make part of the journey
together.

Kindest regards,
Ferenczi

1. Stekel's book, *Die Sprache des Traumes* (see letter 206, n. 1).
2. From their planned meeting in Bolzano (*Freud/Jung*, April 11, 1911, p. 415).

211

Vienna, April 10, 1911
IX., Berggasse 19

Dear friend,

What should I do? He is and remains an uneducable individual, a *mau-
vais sujet* [bad person]; I saw it again in last Wednesday's discussion.[1] Now
I can't decide to make the rejection even clearer, but, heeding your advice,
I will refrain from sending it to him. Your marginal observations are quite
correct, but I will refrain from expressing everything that is wrong between
us.

Kovács's[2] paper is interesting and worth publishing. One could certainly
go into the matter more deeply, but I am not competent in these things. I
have no room in the "Schriften zur angewandten Seelenkunde" for the next
three quarters of a year. You will hear about what is in preparation. But I
will make an effort to put together a literary issue of the Zentralblatt in
which this paper can find acceptance. Must talk with Max *und* Moritz
about it. This Wednesday is free. Rank is traveling in Greece.

I am thinking of leaving on *Friday the 14th at 8:05* with the Southern
Railway and arriving in Bolzano at 12:55. If you are going by way of
Marburg (5 o'clock), get on with me at 1:33 in the morning. But perhaps

you will choose another time to travel. Let me know in a timely fashion. I think, if the weather or other enchantments are not too spectacular, I would be satisfied with returning on Tuesday. I actually should, since my wife and Sophie are going to Karlsbad Tuesday evening. It would make sense to travel on Thursday evening only if we want to be more comfortable, and it is certainly 300 crowns more at a time when money is at a premium.

I await news from you and send cordial regards. *Auf Wiedersehen.*

Yours,
Freud

1. In the session of April 5, 1911 (*Minutes* III, 217–226), Freud and Stekel had presented differing interpretations of specific dreams and approaches to them.
2. See letter 208 and n. 3.

212

Budapest, April 11, [1911]
VII., Erzsébet-körút 54

Dear Professor,

I. I don't have to earn so terribly much money as you; for that reason I am starting my Easter vacation already on Wednesday afternoon and am leaving here on Thursday afternoon, in any case. If you are likewise leaving on Thursday, then I ask you to let me know by telegram (telegraphic communication would be desirable in any event). I am thinking of getting off in *Villach*, spending Friday there, and getting on your train on Saturday morning at 5:*11*.

II. But if you should decide to leave on *Thursday*, then I will go to Vienna on Thursday afternoon and we will make the entire trip together.—I can reserve a sleeping compartment here.

III. Third possibility: You leave *Thursday*, I catch up with you in Marburg (1:*33*), but leave you in peace until Villach (5:*11* o'clock).[1]
The second travel plan would be the most convenient for me; it costs me only two hours more than the direct route from here to Bolzano; there is also no sleeping car direct from here to Bolzano, which I can hardly do without, however.

It is even possible for me to take a detour by way of Vienna, even if I am traveling alone.

I will leave all this up in the air until I receive news from you by telegram. If there is still time, then I will reply to your telegram.[2]

Kind regards,
Ferenczi

1. Ferenczi probably numbered the paragraphs after writing the letter in order to differentiate more easily among the various travel plans.

2. Freud and Ferenczi spent April 16 and 17 together in Bolzano in the South Tyrol.

213

Budapest, April 24, 1911
VII., Erzsébet-körút 54

Dear Professor,

As in a dreamland, that's the way I think of the mountain landscape of Bolzano; also the joy of being able to spend two days with you again in intimate conversation, free from the obligations of work, seems to me here in my isolation to be so improbable that the impression of the fairy-tale-like quality of our splendid excursion is enhanced even more by it. Incidentally, I never depart from you without benefit. I mean by that not an increase in my understanding of mental activity in general but rather a deepening of insight specifically into my own mental life, without which there can be no true knowledge—but especially no true *faith*. The relationship between *knowledge* and *faith*[1] that has occupied people for so many centuries is only being made clear by means of analysis. Without self-analysis the most realistic truth can appear incredible. If one hears something new, then one is really obligated analytically to test one's personal relationship to the herald of the new doctrine in the most conscientious manner before one can make a decision as to the real value of that statement. An instructive but unpleasant example of this was recently delivered to me by two "analysts" who are evidently suffering under the effects of the unfriendly reception that you gave them. *Décsi* went so far as to claim in front of the friend of a patient that I (your friend) "was the biggest charlatan, who inaugurates two-to-three-year treatments." At the same time, his journalistic accomplishments teem with homosexual love-enthusiasm for *Jung*, whom he terms the "father of psychology" (but without giving his name). The other doubting Thomas is *Dr. Eisler*,[2] whose work on Anatole France you once rejected. A rebellious patient once went to him during Easter vacation out of revenge for my leaving him, and he (Dr. E.) pointed to his library and said, "You see, I know these things; I've occupied myself quite a bit with them. But these are things that are good for women with imaginary diseases. A man like you has to be able to pull himself together." Now it is possible that this Mr. Eisler will become my assistant physician at the Health Service. The prospect is not very refreshing.

I want to complete translation of the Five Lectures[3] in a few (two to three) weeks; to be sure, I got only to page thirteen, but I actually worked more diligently yesterday (Sunday).

Frau G. and her (recently operated-on) sister are well. A brief but sunny and cheerful Sunday promenade had to compensate us for so many depressing things.

You are right again! My erythrophobe—the one who once really had syphilis—recently dreamed about a *trial for damages* "for a stiff arm" in which he himself is accused by someone of standing around in the hay *with a burning cigarette*—even though he is the one suing for damages. [His first sexual experiences are connected with hay; so he wants to *infect*[4] this hay (with fire).][5]

If I summarize my observations thus far in this and other erythrophobes, I believe that syphilis leads to erythrophobia only in those people who in childhood had to energetically suppress their rage toward their parents because of unjust punishment [especially because of punishment for *enuresis*]. The dream about fire and the "compensation" for it also leads in this patient to his enuresis, which he didn't master for a long time. Syphilis is just as unjust a punishment (—of God—) as being beaten after wetting the bed. The child thinks to himself: Why only I and not the others! And even if so, am I to be punished for that?

The two motives of erythrophobia: rage and shame, which presuppose it,[6] hold true in like manner for enuresis and syphilis.

Kind regards,
Ferenczi

1. See Ferenczi, "Glaube, Unglaube und Überzeugung" [Belief, Disbelief, and Conviction] (1913, 109; *F.C.*, p. 437).

2. Joszef Mihály Eisler (?-1944), Hungarian neurologist. In 1919 he became a member of the Hungarian Society and worked as an analyst. Eisler was the first practicing psychotherapist in a polyclinic. He died in a concentration camp in 1944.

3. Freud, *Pszichoanalizis;* trans. with foreword by Ferenczi (1912, 99) (Budapest, 1912, 1915, 1919).

4. The interpretation of this dream depends on the German verb *anstecken,* which means both "to ignite" and "to infect" [Trans.].

5. Enclosed in brackets in the original, as is the phrase in the next sentence.

6. See letter 33 and n. 2.

214

Vienna, May 2, 1911
IX., Berggasse 19

Dear friend,

Thanks for your interesting letter. Erythrophobia is quite transparent, but it is particularly difficult to cure. Perhaps the difficulty lies precisely in the transference.

I have had very good times since Bolzano, also some relief in my practice. Just today I had my first spell of tiredness, to which you owe this letter. You see, I have been working in my good evenings: the second edition of the "Dream" for Bergmann[1] and the little folkloristic thing with Oppenheim[2] (not the one from Berlin).[3] Now, writing the program for the Australian Congress will occupy me this month.

Rank returned from Greece sunburned and happy, and he is now energetically advancing the Interpretation of Dreams. The Jahrbuch is going quite slowly. From a Dutch warship in Patang[4] I recently received an enthusiastic letter from a Dr. v. Römer,[5] who wants to come to Vienna in October. You will recognize the name from a few good papers in Hirschfeld's Jahrbuch für sexuelle Zwischenstufen.

Dr. Drosnes[6] from Odessa arrived today and reports that he will form the first Russian group in the fall with two Muscovites—Ossipow[7] and Wirnbow (?).[8] From Jung, who was in Stuttgart, I am expecting news any day now about the congress there,[9] which will hardly have yielded anything special.

A number of things have also happened here. Stekel has come forward and concluded a separate peace; he assures me that his association with Adler at the Zentralblatt has ended. I must therefore keep him, for manifold personal reasons and because it is incalculable what kind of trouble he will cause if we kick him out. He is also basically good-natured. I read aloud the critique of his dream book, with which you are acquainted, at the last session, and he claimed—it had rained lightly.[10] Nothing has changed with the other one, and there I am waiting for an excuse to ship him out—if he gives me that excuse.

So, we really rented a place from Hofer in Upper Bolzano. I plan to finish up here on July 8 in order to have time to enjoy something of the beautiful high plateau after Karlsbad.

Kind regards to you and Frau G.

Yours,
Freud

1. Freud, On Dreams (1901a), 2d ed. (Wiesbaden, 1911).

2. Freud, with David Ernst Oppenheim, Träume im Folklore (1958a [1911]), in Nachtragsband, pp. 576–600; see also the editor's preface, pp. 573–575. Oppenheim (1881–1943) was a teacher of Greek and Latin at the Academic Gymnasium in Vienna. He later became an adherent of Adler's. He died during the Second World War in the Theresienstadt concentration camp.

3. See letter 186, n. 3.

4. On Sumatra; at that time the Dutch East Indies, now Indonesia.

5. Lucien Sophie Albert Marie von Römer (?–?), Dutch neurologist. He was the author of many works, especially about homosexuality in the Netherlands, published in Hirschfeld's Jahrbuch für sexuelle Zwischenstufen, and he collaborated on a psychoanalytic questionnaire that had been published in the latter's Zeitschrift für Sexualwissenschaft 1, no. 12 (1908).

6. Leonid Drosnés (1880–19?), the Russian psychiatrist who took care of the patient who became known as the "Wolf-Man" and who brought him to Freud in Vienna in January 1910 (see letter 110 and n. 5); a member of the Vienna Society since January 18, 1911, later active as a psychoanalyst in St. Petersburg.

7. On account of political arguments at institutions of higher education, a few professors and nontenured faculty, among them N. E. Ossipov, resigned their positions at the university and met privately at so-called "Little Fridays," where psychoanalytic papers were read and discussed. René Fischer and Eugenie Fischer, "Psychoanalyse in Russland," in *Tiefenpsychologie,* ed. Dieter Eicke, vol. 2 (Weinheim, 1982), pp. 699f. The founding of an official society in Moscow was not reported in the *Zeitschrift* until 1922; see *Zeitschrift* 8 (1922): 236, 525.

8. N. A. Wyrubov (?–?), Russian neurologist and professor in Moscow; founded the journal *Psikhoterapiya* in 1909.

9. The annual meeting of the German Society for Psychiatry, held April 21 and 22.

10. An ironic statement perhaps indicating that Stekel had accepted the critique.

215

Budapest, May 3, 1911
VII., Erzsébet-körút 54

Dear Professor,

Progress in the area of induction.

1.) Yesterday Frau G. thinks of the words *poppy-seed noodles (mákos nudli).*[1] I associate: papaver, papa—ver (= father hits), *poppy-seed—poppy cake.* [Otherwise nothing!][2]

Right away, another experiment:

Frau G. thinks: *Spider* (= Pók). I: Palliative. Preservative. Prophylaxis. Péczely [= a doctor who diagnoses from the eyes and prescribes masturbation as a curative]. A Swedish woman (Ingeborg Kuncze), who had lent me a "map for eye diagnoses." Palugyai. Pálos. Palus (swamp). Potrohos (= rotund). Pók[3] (spider).

[Supplement: Frau G. has "eye phobia" and some spider anxiety (she told me the latter only after the experiment). As I told you, I relate both to suppressed sadism. I looked Frau G. in the eyes before the experiment.]

––––––

2.) Encouraged by these experiments, I became daring. Today I took an evening walk into the city woods,[4] then rode back into the city on an omnibus. Sitting inside were: a boy, a pretty girl, an old gentleman, a chambermaid, and a soldier [platoon leader]. I thought to myself: Now I will look at each one individually and free-associate; I must guess their thoughts. Of course, I will never learn if it's correct and *what* is correct about it.—

At the soldier the following comes to my mind: Konrad, Konopist—in the end, his name is *Kohn*. But he doesn't look very Jewish! On getting off I ask: Are you Herr Kohn?—*Yes*, he says astonished. *Johann Kohn.* How do you know me?—I got off! [The name Kohn is very rare here now.][5]

I felt quite dreamy after this score.

Since I don't know any prophetesses, I have to be content with experiments of this sort.

Kind regards,
Ferenczi

A patient of mine collected the enclosed drawings[6] from a humoristically obscene weekly. They depict comical dreams. Some very characteristic.

1. An Austro-Hungarian specialty.
2. Enclosed in brackets in the original, as are other similar remarks throughout the letter.
3. Underlined three times in the original.
4. Városliget, the city park in the heart of Budapest, where Ferenczi liked to walk.
5. Many Hungarian Jews Magyarized or changed their names out of a need for assimilation under the influence of nationalism and as a reaction to increasing anti-Semitism.
6. These drawings are missing; see letter 216 and nn. 1 and 2.

216

Vienna, May 11, 1911
IX., Berggasse 19

Dear friend,

The illustrated dreams are magnificent. The artist apparently understands dreams much better than Bleuler, Havelock Ellis, et al. Your observations are quite right. The nicest page seems to be the one by the Frenchman Bonne,[1] and the most important one is your conclusion appended to it. But now a question. Who is the artist? Is he definitely a Hungarian and not a German? In the latter case the evidence seems to be missing.[2]

Your experience with Herr Kohn is also singularly beautiful. But are you certain that it isn't a cryptomnesia? Didn't you perhaps recognize the man from family resemblance? Is he supposed to carry around the visual picture of his own name with him while he rides the tram? Do you admit that this success also can't be explained by means of thought transference?

Jung writes that we must also conquer occultism and requests permission to undertake a campaign in the realm of mysticism. I see that the both of you can't be restrained. You should at least proceed in harmony with each other; these are dangerous expeditions, and I can't go along there.

Brill complains that he hasn't heard anything from you for so long. In the same letter he reports that his wife[3] was dangerously ill post partum, had to be operated on twice, but is now convalescing at home. Their little daughter is said to be thriving.

Not much new with me. The sick list has been lengthened by Ernst, who has been diagnosed as having an ulcer or a fissura gastriduodenalis.[4] He was put on a milk diet but is supposed to make his *Matura*[5] before he undergoes a rest cure. He is taking it with great understanding.

The next issue of the Korrespondenzblatt is supposed to give information about the Congress, etc.

Regards to you, uncanny one.

Cordially,
Freud

1. Freud discussed this cartoon, taken from the Hungarian humor magazine *Fidibusz*, in the fourth edition (1914) of *Interpretation of Dreams* (1900a, pp. 367f) and showed it on May 17 in the Vienna Society along with other drawings sent by Ferenczi (*Minutes* III, 266).

2. See Freud 1900a: "For instance, according to Ferenczi . . . a ship moving on the water occurs in dreams of micturation in Hungarian dreamers, though the term *'schiffen'* ['to ship'; cf. vulgar English 'to pumpship'] is unknown in that language" (p. 352, n. 2).

3. K. Rose Owen Brill (1877–1963); the daughter, Gioia, is now Mrs. Philip G. Bernheim.

4. Ulcer or fissure in the stomach (duodenum).

5. University qualifying examination.

217

Budapest, May 11, 1911
VII., Erzsébet-körút 54

Dear Professor,

I obviously didn't want to burden you with my depressed mood, and that is why I have been writing to you so infrequently. Reason: serious illness of my eldest brother.[1] He is suffering from tabes dorsalis and had a positive "Wassermann".[2] Two months ago, under *strong* bleeding, a small tumor of the palate broke out. Diagnosis of syphilis was made, given two injections of Salvarsan.[3] No success. Weight loss. Suspicion of Cc![4]

Today my brother is coming to Budapest. I am very pessimistic about the case, and although I am outwardly *quite* calm, I notice from countless little incidents how deeply the matter affects me.—Even the translation of the Five Lectures has come to a halt.—But I am taking care of analyses, office hours, and court agendas in a normal fashion.

When are you thinking of going from Karlsbad to Bolzano?—and (if you are thinking about my coming), what time do you have in mind? I certainly don't need to assure you that I will gladly and definitely come. (As an employee of the Health Service, I have to specify the time of my vacation by May 20.)

Let us hope my brother's illness will not hinder me.

Kind regards,
Dr. Ferenczi

Frau G. sends thanks for your greeting. She requests some confidential information from you. A young man by the name of *Lorschy* made an appointment to see you some time ago (March?); a philologist, whom you will probably recognize from his peculiarly halting manner of speech and from the fact that you sent him to Nepallek.[5] He is the "first case" of Frau G.'s daughter—Elma. Now, Frau G. would like to know what kind of an impression he made on you. Incidentally, this is only of theoretical significance, since Elma is steadfastly clinging to the "second case" (the young journalist).—

1. Henrik Ferenczi, born March 27, 1860, died in 1912 of cancer of the palate. A bachelor, he was a functionary and president of the guardianship tribunal in Miskolcz.

2. The serum reaction to syphilis, named for August P. von Wassermann (1866–1925).

3. See letter 164, n. 2.

4. Carcinoma (cancerous tumor).

5. Richard Josef von Nepalleck (1864–1940), Doctor of Laws and Medicine, practicing physician and forensic expert in Vienna. Recommended by Adler, he was a member of the Vienna Society from May 11, 1910, and its treasurer from 1919 to 1927. By his arrangement the famous composer Gustav Mahler, whose wife was a relative of Nepalleck's, had consulted Freud in 1910 during the latter's vacation in Holland (Jones II, 79–80).

218

Budapest, May 13, 1911
VII., Erzsébet-körút 54

Dear Professor,

In the case of "Kohn," cryptomnesia can naturally not be excluded (as, by the way, is hardly ever the case), but it is highly improbable. He is a young soldier (platoon leader), probably from the provinces. I haven't spoken to soldiers for many years, and it is not very probable that I may have had something to do with him before he became a soldier. But he is from Budapest, so I could have treated him (or a member of his family) in the polyclinic of the Workers' Health Service. Too bad I avoided a conversation with him.—Transference can't be excluded. Still, I consider it possible that certain strongly feeling-toned ideational complexes are in a *constant* state of arousal, among them the determinations of one's own ego come into primary consideration. You know, of course, how one is inclined to hear one's own name being called out of all kinds of noises. [The joke in which someone calls out "Kohn" and punches an innocent Kohn who happens to stick his head out of a train window is also familiar to you.—][1] If it can be confirmed that this is really the case, then a certain connection between this constant complex arousal and the *tendency to projection* can be assumed.—The assumption that I once ventured to make in Italy—namely, that the *paranoid really* learns certain things with the aid of induction—, should be dropped and modified as follows: the paranoid is inclined toward projection and complex *emanation,* the hysteric toward introjection and complex *resonance.*[2] These are, to be sure, nothing but fantasies, but they should not be dismissed as impossibilities.

I consider the fight against occultism to be *premature,* but I am inclined to cooperate with Jung, if he wants to come out already. It would be desirable if I could discuss this with Jung personally and if, in general, we proceeded together. Two psychoanalysts must certainly be capable of working for the cause by putting aside their personal ambition. Still, working together requires, in addition to good will (the conscious), also the feeling of belonging together, i.e., personal liking for each other and friendship. As far as I am concerned, the matter should work perfectly. But I don't know how it stands with Jung.

Since I consider this matter consequential for the entire psychoanalytic cause—and in the event of failure or going astray, even fateful—I think it would not be superfluous if you got Jung to come to Vienna, where we could work out the plan of action with your help and under your control, so to speak, and we could divide the work among ourselves. Personal contact and a renewal of friendly relations between Jung and me would be an important secondary outcome of this encounter.

I know your diplomatic sense of tact, by the way, and so I leave this whole matter for you to decide.—You know only too well that the "complex of the hostile brother" is strongly developed in me. But I believe that in the last few years I have learned how to master this complex to a large extent.

The specialists who examined my brother consider the case *syphilis,* which has considerably improved my state of mind. The results of the histological examination of the ulcer are not in yet, however.

I was very sorry to hear about dear Ernst's indisposition. You certainly have much to do along with it and often have to call on Saint "Ἀνάγκη."[3]

In your letter I received no answer to the question of when you are going to Bolzano.

Kind regards,
Ferenczi

1. Enclosed in brackets in the original.

2. See Ferenczi, "Zur Begriffsbestimmung der Introjektion" [On the Definition of Introjection] (1912, 84; *Fin.*, p. 316).

3. See letter 141 and n. 3.

219

Vienna, May 14, 1911
IX., Berggasse 19

Dear friend,

You were unjustifiably disappointed if you missed the answer to your question about the stay in Bolzano. My letter was not yet the answer to your last one but rather crossed it. I can now tell you that I will go to Karlsbad on July 9 and expect to arrive in Bolzano on August 1, that we plan to stay there for two weeks,[1] perhaps somewhat longer if the others are still in the mood to stay. From the middle of August until the middle of September (now comes the hasty sentence!)[2] would be the time for the second vacation, perhaps at Lake Caldonazzo. It would be useless to give you more specific details, since no more can be determined now. But I think you know what you should consider for determining your own vacation.

You will see from the enclosed Korrespondenzblatt that Jung has suggested two dates for the Congress. I will have to write him that the earlier ones, the 16th/17th of September, are difficult for me to accept for the private reasons known to you.[3]

It also appears to me that you have chosen the more pessimistic assessment for your brother. An ulcer on the palate is not a direct indication of syphilis. Is he the one from Berlin, whom I know? I think not.—Unfortunately, I can't remember a Herr Lorschy, even from the indications given. In any case, he wasn't with Nepallek, and I didn't hear anything more from him.

It also seems to me that you and Jung ought to proceed together, or you at least ought to know about each other; I wrote to him to that effect a few days ago.[4] But the understanding between you ought to come without my intervention, otherwise it would be incapable of surviving. I am in agreement with your judgment about being premature. Your explanatory remarks about the little Kohn made an impression on me. I think that is a point of departure from which we will get somewhere.

I wish you brighter spirits and send kind regards.

Yours,
Freud

1. After this word the phrase "since our anniversary is on September 14" is crossed out.

2. See n. 1.
3. The Freuds' twenty-fifth wedding anniversary on September 14.
4. There is nothing, however, in the Freud-Jung correspondence in reference to this.

220

Budapest, May 15, 1911
VII., Erzsébet-körút 54

Dear Professor,

This time I will reply very briefly and epigrammatically, since I would still like to mail this letter today.

1.) I am gladly prepared to get in touch with *Jung*, even without your intervention, and perhaps spend a part of my vacation in Zurich. The question is only whether I should offer to collaborate with him—or wait for his invitation. Perhaps (after your letter) he will give some sign of life. In any case, I have the best intentions with regard to cooperation.—What do *you* think?

2.) You forgot to enclose the Korrespondenzblatt; for that reason I don't know the *later* date that Jung has proposed. I presume the 25th to the 27th of September, or the like.—I, too, opt for the latter.

3.) I could arrange my vacation time as follows: I would come to you (Lake Caldonazzo?) *at the end of August,* stay ten days, then go to *Jung's* around the 6th–7th of September (if the understanding between us comes about), stay there *until* your arrival with your wife, leave you alone for a while with Jung and endeavor to spend another 1–2 days before the Congress with you (—perhaps with *Jung*, which would make three of us).

4.) Part of my concern for my brother is certainly a death wish toward the eldest; part has turned out to be real: the microscopic examination showed *syphilis* + an epithelial growth, about which it can't be determined with certainty whether it is leukoplakia or epithelioma.[1]— He is *not* the one from Berlin,[2] but the one in Miskolcz who lives with my mother, the 50-year-old president of an orphans' agency, Doctor of Laws.—

Nothing special to report about transference experiments; something like the following: A Gypsy woman prophesied to a hysteric suffering from a wish to have children that she would have children. She responded: "I have one already"—and pointed to an adopted girl. "She isn't your own", said the Gypsy, even though that was a "closely guarded secret of hers, unknown to everyone in the house."—(Perhaps it isn't such a closely guarded secret as she thinks.)

I am on the trail of a new "prophetess."

An interesting solution to *masochism* in a patient: *He has himself beaten, would like to be humiliated, etc., in order to achieve the feeling of debasement which is necessary for him to break out and avenge himself and which is otherwise lacking in him; the more deeply he debases himself—the nearer he feels himself to be to the frontier where his capacity for suffering ceases and he amasses the courage necessary for a sadistic outbreak. But this frontier has moved away from him into an asymptomatic distance—he can approach it only now and then in dreams.*

Cordially,
Ferenczi

1. Leukoplakia = an often precancerous formation of lesions; epithelioma = a tumor consisting of epithelial cells.
2. Zsigmond, the brother who lived in Berlin (b. 1862), was a chemical engineer.

221

Vienna, May 21, 1911
IX., Berggasse 19

Dear Professor,

I hope you have become convinced in the meantime that your concern for your brother has really grown out of soil in this world rather than in the other. Being ill is normally an omnipresent part of existence (like C H O N S[1] in chemical analysis).

My wife came back today with Sophie,[2] both recovered, and the latter, I hope, improved for a rather long time. I now have 4–5 difficult weeks ahead of me because of new patients, then probably a soft landing until the end of the term.

Your cooperation with Jung, if it comes about at all, should be the result of mutual needs, totally independent of me, and long in the making. You see, I think he is basically a nongregarious worker. So, you should review the points of your program that relate to your stay with him in Zurich with that in mind. The dates that you have set for your visit with us at the end of August are *very* agreeable to me. We will probably no longer be in Upper Bolzano by then. I can reveal to you that my wife doesn't want to go to Zurich, or at least she doesn't want to participate in the visit with Jung, for which I have set aside the last week, the one after the Congress, if it can be postponed until the 21st/22nd of September. Further, I am sure of your discretion when I reveal to you that we were married on September 14, twenty-five years ago. On the whole, it has worked out very well, unusually well in some respects. The details of our plans for the middle of September can't be firmed up yet.

The Korrespondenzblatt (which I didn't forget but found to be too thick for the letter) should have gotten to you *rite*[3] in the meantime. Actually I didn't want to write to you before I could tell you that Adler and perhaps some others had reacted to a forceful request on my part by resigning.[4] But since this hasn't happened yet, I didn't want to postpone the letter any longer. In order to understand my growing intolerance and my conviction that there is no great loss to be shared, just read the review of his last lecture in the Korrespondenzblatt.[5]

Forel has presented me with the 6th edition of his "Hypnotism";[6] but what is in there about ΨA is, regrettably, dim-witted and represents the decidedly not dim-witted biases of Frank[7] and O. Vogt,[8] whose great services—I don't know what they are—he can't praise highly enough—they are puny Johnny-come-latelys, nothing more. His arguments, e.g., against sexuality, are really depressing for a man who has written a fat book about the sexual question.[9] It really put me out, for once.

Otherwise, nothing is happening here; rather, we are waiting for the appearance of what is ahead. I finally saw your paper about obscene words with the remarkably deep conclusion[10] set for Nuremberg.[11] You probably already have it for proofreading.

Incidentally, I hardly know a more deceptive and more complicated problem in our field than that of masochism. The result is that most people probably satisfy [the demands of] masochism and sadism simultaneously. What they themselves talk about is never really decisive.

We are now collecting interpretations of symbols, because we see that we have to do Stekel's important work anew with a better critique, and we are also asking for your contributions (to be directed to Rank). He [Stekel] is probably correct in most cases, but in his well-known slipshod, unscrupulous manner.[12]

Today I am tormented by the secret of tragic guilt,[13] which will certainly not resist ΨA, but I don't want to get distracted now.

Best regards,
Freud

1. The chemical symbols for carbon (C), hydrogen (H), oxygen (O), nitrogen (N), and sulphur (S), which are the most common elements associated with organic matter. The same comparison is made in regard to bisexuality in the study of Woodrow Wilson by Freud and William Bullitt (in which the extent of Freud's influence on the published text has been debated): "Psychoanalysis has established this fact [bisexuality] as firmly as chemistry has established the presence of oxygen, hydrogen, carbon and other elements in all organic bodies." Sigmund Freud and William C. Bullitt, *Thomas Woodrow Wilson, Twenty-Eighth President of the United States: A Psychological Study* (Boston, 1966), p. 37.

2. From Karlsbad (see letter 211).

3. Latin for "in the usual orderly fashion."

4. See letter 223 and n. 3.

5. Rank's report of the session in *Zentralblatt* 1 (1910–11): 371 on Adler's lecture of February 1 at the Vienna Society (see letter 199 and n. 4).

6. See letter 184, n. 3.

7. See letter 131 and n. 5.

8. Oskar Vogt (1870–1959), director of the Kaiser Wilhelm Institute for Brain Research in Berlin. In 1909 he, Auguste Forel (whose assistant he had been), and Horace Frank had founded the International Society for Medical Psychology and Psychotherapy. In 1925 Vogt, a member of the Academy of Sciences in Moscow, established the Institute for Brain Research there. He was a critic of psychoanalysis (see Jones II, 118).

9. Auguste Forel, *Die Sexuelle Frage* (Munich, 1905).

10. "Über obszöne Worte, Beitrag zur Psychologie der Latenzzeit" [On Obscene Words] (1911, 75; *C.*, p. 132); at the end of this essay Ferenczi expresses the hope that ethnographic investigation may support his assumption that obscene expressions are "infantile" and therefore of an abnormally motor and regressive character.

11. Nuremberg was being discussed as the site for the next Psychoanalytic Congress.

12. See Freud's notes on symbolism in dreams and on Stekel's contributions in later supplements to the *Interpretation of Dreams* (1900a, pp. 350ff).

13. The question of the "tragic guilt" of the hero of a tragedy was already hinted at in the *Interpretation of Dreams* (1900a, p. 262) and analyzed in *Moses and Monotheism* (1939a [1934–38], p. 87). This passage could be the first indication that Freud was beginning to work on *Totem and Taboo*; see also letter 223.

222

Budapest, May 27, 1911
VII., Erzsébet-körút 54

Dear Professor,

Many thanks for your detailed letter; I would like to take up its points in order.

You seem to be judging the cooperation with Jung pessimistically (as I gather from your statements in regard to it). You are probably right when you take him to be a nongregarious worker. But if that is the case, then I will have to go public with my results independently of him. But I consider publication to be premature—all the more so considering I suspect it will be possible for me to establish induction with experimental certainty.

According to what you said, I must assume that, under revising my program with regard to the trip to Zurich, you understand giving up the visit with Jung. It has a depressing effect on me that psychoanalysis cannot enable two men to cooperate in common cause while setting aside—more correctly, mastering—personal sensitivities. Indeed, I demonstrated that myself when I so brusquely withdrew from our collaboration on paranoia.[1] But this incident made me wiser, and for my part there would be no hindrance put in the way of working together honestly with Jung.

But if Zurich stays out, then I would come to your place at the end of August and would stay there until your wedding trip. I should be able to make some use of the time between September 14 and the Congress. Then the Congress would come, and the trip home would connect directly with it.

Strangely enough, I have lately been seeing many cases that correspond to the Adlerian mechanism *to a certain degree;* cases of bodily inferiority and compensatory grandiosity. The *motive,* however, that has driven these people to renounce love was certainly disappointment and despair *in love;* this love was completely *genuine.*—To be sure, one of my patients has given up his daily pollutions and his cruel chasing after innocent girls since he gained the insight that he thereby wanted to prove his own potency (which he doubts). But these are superficial things; deep down, he is a poor, disappointed creature, who, because of his bodily inferiority as a child, despaired of being loved by his mother. Perhaps this would be a theme for the Congress.—

I was happy to hear that you liked my paper on obscene words. My solutions to masochism don't totally satisfy me, either. Still, I believe one first has to try with all means at one's disposal to explain a psychic state *psychologically,* and only then, when everything fails, take refuge in the organic.

Yesterday I received Abraham's Segantini.[2] The first chapter, which I read, is good, but not very deep.

Smaller happenings:

A very talented young law student, who recently became a medical student in order to learn psychoanalysis, is now residing in *Bonn* and is doing experimental psychology with *Verworn.*[3] When the latter spoke about dreams, our friend (his name is Radó)[4] got up and spoke enthusiastically about your Interpretation of Dreams. (It was during the "discussion hour.")

Verworn responded angrily, "Ah, you mean the *Freud* with his sexuality? Of course, some of his claims are correct, but, then, he has exaggerated everything in such a way that hardly anybody, besides his personal adherents, gives him any credence. After all, if one diddles around long enough with these things, one can always get something sexual out of them." During this discourse he is said to have had an expression on his face of a man who is talking about something disgusting.

The young lawyer is so naive as to believe he will still convert Verworn.

Décsi recently gave a lecture on ΨA in the "Physicians' Association"; he spoke quite respectably, so that I was able to praise him.[5] If he weren't in Stein's hands, something could come of him—but as it is, it is out of the question.

Best regards,
Ferenczi

May 30

A postscript that I wanted to append to this letter and in the end still neglected to write has had the effect of delaying its mailing. In the meantime your letter came, which diverted my interest from personal things and directed it toward matters of fact. The events in Vienna are taking place all at once; I can totally concur with your dispositions and am happy that the situation is getting cleared up. Adler's opposition must also have had a paralyzing effect on my power, that is to say, desire for work. I feel more at one with the Zentralblatt since his influence on it has been gradually diminishing. Sachs and Rank are right. Medicine alone will fill the volumes of the Zentralblatt for a long time to come; literature is making ever-increasing demands—psychoanalysis's campaign of conquest is unstoppable.

It is not *now* my intention to continue the work on obscene words; I would gladly relinquish it to a linguist. Instead, I think I have found two mythological solutions (Samson + Hercules),[6] about which I would like to report to you personally. What are you doing on Whitsun? Should I visit you? Please answer in passing, if only by correspondence card. I would also like to relate to you in person the above-mentioned postscript, which I have not pursued here. But don't let me disturb you if you have other plans! The enclosed letter[7] came today from Stekel. I responded to him quite openly, but in a very friendly manner. I told him that I often had to speak my mind in opposition to the all-too-optimistic presentation in his book (Anxiety Hysteria)[8] in front of my patients who referred to it.

Best regards,
Ferenczi

Jung will write one of these days.

1. During their trip together in Sicily; see letter 169, n. 3.

2. See letter 188 and n. 8.

3. Max Verworn (1863–1921), in 1901 professor of physiology in Göttingen, and from 1910 on in Bonn. He was editor of the *Zeitschrift für allgemeine Physiologie.*

4. Sándor Radó (1890–1972), lawyer and physician; first secretary of the Hungarian Society (1913). In 1922 he went to Berlin, where he underwent analysis with Abraham and became a member of the Education Committee of the Institute. In 1942 he became chief editor of the *Zeitschrift* and in 1927 of *Imago.* In 1931 he was invited by Brill to set up an educational institute in New York modeled on the one in Berlin. He gradually distanced himself from Freud, left the New York Society, and, with Carl Binger, Abram Kardiner, and others, organized his own analytic institute at Columbia University, which was finally recognized by the American Psychoanalytic Association. Radó represented a behavioristic view within psychoanalysis; he is especially well known for his works on toxicomania.

5. Ferenczi summarized Décsi's lecture of May 22 in *Zentralblatt* 1 (1910–11): 522: "Dr. J. *Décsi* gave a lecture on the *Program of Psychotherapy,* in which he came to the conclusion that psychoanalysis and the instruction which is based on it are the only

rational means of control and prophylaxis. Nevertheless, the lecturer also approved of suggestive measures. The lecture was received with applause. In the discussion, *the reviewer* emphasized the necessity of excluding all forms of suggestion from psychotherapy. He referred to the stultifying influence of today's education on children, and he demanded that we finally place a high value on the power of youth instead of age. Elders are of undeniable value as moderating, inhibiting factors. But they ought not to abuse this capability of theirs."

6. No references could be found in Ferenczi's works to the biblical hero Samson and the myth of Hercules. Freud had addressed the latter in the *Interpretation of Dreams* (1900a, pp. 469–471) and returned to him in "The Acquisition and Control of Fire" (1932a [1931], pp. 188, 191f).

7. This letter is missing.

8. Wilhelm Stekel, *Nervöse Angstzustände und ihre Behandlung* (Berlin, 1908). See also letter 12 and n. 6.

223

Vienna, May 28, 1911
IX., Berggasse 19

Dear friend,

It was not until it was in print that I was able to acknowledge your paper on obscene words and appreciate the meaning with which you are able to endow my suppositions. I am very enamored of your idea and would only wish that you could present the most detailed proof of it yourself or through a linguist.[1] An article that came to my attention yesterday in Jung-Ungarn[2] [Young Hungary] showed me that your activity in Budapest is making an impression on the best forces in your homeland. You should console yourself if it happens to be physicians who behave in a refractory manner; it doesn't much matter.

When I finally have the Zentralblatt entirely in my hands it will no longer come to pass that a work of yours will wait so long for publication. All indications are now to that effect. To be sure, I no longer know what I have already told you and what I haven't. My head has become unreliable in the face of the difficulties of the last few weeks. As the matter now stands, Stekel has reconciled with me completely and has performed a very good service in containing the others. After I served Adler with the *consilium abeundi*, he contented himself with a qualified explanation and has remained in the Society along with his faithful for the time being.[3] For the first time in a long while everybody has behaved properly. Stekel promises that secession, if it comes about at all, will do so in an orderly manner. In the meantime I have gone ahead with the operation and demanded directly of Bergmann that he remove Adler from the editorship.[4] I will come out ahead with Stekel as the sole editor and be able to influence him better. I will put up with him; his fund of good-naturedness makes this possible. Of course, this is totally lacking in Adler, the paranoiac.

In the meantime Dr. Sachs and Rank have suggested a new journal to me, which should be totally removed from medicine and dedicated to the literary, mythological, and philosophical applications of ΨA. I don't know if this is yet the time for it, but I am counting on your most intensive collaboration in the event that it is undertaken. I will discuss it with both of them tomorrow evening. It would be the companion periodical to the *Schriften zur angewandten Seelenkunde*.[5]

My head is finally refusing to accomplish anything new. Various themes, all of a nonmedical nature, have arisen and are recommending themselves for the days of solitude in Karlsbad, as is the case with the uncanny and tragic guilt;[6] but the necessity of reading much by others is scaring me away and makes it impossible to work on this in Karlsbad. So I will probably not satisfy these cravings. Overwhelming inspiration has continued to abandon me during all these weeks.

I can't tell you anything more about our summer plans that goes beyond what has already been decided.

I have pondered your relationship with Jung once more, and I think you should pay a visit in Zurich at a time when I am not along, to present him with material and discuss things further with him.

In the meantime I hope you are calmer about your brother. Ernst is not doing badly. Just today he caught some influenza or fever with sore throat; he is behaving quite sensibly as a patient.

Things seem to be stirring in Holland. A Dr. *Stärcke*[7] from the vicinity of Utrecht is requesting admission into the Society; he claims to have represented ΨA orally and in writing since 1905. I have here a very intelligent man from Leyden, Dr. *van Emden*,[8] who is teaching himself ΨA and will then practice it on patients. Other Dutch physicians have turned to Stekel. Marcinowsky, the apostate, seems to be not at all well, asked for permission to attend the Congress, and received the reply that he should apply for acceptance in Berlin.

I send kind regards and hope to hear from you again soon.

Yours truly,
Freud

1. Ferenczi, proceeding from Freud's observation that "the utterance of the obscene words . . . compels the person who is assailed to imagine the part of the body or the procedure in question" (Freud 1905c, p. 98), had expressed the opinion that in obscene words in particular, but basically in all words, there resides "the capacity of compelling the hearer to revive memory pictures in a regressive and hallucinatory manner" (1911, 75; *C.*, p. 137; *Schriften* I, 62).

2. Jenö Hárnik, "Zur Psychologie des Propagandisten," *Jung-Ungarn*, Bruno Cassirer, editor. See also the review by J. T. v. Kalmár, *Zentralblatt* I (1910–11): 510.

3. It is not clear from the *Minutes* what Freud is alluding to here with the term *consilium abeundi* (the advice given to a student to leave an institution of learning in order to avoid being expelled). In the session of May 17, at which Adler was not present, Paul Klemperer had interpreted a dream following Adler's method. Freud replied that it was "better to look at things in order to find out what they say, rather than what Adler has said and whether he is right" (*Minutes* III, 263). Karl Furtmüller, another of Adler's adherents, thereupon rejected "as unjustified Freud's overall reproach of a partiality that is not becoming to a scientific discussion" (ibid.). On May 24 Adler played up this incident but claimed to be quite satisfied with the resolution of the plenum that his views were not in contradiction to those of Freud (ibid., p. 268; see letter 204, n. 1).

4. Adler was—along with Stekel—still the editor of the *Zentralblatt*.

5. From this idea of Rank's and Sachs's there arose *Imago, Zeitschrift für Anwendung der Psychoanalyse auf die Geisteswissenschaften* (named after the novel by Carl Spitteler; see letter 131, n. 2), the history of whose founding is discussed in many letters later in this volume.

6. Eight years later Freud published "The 'Uncanny'" (1919h) in *Imago* 5 (1919): 297–324.

7. August Stärcke (1880–1954). In 1921 he received the Freud Prize for his work *Psychoanalyse und Psychiatrie* (Vienna, 1921).

8. Jan E. G. van Emden (1868–1950) from The Hague; served as president of the Dutch Society. He and his wife soon became friends of the Freud family.

224

Vienna, June 1, 1911
IX., Berggasse 19

Dear friend,

So, I will spare us all discussions about our conversations at Whitsun and am very pleased about your fortunate idea. I ask you only, don't come on Sunday but rather on Monday, for I have been very tired since a severe migraine on May 29 (May 6 + 23),[1] and I want to get a good rest on Sunday, i.e., sleep through the morning and be completely inactive.

But don't exaggerate discretion to the extent that you call it off.

Auf Wiedersehen.

Cordially,
Freud

1. Freud is referring to the male rhythm of twenty-three days postulated by Fliess (6 + 23 = 29). May 6 is Freud's birthday.

225

[Budapest,] June 1, 1911

Brief Additional Communication

The spoken expression *"sich etwas herunterreissen"*[1] is *certainly* not the cause, but rather a consequence of the deep psychological connection between masturbation and tooth pulling.

The actual connection is explained by the *castration complex. Sich einen herunterreissen* [to tear one down] means: to do something for which something else (tooth, penis) is torn off one.

Two patients who never heard the expression *"herunterreissen"* dreamt about pulling teeth; one *became very ill from anxiety* after having a tooth pulled. The analysis yielded a colossally strongly pronounced castration complex. The same explanation held true for the second patient.

The two fears, of losing tooth or penis, obviously coincide chronologically (second dentition) and represent each other in the psychic material.

I consider this determination important and regard it as a confirmation of our view on *symbol formation.* The following on this:

1.) Things that are *similar* to one another are *equated* with one another by the child (penis = tooth, castration = tooth pulling). That corresponds to the way in which the ucs. deals with images in general (dream, joke).

2.) Things that were identified with one another in childhood on the basis of their similarity (penis = tooth, butterfly = vagina) can *later* represent themselves as symbols [tooth for penis, butterfly for vulva].[2]

3.) As a consequence of the *repression* of the sexual (latency period), the objects which are equated with them in infancy undergo *symbolic overemphasis* [a kind of "return of the repressed"].

Kind regards,
Ferenczi

1. See letter 21.
2. Enclosed in brackets in the original, as is the phrase in the next paragraph.

226

Budapest, June 3, 1911

Dear Professor,

On Monday I have a court proceeding. So I will postpone my trip to Vienna until the next Sunday. At least you will be able to have a good rest, which you deserve after the trials of the last few weeks.

The idea about symbol formation is taking shape more and more.[1]

All at once it becomes clear to me why children don't understand symbolism (they don't need any yet), why they have no sense for jokes, why their dreams are pure wish-fulfillment dreams; finally, why children and adults do not understand or misunderstand one another.

As long as one is naive (native), i.e., not repressed, one needs no indirect language. On the other hand, the child neglects small differences, that is to say, it remodels its world according to its desire (pleasure principle). Only "the necessity of life" teaches the child also to pay attention to small differences (reality principle).

This developmental process is disturbed by education (repression), however, and, as a consequence of this, it is uneven. Certain ideas are disturbed in their development (see: Obscene Words).—*In place of them, the ideas which are equated with the repressed in infancy undergo symbolic overemphasis. Hence, the domination of symbolism in the ideational sphere of the sexual.*

In order for the symbolic alignment of two ideas to come about, in addition to physical homogeneity (similarity), the same feeling-tone of the two ideas (tooth pulling, castration) is probably also necessary. Perhaps even the latter is the more important, and two things which are quite dissimilar in their physical manifestation can be symbolically equated if they are toned by the same feeling.

Kind regards,
Ferenczi

I have written to Jung.

1. See Ferenczi, "Zur Ontogenese der Symbole" [On the Ontogenesis of Symbols] (1913, 125; *C.,* p. 276).

227

Vienna, June 5, 1911
IX., Berggasse 19

Dear friend,

I had rested up yesterday, and your cancellation was a disappoinment to me. Now you should keep hold of next Sunday, when we have a lot of things to talk about.

In matters of symbolism I now have one thing to counter you with. You explain "why children don't understand symbols"; I call to your attention the fact that children use symbols from the outset, for example, Little Hans with his horses and wagons.[1] So that is not correct. Symbolism is there earlier than are the motives for its use. Up to now I see only one thing in this obscure matter (and even that very obscurely): symbolism seems to be the beginning of concept formation, the concept formation of the undifferentiated ucs. I think I have noticed myself that in this primitive abstraction the child allows himself to be led by commonalities which we later set aside, e.g., in a very special way by impressions of movement. Here we will have to observe and collect for a very long time.

I recently found in a Dutchman the same (women) = room symbolism as in the Germans, even though his language has no such thing![2] Unfortunately, I don't speak Dutch, but he speaks German well. We will have to wait until we can treat in foreign languages. The same doubt also exists with your cartoonist in the Fidibus.[3] I am confirming Stekel's new symbols daily, as was the case today, with the twins for testicles. (She is carrying twins in her arms, one slipped away from her, so she is afraid he could fall. Cf. the hat dream in the Zentralblatt.)[4] This is the patient in whose history everything depended on whether her husband's orchitis[5] was one- or two-sided.

I say again: *Auf Wiedersehen.*

Cordially,
Freud

1. According to Freud's interpretation, for Little Hans the "falling horse was not only his dying father but also his mother in childbirth" (Freud 1909b, p. 128), loaded wagons were "stork-box carts" (p. 81), or pregnant women.

2. Here Freud is referring to the German colloquialism *Frauenzimmer* (literally, "woman room"), which has no equivalent in English either [Trans.].

3. See letter 216, n. 1.

4. "The Hat as a Symbol of a Man (or of Male Genitals)," in "Nachträge zur Traumdeutung," *Zentralblatt* 1 (1910–11): 187; this text was taken up by Freud in the third edition of *Interpretation of Dreams* (1900a, pp. 360f).

5. Inflammation of the testicles.

228

Budapest, June 7, 1911

Dear Professor,

I want quickly to dispel a misunderstanding.

I didn't mean that children don't understand symbolism because they don't *have* any yet; *they have nothing else,* and that is precisely why they don't feel anything *special* with symbolic manners of speaking. It is only with repression (latency) that symbols take on a special meaning—symbolism represents the repressed sexual.

Little Hans was already a neurotic—so he could already not only form symbols but also understand them.

I will definitely appear on Sunday morning and will also have to tell you some personal, as well as factual, things—.

Kind regards,
Ferenczi

I am still awaiting Jung's reply.

229

Budapest, June 19, 1911
VII., Erzsébet-körút 54

Dear Professor,

I came home refreshed and eager for work, and I have already written the little contribution that I promised *Stekel* for the Zentralblatt (Paranoia as a Consequence of Rectal Fistula),[1] and am otherwise somewhat more diligent.

In one case I was *already* able to verify your supposition that obsessional ideas mask erections. More about that next time.

Based on Frau G.'s sensible suggestion, I want to take my summer vacation in the month of *August* and take a little, special vacation for Weimar.[2] My visit to Upper Bolzano, which I imagine will last two weeks, will take place during the month of August. But since you won't get to Bolzano until August 1, and since I would like to let you rest for a while undisturbed in the bosom of your family, I probably won't arrive in Upper Bolzano until about August 10–12. I will await more precise information from you on this. You know I can come any time in the month of August, so you can decide when.

The response from *Jung* has arrived. Very friendly, very forthcoming. But with respect to what we decided at Castle Kobenzl, I will content myself with a kind word of thanks, and I will dispense with the visit. I am enclosing the letter.[3] But please handle it discreetly with consideration for *Jung's* special wish. I.e., I don't want it official that I shared with you the passage about the "secret arts."

I am in great suspense about Adler's tricks. Let us hope everything is now settled and the troublemaker has been put on the spot.

Jones is writing me very friendly letters. I still have to mollify *Brill* with a letter before the Congress.[4]

Kind regards,
Ferenczi

Please return Jung's letter.

1. Ferenczi, "Reizung der analen erogonen Zone als auslösende Ursache der Paranoia, Beitrag zum Thema: Homosexualität und Paranoia" [Stimulation of the Anal Erotogenic Zone as a Precipitating Factor in Paranoia] (1911, 77; *Fin.*, p. 295), *Zentralblatt* 1 (1910–11): 557–559.

2. The Third Psychoanalytic Congress in Weimar, September 21–22, 1911.

3. This letter is missing.

4. See letter 216.

230

Vienna, June 20, 1911
IX., Berggasse 19

Dear friend,

Jung's letter enclosed. He is very kind. Stay warm with him. I know about his astrological studies, by the way.

Your visit during the time indicated is very agreeable to me, as it would be at any other. We may have difficulty in providing accommodations for you, so please notify us in a timely fashion!

The affair with Adler is now acute. Through his lawyer he has tied his resignation from the journal to conditions that are ridiculously presumptuous and quite unacceptable.[1] At the same time, after his resignation from the Society a legal action is being taken against me that is supposed to culminate in a declaration and discussion in a special plenary session, with my possible resignation.[2] I am inclined to be as intransigent as possible and at this opportunity rebuff everything that is disturbing. I don't know whether the majority will follow me. In any case, the whole mythology is there: aggression, covering one's behind, rabble-rousing, up and down[3] are being staged, and with me the main thing is my resolve to maintain the Society and the journal. I have announced a gathering in the Prater for the 28th.[4] By then most things will have been decided.

Otherwise not much new; I am counting the days until vacation, and they are passing slowly. The Interpretation of Dreams is finished[5] and is already supposed to be published and distributed before my departure.

Kind regards,
Freud

1. Freud had written to J. F. Bergmann, the publisher of the *Zentralblatt*, that he had to choose between Adler and himself (see letter 223). Bergmann brought this letter to Adler's attention, and in June the latter drew up a declaration announcing his resignation from the editorship (*Zentralblatt* 1 [1910–11]: 433).

2. "I have finally [in the original *endlos*, "endlessly," rather than *endlich*] got rid of Adler," Freud had written to Jung on June 15 (*Freud/Jung*, p. 428). Along with Adler, David Bach, Stefan von Maday, and Baron Franz von Hye also left the Society. On the

same day on which Freud wrote this letter, Karl Furtmüller, Margarete Hilferding, Franz and Gustav Grüner, Paul Klemperer, David Oppenheim, and Josef Friedjung wrote a declaration in which they termed Adler's resignation "unquestionably provoked" and condoned his actions; but they further expressed the wish to remain "eager members" of the Society. See Bernhard Handlbauer, *Die Adler-Freud-Kontroverse* (Frankfurt, 1990), p. 157. At the special general meeting of October 11 it was decided to declare that membership in the Society for Free Psychoanalytic Investigation, which had been founded in the interim by Adler, and in the Psychoanalytic Society were incompatible, whereupon the second group (with the exception of Friedjung) announced their resignations (*Minutes* III, 281–283; see also letter 242).

3. Aggression and striving for power were viewed by Adler as central motives for human action, whereas "the sexual was to be understood as a jargon, a *modus dicendi*." Alfred Adler, *The Neurotic Constitution* (New York, 1917), p. x. Neurotics were striving to create for themselves a fall-back position in social relations (ibid., p. 310), and in every symptom one recovers "the feeling of effeminacy, of inferiority, of being 'down,' and the masculine protest, the fictitious manly goal, the feeling of being 'above'" (ibid., p. 353).

4. In the attendance book in the *Minutes* there is a note of a "pleasant gathering on June 28, 1911—Konstantinhügel." Adler and his adherents were not present (see *Minutes* III, 267). The attendance book itself has not been reproduced in the English-language edition [Trans.].

5. The third edition.

231

Budapest, July 3, 1911
VII., Erzsébet-körút 54

Dear Professor,

It is also gradually getting to be summer here. Many patients are staying away, and if I were not bound by official duties, I would follow their example and go on vacation. But as things are, I will wait until August 1. It's hard for me to do, since I am already quite tired.

In this mood the publication of the third edition of the "Interpretation of Dreams" had an electrifying effect on me. I am very, very thankful to you for that. A cursory inspection already reveals the presence of a rich accrual, as well as the conscientious collaboration of our Rank.

I already have a publisher for the "Five Lectures"[1] in Hungarian and for a second volume of "Lélekelemzés."[2] He is not disinclined to publish more of your works by and by. In two years a small "Freud Library" will have been published.

The lady (Pollatschek the elder), who is now doing psychoanalysis with Bircher and to whom I promised your "Everyday Life"[3] in Russian, is now requesting what was promised. But I forgot to take it along from your place. Would you be so kind as to send it to her? She is now called Frau L. *Polányi*[4] and is living in Bircher's sanatorium "Living Force."

I have been informed of the Adlerian affair up to his unacceptable demands. *What happened then?*

This is obviously my last letter before your departure for Karlsbad; I wish you undisturbed rest—inward and outward—for your stay there.

Cordially,
Ferenczi

1. See letter 213, n. 3.
2. See letter 122 and n. 3.
3. See letter 156 and n. 1.
4. The Magyarized name of Cecilia Pollacsek (see letter 184 and n. 4).

232

Vienna, July 5, 1911
IX., Berggasse 19

Dear friend,

This is also my last letter before Karlsbad (Haus Kolumbus). A few days ago I composed another letter for you that was not mailed. I don't know whether my tiredness in this made me perceptive or simply depressive. The letter was preoccupied with inner changes in a deeply tragic way and was left lying until the *lendemain*[1] because of the aforementioned doubt.

It would take too much to explain now in all its details how the Adler affair has developed further. On to Bolzano! Suffice it to say, he is now out of the Society and the newspaper, and I am on very good terms with Stekel, who has proved himself to be consistently loyal. I hope that your more active participation in the journal will be one of the desired consequences of this change.

The new journal[2] has encountered difficulties. Bergmann doesn't want it; he claims it will harm the Zentralblatt, and since I need him for entering the journal into the service of the I.P.A., I will probably postpone the founding by a year.

I will look for the book for Frau Polányi, and, when I find it, I will send it off.

Dr. van Emden is becoming very attached to ΨA, which he wants to make his life's calling. He and his wife are going to Karlsbad, where I will dedicate an hour to him on an afternoon walk. So I really do have some understanding and kind company.

How is your brother, and what is Frau G. doing (to whom I ask you, please, to send kind regards)? I am still so busy that I won't get to pack before half past seven on the day of departure.

I'll see you again in Bolzano, when I will again be at full strength, but I look forward to hearing from you frequently while I am gathering strength.

Yours truly,
Freud

1. The following day.
2. *Imago.*

233

Today only the fourth day, so let's postpone all judgment. A cure like this is downright unrefreshing. One doesn't have any resistances to overcome.

Kind regards,
Freud

1. Picture postcard. The caption reads: "Karlsbad. Mühlbrunnen-Kolonnade."

234

Budapest, July 14, 1911
VII., Erzsébet-körút 54

Dear Professor,

I certainly hope that the deeply tragic mood about which you wrote to me in your last letter has finally lifted, and I was happy that your ucs. already surmised this in advance (as the symptomatic forgetting showed). But, on the other hand, I have to admit that I would like to have read that letter, possibly out of egoistic and infantile motives for the most part, but it can't be completely denied that perhaps a trace of wanting to sympathize sprang from more honest sources.

You have a difficult year behind you; the "Adler" episode has caused you much unnecessary struggle. I think we have yet to struggle with some Adlers; the paranoid manner of reaction to psychoanalysis will run its course everywhere; I fear that I have already properly worked in an Adler (and a less talented one, to boot)—*Eisler,*[1] whom you already know. Having been warned by the events in Vienna, however, I will keep a close eye on him, since I can no longer get rid of him.

My brother's suffering is getting worse. I have inwardly "settled" this case a few times already, but every new phase of the illness shakes up my old complexes again—and causes me a day of depression. The fear that it is indeed a cancerous illness becomes more certain every day.

Frau G. thanks you for the greeting and returns it cordially. Just think, I decided to take her daughter (Elma) into psychoanalytic treatment; the situation, you see, was becoming unbearable. For the moment, the thing is working, and the effect is favorable. Of course, she has to talk much more about me than other patients do, but that is not turning out to be an absolute hindrance. She is *consciously* overcompensating (in Adler's sense);[2] naturally I look for and find the most natural drives repressed behind this.

Kind regards,
Ferenczi

1. See letter 213 and n. 2.
2. According to Adler, neurotics often overcompensate for feelings of inferiority with the aim of achieving superiority over others.

235

Karlsbad, July 20, 1911

Dear friend,

The tragic letter that you wished to read is lying in my drawer in Vienna and can't be handed over to you until October.

The first thing I am experiencing here—as in a ψα cure—is the emergence of all my bodily ailments and along with them a deep discord with interesting symptoms that give me something to think about but don't reveal any solution. Only my heart stays well behaved. At times I was able to compete with the late Lazarus.[1] I again had a thought that has to do with the instinctual origin [*Triebherkunft*] of religion, and I will perhaps work it out.[2]

I was very pleased to see your articles[3] finally in print. Now that I am no longer powerless, you should take your proper place in the Zentralblatt. During the next year Adler will have to be held down with cold ruthlessness. It will be be good for all concerned.

The lack of space on the Ritten has caused my people there to make a small move. So you will visit me in the Hotel Klobenstein, not in the Hoferhaus. You will receive more specific information at the proper time.

I greet you and Frau Gisela cordially and wish you much practical success in the new enterprise with Fräulein Elma, but, of course, I fear that it will go well up to a certain point and then not at all. While you're at it, don't *sacrifice* too many of your secrets out of an excess of kindness.

Cordially,
Freud

1. Biblical figure who, after his death, was brought back to life by Jesus (John 11:1–44).

2. Another reference to the forthcoming work on *Totem and Taboo* (see letter 221 and n. 13).

3. Probably "Über obszöne Worte" [On Obscene Words] (1911, 75; *C.*, p. 132) and "Anatole France als Analytiker" (1911, 76), both published in the *Zentralblatt*.

236

Budapest, July 24, 1911
VII., Erzsébet-körút 54

Dear Professor,

After long and painful deliberations with the surgeons et al., and also with Eiselsberg[1] in Vienna, whom we saw last Wednesday, we have, after all, decided on an operation on my brother's palate. My brother has successfully withstood the terrible intervention (removal of almost all of the hard palate, the right upper jawbone, all three right nasal turbinated bones, the septal cartilage, and the neck glands). Prof. Herczel,[2] who is known to you by name, performed the operation. The feared complication (pneumonia) did not occur, so we can hope that *this* phase of his suffering has been successfully overcome. Of course, we have to reckon with the probability of a recurrence; but if the intervention has succeeded in prolonging my brother's life somewhat, then we have accomplished our goal. I often had to say your password, "Ανάγκη."[3]—

Frau G. has also now proved herself to be a true life's companion; she thanks you for your kind greeting.—Elma's treatment is going along normally for the time being. In the meantime I will be able to report to you orally on her case.

Since I don't want to travel until my brother is in Budapest, my vacation time will last from about August 8 until September 11; so my stay in the Tyrol would be at about the end of August and beginning of September. Is that all right with you?

Brill writes me that he wants to embark on August 31 in New York, and afterwards be together with me, and, if possible, also with you. I will share my itinerary with him.

I now have little to do, except for my brother. But I am also already quite tired of the treatment.

Kind regards,
Ferenczi

1. Anton Freiherr von Eiselsberg (1860–1939), titular associate professor at the University of Vienna since 1901 and head of the first surgical clinic there; one of the most respected surgeons of his time.

2. Baron Emanuel Herczel (1861 or 1862–1918), lecturer at the University of Budapest; one of the pioneers of modern surgery in Hungary.

3. See letter 141 and n. 3.

237

Klobenstein, Hotel Post[1]
July 31, 1911

Just arrived here, where you will be cordially and *warmly* received at any time.

Yours,
Freud

1. Picture postcard. The caption reads: "Rittenbahn Klobenstein."

238

Budapest, August 3, 1911
VII., Erzsébet-körút 54

Dear Professor,

The healing of my brother's wound is progressing normally, so I expect to be able to begin my vacation on Tuesday, the 8th. I want to fritter away the first eleven days here in Hungary, a few days with my sister in the country,[1] then two days in Eperjes,[2] a town in northern Hungary, where they can supposedly show me two mediums who work miracles; I would like to look at them from the standpoint of induction. My friend Berény,[3] a talented young painter, is accompanying me on this expedition. Then come a few days in the Tátra, so I will be in Bolzano around the 19th-20th and will be able to spend the rest of my planned four weeks of vacation near you.

The depressive impressions of the last month have paralyzed all scientific activity in me. Symbolism, induction—everything is resting, or silently ripening, but I don't know anything about them. I am utilizing this period of intellectual paralysis to translate some of my German writings into Hungarian and to prepare the second edition of "Lélekelemzés," which will be published in the fall. At the same time I am having your Five Lectures published in Hungarian; I am just now publishing the last of these lectures.—Recently I was unable to withstand the temptation just once to oppose our Hungarian opponents from the university. I did that by publishing my Nuremberg lecture about the founding of the IPA.[4] I also wanted to show the people how well things are going already in ΨA., and I put together the list of our branch societies in a notice.—The youth and the intelligent public have, by the way, already been won over, but they are easily led astray in the matter by the vituperation of the professors.

I will inform you about the places where I am staying as I go along, and I await a reply as to whether the time of my visit is appropriate.

Kind regards to everyone.

Yours,
Ferenczi

1. Possibly his sister Ilona (b. 1865), who was married to Jószef Zoltán, a landowner in Kótaj (County Szabolcs).

2. Approximately 170 kilometers from Budapest.

3. Robert Berény (1887–1953), a member of the "Group of Eight," a group of artists who introduced modern art into Hungary and wanted to bring down the bastions of academic art. Berény was forced into exile because of his participation in revolutionary movements—he was a member of the art directorate of the socialist republic—and he settled in Berlin but returned to Hungary in 1926. Together with Olga Székely-Kovács, he drew caricatures of the participants of the Eighth Psychoanalytic Congress (1924) in Salzburg (see *Caricatures of 88 Pioneers in Psychoanalysis* [New York, 1954]).

4. See letter 173, n. 6.

239

Klobenstein
Hotel Post, August 4, 1911

Dear friend,

My recollection tells me that I was not sparing with complaints from Karlsbad, and so I am now pleased to inform you that I have been sitting here in complete comfort since July 31. The only thing missing is that my wife should get out of bed after coming down with a summer diarrhea, and that it should rain, so that mushrooms can sprout in the magnificent woods. Air, view, accommodations, and service are ideal, and the worries about room for the accommodation of guests or newly arrived family members that plagued us in Upper Bolzano are not present here. We are not considering staying anywhere else, and we expect that fall will take shape here more pleasantly than summer, which was too hot anyway. With that we await you here at the time you indicated and ask only that you inform us of the day so that we can reserve a room for you.

Martin is staying in Millstatt for the time being, and Ernst, after terminating his treatment in the last few days, is going to visit Mathilde in Aussee. Quite a few illnesses, as you can see.[1]

You have also lived through some of this in your neighborhood recently. I wish you good recovery until you come to us.

My intellect, or whatever one usually works with, is also on vacation. I am reading the history of religion and have ordered some books that haven't come yet. In the meantime I have the results of the work in advance and a nice little place in the woods close by where one can read and take notes; so my knees are more or less bare from my alp outfit.

Karlsbad was made bearable for me by the pleasant company of van Emden, who is being completely converted to ΨA. Now I am looking forward to our being together. Perhaps the woods of Klobenstein will also see things come into being which I—or perhaps you—will later be able to present to the world.

My hearty congratulations for Lélekelemzés II.

Auf Wiedersehen and much news in the meantime.

Yours,
Freud

1. Martin was still convalescing after his accident on the Schneeberg (see letter 195 and n. 4), and Ernst had to undergo a rest cure for his stomach and intestinal ailments (see letter 216 and n. 4).

240

Klobenstein
August 11, 1911

Dear friend,

I am replying immediately[1] because I can't determine when this letter will get to you. We are already very much looking forward to your arrival. Unfortunately, it is still too hot; let us hope you will bring cooler weather with you. We have belatedly but quickly become friends with your brother from Berlin; Röschen is a charming child.[2] Your brother is an optimist and claims the weather will be right when he gets to Berlin. He is leaving this morning from Upper Bolzano.

If Dr. Spitz[3] is to be taken seriously, I am ready. But that is a condition for treating him; otherwise it would be too unpleasant to take on a physician as a patient. Since you recommend him warmly, it certainly seems to be in order.

Don't forget to announce your arrival so that we can reserve a good room for you.

I am totally totem and taboo. Get a good rest.[4]

Cordially,
Freud

1. A communication from Ferenczi is evidently missing here.
2. Zsigmond Ferenczi and his adopted daughter Rosa, who later married Werner Richter, first an officer, then a journalist. One of her sons would assume the name Ferenczi.

3. René Arpád Spitz (1887–1974), the famous psychoanalyst and developmental psychologist. Born in Vienna, he spent his childhood and school years in Budapest, where in 1910 he concluded his study of medicine. His analysis with Freud was perhaps the first "training analysis." In 1922, after the First World War, he again came into contact with the Vienna Society, and in 1930 he became a member of the Berlin Society. In 1932 he went to Paris, and in 1938 he emigrated to the United States, where he became a professor, first in New York, then, from 1957 on, in Denver. During the 1950s he published his pioneering works on the origins of the first object relations and the consequences of the separation of the infant from its mother. Between 1963 and 1969 he again taught in Europe, principally in Geneva, then subsequently returned to Denver.

4. On August 20 Ferenczi arrived in Klobenstein and remained for two weeks. In the middle of September Freud went alone to Zurich and spent three days at Jung's house in Küsnacht, then continued on—probably in the company of Jung and his wife—to the Third International Psychoanalytic Congress in Weimar (September 21–22). There he presented a brief "Nachtrag zur Analyse Schrebers" [Postscript to the Case of Paranoia] (1912a [1911]). Ferenczi—"prodded" by Freud in Klobenstein (*Freud/Jung*, September 1, 1911, p. 441)—spoke "about homosexuality." These and the other lectures were reviewed by Otto Rank in *Zentralblatt* 2 (1911): 100–105. Jung and Riklin were reelected by acclamation to their posts as president and secretary, respectively, of the IPA; and the *Korrespondenzblatt*, which had so far been published independently, was incorporated into the *Zentralblatt*. Furthermore, the American Psychoanalytic Association was recognized as a branch society of the IPA, along with the New York Society. After the Congress Freud remained briefly in Weimar in order to be able to talk with Abraham (Jones II, 90; *Freud/Abraham*, October 29, 1911, p. 109).

241

Budapest, October 2, 1911[1]

Dear Professor,

I greet you in your home and wish you health and good spirits for the ongoing work year.

The lymphangiitis[2] that I acquired in Weimar left me bedridden for four days. Now I am already completely restored and fully occupied.

Dr. Spitz wants to see you tomorrow and the day after. He requests that you reserve one hour a day for him. I was to blame for the misguided assumption that you would perhaps also give him three hours.

Best regards,
Ferenczi

1. Sealed postcard.
2. Inflammation of the lymph vessels.

242

Vienna, October 5, 1911
IX., Berggasse 19

Dear friend,

I don't want to make my reply to your letter dependent on Dr. Spitz's appearance, and I thank you for your greeting in the opening, which I return.

Your lymphangiitis corresponds to my periostitis,[1] which is now abating. In its place I have caught a horrible cold in Vienna.

Nothing much is happening. I am working with five patients; most resumptions have been scheduled for a later date.

The publication of the new journal by Deuticke has been assured. Next Wednesday is the first session of the Society and the attempt to force out the Adler gang.

Ernst returned from Lake Garda this morning, nicely recovered. A new family doctor will take care of both patients. Oli gives the impression of being content.

A new periodical for "pathopsychology," which has behaved ambiguously in its foreword, is offering by letter to be a confederate (Specht[2] in Munich).

In anticipation of everything that this year will bring, I am

Cordially yours,
Freud

1. An inflammation of the covering of the bone.

2. Wilhelm Specht (1874-?), German psychiatrist, had worked since 1907 with Kraepelin in Munich and in 1914 became associate professor of psychiatry at the university there. He was founder and editor of the *Zeitschrift für Pathopsychologie* (Leipzig), the first issue of which was published in August. His letter had been sent by Freud to Jung, who commented on it in his reply (*Freud/Jung*, October 6, 1911, pp. 445f). In his foreword Specht raised the objection that Freud's theory stood in contradiction to "the certain experiences of clinical psychiatry. And it is certain that he [Freud] constructed the basic psychological concepts that he uses on his own, without contact with psychology." See Rudolf Reitler's review, *Zentralblatt* 2 (1911-12): 407-409.

243

Budapest, October 11, 1911
VII., Erzsébet-körút 54

Dear Professor,

Many thanks for your communication, which is rich in content. I prophesy a brilliant success for the "Zeitschrift (Zentralblatt?) für angewandte

Seelenkunde," but only after an unavoidable incubation period.—Specht's suggestion came as a surprise to me; probably the first accommodating step from the opposition.—What did you reply to him?

Did a Wednesday meeting take place in the meantime? I am very eager to know about what transpired.[1]

I am appending another last wish to this long series of requests: The "Society for Psychical Research"[2] is requesting that I send in the enclosed declaration of membership and wants you to sign it. Please do that and send the declaration, along with the enclosed letter, to the Society. Excuse the effort and expense that I am costing you thereby. I hope I won't have to bother you with this matter anymore.

I am fully booked and eager for work—but preoccupied with family matters (brother).

Kind regards,
Ferenczi

Perhaps I can take young *Kramer* (homosexual), whom you sent to me, into treatment in November (or December).

1. See letter 230, n. 2.
2. Since the beginning of 1911 Freud had been an honorary member of the Society for Psychical Research (Jones II, 88).

244

Budapest, October 18, 1911
VII., Erzsébet-körút 54

Dear Professor,

Thanks for taking care of the letter from the Psychical Society and for the report on the resignation of the Adlerians.[1] I admire your rigor and intransigence, which I approve of completely but out of weakness would not have been able to exercise with such consistency had I been in your shoes. Aside from the usual (constitutional) factors, I think you owe this ability to the daily purifying bath (I mean daily analysis) which protects your soul from the accretion of inhibiting influences.

The work of analysis is going smoothly; I sent away the impotent millionaire, and in his stead, as well as that of other unpleasant clients, I have obtained better ones.

I am less diligent in scientific work. I am reading quite a bit about "occult" things. Among analytic writings I am *exceptionally* pleased with Rank's Lohengrin.[2]

The other news is rather sad. My brother, inasmuch as his second operation was also not radical, is now inoperable and is nearing his end.

The analysis of Frau G.'s daughter (Elma) was already making very nice progress when one of the youths in whom she was (neurotically) interested (actually the only one who was worth anything) shot himself on her account a week ago. It is very questionable how the matter will go now.

It is possible that I will go to Vienna for the second debate on masturbation.[3]

Kind regards,
Ferenczi

1. A letter from Freud is evidently missing.
2. Otto Rank, *Die Lohengrinsage, Ein Beitrag zu ihrer Motivgestaltung und Deutung*, vol. 13 of *Schriften zur angewandten Seelenkunde* (Vienna, 1911).
3. Ferenczi is referring to the second session (December 6, 1911) of the series of discussions by the Vienna Society on masturbation, which had begun on November 22 (*Minutes* III, 320ff); his presence was not recorded. The series was published, along with Freud's contributions (1912f), under the title *Die Onanie, Vierzehn Beiträge zu einer Diskussion der "Wiener Psychoanalytischen Vereinigung,"* vol. 2 of *Diskussionen des Wiener psychoanalytischen Vereins* (Wiesbaden, 1912).

245

Budapest, October 19, 1911
VII., Erzsébet-körút 54

Dear Professor,

One is so very much under the influence of deeply rooted feelings of obligation that I hesitated for a moment about whether or not to send you the enclosed letter from Frau Jung,[1] despite direct instructions not to do so. But my hesitation didn't last more than a minute, for I saw immediately that the only instrumental thing is to compose the answer to the letter in collaboration with you, that is to say, seek your advice about it.

My suggestion would be that I write Frau Jung a calming letter in which I assure her (and with a good conscience) that I have noticed *nothing* in the way of resistances from you, and I will encourage her at the same time to direct herself to you, without subjecting herself to the risk of being misunderstood.

But, if necessary, I request your *immediate* response as to what, if anything, I should change in the text of this planned letter.

I presume that Jung is now going through a period similar to the one I experienced in Sicily: the dissatisfaction with the *incomplete* intimacy with his teacher (father). Frau Jung, who, by the way, really thinks and writes in a kind and at the same time perceptive manner, could be partly right in her assertions (where she talks about your antipathy toward giving completely of yourself as a friend). It is certainly false that it is your "authority" that you want to protect.[2] More likely the deep aftereffects of the Breuer-Fliess experiences could be responsible for it.

But it is a fact that a piece of sexual curiosity is in play in me and Jung. But shouldn't it be permitted in this sublimated form?

I see some transference to you in this "exercise of statesmanship" on Frau Jung's part.

Objectively, Frau Jung may have discerned something of your disapproval of Zurich occultism and perhaps also your not total satisfaction with Jung's paper on libido.[3]

Kind regards,
Dr. Ferenczi

It is self-evident that you must guard the secret of my indiscretion strictly and for all time.

P.S. Naturally I have nothing against the publication of Bleuler's attack.[4]

1. Jung's wife, Emma (née Rauschenbach; 1882–1955), feared—correctly, as it turned out—an estrangement between her husband and Freud, and had written to Ferenczi for that reason. Upon his reply, which he had composed following Freud's advice (see letters 246ff), she then evidently wrote directly to Freud on October 30, 1911 (*Freud/Jung,* pp. 452f). Her letter to Ferenczi is missing.

2. In his autobiography Jung later cited as the main reason for his break with Freud the fact that the latter had placed "personal authority above truth." In this regard Jung referred to an episode during their trip to the United States when he had tried to interpret a dream of Freud's and the latter, according to Jung, had refused to share "details from his private life." Freud's response, "'I cannot risk my authority!' . . . burned itself into my memory." Carl Jung, *Memories, Dreams, Reflections* (New York, 1973), p. 158. See also John M. Billinsky, "Jung and Freud (The End of a Romance)," *Andover Newton Quarterly* 10 (1969): 39–43.

3. Carl Jung, "Wandlungen und Symbole der Libido," *Jahrbuch* 3 (1911–12): 120–227, and *Jahrbuch* 4 (1912–13): 162–464.

4. He is referring to the publication of Bleuler's polemic against Ferenczi's paper "Über die Rolle der Homosexualität in der Pathogenese der Paranoia" [On the Part Played by Homosexuality in the Pathogenesis of Paranoia] (1911, 80; *C.,* p. 154), *Jahrbuch* 3 (1911–12): 848–852. Ferenczi responded with a countercritique (1911, 81) in the same volume (pp. 853–857). See also letter 307 and n. 1 and *Freud/Jung,* November 13, 16, and 24, 1911, pp. 460, 464f, and 466.

246

Vienna, October 21, 1911
IX., Berggasse 19

Dear friend,

That is very amusing. I see how you want to triumph, but I will see to it that you will not succeed. Above all, it does not seem to me at all a *fait accompli* or supported by the text of the letter (which will be returned) that Jung himself has this impression. That would yield the analogy to you, which is so clear to you. If it is merely a product of the little woman, then the similarity dissolves altogether. But I do admit the probability that she is being supported by statements from him.

I am in complete agreement with the wording of your letter to her; you can also strike the reference to astrology and the paper on libido, because my discomfort with the first instance is not personal, and my objections to the paper on libido are very slight and very clear. In addition to that, you can add that she would certainly not spoil anything, for she should know how much I like her and how highly I esteem her intellectual participation.

On the whole, the matter is not very flattering. If I were not obligated to ΨA, then I would only smile; as it is, however, I want to be careful and wait for material to be presented for signs as to whether I can learn something new about myself.

Eternal discretion goes without saying!

It also occurs to me that Jung went to St. Gallen right after the Congress, and she went to Schaffhausen. The couple probably haven't spoken to each other for weeks.

—As for other news, I can only report that I am in all kinds of little difficulties, e.g., with the new journal. Deuticke has withdrawn; Urban and Schwarzenberg, whom I went to later, have turned us down for understandable reasons, and J. Amb. Barth[1] has postponed making a decision. It annoys me that the thing won't come about.

Ernst is doing well, and nothing has been decided with Sophie.

I greet you cordially, in a hurry.

Yours,
Freud

1. A renowned publisher in Jena.

247

Budapest, October 23, 1911
VII., Erzsébet-körút 54

Dear Professor,

I wrote to Frau Jung along the lines of my last letter to you, touched on occultism and transformation of libido, and animated her to write letters to you.

I also considered the possibility that Jung suspects nothing of the whole matter, but I finally arrived at the presumption that his wife couldn't have produced the matter out of thin air.

I didn't want to triumph over you. Even if Frau Jung's impressions coincide with those of Jung, the both of us (Jung and I) could certainly be mistaken and consider our infantile needs to be our right. If Jung had the same complexes as I, that would still be no reason on my part to triumph over you. At most it would be an indication of how hard it is for one to renounce the communality of thought [*Gedankengemeinschaft*] with a being akin to a father.

At this point in my letter I have to draw a line and report a complication that I am unconsciously guilty of causing. I just read through your letter once more and notice, deeply ashamed, that I have carried out your instructions quite incorrectly.

The first misunderstanding was caused by *you* in reading *my* letter; I remember exactly that I did not have the intention at all (and also did not reveal the intention in the letter) to write to Frau Jung about your dissatisfaction with Jung's occultism and work on libido; I was only writing about my personal view! So I was somewhat surprised when I read in your letter this morning that I should *touch on* [*streifen*] the business with occultism and the paper on libido in my letter to Frau Jung. But I (as an obedient pupil) did it anyway, to be sure, in such a way as to talk about it as if it were an unsupported *supposition,* and I emphasized that I never have heard anything disparaging from you about Jung.—

You can imagine my unpleasant surprise when I now, *naturally* after mailing the letter to Frau Jung, read through the letter once more and see that, instead of *touch on* [*streifen*], I read *strike* [*streichen*]! It is strange that I also understood how to rationalize your other remarks about Jung's occultism and libido paper, which are not at all suited to *touch on.*

So this shows that you *justifiably* misunderstood me, i.e., that in your response you wanted to neutralize an intention that was unconscious to me but must have been present in me. But you didn't succeed; my intention utilized precisely your misunderstanding in order to get its way.

It's a good thing that I did it in such a way as not to obligate you to anything. You can go ahead and deny everything that I uttered as a supposition.

The matter doesn't exactly look like a triumph for me!

Kind regards,
Ferenczi

248

Vienna, October 25, 1911
IX., Berggasse 19

Dear friend,

The matter is becoming very interesting. To your misunderstanding should also be added the act of false obedience, in that you drew a line [*Strich*] in the middle of the letter and called it that. I did, after all, ask you to "strike" both points.

I certainly didn't understand anything but that both objections originated from your private conception. There was no mention of them in the enclosed letter. We will see what she does or causes to have done now.

I am enclosing a clipping for you today in which "Schottländer"[1] thinks kindly of you. Keep it!

A Prof. Jul. Polgár from the Graduate School of Business has expressed a desire to me in writing to translate the Worcester lectures. I naturally referred him to you and suggested to him that he should get in touch with you in general.

I send kind regards from domestic cares and my own miserable cold.

Yours,
Freud

1. Adolf Friedländer, who had announced himself as "Professor Schottländer" on the occasion of a visit to Freud (see letter 78; Jones II, 117). It has not been possible to identify the clipping.

249

Vienna, November 5, 1911
IX., Berggasse 19

Dear friend,

Here is the letter back from Frau Jung. She has written to me in the meantime, and I responded tenderly and in detail, but without actually understanding the matter. Understanding is only just now dawning on me, since my failure to mention the *"Wandlungen"* comes to the fore as the only incriminating evidence. Since I am now writing on the same subject, I may have aroused mistrust through some idiosyncrasies that have to do with the roots of my work. I will in any case very carefully conceal the signs of wanting-to-find-everything-alone and hand over what is permissible. My "Postscript",[1] which seems suspicious in this light, was finished in Klobenstein *before* the arrival of the Jahrbuch.[2] I will report more on the subject to you when Emma Jung's reply arrives. In any case motives like yours,—of wanting to know more about the father—are quite remote from her.

I am not satisfied with anything here now; physically and mentally I am in the condition that customarily accompanies intensive inner labor—or, better said, the preparation for it. It is a kind of misery; when I am well, I am seldom productive. I read, read, and it ferments; I don't know whether I will come to anything.

Only now is my practice rising over the level of two thirds. Dr. Spitz is very interesting; the window dressing is over, and he is behaving quite properly neurotic, with strong resistances. A "countess,"[3] who has been in the news much lately, is supposed to enter treatment tomorrow. We are going to establish the new journal with Heller tomorrow. This is still the only chance. Stekel is sometimes so disgustingly banal that I have difficulty keeping to my decision with respect to him.

Nothing new in the world, except that the secretary from Sydney[4] reports that the communications from Jung, Ellis, and me were received with "unusual" applause. He also sent offprints.

Kind regards,
Freud

1. "Nachtrag zu dem autobiographisch beschriebenen Fall von Paranoia (Dementia paranoides)" (1912a [1911]), Freud's lecture at the Weimar Congress.

2. *Jahrbuch* 3, 2d half-volume (August 1911), in which the first part of Jung's work had been published.

3. Probably Claire Wallentin-Metternich (see letter 255 and n. 3).

4. Andrew Davidson, secretary of the Australasian Medical Congress (see letter 204 and n. 6).

250

Budapest, November 9, 1911
VII., Erzsébet-körút 54

Dear Professor,

Yesterday I received the enclosed letter[1] from Frau Jung; You should also have received her communication in the meantime. So I have apparently not done anything bad—despite the symptomatic action.

Dr. Polgár (the high school teacher) visited me recently; I will have a longer conversation with him today.

I gave up the weekly gatherings with our local disciples, who, with few exceptions, have failed completely to prove their worth. Instead I am again turning to a broader segment of young students and will give a lecture for them every Monday, probably from next week on. I will read your Five Lectures in Hungarian, with commentary. The translation is in press.

My time is divided up among analytical practice and smaller—larger cares and inner conflicts.

Kind regards,
Ferenczi

1. The letter is missing.

251

Vienna, November 13, 1911
IX., Berggasse 19

Dear friend,

I am hurrying to notify you still today that the new journal[1]—probably "Psyche"—has come into being between Heller and us. Its first issue is supposed to come out in the middle of March. Naturally we are strongly counting on your participation and propaganda. I am very glad, for the difficulties have weighed very heavily on me.

A second letter came from Frau Jung,[2] which was more diffuse than the first; it confirmed that, aside from not mentioning the *"Wandlungen,"* I gave no other suspicious signs about myself, and otherwise it seemed really to be fed more by personal interest. The correspondence will probably be ended with my reply.

I am again busy from 8 to 8; but my heart is totally with Totem, with which I am progressing very slowly.

On Wednesday we don't have a holiday but instead a session to interview a candidate.[3] The masturbation debate begins next Wednesday. *Avis au Voyageur.*[4]

Kind regards,
Freud

1. *Imago;* see letter 223 and n. 5.
2. See *Freud/Jung,* November 6, 1911, pp. 455–457.
3. Theodor Reik, a Ph.D. candidate, had been notified by Stekel on October 11 that he was to give a trial lecture (*Minutes* III, 281), which he delivered November 15 under the title "Death and Sexuality" (ibid., pp. 310–319). After the lecture Reik was unanimously elected to membership. Reik (1888–1969) was born in Vienna and studied psychology, German, and French literature at the university there. In 1914–15 he was able to undergo a cost-free training analysis with Karl Abraham. In 1915 he became Rank's successor as secretary of the Vienna Society and retained this function until he moved to Berlin in 1928. In 1934 he emigrated to Holland, and in 1938 to New York, where, as a nonmedical analyst, he was "strongly admonished" by the Psychoanalytic Society there "against practicing, or rather forbidden to practice, psychoanalysis." Theodor Reik, *The Search Within: The Inner Experiences of a Psychoanalyst* (New York, 1974), p. 656. Reik worked as an analyst anyway, and in 1948 founded his own group, the National Psychological Association for Psychoanalysis.
4. French for "advice to the traveler."

252

Budapest, November 14, 1911
VII., Erzsébet-körút 54

Dear Professor,
    You must have already noticed a long time ago that for a long time my letters have been less frequent and more devoid of content than before. You once even made a remark to this effect when you asked if we don't have anything more to say to each other. I left the matter somewhat in disarray, was reluctant to cleanse myself from the inside, until today, under rather distressing circumstances (when will they finally cease with me?!), something became clear. It seems that I wanted to commit a terrible act of violence. Dissatisfied with both parents, I wanted to make myself independent! I noticed that you interpreted my inclination toward you as transference and (evidently out of educational considerations, perhaps also because in your few free days you were longing for a *free*, not an infantile, person) didn't want to give too much opportunity for this transference. That was my "impression," but one that I consciously considered exaggerated.—The reaction to this impression was the decision to make myself independent. (I don't want to be infantile, don't need a father confessor,

want to be rid of sexual curiosity, want to come to terms with myself on my own, etc.)

As a parallel process an apparent detachment of libido from Frau Gisela was playing itself out in me. An occasion for this was offered by the treatment of her daughter, who is in treatment with me and in the stage of transference. I thought seriously that I am true to Frau G. only out of piety, and had fantasies about marrying Elma. (Recurrence of a similar condition in the spring.)

A talk with Frau G. today (with tears *on my part*) showed me that I overestimated myself colossally when I considered myself capable of loosening the strong bonds of fixation on her; I recognized my strong interest in young, pretty creatures in the last few months to be arrangements that were supposed to mask this fixation. (Of course, there was also something *genuine* in it.)

At the same time—after a last welling-up of the striving for independence with respect to you—I recognized that your friendship—yes, even your fatherly advice—is indispensable to me.

The result of all these events is this letter to you, from which you see that I haven't gotten very far with independence. But perhaps I can at least better control my mood and my actions with this knowledge. I hope that my desire for work will also increase.

Yesterday I began a cycle of five lectures. I am freely delivering *your* Five Lectures[1] and am having much success with them.—Please share with me soon your impression of the content of this letter. Without *any* reservation, of course!

Yours truly,
Ferenczi

Postscript: Today I wrote down a whole series of "free associations" about myself; the nicest one was this:

> "I remain a 'son'
> Have religion."!

November 15

I preferred not to send this letter off hot off the press. I thought the complete course of the reaction would necessitate a later report. On the whole, however, I have little to change in what has been said; at the most, what amounts to the fact that I am conscious that the events described should be regarded as a phase of my struggle for freedom, which, amid numerous vacillations, could last a long time.

Now to matters of fact. I thank you for the pleasant news about the founding [of the new journal]; I will not refrain from attempting to be active as a collaborator in it; success should be anticipated.

Pólgar, the high school teacher, introduced himself to me. He is quite a capable person, who still knows little ΨA, but what he has read he has correctly understood. He also introduced me to his friend Dr. Varjas[2] (both Jews, naturally). I like the latter less; he is, to be sure, smart, but too conceited. Incidentally, both are first and foremost *logicians,* who are doing *absolute logic,* which has been revived by *Husserl*[3] (supposedly already in existence in embryonic form since Aristotle). This logic is supposed to be independent of all psychology, that is to say, inaccessible to any psychological analysis; thus it is also independent of psychoanalysis. Both concede that ucs. mechanisms are concealed behind logical mental activity in general, but they are evidently primarily interested in the laws of functioning of the organ of consciousness. Despite this attitude they want to "have peace and quiet" and correct, expand, limit, and systematize psychoanalysis, with which they have no personal experience as yet. There is—I think—more to be expected from Polgár, who is somewhat more modest, than from his friend. So: still not the right co-workers! [Since the cs. is the organ for the recognition of reality, the laws of thinking must somehow agree with mathematics, i.e., with the abstract laws of reality. The proof of this connection between logic and mathematics shouldn't impinge on psychoanalysis for the foreseeable future, however.][4]

Cordially,
Ferenczi

1. *Five Lectures on Psycho-Analysis* (Freud 1910a, [1909]).
2. Sándor Varjas (1885–1939), a philosopher who was concerned with logic, epistemology, and aesthetics as well as psychoanalysis. As a member of the Social Democratic party, he participated actively in the revolution in the late fall of 1918, and during the republic (1919) he taught at the University of Budapest. After the counterrevolution he was arrested and in 1922 was sent to the Soviet Union in a prisoner exchange.
3. Edmund Husserl (1859–1938), founder of phenomenology, graduated in 1883 as a Doctor of Philosophy from the University of Vienna. From 1884 to 1886 he attended the lectures of Franz Brentano, on whose recommendation he qualified as an associate professor of philosophy at the University of Halle in 1887. From 1901 on he was a professor of philosophy at the University of Göttingen, and from 1916 to 1928 at the University of Freiburg. In January 1936 he was denied the right to teach by the Nazis. Varjas and Polgár were referring to Husserl's position in his early work *Logische Untersuchungen,* 2 vols. (Halle, 1900 and 1901), in which he criticized logical psychologism and developed a conception of logic as a formal scientific doctrine.
4. Enclosed in brackets in the original.

253

Vienna, November 17, 1911
IX., Berggasse 19

Dear son,

You demand a quick response to your affective letter, and I would like to work a little today. I am pleased about good news that I will share with you later. So, it will come out brief and not tell you much new. Of course I know your "complex ailments" and gladly admit that I would rather have an independent friend, but if you make such difficulties, I have to accept you as a son. Your struggle for liberation doesn't need to take place in such alternation of rebellion and subjugation. I think you are also suffering a little from the fear of complexes that has attached itself to the Jungian complex mythology. Man should not want to eradicate his complexes but rather live in harmony with them; they are the legitimate directors of his behavior in the world.

By the way, you are scientifically on the right track toward making yourself independent. Witness your studies in occultism, which perhaps contain an excess of zeal as a result of this striving. Otherwise, don't be ashamed to be of one mind with me, and don't demand anything more from me personally than I am willing to give. One must be happy when a person, for once, comes to terms with himself on his own. You certainly know the good definition: Whatever you don't have coming to you is *Rebach*.[1]

Now the news: Karger[2] needs the fourth edition of Everyday Life for 1912. Our Frenchman in Poitiers, who has been silent since January, sent me a letter today, a contribution for the Zentralblatt (homosexuality and paranoia with reference to two authors of the Jahrbuch who are known to you)[3] and a reprint of a splendid article in the Gazette des Hopitaux (p. 1845, vol. 84, no. illegible). It is called "Le 'Rapport affectif' dans la cure des Psychonévroses."[4] It is right up to date and singles out an essay by Ferenczi. Try to read it right away. I will write to him that he should send you a copy.

Now, good-bye and calm down.

With fatherly regards,
Freud

1. *Rebbach* or *Reibach*, Yiddish for credit or gain.

2. S. Karger, the Berlin publisher of *The Psychopathology of Everyday Life* (Freud 1901b).

3. Pierre Ernest René Morichau-Beauchant, "Homosexualität und Paranoia," *Zentralblatt* 2 (1912): 174–176. Morichau-Beauchant (1873–1951), professor of clinical medicine at the Ecole de Médecine in Poitiers, had written Freud a letter at the end of 1910 in which he had referred to himself as Freud's pupil (*Freud/Jung*, December 3, 1910, pp. 377f; see also Freud 1914d, p. 32). In January 1912 he joined the Zurich group (*Freud/Jung*,

January 23, 1912, p. 482). Through his works "psychoanalysis was 'officially' introduced to national [French] soil." Elisabeth Roudinesco, *La bataille de cent ans, Histoire de la psychanalyse en France*, vol. 1, *1885–1939* (Paris, 1982), p. 234.

4. P. E. R. Morichau-Beauchant "Le 'rapport affectif' dans la cure des psychonévroses," *Gazette des Hôpitaux*, November 14, 1911, pp. 1845–49. Ferenczi was in agreement with this article, which he cited in "Zähmung eines wilden Pferdes" [Taming of a Wild Horse] (1913, 104; *Fin.*, p. 336; *Schriften* I, 134).

254

Budapest, November 26, 1911
VII., Erzsébet-körút 54

Dear Professor,

Your fatherly speech had an immediate effect on me. It made me laugh heartily. On the other hand, it made me think, and I had to admit you were right about everything.—*Theoretically*, I knew, of course, that one can't eradicate one's "complexes" (I've taught my patients that for years), but in practice I seem to have sinned against this wisdom: I wanted to be something other than I really am and wanted to have you different than you are. I was evidently demanding an alignment of our personalities: either you come down to me or I have to raise myself to you. Only seldom was I objective enough to see that we can exist well alongside each other, be happy with each other, while at the same time dispensing with this forced alignment; one then joyfully gives and takes as much as one can willingly give and take. I know, by the way, that this insight does not yet mean the definitive end to my "struggle for liberation"; but perhaps I will be successful in removing the element of crisis in this developmental process. In any case, I thank you for your kindness in playing the role of the father, as long as I need such a thing; perhaps I will yet have the experience of extending my hand to you as a free man. (This fantasy, by the way, corresponds to my observation that in a dream *friend* always means *father*, i.e., a father who deigns to live with his son in a bond of friendship.)

I am now so busy that I don't yet know for certain whether I can come to the Wednesday session. If I come, I will let you know in advance.

My public lectures here are attracting some attention; the enthusiastic listeners are making noise all over town; a humoristic periodical is making fun of me and analysis and is getting publicity for me by intimating (derisively) that I charge fifty crowns for a session. The *Äzte*[1] is good!

I am analyzing a young, very intelligent woman with jealousy mania, but who has conscious homosexual interests as well. I am having such spectacular success with her that I am beginning to believe in the possibility of curing her. At this point of cs. homosexuality I can gradually pull out everything she has projected up to now.—Another, equally very pleasant hour of analysis was provided me by a young woman who is so clever that I hardly have to tell her anything—she discovers everything herself, like Breuer's patient. Perhaps she will solve the question of masochism for me.

I am not satisfied with Oppenheim's paper on jealousy.[2] I would like to write a better one about it. Then a paper on *"audition odorée"*;[3] a classic case! I also intend to write the article on technique which you allude to!—But lectures, corrections, fatigue, complexes are holding me up for the time being.

H. Silberer is already knocking on the doors of occultism[4]—let us hope not so strongly that I have to announce my presence. I am not doing anything with it at the moment.—The news from France was very gratifying.

Kind regards,
Ferenczi

1. *Ezzes*, Yiddish for good advice or tip.
2. Hans Oppenheim, "Zur Frage der Genese des Eifersuchtswahnes," *Zentralblatt* 2 (1911–12): 67–77.
3. Synesthetic perception of noises and odors.
4. Silberer's "occult" interests soon found a place in several publications; see e.g., Herbert Silberer, "Mantik und Psychoanalyse," *Zentralblatt* 2 (1911–12): 78–83, and "Lekomantische Versuche," pts. 1–4, *Zentralblatt* 2 (1911–12): 383–401, 438–450, 518–530, 566–587.

255

Vienna, November 30, 1911
IX., Berggasse 19

Dear son,

(Until you object to this form of address.) There are all kinds of annoying things going on in the world that require writing about. Bleuler is intolerable. He wrote to me that he has again resigned from the Association.[1] I cursed him out for that, and now I am awaiting further reports from the theater of war.

Jung is sending you the enclosure to this letter and asks you "to react without affect to it and perhaps emphasize the ethically neutral position of ψα interest with regard to the practical-hygienic efforts." The paper, as well as your reaction to it,[2] are designated for the Jahrbuch and should get back either to Jung or to Deuticke. You should ask Jung himself about that.

The work on totem is a mess. I am reading fat books without any real interest, since I know the conclusions already; my instinct tells me so. But all the material has to be ground through, and in the meantime the insights become clouded. There are many things that don't want to make sense, and yet shouldn't be forced, and I don't have time every evening, etc. Sometimes I feel as though I only wanted to start a little liaison and at my age discovered that I had to marry a new wife.

I am working diligently from 8 to 8 o'clock, but I have very little time for the boys, and they get rowdy very quickly if they're not busy with something.

Dr. Spitz made a bit of a play of grandiosity and was penalized for it by being deprived of three hours, and since then he seems to want to take it more seriously. The mainsprings have been weakened considerably, since he wants to give in to his father and doesn't want to remain a physician. Still, he is quite nice.

My most interesting patient is now Wallentin-Metternich,[3] but unfortunately only for a short time.

I send kind regards, with complete understanding for all the complications under which you now stand.

> *Weiber, Widersacher, Schulden!*
> *Ach, kein Ritter wird sie los.*[4]

Yours,
Freud

1. In a letter of November 27 (Library of Congress), Bleuler had written to Freud that he had to resign from the Psychoanlytic Association because his assistant physician had been denied participation.

2. This is a reference to Bleuler's critique of Ferenczi's paper on homosexuality and paranoia and Ferenczi's countercritique (see letter 245 and n. 4).

3. Claire Wallentin-Metternich (1879–1934), Viennese actress, married to Gisbert Graf Wolff-Metternich zur Gracht until their divorce in 1915.

4. "Women, adversaries, debts! / Oh, no knight gets rid of them." Final stanza of Goethe's ballad "Ritter Kurts Brautfahrt" (1804), in *Sophienausgabe* I, 176f.

256

Budapest, December 3, 1911
VII., Erzsébet-körút 54

Dear Professor,

I still have no right to declare myself mature—the pressing need to report to you about personal events that concern me is a sure sign of my infantile attitude.—It was sufficient that you wrote a word about your understanding of my difficult situation, and already I have to tell you everything.—

Things are proceeding more rapidly than I imagined they would. I was not able to maintain the cool detachment of the analyst with regard to Elma, and I laid myself bare, which then led to a kind of closeness which I can no longer put forth as the benevolence of the physician or of the fatherly friend.—I know and share your view of the Janus character of the neurotic, and it is precisely this conviction that toughened my resolve, again and again, to resist temptation. Perhaps in the end my sight was clouded by passion—in any event, I can't perceive anything in Elma's character that would have prevented me inwardly from approaching her. My situation is made easier—and more difficult—by Frau G.'s incomparably kind, unstintingly kind and loving attitude toward me—she has been told everything. I harbor the most tender feelings toward her—I feel terribly sorry for her.

She knows that I am writing to you and asks you through me to compel me to make a quick decision.

From an analytic point of view I have to conceive of the matter in such a way as to conclude that Elma became especially dangerous to me at the moment when—after that young man's suicide—she badly needed someone to support her and to *help* her in her need. I did that only too well, even though I held my tenderness in check with difficulty for the moment. But the path was cleared—and now, to all appearances, she has won my heart.

You know me, my wish for a family; you also know Frau G., her good qualities, and her only disadvantage[1]—as well as the weak point of my organism (albuminuria).[2] Perhaps you can call my attention to something that could be of use to me in my struggle to decide.

I thank you for your understanding—

Lovingly yours,
Ferenczi

1. That is, her age. Ferenczi "was afraid . . . that at a possible subsequent birth the woman [Gizella] might be damaged as a consequence of the narrowed genital canal" (Ferenczi 1915, 160, p. 306).

2. Protein excretion with the urine, either harmless or an indication of a chronic kidney ailment.

257

Vienna, December 5, 1911
IX., Berggasse 19

Dear friend,

First break off treatment, come to Vienna for a few days (Wednesday evening through Sunday (holiday in between)[1] would be a good arrange-

ment), don't decide anything yet, and give my regards many times to
Frau G.

Cordially,
Freud

1. Enclosed in parentheses in the original.

258

Vienna, December 17, 1911
IX., Berggasse 19

Dear friend,

Thank you for your detailed communication, and I now want to adhere
to the contract from my end by saying nothing further.

Frau G. has asked for a statement from me, which, on account of incognito, I can only send to her address via you.

On the day of your departure a wine arrived from Tokay, which everyone
enjoyed and for which I—innocently—thank you very much.

If you aren't able to use Ernst, I hope that you told him so and didn't
force yourself.

I had a difficult week in which I wasn't able to work at all.

When you next come to Vienna for a holiday or a debate on masturbation,
I will show you the Encyclopaedia Britannica.

Best regards,
Freud

259

[to Gizella Pálos]

Vienna, December 17, 1911
IX., Berggasse 19

Dear lady,

What I am writing to you today will remain completely between us and
is totally sincere, without any embellishment, as is commensurate only
with my esteem for you.

Our friend has hurt me very much and has forced me, myself, to give
advice in which my feelings do not participate. When, years ago, I first
learned of the relationship that he had lodged himself in, I made a face and
made it very clear to him that I wished something else for him. When I
then became acquainted with you, I quickly learned to esteem you and was
able to concede to him that, in comparison to other husbands and lovers,
he possessed incomparably more than what he had renounced. Since then,

not a word or a gesture has issued from me that could have weakened his attachment to you.

His efforts to separate from you originated and proceeded quite independently, and I have seen with deep regret that nothing can be stopped. I understand the tragedy of aging; it is, after all, mine as well. The hard truth is that love is only for youth and that one must renounce; as a woman, one must be prepared to see one's sacrifices repaid with ingratitude. No reproach for the individual, a natural fate, as in the story of Oedipus. In addition, it is the case with *him* that his homosexuality imperiously demands a child and that he carries within him revenge against his mother from the strongest impressions of childhood. But you know all that. I am telling you nothing new, with the possible exception of one thing, namely, that I was certain that *the* woman would understand it, know how to bear it, and make it still easier for him. ΨA may have accelerated this inexorable development still further.

Now, the other part, in which my behavior will certainly be less comprehensible to you. He is turning away from the mother to the daughter and expects from me that I should recognize this trade as one that holds out a promise of happiness. In the process, the wounded woman will experience a blossoming of the beautiful consolation of being allowed to withdraw to the role of happy mother. And here my doubts begin, as well as those about your lucidity. You have shown me this daughter. I did not find that she could place herself alongside her mother, and I remember the quiet intimations with which you endorsed my concerns. Indeed, if it had been the case that the girl had fallen in love with her mother's youthful friend, pined for him, and suffered in the process until both of the others discovered the secret, it would have been a beautiful novel with a touching conclusion, as so often happens in real life; but neurosis would not have been allowed to play any role in it. It is enough that his choice is depreciated by the consideration that he is automatically swinging from his mother to his sister, as was once the case in his earliest years. But the girl should not have been allowed to show so clearly that she wants to repress her mother just as she did when she was a child, and that she wishes nothing but this. She would have had to pass the test that would have been put to her under the otherwise most favorable conditions, of longing for the man for a few years without betraying a mental inability to resist and a very sensitive narcissism (see the effect of the feared distortion in her face!). The suspicion has to arise that to the man she will become a poor substitute for the mother and that she will ill withstand the difficulty of the situation once it arises.

The main difficulty is this: Does one want to build this alliance for life on concealing the fact that the man has been her mother's lover in the fullest sense of the word? And can one rely on the fact that she will take it well and overcome it in a superior manner when she knows it? That requires a high degree of mental freedom, not a piece of infantilism; in short, she would have to be more like her mother and not have betrayed that strange inclination to flee into illness.

In such painful uncertainty I decided, as a friend, to be as sincere and unsparing as possible in the hope thereby of mitigating my responsibility as much as possible. I also told him nothing new, only gave expression to voices that he had heard very clearly. One has to leave the poor mother to her twofold suffering; it makes no sense, in order to spare her, to *hasten* a decision which could lead to chronic suffering for everyone. But one may subject the girl to a test as to whether she shows herself to be improved, more independent, more able to withstand abstinence, equipped with more trust in her own feelings as a consequence of the new love. In the meantime one can clarify for oneself whether something is left over from the new object choice if one takes the displacement from the mother to the sister away from it. If everything goes well, one can then venture to build the new reality on the old fantasies. Otherwise it is better to renounce, better to estrange oneself entirely. Look for happiness somewhere else, if it can still be found at all, rather than blindly follow the seductive demons. That is what I advised him, and I think I had penetrated completely into his own best impulses.

I became so hard-hearted out of sympathy and softness. It should not be difficult for him to rid himself of my advice, but his thoughts are along the same lines.

Now help us and spare yourself. You will certainly have conquered the loving woman more easily, but you should also restrain the tender mother. You should be expected to accomplish this as well.

I greet you kindly, and I hope that enough of our relations will weather the storm.

Yours,
Freud

260

[Budapest]

Bulletin[1] of December 18, 1911.
Patient spent yesterday in considerable turmoil. There was a moving talk with Frau G., which evidently dissolved the apathy. Simultaneous with the awakening of mourning over the loss of Frau G. (that is to say, over the end of the relationship), clearer insight into his own intentions. Marriage

with Elma seems to be decided. What is still missing is the fatherly bless-ing.

Frau G. (the other, more severely ill patient) is suffering greatly. Alleviation of her suffering by means of more energetic measures would be indicated.

Kind regards,
Ferenczi

1. Ferenczi uses the English (or French) word *bulletin* in the original.

261

Vienna, December 26, 1911

Dear friend,

Perhaps you are surprised that, especially under these conditions, I don't write more, and more often. But that is intentional; I have no more to say, perhaps I have said more than was justified, and I don't want to spoil your future completely. So I will congratulate you wholeheartedly when you let me know that the time has come.

There is one good thing about your foreseeable decision which I cannot dispute. You will remain in contact with Frau G., whom you otherwise would have lost.

I ask you to thank Frau G. very much—the letter does have to go through your hands—for her second letter, and to ask her pardon for everything gray and black that I thought I had to say to her, and to give her very special thanks for the reception that she gave to Ernst. I am again obliged to you for the same reason. The boy enjoyed it very much.

These days I have been writing without the proper mood: On Types of Onset of Neurosis (Zentralblatt),[1] On the Universal Tendency to Debase-ment, etc. (Jahrbuch).[2]

Very cordially,
Freud

1. "Types of Onset of Neurosis" (Freud 1912c), *Zentralblatt* 2 (1911–12): 297–302.
2. "On the Universal Tendency to Debasement in the Sphere of Love" ("Beiträge zur Psychologie des Liebeslebens," pt. 2) (Freud 1912d), *Jahrbuch* 4 (1912–13): 40–50.

262

Budapest, December 30, 1911
VII., Erzsébet-körút 54

Dear Professor,

It is now already late at night—and a detailed recounting of everything that is happening and has happened would be too complicated. But before the end of the year I would not like to withhold from you my good wishes, and, while I send them to you and to your loved ones, I will tell you that the—certainly positive—decision about my marriage to Elma will probably not be long in coming. This decision is made possible only through the incomparable love and kindness of Frau G., who has recovered from the heavy blow and has joyfully placed herself in the service of our happiness.

I am sending you herewith the "Five Lectures"[1] in Hungarian and the second collection of my works, called "Psychic Problems in $\psi\alpha$. Light."[2] Once again: a toast to the New Year!

Cordially,
Ferenczi

1. See letter 213 and n. 3.
2. See letter 122, n. 3. The volume contains these works: "Introjektion und Übertragung" [Introjection and Transference] (1909, 67; C., p. 35); "Über obszöne Worte" [On Obscene Words] (1911, 75; C., p. 132); "Anatole France als Analytiker" [Anatole France as Analyst] (1911, 76); "Die Psychoanalyse des Witzes und des Komischen" [The Psycho-Analysis of Wit and the Comical] (1911, 78; F.C., p. 332); "Zur Organisation der psychoanalytischen Bewegung" [On the Organization of the Psycho-Analytic Movement] (1911, 79; Fin., p. 299); "Über die Rolle der Homosexualität in der Pathogenese der Paranoia" [On the Part Played by Homosexuality in the Pathogenesis of Paranoia] (1911, 80; C., p. 154); "Zur Erkenntnis des Unbewussten" [Exploring the Unconscious] (1911, 81a) and "Suggestion und Psychoanalyse" [Suggestion and Psycho-Analysis] (1912, 94; F.C., p. 55).

263

Budapest, January 1, 1912
Grand Hotel Royal
Nagy Szalloda

Dear Professor,

I can't wait for the reply to my New Year's letter—and I have to report in all haste about great changes.—

Everything seems to be settled—Elma and I in agreement with each other and with ourselves; my attempts to interpose a hiatus failed at Elma's and Frau G.'s urging—as well as at the weakness of my resistance. At the last minute, when the already completed plan was presented to Elma's father, he made a few hesitant objections by alluding to Elma's earlier engagement, which had been called off a few years ago. At that, to my amazement, certain doubts crept into *Elma's* mind. That made me suspicious. I inquired further and learned from her (what I certainly should have learned in her analysis) that *every time* she wishes something especially strongly, she inwardly feels an inability to wish (as well as to hate) without reservation. *That* always made her so unhappy.

She then sought to soften the impression, and I have to admit that she can show a degree of devotion and tenderness that we and she herself earlier thought her incapable of. But the scales fell from my eyes, and when, even after this scene, her presence did not fail to arouse feelings of tenderness in me, I had to recognize that the issue here should be one not of marriage but of the treatment of an illness. Of course, I myself cannot continue the treatment. After many bitter tears (which certainly had partly to do with her own fate) she consented to go to Vienna and enter treatment with you. I and Frau G.—we could hardly decide to entrust her with anyone else. The family has been advised of the fee.—If I get a positive response from you—which I very, very much wish—I will go to Vienna on Saturday evening, she will leave a day earlier, and on Sunday I can turn her over to you.—I have little doubt about the outcome of the matter—I have also attempted to prepare Elma for the possibility of breaking the engagement. I will naturally stand aside until the departure.—You can imagine Frau G.'s state of mind.—

I am hoping confidently for your assent and await your prompt reply. I won't write much now about myself. The feeling of having perhaps escaped danger mitigates the pain of disappointment.

Awaiting your reply, I am

Yours,
Ferenczi

264

Vienna, January 2, 1912
IX., Berggasse 19

My dear friend,

How bitterly I feel being perhaps more perceptive and freer of illusion than others, and having to be right. When your express letter arrived, I naturally thought it would contain the news of your engagement, and I recapitulated in myself the intentions of showing no sensitivity now that you neglect the sullen old man in favor of the charming young woman, and of waiting until the both of you have forgotten my advice to the contrary. Then I read it, and now I don't know whether I should be more satisfied. You speak of a drastic change in yourself, as if the scales had fallen from your eyes. I know that I have done nothing to bring that about and would rather have remained grossly wrong.

Now, to the matter of the treatment! If you don't ask about my inclinations and expectations but rather *demand* of me that I undertake it, then I naturally have to assent. Actually, I don't have an hour free; a patient who caused her husband to urge her to break off treatment on December 31 wants to come back tomorrow, and that was my last free hour. I could hold her up until you have decided, for I don't believe that the decision which was made in the first instance is the final one. Just imagine under what unfavorable auspices I am supposed to begin. After withdrawing the bonus that can spur her on to recovery, with the knowledge that I was not in sympathy with her intentions, and with the vague desire for revenge against you, the one who is sending her into this treatment! In this humor, a woman can hardly be woo'd![1] In addition, if things don't go well, there is the silent ill will between us, or at least between the both of us and the noble woman, the superfluousness of my having to peer so deeply into your very own affairs without having accomplished anything for the effort. Is the attempt worth these stakes? I leave it up to you to decide. Send me a telegram if you go back on your intention. It pains me that I can't be with you now. I was depressed the whole time and anesthetized myself with writing—writing—writing.

Very cordially,
Freud

1. "Was ever woman in this humour woo'd? / Was ever woman in this humour won? / I'll have her; but I will not keep her long." Shakespeare, *Richard III*, act 1, sc. 2.

265

Dear friend,

I thank you from the bottom of my heart for your letter. In the trials and confusion of the last few days the memory of the cheerful and dispassionate hours of our relations of friendship was my only unalloyed joy. With respect to Frau G., the joy was mixed with sadness; with respect to Elma it was mixed with concern and regret.

I cannot spare you the effort and trouble of taking Elma into treatment. There is no other way out. She wishes to be treated by me—that is naturally out of the question; if we leave her to herself, then we will jeopardize her stability. We will take into account the probability that more significant success will not be achieved here.

I have not expressly withdrawn the bonus (marriage); only I feel inwardly and I believe that Elma's absence will dissolve the transference relationship in me, and the treatment will do the same in her. I will have to and be able to tell you more about that in person. I will come at the usual hour on Sunday morning.

I threw myself with youthful bravado into this adventure, the last thing that brought me close to the realization of the family romance. Now I have become a modest man.

I took it upon myself to fatally insult dear Frau G. and to suppress a lot of other scruples of conscience. Burdened in this way, I approached Elma as a suitor. But when, at this moment, she showed not the pure joy of a lover but rather the pain of her emotional wounds, the endurance test failed.

For the moment I don't feel *all too* depressed. Only a sad regret when I see Frau G. and Elma—otherwise a kind of relief. I am often reminded of your principle about *Rebach*, which you don't have coming to you.[1]

I thank you repeatedly for your letter, which did me much good.

Thankfully yours,
Ferenczi

Elma does not suspect that you were opposed to our marriage.

1. Freud had expressed it differently (see letter 253): "Whatever you don't have coming to you is *Rebach*"—therefore gain.

266

Vienna, January 13, 1912
IX., Berggasse 19

Dear friend,

I can imagine how anxiously you are awaiting news from me. But I can't tell you much. There is nothing up to now that would justify unfavorable conclusions, but also nothing decidedly favorable. She is quite inhibited, obviously wants to be the good child, to please, to be treated with tenderness; fears loss of love if she admits something. Consciously she is quite well behaved, but the ucs. portions are not coming out right. We are in the processes of raising a long-buried propping by the father [*Vateranlehnung*].[1] She is one of those children who, very spoiled by the father in the first few years, have felt the unavoidable loss of intimacy as neglect. It seems that all her attitudes and desires go back to this factor; hence, the yearning to show herself naked, the sexual curiosity to see something male. The break-ing of the habit of masturbation in early years has already been secured; her consciousness of guilt is connected with her illicitly acquired knowl-edge of the male genital. Hence, her having to conceal, to play a role, etc. I have not yet been able to get a picture of the extent to which her remain-ing stuck in narcissism and her urge for her own masculinity is connected with her father fixation.

Up to now I have found nothing that could not dissipate in the face of a fortunate reality. Certainly her love for you is based on her attitude toward her father and the competition with her mother. Her reaction to the knowl-edge of your relations with her mother is still completely absent and could easily establish itself in marriage as a revenge for her father.

It's nice that she has an inclination to forget and to confuse the words for east and west in all languages except Hungarian. Her second language was French: *le lever et le coucher du soleil.*[2] The sun is naturally her father,[3] who probably took her to bed with him in the morning, and then got up in front of her, and with whom she would like to go to bed at night.

She falls in love compulsively with doctors, i.e., with persons who see her naked, physically, and now mentally.

So wait, not without good expectations.

Cordially, and with regards to the dear mother.

Yours,
Freud

1. The German word *Anlehnung* has been translated by Strachey as "anaclisis" [Trans.].

2. Sunrise and sunset. The French verbs *coucher* and *lever* also mean to go to and get up from bed [Trans.].

3. In the analysis of Schreber (1911c [1910], pp. 53ff) and in the postscript to it (1912a [1911], pp. 80ff) Freud had described the sun as a father symbol.

267

Budapest, January 15, 1912
VII., Erzsébet-körút 54

Dear Professor,

Many thanks for your communications, which I can't respond to now, because I now—in haste—want only to report some news. Elma's father (a very eccentric, self-centered person), who was somewhat upset by the details of the analysis, which Elma, incomprehensibly, shared with him and which he doesn't have a clue about, wants to write you a letter. He doesn't say what kind. Please don't allow yourself to be influenced in the slightest by his remarks. I don't think he wants anything but to show that *he*, too, is there, and I think he would consider himself happy if you replied to him and perhaps dropped a flattering phrase about his intellect or his style of writing.

More next time. Again, many thanks.

Yours,
Ferenczi

268

Budapest, January 18, 1912
VII., Erzsébet-körút 54

Dear Professor,

It was evidently prudence on my part that I am deciding only after such a long time to report about myself. My moods have been changing so suddenly that a picture of any given moment would only render an incomplete account of my *status psychicus.*—The last evening in Vienna[1] depressed me inordinately. I interpreted every reaction of Elma's in the context of her inability to love (dementia praecox) and saw the future in the gloomiest light. I had almost taken it for granted that nothing would come of this marriage, and I began to console myself with the fact that I would find sufficient compensation for the loss of family happiness in the understanding and loving company of Frau G. and in scientific intercourse with you.—It took almost a week before this view of mine began to moderate. Elma's letters and your not unfavorable report eased my mood, the impressions of pathology in Elma's being were partly eradicated, memories of scenes that seemed to prove to me her ability to love emerged more frequently, and I began to reckon with the possibility of a positive solution. In the meantime I visited Frau G. daily; she proved to be—even in her own sad state—a consolation. So much ability to love, such intellectual and emotional ability to achieve and to sacrifice is, to be sure, a painful reminder of what could have awaited me with Elma. And yet I must, in truth, confirm that, in being together with Frau G., despite all these confirmations—despite all conscious substantiations of her attractiveness, her intellect, her spirit—I don't feel that same enthusiasm, that carefree, joyful, natural élan that Elma brought out in me. Love is irrational!

In summarizing my moods and my intentions I can say that I feel strong enough to overcome the irrational in me and am *much sooner inclined to renounce the possibility of happiness* than to subject myself and Elma to the dangers of a marriage that has *too much* risk attached to it. Among the dangers that threaten me, the possibility of a belated revenge for her father is, in my opinion, no slight one.

(In order to give you an idea of the ambitendency [*Ambitendenz*][2] that prevails in me, I will add here that, while I was writing the words "that I feel strong enough"—doubts about this strength arose in me.

Meanwhile, I am also exerting myself over a difficult possibility: to ensure for myself Frau G.'s love also in the event of my marrying Elma. It is painful to me to see her unhappy, and I obviously wish that she should share in our joy.—

So this means: wait patiently and make everything dependent on the results of the analysis.

Since Elma is inclined to hide things, or, more precisely, to reveal them elsewhere, in the interests of her analysis, I want to share with you the content of today's letter from her.

"Mama's letter to me would have been sufficient; it was superfluous for Sándor to write to Freud immediately. Prof. Freud declared, to my regret, that he would rather that I didn't tell anyone at all about the analyses."

[She promises to be obedient in this as well, in order to further the cure; she is already very impatient—especially since the last hour was "bad" and she was not able to talk at all.][3]

She wants to know *positively* what you have written to me about her, whether you are satisfied with her progress. [Frau G. responded to her in a reassuring manner.]

"Let Sándor know that I am almost always thinking about him. I wish so much to see him happy and myself with him. I certainly hope very, very much that everything will turn out well—but today I am anxious about the future. My character is so unbalanced, such a terrible chaos is reigning in me that it would be a risk for anyone to take me as a wife. Even if the analysis clarifies the situation, I will still be the same old way and the bad things can begin again at any occasion. The only possibility to live will be by avoiding such occasions. Sándor can have neither the desire nor the patience to take me by the hand every step of the way [literally: "lead me every step of the way"]—. . . I fear I will only create worry for everyone who takes me" . . . [There follow a few lines about the hope that it will turn out well.] Then: "Dear Mama, you never write about yourself. If you have reached an agreement with Sándor that you cannot live without each other, then write me that honestly. As long as you feel yourself so deeply affected by the loss of Sándor, Sándor will neither tear himself away inwardly from you, nor will I be able to accept his love without misgivings. We are aware of your suffering, of course, even if you want to hide it; It would be better if we are honest. Your untroubled feelings deserve to be spared more than mine. My future is a series of difficulties anyway; more or less renunciation doesn't count much with me."

[At the end, again a fantasy: I would come and get her and take all difficulties onto myself.] "Naturally, I can't ask for that."

In passing, there occurred to me a peculiarity that I have observed with Elma and other narcissists.

It has often occurred to me that narcissists—despite their grandiose fantasies—prefer *conceited* people to *really significant* or modest ones. [Elma's raptures always applied to those conceited people whom she recognized as such!] The explanation is, 1.) that *conceited* people play the role of the "great one" better than people who are really significant but self-critical, 2.) that it is easier to feel superior to a conceited person (the former factor is more important), 3.) that in such people she loved *herself* (the one who is conceited).

On the theme of the *ambivalence of majesty*[4]:

    1.) The expression "noblesse oblige."[5]

    2.) The story of a Spanish queen whose dress caught fire but who couldn't be saved because etiquette forbids touching the queen: *"Non tocar la reina"* [These are not the *exact* words.]

I now have a sensational case, significant enough to be a brother of "Little Hans."[6] A boy who is now five, *Bandi*, was bitten on his penis by a rooster when, at age 2 1/2, he urinated into a poultry cage (bleeding, pain, bandages). *Since this moment* the boy's entire psychic life revolves around chickens and roosters. He plays only with imaginary chickens, the necks of which he cuts off, or which he *kisses*. He was already speaking quite well, but after the incident he was only *crowing* and *clucking* for months, so that his parents were having serious fears that he had lost the ability to speak. He gradually began to talk again, of course, mostly about poultry; he imitates their voices fabulously and uses his musicality to sing songs to himself for hours which have to do with rooster, turkey, etc. His interest in chickens gradually extended to other birds, then also (but to a much lesser extent) to quadrupeds. He is a colossal sadist and masochist.—

The little one was often threatened with castration for masturbation. He calls his father a *rooster* and has condensed the figures of the father and the dangerous rooster.

    Kind regards,
    Ferenczi

1. Before the beginning of Elma's analysis with Freud.

2. Ferenczi's expression "ambitendency" was later used by Margaret Mahler—who became interested in psychoanalysis through Ferenczi—and, as with Ferenczi, (see letters 271 and 273) was used to designate a not yet internalized conflict. Margaret S. Mahler,

Fred Pine, and Anni Bergman, *The Psychological Birth of the Human Infant* (New York, 1975), pp. 94ff, 107f, 214, 217.

3. Enclosed in brackets in the original, as are other similar remarks by Ferenczi throughout the letter.

4. Freud was developing this theme for *Totem and Taboo* (1912–13a), especially in chap. 2b, "Taboo and Emotional Ambivalence: The Taboo upon Rulers."

5. The obligation associated with high rank or birth.

6. Ferenczi published this case, which had been reported to him by Frau Dezsö Kosztolányi while she was in analysis with him, under the title "Ein kleiner Hahnemann" [A Little Chanticleer] (1913, 114; *C.*, p. 240); Freud cited it in *Totem and Taboo* (1912–13a, pp. 130ff and 153; see letter 270).

269

Budapest, January 20, 1912
VII., Erzsébet-körút 54

Dear Professor,

The reports about Elma actually don't surprise me. I feel that I have seen, in part, *almost* everything that you tell me about her and have in part had vague intimations about it but (probably in order to be able to keep her with me) have not been able to admit it to myself clearly and analytically and didn't want to have her confess it to me. About what you call peccadillos, I have often posed direct questions to her without having received proper answers. She brought me, among other things, a dream in which that dentist embraces her and she acts as if she were shocked by it, even though she wasn't. The associations led from this fragment of a dream to the theme of feigned virginity, and in regard to that she came up with the association that she had read a lascivious novel by Willy,[1] in which a girl's first sexual intercourse with a man was described. *"Elle ne cria pas"* [she doesn't cry]—is written there, which she claims to have understood only later. In the same dream there were allusions to bleeding on defloration (red roses).—My therapeutic plan with Elma was such that I would counter her coquetry with polite refusal and in that way force her to come out with her true affects. In this stage of the treatment the misfortune occurred that the reins of my self-control fell out of my hands.

It doesn't actually surprise me *now* that Elma is not behaving like a bride. I know, of course, that by far the greatest part of her love for me was father transference, which easily takes another as an object. You will hardly be surprised that under these circumstances I, too, can hardly consider myself a bridegroom any longer.—I believe that Elma will profit greatly with you; it is truly fortunate for her that she could come to you; I hope along with you that she will overcome a portion of her infantilisms—among them also the fantasy of becoming my wife.—

That is how I see her future now. As far as I am concerned, the matter also doesn't look so desperate as one might have thought in the beginning. I will, of course, finally have to give up the family romance. Friend, lady friend, and science remain with me, and I must say that I seem to myself to be very rich in possessing these.

Strangely, the infantile curiosity to experience fatherly intimacies has subsided noticeably in me lately. The main thing that I was curious about was whether the father loves me. The great and heartfelt sharing that you brought to me in these difficult days seems to have calmed me down with respect to this.

For that reason I can now think and write about Jung entirely without brother envy. I suspect that he has—in addition to the money complex, which you emphasized—an unlimited and uncontrolled ambition, which manifests itself in petty hate and envy toward you, who are so superior to him. The case of Hirschfeld[2] is proof of that. His unsatisfied ambition makes him *dangerous* under certain conditions.

He is also not very tactful in choosing his methods; the manner in which he responded to you is very significant.

Even so, it would be a mistake for you to be too resentful of him on account of this *"gaminerie."*[3] The best solution would, of course, be a free discussion (with ψα. openness). For this it would also certainly be necessary to take Jung into psychoanalytic treatment from now on.

All in all, I think that some *caution* is indicated with respect to Jung. But in my opinion he doesn't deserve having the Fliessian *mistrust* transferred to him.

There is no alternative: you have to do everything yourself all your life. Your successor has not yet arrived; by that I mean that among us analysts there is still not a single one who, having completely mastered his personal weaknesses, particularly his egoism, could work for the cause and also has the necessary talent and endurance to do so.

This is small consolation for you, but what use is there in denying it!

I thank you for your letter once again and await a reply—but I don't want to force you to it.

Yours truly,
Ferenczi

Frau G. knows nothing about the content of your letter.

1. Willy, pseudonym of Henri Gauthier-Villars (1859–1931), author of numerous erotic novels and husband of Colette (1873–1954).
2. See letter 118, n. 4.
3. Mischievousness.

270

Dear friend,

Your rooster-man[1] is precious. I will probably ask you to give me the observation for the work on Totem or to publish it without reference to the Totem. Scientific handiwork has a need for little things like that.

It is my intention with Elma not to let myself be restrained by any danger of influencing her by the truth when I report to her, especially since I know that a decision will be possible for you only after the end of the treatment. We have accomplished little for the time spent up to now (two weeks). She still presents the mask of the poor child who accepts everything I tell her, but has no interest in it and therefore doesn't produce anything. But resistance is already clearly shimmering through. It says: Just get out of the treatment as soon as possible. One can also get married without having any clear feelings beforehand and still be happy. She takes as a precedent for that the example of her cousin here. But that could be the transference of the driving situation in her life up to now, flight from her father, on whom she is fixated, to all kinds of young people who have been selected in such a way that she can't marry them, so that she stays home again until her father renews the infantilely fantasized seduction. The affective and intellectual superstructure over this complex skeleton seems to be quite poor, although I won't be able to pass judgment until I get further.

The affair with Jung is as follows.[2] Two weeks ago I earnestly inquired about how he was when I learned about his injury[3] through Pfister. He didn't reply, and has written only once in the meantime about editorial matters, whereupon I responded matter-of-factly under the heading "business," as is customary with us. I am not writing spontaneously now, and I urgently request that you not intervene. It cannot be a matter of $\psi\alpha$ openness on my part, since he is silent and hasn't been giving honest information, and I am not inclined toward "treatment." You now see that his wife's letter to you at that time really did contain a projection of ill will toward me. What annoys me is that in my responses in letters to you [them][4] I again became very warm in foolish devotion and that I told him about all the results of my research on religion,[5] just as I did to you. He who has the stuff in him to be a sensitive ass never ceases making a fool of himself, even when he has gray hair. But I will not give rise to anything that indicates that I am taking offense; I will gladly forgive, only I can't keep my feelings unchanged. The $\psi\alpha$ habit of drawing important conclusions from small signs is also difficult to overcome. His ambition was familiar to me, but I was hoping, through the position that I had created and was still preparing for him, to force this power into my service. The prospect, as long as I live, of doing everything myself and then not leaving behind any sterling successor is not very consoling. So I admit to you that I am by no means cheerful and have a heavy burden to bear with this triviality.

Now I am leaning on you again, and I confidently hope that you will not disappoint me. But perhaps you are embarking on unhappy times.

Today I wrote a brief postscript to Gradiva for its second edition.[6] My sister-in-law is reading Jokes; it is likewise supposed to be published unaltered.[7] The next thing is an English essay on the "Unconscious"[8] for the Society for Psychical Research.[9] Unfortunately, I don't get home from work until 9 o'clock in the evening. An essay against my "Formulations"[10] which Bleuler sent me—his lecture in Weimar[11]—is not good and a decided relapse into the old ψ description. I could now easily settle the only objection that made an impression on me then. Your contribution on masturbation is not going to be read until tomorrow.[12] We have taken over a new place, with our earlier innkeeper, the Doktorenkollegium. I send kind regards in these dark days.

Yours,
Freud

1. Ernest Jones translated Ferenczi's description of this case, "Ein kleiner Hahnemann," into English as "A Little Chanticleer." A literal translation would be "A Little Rooster-Man," which suggests an analogy to the "Rat-Man" *(Rattenmann)* and the "Wolf-Man" *(Wolfsmann)* [Trans.].

2. Jung had written to Freud only occasionally for several weeks. He was working on the second part of "Wandlungen und Symbole der Libido" *(Jahrbuch* 4 [1912–13]: 162–464), which made the scientific break with Freud obvious.

3. Jung had been bitten by a dog.

4. The original reads "letters to you" *[Briefe an Sie]*. Ferenczi calls attention to this slip in letter 271.

5. See e.g., the letters of October 13, 1911 *(Freud/Jung*, pp. 448f), and December 17, 1911 (pp. 472f). On November 12, 1911, Freud himself had written about his ambivalence over telling Jung what was on his mind: "Why in God's name did I allow myself to follow you into this field?" (p. 459).

6. "Postscript to the Second Edition" *[Delusions and Dreams in Jensen's "Gradiva"* (1907a)] (Freud 1912k).

7. *Jokes and Their Relation to the Unconscious* (1905c); he refers here to the second edition (1912).

8. Written in English in the original.

9. "A Note on the Unconscious in Psycho-Analysis" (1912g), *Proceedings of the Society for Psychical Research*, Supplement, 26 (1912): 312–318. Published in German in the translation by Hanns Sachs in *Zeitschrift* 1 (1913): 117–123.

10. Freud 1911b.

11. Eugen Bleuler, "Zur Theorie des Autismus," lecture delivered at the Third International Psychoanalystic Congress, in Weimar, September 21–22, 1911; presumably identical with "Das autistische Denken," *Jahrbuch* 4 (1912–13): 1–39.

12. At the fourth discussion on masturbation at the Vienna Society, January 24, 1912 (*Minutes* IV, 20f); see also letter 272.

271

Budapest, January 27, 1912
VII., Erzsébet-körút 54

Dear Professor,

For a ψ. understanding of Jung's attitude one must perhaps also take into account the reaction that could have been elicited by the somewhat disparaging remarks that you made in the Vienna Society about Jung's paper on libido and which Fräulein Spielrein[1] may have told Jung about.—Otherwise I have no other ideas about this subject now.

The way I feel, I will fulfill the expectation that I won't disappoint you—provided that you don't raise your expectations too high. As far as my relation to you as a person and to ΨA is concerned, I am sure of myself. Unfortunately, I am also conscious of the fact that my powers as well as my personal and social position do not make it possible for me, as a worthy successor, to continue the work which you have begun, at least not to the extent that I could be the "sterling successor." (You also don't expect that of me!) I certainly hope that, with increasing inner freedom and under favorable external conditions, I will be able to contribute something to the advancement of our common cause.

I think that you will also remain true to your principle "Αναγκη"[2] in the matter of your successor and—if necessary—resign. A significant intellectual movement such as this is often interrupted by a temporary setback. What you have accomplished up to now and what we still expect from you can, however, no longer be suppressed—even without a direct successor. In a fairly large city such as Budapest one has a greater opportunity to observe how society becomes saturated with new ideas. These ideas pave the way for themselves by means of their own specific gravity—it is sufficient for them to be expressed *once* in a generally comprehensible way.

In order that you may see that I have learned from you the art of concluding greater things from small signs, I will cite a passage from your last letter. You write to *me* about Frau *Jung:* "What annoys me is that in my responses in letters to *you*[3](!!) I again became very warm in foolish devotion."

I am also sorry that you shared the themata about the psychology of religion with Jung. It's possible that part of his resistance is rooted in envy over this discovery of yours.

II.   January 31

Strong swings of feeling have kept me until today from consolidating my thoughts by letter about the case of Elma. Your letter today brought with it a certain relief from these tensions. The role that you play in this important matter in my life makes it necessary for me to raise honesty to a peak and to tell you things about myself which you would perhaps rather be spared knowledge of.

I mean my relations to Frau G. When I almost gave up Elma for lost (and *this* prospect has also not disappeared completely)—my efforts were directed at ensuring Frau G. for myself in the future, in order to avoid the unbearable isolation that is normally my lot. She wanted to remain completely on the ground of the sublimated—but I (in order to flee Elma) pressed for a resumption of the old relations. It did *not go well.* It was becoming more and more apparent that I haven't entirely given Elma up and that at least a part of my sexual desires were not genuine. My attempt at intimacy ended with sadness and depression on both sides. (What is scientifically interesting in this is the fact that twice, *after consumption of alcohol,* my actual impoverishment of feeling became conscious: sure proof of my supposition that untrue expressions of feeling (dementia praecox)[4] disappear under the influence of alcohol. One ought to treat excited dementia patients with alcohol.)

Frau G. is behaving with nobility, kindness, and generosity. I am inexhaustibly in cs. awareness of her good qualities; her love for me is inexhaustible—even though she knows everything that is going on within me. If the matter with Elma doesn't work out (which I still consider to be much more probable, since I don't want to get into a risky undertaking), then I will find in her a support for the rest of my life and will always be able to count on her for understanding and love.—I also think that when the prospect of Elma is extinguished in me *once and for all,* a reawakening of the old, irrepressible intimacy with respect to Frau G. will also be possible.

But I will not conceal the fact that I am totally dominated by the reports that you give me about Elma, that, for instance, your letter of today, which sounds more favorable, has pleased me very much.

Pardon me if I burden you so much with my cares and anxieties.—

I recently began a paper on "Transitory Symptom Constructions during Analysis" (transitory conversions, obsessions, projections, "hallucinations," etc.) with many examples. That is also something semitechnical; at your request I want to finish the paper more quickly.[5]

I am sending you enclosed the "Rooster-Man," which I ask you to use as you see fit. I would be very pleased if you can use it for the paper on taboo.

I find it excellent and correct that taboo-totem is an expression of ambivalence (more precisely of ambi*tendency* [*Ambitendenz*]).

But what is the ultimate source of ambitendency itself?

I think it is the conflict between the *ego instincts* and *sexuality,* which, despite their opposition, still exist *side by side* in more primitive stages and in neurosis, while *repression* and *compromise formation* ordinarily remove the conflicts.

Thankfully yours,
Ferenczi

Postscript

Dear Professor,

I had my letter of today, along with the enclosure (seven written half-sheet pages), mailed by a servant. In the afternoon the post office telephoned that a letter with my printed address without an envelope had been found among the packages. Thereupon I sent an envelope addressed to you to the post office and had the letter sent to you by registered mail. There is no report of the enclosure (which contains the description of the Rooster-Man). In the event that the enclosure has been lost, you will soon receive a copy of it.

Kind regards,
Dr. Ferenczi

1. Sabina Spielrein (1885–1941) was born in Russia. Beginning in 1905 she studied medicine in Zurich, and became a member of the Vienna Society on October 11, 1911. From 1912 on she lived in Berlin, Munich, Lausanne, Châteaux d'Oex, and Geneva, where Jean Piaget was in analysis with her for eight months in 1921. In 1923 she returned to the Soviet Union and became a member of the Society there. In 1941 she was murdered by the Nazis, along with her two daughters. She anticipated Freud's concept of the death instinct in her essay "Die Destruktion als Ursache des Werdens" [Destruction as the Cause of Coming in to Being], *Jahrbuch* 4 (1912): 465–503. From 1904 until 1909 Spielrein was in treatment with Jung for what was diagnosed as "psychotic hysteria"; their relationship led to a love affair, about which Freud was informed. See Aldo Carotenuto, ed., *A Secret Symmetry: Sabina Spielrein between Jung and Freud* (New York, 1982).
2. See letter 141 and n. 3.
3. Underlined three times in the manuscript. See letter 270, n. 4.
4. Enclosed in parentheses in the original.
5. S. Ferenczi, "Über passagère Symptombildungen während der Analyse; Passagère Konversion, Substitution, Illusion, Halluzination, 'Charakterregression' und 'Ausdrucksverschiebungen'" [On Transitory Symptom Constructions during the Analysis] (1912, 85; *C.*, p. 193).

272

Vienna, January 28, 1912
IX., Berggasse 19

Dear friend,

I am writing to you again because I can imagine your lively interest in a piece of my work. The analysis is going forward in a lively manner, and the masks are gradually falling away. The jealousy toward the favored sister with death wishes toward her is being woven into the context, and the associations are less forced. I will report to you again when there is something decisive.

Jung has finally written and apologized for the fact that he is presently incapable of expending his "libido" by stating that his work on libido is taking up too much of his time. I responded just as briefly on the factual content and the business of editing, and so things are now leveling off without the further clouding of an interruption of the correspondence. I also have things to do and now know how to maintain what is valuable to me.

Today I completed the seventh (!) treatise of this season, the essay on the "Unconscious" for the Society for Psychical Research.[1] I wrote it in English; it was not easy. Now I can again dedicate myself to my savages in order to trace taboo to ambivalence.

It would appear quite useful to me if you wanted to utilize your present emptiness of feeling to write an article on technique for the Zentralblatt. I have to break off after two of those,[2] and I don't want to see technique in Stekel's hands.

Rank's paper, for which he has used the Hungarian dream drawings,[3] has again turned out very good. Your contribution on masturbation was read aloud on Wednesday, and most were very much in agreement with it, as was I; Stekel objected to it strenuously.

Yesterday Martin was finally officially declared an invalid, and he is rejoicing.[4]

I greet you and Frau Gisela cordially.

Yours,
Freud

1. See letter 270 and n. 9.

2. "The Dynamics of Transference" (1912b) and "Recommendations to Physicians Practising Psycho-Analysis" (1912e).

3. Otto Rank, "Die Symbolschichtung im Wecktraum, und ihre Wiederkehr im mythischen Denken," *Jahrbuch* 4 (1912–13): 51–115. The drawings of dreams (see letters 215 and 216) are reproduced and discussed (pp. 98–101).

4. Martin was declared unfit for military service after his skiing accident (see letter 195 and n. 4).

273

Budapest,
[undated, presumably
beginning of 1912][1]
VII., Erzsébet-körút 54

Dear Professor!

Among some old notes I found the following little write-up about an interesting case of ambitendency in a 2 1/2-year-old boy.

The little boy had the remarkable habit of continuing to do things that were forbidden him, but always adding: "One is not allowed!" [*Man darf nicht*] (e.g., He puts something dirty into his mouth and says: "One is not allowed." ("*Nem szabad!*")[2]) etc.

The analogy with manifest ambitendency in savages is striking.

Kind regards.

Yours,
Ferenczi

1. The letter gives no clear indication of chronology; Balint suggests placing the letter here.
2. Enclosed in parentheses in the original.

274

Vienna, January 31, 1912[1]

Everything arrived. Many thanks.

Yours,
Freud

1. Postcard.

275

Vienna, February 1, 1912
IX., Berggasse 19

Dear friend,

I have not received a letter for a long time in which the truths have pressed as much as they have in your last. Fortunately, they are not a lot of sad ones.

So, first your Rooster-Man. It is simply exquisite and will have a great future. But I hope you will not believe that I simply want to confiscate him for myself; that would be too low (of me). Only, you shouldn't publish it until I can come out with the return of totemism in childhood so that I can refer to it there. You will I hope still fill the gap about whether the threat of castration occurred *before* or *after* the adventure.[1] It is very significant. I have had similarly audacious thoughts about castration as you have. We would certainly like to know whether the jealous little father-man of the Darwinian primal family really castrated the boys before he contented himself with chasing them away.[2]

Your plan of work seems to me to be very practicable, and I hope to see its execution follow soon.

What you report to me about the changes in your relationship with Frau G. was not surprising at all. I had presumed that it would go first one way and then the other. There is nothing to be ashamed of in that, even though it is not right. With Elma, something is, in fact, happening. We are getting further, are succeeding in penetrating and breaking through the father identification, which, in the form of prudery, was the main obstacle to the work and also constitutes a large portion of the manifest narcissism. Today I was able to observe the first sign of her ability to take part in independent thinking, with an excellent insight right away. If we succeed further and she gives up her infantilism (that is, after all, the only legitimate diagnosis), then a new situation will arise that in no way has to be connected with the old. You will also have to decide anew and to reckon with an additional factor. I do not have a high opinion of her love for you up to now; I don't know whether it will stand up to analysis.

What you write to me about Jung and the questions about the future did not fail to have an effect on me. But it contains enough that is flattering to recommend it to logic. Nothing has actually happened. If, after the suspension of our correspondence which he has decreed, he again begins to write, then everything will be on track. But it is different with me. I am trying to reconcile myself to the idea that one also has to leave this child to Ἀνάγκη,[3] and I will draw a piece of exposed libido back to myself and cease strenuous efforts to move forward. What I can still effect will take place without any personal consideration. Our common interest will see to it that we stay together, even without developing intimate relations of feeling. There is no rancor in me. An enlargement of my ego is certainly always painful to me; I bear it as badly as I do satisfying my ambition (*vide* New York). Must *I*[4] really always be right, always be the better one? In the long run it becomes downright improbable to one.

It has not escaped you that my mistrust is revealing itself anew in this at the moment when I am trying to compensate myself with a new arrangement.

The question of taboo ambivalence suddenly came together a few days ago, almost snapped in with an audible "click," and since then I am practically giddy. My interest has been extinguished for the moment, and I have to wait until it gathers itself together again. I still have left hanging the last ψ formulation of the relationship. Another conception that seems more attractive to me is struggling with the one that you present (again the conflict of the two instincts). It is not yet quite ripe for articulation.[5]

I already sent off an article about the unconscious to the Society for Psychical Research. You will receive the January issue of the Zentralblatt right away; mine arrived today.

A storm is now raging against ΨA in the Zurich newspapers.[6] (Didn't I already write to you about it?) I know about it only by coincidence; Sadger got the issues from a patient. Maeder informed me yesterday that they intend to put out a public statement defending it. My name is not being mentioned in Vienna as a matter of principle despite various opportunities to do so lately (Appel's dream play based on Berger's novella),[7] and that is much more pleasant for me.

Kind regards in anticipation of your report.

Yours,
Freud

1. Ferenczi did not succeed in establishing the chronology. See his discussion of this point in "Ein kleiner Hahnemann" [A Little Chanticleer] (1913, 114; C., p. 243; *Schriften* I, 166).

2. See *Totem and Taboo* (1912–13a, 125f).

3. See letter 141 and n. 3.

4. It is unclear whether this word is underlined in the original.

5. In *Totem and Taboo* Freud writes that we know "nothing of the origin of this ambivalence" and that it could be "a fundamental phenomenon of our emotional life" or "acquired by the human race in connection with their father complex" (1912–13a, p. 157).

6. See *Freud/Jung*, January 23, 1912, p. 482, and Ellenberger, *Unconscious*, pp. 811ff.

7. Presumably Wilhelm Appel (1875–1911), whose drama "Hans Sonnenstössers Höllenfahrt" (1911), which was performed in 1912 in the Vienna Volkstheater, is considered to be the first "dream play" [*Traumspiel*]. Alfred Freiherr von Berger (1853–1912) was a writer and professor of aesthetics at the University of Vienna and, from 1910, director of the Burgtheater. In 1896 he had published a positive review of *Studies on Hysteria* (Freud and Breuer 1895d). His novella was titled *Hofrat Eysenhardt* (Vienna, n.d.).

276

Budapest, February 7, 1912
VII., Erzsébet-körút 54

Dear Professor,

Actually, I didn't want to reply to you until tomorrow or the day after, but a telegram announcing the sudden catastrophic worsening of my brother's condition forces me to hurry, since I will probably have to leave tomorrow or the day after. I am still on the fence as to whether I shouldn't yet go to Miskolcz today in order to support my mother in the difficult hour of the final farewell.

———————

Your reports about Elma always evince in me the appropriate reactions, not least your remark that you do not have a very high opinion of her love for me. I knew that, of course, and have written to you about that a few times—but I don't seem to have believed it entirely, otherwise your communication wouldn't have depressed me. In spite of all that I still can't make a final decision and have to postpone making one.

What strikes me in Elma's letters is the aggressive tone in which she has been writing about her uncle Ludwig (whose guest she is);[1] she also didn't like this uncle very much before—presumably because he cared about her too little. I thought I should call your attention to that.

A small extract from the picture of my personal condition: I am not sleeping very well now and don't feel rested in the morning.—Last evening Frau G. (who usually has an almost unbelievable capacity to understand and to forgive) was somewhat cold and distant to me, which hurt me.—But the following night I slept better than I have in a long time. Evidently I don't feel well when a punishment that I deserve is being withheld!

———————

I fear that—in ceasing your "strenuous efforts to move your libido forward" you will easily go to the other extreme and could also punish innocent parties with your mistrust. Naturally, I am thinking of myself first.—Otherwise, I have to concede that you are right, inasmuch as I, too, am of the opinion that the interest in ΨA should be strong enough to ensure keeping its representatives together even without personal intimacy.

———————

I hope soon to be able to fill the gaps in the life history of little Árpád.[2]

———————

Your paper on transference[3] is *uncommonly* instructive (only a very few will understand it). Your statement about suggestion and analysis[4] will be used against us by our opponents. "So, suggestion, after all"—they will say, and they will think that one can then very well stay with the old procedures.—

A storm like the one in Zurich was about to break out here on the occasion of a suicide whose victim was erroneously said to have been my patient.[5] I used this to my advantage with an energetic excursion against attacks of this sort. But I don't have any illusion that that will be of much use for the future.

I get very annoyed when I read *Scheler's* essay on "Resentment" in the "Zeitschrift für Pathopsychologie."[6] To be sure, he says in one place that he has the *expression* repression from you, but he acts as if *he* himself were the discoverer of the process, and neglects to name you when he talks about "displacement," "tearing away of affect from its object," and the like. I would very much like to reproach him for that in the Zentralblatt. Scheler will probably feel obliged, on account of his name, to be a *Scheeler*.[7] (Hence his predilection for the theme of "resentment.")—Messrs. the pathopsychologists are proving to be very active in the field of intellectual theft in other ways as well. The whole of "pathopsychology" is now nothing but psychoanalysis sailing under the wrong flag. Whatever else they come up with is insipid and sterile.

A young colleague who was in Berlin was telling me (a point of light in an otherwise cloudy sky) that the clinician *Kraus* last semester dedicated two entire lectures to analysis and came out in favor of it in the most enthusiastic way.

I have just received the news that my brother is now doing less badly and that he may stay alive a few more days.

Kind regards,
Ferenczi

1. Probably a brother of Géza Pálos, Elma's father.
2. The pseudonym chosen for the "Little Chanticleer" (Ferenczi 1913, 114; *C.*, p. 240).
3. "The Dynamics of Transference" (Freud 1912b).
4. Freud "readily admit[ted] that the results of psychoanalysis rest upon suggestion; by suggestion, however, we must understand, as Ferenczi (1909) does, the influencing of a person by means of the transference phenomena which are possible in his case" (1912b, p. 106).
5. Evidently the suicide of Mor Magyar, a Budapest businessman; see *Budapesti Napló*, January 12, 1912.
6. Max Scheler, "Über Ressentiment und Moralisches Werturteil," *Zeitschrift für*

Pathopsychologie, nos. 2–3 (1912). Scheler (1874–1928) was a German philosopher who applied the phenomenological method to the study of values. From 1901 he was docent in philosophy at Jena and from 1906 at Munich; then from 1918 he was a professor at Cologne and from 1928 at Frankfurt. He was co-editor of the *Jahrbuch für Philosophie und Phänomenologische Forschung.* Among German philosophers of the time it was Scheler who most often took issue with psychoanalysis.

7. "One who looks askance" [Trans.].

277

Budapest,
February 9, [1912,] at night.
VII., Erzsébet-körút 54

Dear Professor,

I just received news of my brother's passing.

I will leave tomorrow (Saturday) morning for Miskolcz and will probably return on Monday.

Kind regards,
Ferenczi

278

Vienna, February 13, 1912
IX., Berggasse 19

Dear friend,

I think you have overcome the painful impression against which our human logic always shows itself to be so frail, and you are now again ready to hear about our common interests.

So, with Elma I am moving decidedly forward, and, after mighty struggles with her father's prudery, I recognize in her the familiar human and feminine characteristics. Just now she emphasized her love for you, but I maintain that everything must first pass through the crucible of the treatment, and she is agreeable to that. Just today we came upon important things, the outcome of which could become decisive for success. I am gradually getting used to the idea that you could take your summer trip with her instead of with me, although, if it comes to that, you certainly won't have *me* to thank for it. On the contrary, I will put as many difficulties in her way as possible.

You will recollect that I traced her father fixation to his efforts to break her of the habit of wetting her bed. Now, a few days ago she brought me the fantasy about Brunhild[1] in connection with a dream. That goes along with it.

With regard to your indecision, I would like to note that masochistic impulses very frequently take their course in an unfavorable marital choice. One then gets one's misfortune, is punished by God, and doesn't have to worry anymore. Note that in saying this I am in no way taking sides against Elma. It suffices that you consider her so in order to have one more masochistic motive in your motivational equation.

If you want to review Scheeler,[2] I ask you only to inform Stekel of your intent. The March issue will again be very good, February less so. "Imago" is almost set. I am working on Taboo, which gives me much pleasure, and on the second editions of "Jokes" and "Gradiva."[3]

Jung was kind enough to write the day before yesterday; no sign of conflict; nothing has changed with me.

I am supposed to express to you the heartfelt condolences of our entire family and am pressing your hand in my own thoughts.

Yours,
Freud

P.S. There is a chance that I will be in Györ[4] on Thursday. If so, I will send a telegram in any case.

1. Brunhild, Queen of Iceland, a heroic maiden endowed with superhuman strength and daring, wanted only to marry a man who could vanquish her in battle and in bed. Since her suitor Gunther, King of Worms, was too weak for the task, his friend Siegfried slipped into his role, but could accomplish the task only with the aid of a magic hat, which made him invisible and invested him with sevenfold powers. The intrigue of the two men was later uncovered, and Brunhild had Siegfried killed by Hagen.

2. Spelled this way in the original.

3. Freud 1905c and 1907a. The second edition of each was published in 1912.

4. A city on the Danube, about halfway between Vienna and Budapest.

279

Budapest, February 18, 1912
VII., Erzsébet-körút 54

Dear Professor,

I have so completely abreacted the mourning for my brother during the course of his illness, which was replete with dashed hopes, that his death and burial could arouse only emotion in me, but no despair or deeper mental anguish. I can therefore accept the expression of sympathy that you and your family conveyed to me only in regard to the pain that I have endured for his sake in years gone by. Please thank them in my name for their concern.

The matter with me is now as follows: I have not repeated the failed attempts to restore the old relationship with Frau G. I visit her every day now and talk to her about scientific things, about Elma and her condition, etc.—but I resist the temptation to want to console her with tendernesses. She is noble, good, and kind, as always. Since she noticed that she can't satisfy my libido with all her devotion, her earlier despair has abated and been replaced by a more melancholy, gentler sadness—but she has evidently also been injured in her femininity by my attitude, and she has withdrawn a large piece of libido from me. Her motto is she "wants no alms." When I am with her and observe her incomparable spiritual qualities, it now seems impossible to me that I could not totally and completely love this exceptional woman, the best and noblest whom I have ever known. And yet circumstances speak in favor of this. Since I initiated the frantic exertions to restore our old relations, I have been feeling physically better. I sleep better, and I can work again. (I finished writing the paper on "transitory symptom construction during analysis.")[1]

I have absolutely no idea what I will do with my regained freedom. I can't say anything definite about my intentions with Elma. But I also feel freer with respect to her, and I am *now* much more accessible to sage advice than I was then, when I was dominated by attempts at liberation in addition to Elma's attraction. I also haven't given up for lost *the* possibility that, once I have totally given Elma up, I will be satisfied with a less intense, *more intellectual* association with Frau G.

If you have no objection I will go to Vienna next Sunday to discuss this and other matters with you; Elma must know nothing about my presence in Vienna—by the way, I will leave that for you to gauge.

I will be pleased to hear about the progress of the taboo theory; my interest in ΨA has now totally and completely returned, and a number of quite usable topics for papers are in process in me.

Elma wrote me two letters. I consider it appropriate to translate some passages from the first letter (received today) for you.—

You are right about masochism as one of the driving forces of an unfavorable choice in marriage to the extent that *I* consider this marriage choice unfavorable—especially in comparison with Frau G.'s qualities. (The *fear* that Elma will be unfaithful to me if she feels herself injured or disappointed by me—could also contain masochistic elements.)

But now—as I said—I feel strong enough to vanquish irrational tendencies in me; I must therefore ask you also to share your objective views with me in the future, openly and without reservation.—

To reiterate: the wish to see Elma again, to be with her, rarely emerges in me (consciously), and when it does, it is not very intense. The disap-

pointment that she had in store for me may play a part in that.—Certainly
I don't feel sexually aroused by anything else, and I don't know if it would
be different with me if Elma were normal and healthy and I didn't doubt
her ability to love.

Forgive me if today I don't write about anything more important than
my personal affairs. I am conscious of the fact that I am troubling you with
matters that I should actually take care of myself. But—you know!—I am
still the son—albeit one who is involved in painful struggles for his independence.

Kind regards,
Ferenczi

From Elma's letter of today:
"I know that you wish only the best for me . . . and would gladly give
me the tenderness I need"—[She inserts parenthetically here that she erroneously wanted to write "weakness" here in place of the word "tenderness," which is formed in Hungarian from the stem "weak." (From that I
conclude that it matters to her mainly to see me as weak and to triumph
over me.)][2]

————————

"I fear that I will never learn to bear sacrifice and deprivation without
bitterness." (*That* prospect is certainly not enticing.)

————————

After she praised you and analysis, she says that she hopes the analysis
won't examine the deepest layers in her, which is due to the weakness of
her intellectual abilities.

————————

She then writes (as if she wanted to condemn you) that you don't tell her
any more about analysis than is necessary to explain *her* case. I think that
behind this is the wish to be treated by you as she once was by me. At the
same time, fantasies of being equal to you (wish to be a man, a scholar).

"I learn about the science of analysis only things that have to do with
me; however interesting that may be—new perspectives aren't opened up
by it."

"It appears to me as if we are going around in circles and are not making any progress now."

"I am not talking out of dissatisfaction; I only want to talk truthfully about my feelings."

"Many sensations in me have certainly not yet been explained, *and I also don't have the courage necessary for the truth.*" (Evidently she is still withholding some of her associations.)

"I am no longer 'ill'—but I am still living much too much in fantasies and exaggerations, so I can't go home."

In conclusion: "I kiss you and Mama with much love," and the remark: "With this last sentence I had to think for a long time how one writes it correctly in Hungarian." (Certainly her doubt about the reality of these "many loves" is being expressed in this grammatical uncertainty.)

----

1. Ferenczi 1912, 85; *C.*, p. 193; see letter 271 and n. 5.
2. Enclosed in brackets in the original.

280

Vienna, February 20, 1912
IX., Berggasse 19

Dear friend,

So, come by all means. This time it will also fulfill a need in me. I am right in the middle of a section of the paper on taboo and can present to you about half of it as finished. *I* will tell Elma nothing about your trip; otherwise you would have to go to her. I am not sure about the outcome with her. After the last attempt we came to the main resistance, her desire for revenge (transferred from her father), and it has been hard going ever since. Today I was tough, and she went away with a very angry expression on her face. I knew about the letter to you. It is entirely dictated by the same desire for revenge, over which a thick veil is naturally still lying, as is the case with everything that comes up. I am making an effort to tear it.

I will refrain from writing about the various novelties in science, since I will be speaking to you in a few days.

I have the impression that the cause is progressing inexorably. In the last few days I delivered the second editions of Jokes and Gradiva,[1] and now it's the fourth of Everyday Life's[2] turn.

Jung has written without guile for the second time. So there won't be any storm there. In my last reply I let him hear some distant rumbling. Pfister confesses that he has found a girl, for whose sake it is worthwhile for him to seek a divorce.[3]

I am being tormented by a miserable cold. Everything is well at home. I await news from you before your arrival.

Kind regards,
Freud

"Imago" is enclosed.

1. See letter 278, n. 3.
2. That is, the fourth edition of Freud 1901b (Berlin, 1912).
3. Pfister had notified Freud in October of the previous year that he wanted to get a divorce, whereupon Freud had "strongly urged him to go through with it" (Freud/Jung, October 12, 1911, p. 448). Pfister, however, remained married to his wife, Erika, née Wunderli, until her death in 1929, and then he married his widowed cousin Martha Zuppinger-Urner.

281

Budapest, February 29, 1912
VII., Erzsébet-körút 54

Dear Professor,

After a number of people declared the manuscript of my article on transitory symptoms to be readable, I have decided to send it in its original form and spare myself the displeasure that I would have had in writing out a fair copy.

Rarely has a visit with you given me such undisturbed intellectual and emotional satisfaction as the one last Sunday. The fault on some other occasions (Palermo!)[1] lay not in you, of course, but in me. For some time, however, I have been feeling so absolutely free of inhibitions and resistances of any kind with respect to you that I can direct my interest unreservedly to our common intellectual and personal affairs. The striking and beautiful solution to the question of *taboo* (fear of temptation)[2] has naturally made the greatest impression on me. The question of the differentiation of symbol, reaction, and substitutive formation still concerns me as well.—

This trip was significant for me personally, inasmuch as my doubts about the solution to the affairs of marriage have been laid to rest. What from now on speaks against marrying Elma, outside of the logical reasons, is also my inner voice, so from now on I am also *affectively* convinced that this plan should be dropped.

The editorial section of the enclosed newspaper[3] (one of the most respected in Budapest) talks about you in dithyrambic phrases on the occasion of the publication of the Five Lectures in Hungarian; it talks about me as well. The beautiful Frau Dr. Stricker[4] (who once looked you up in Vienna) is going to give the teachers a lecture on Ostwald, Payat (?),[5] and you. In so doing, she is advertising her private school, in which teaching is being done according to your principles, and at the same time nudism and love of art are being advanced.

I read the galleys of "Imago" with pleasure. Robitsek's article about Kekulé[6] was very interesting.

Kind regards,
Ferenczi

1. The incident on their trip together; see letter 169, n. 3.
2. See *Totem and Taboo*, according to which "the basis of taboo is a prohibited action for performing which a strong inclination exists in the unconscious," and "the magical power that is attributed to taboo is based on the capacity for arousing temptation" (Freud 1912–13a, pp. 32, 35).
3. The identity of the enclosure cannot be established.
4. See letter 169, n. 10.
5. This reference cannot be identified.
6. Alfred Robitsek, "Symbolisches Denken in der chemischen Forschung," *Imago* 1 (1912): 83–90; cited by Ferenczi in his "Kritik der Jungschen 'Wandlungen und Symbole der Libido'" (1913, 124; *Bausteine* I, 250). Robitsek, (1871–1937), who had studied with the chemist Friedrich August Kekulé (1829–1896), interpreted in this essay the dreams or fantasies through which Kekulé discovered the tetravalence of carbon and the ring structure of benzene, which made him famous.

282

Vienna, March 3, 1912
IX., Berggasse 19

Dear friend,

Thanks for your paper. It was immediately conveyed to Stekel together with my Recommendations,[1] which have been completed in the meantime. Your feelings during last Sunday correspond to mine. So we have finally met on equal terms. The strange spring weather makes one think that it will be Easter Sunday in five weeks. Perhaps we will make the project of the brief Easter trip a reality. In his last letter Jung hinted that I must be angry with him, whereupon in my reply I came out of my reserve somewhat and scolded him.[2] It does seem to me that he is rather neglectful of the interests of the Association. It is impossible to get a Korrespondenzblatt from the Central Office. The January issue is the only one to come out in the last six months. The groups learn nothing about one another and so become more and more isolated. He is not participating at all in the Zentralblatt and in Imago. Up to now the Jahrbuch has been delayed by 3/4 of a year.

On no account will it be a matter of indifference to you to hear that Elma has taken a great leap forward. Tracing back her compulsive attitude toward being disappointed by her father, her identification with him since, her desire for revenge, her striving to do to others what she has suffered through him, all that has been recognized by her with conviction. Since then she has been speaking and also behaving differently. Now there still remains the origin of the surface current [*Oberströmung*], which has mobilized repression without accomplishing anything proper itself. This probably originated during puberty and is connected with the image of her mother; it is genuinely feminine. The scheme would go something like this:

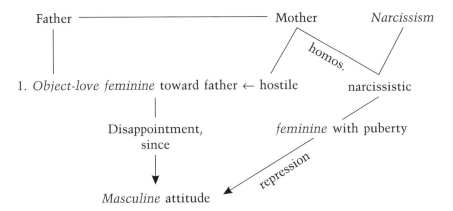

We will come back to this.

Kind regards,
Freud

1. "Recommendations to Physicians Practising Psycho-Analysis" (Freud 1912e).
2. Jung had assumed that Freud was angry at him because of his laziness. Freud had
replied that he had, to be sure, "awaited [Jung's] letters with great impatience and answered them promptly," but that he had "quickly turned off" his "excess libido." Furthermore, he had made the criticism "that the organization is not functioning properly"
(*Freud/Jung*, February 29, 1912, p. 488).

283

Vienna, March 8, 1912
IX., Berggasse 19

Dear friend,

I am sending you the enclosed letter in an—official capacity. I will write
to the author that he should visit you. You will deal with him as you see
fit.[1] There was something crazy in the way in which it was sent—express.

Is it all right with you if I already inquire at Brioni whether we can find
accommodations there over Easter?

Cordially,
Freud

1. See the postscript to letter 284.

284

Budapest, March 8, 1912
VII., Erzsébet-körút 54

Dear Professor,

I must once again write about myself, so that, after settling the personal
matters, I can then uninhibitedly talk about other things.

The Sunday that I spent with you was a turning point for me. (The many
corrections in this sentence, however, prove the uncertainty about it that
still prevails in me.) The fact is that the experiences that came about
through Elma's analysis significantly diminished her value in my eyes, and
that my eyes have again focused on the qualities of Frau G. (from whom I
have turned away up to now with a kind of defiant decisiveness) in such a
way that the comparison must now again doubtless turn in Frau G.'s favor.
At the same time I have been freed from the almost complete inhibition
that has dominated my sexual life for months, and the status quo ante

(being attracted by Frau G.—but also by other females) seems once again to have been restored.

Then came your letter with more favorable news about Elma.—This, too, changed nothing in my ψ. attitude depicted here. Still, it prompted a certain unrest in me that I have to interpret in such a way that inwardly (without being in love with Elma) I have still not given up the idea of founding a family. This is, nevertheless, something different from the energetic, passionate manner in which I wanted to realize the marriage in January. So with me it is now evidently a matter of passing up, not without compelling need, the (obviously last) opportunity to become a father. This theoretical requirement is, however, no longer so intimately bound up with Elma's person that I could not renounce it this time. My first thought on reading your letter was the question of whether your view about Elma's value for me has not changed in the course of the last few days. To be sure, mature reflection made this assumption improbable, since I had to consider that, at best, the treatment would restore her ability to exist but cannot significantly improve her ability to achieve. Still, I seem to yearn to be enlightened by you in this respect so that my abandoning this plan will be less painful.

A dream that I just had in this conflictual mood showed me that I (stimulated by the plan of our Easter trip) would like to flee *both* women by leaning on you and science. But that is certainly only a product of the momentary compulsive situation; I know, of course, that I cannot exist without the favor of a woman.

In the course of the last few months I was actually in Frau G.'s company more often than ever and had the opportunity to actually get to know the magnitude of her soul and her ability to sacrifice, her nobility and her simple, natural love; her exceptional talent of being able to participate in my scientific efforts is also making a big impression on me again.—You were right when, on my first trip to Vienna where I revealed to you my intention to marry, you called attention to the fact that you noticed the same defiant expression I had on my face when I refused to work with you in Palermo.

In the event that I finally break the "engagement" to Elma, I must also naturally take care and manage this refusal in such a way as to cause her as little pain as possible.—I promised her at the time that we would "get to know" each other again after the treatment; but I think it would be more instrumental if she went away from here for a time (perhaps to one of her aunts in Italy). Of course, I have to make my intentions known to her beforehand.

I am very much looking forward to the Easter trip. *Dalmatia* or an *Adriatic island*, perhaps *Venice* would come into consideration. Which days during the month of April would you be free for that? I have to know that even earlier so that I can postpone until the proper time two lectures that have been scheduled for after Easter.[1] I would like to call the condition that is now prevalent in Budapest "analytic fever." Lay circles are talking— and physicians are cursing about nothing else.—A young assistant, Moravcsik's,[2] came to me with an analytical work about Maeterlinck's "Oiseau bleu,"[3] which I haven't read yet, however. Perhaps I will give a course for physicians during the second semester (after Easter). The assistants at the clinic are very eager to learn something, but their boss doesn't let them work. he says that ΨA is not a science *yet*; physicians should rather concern themselves with more serious things, for instance, he gave one of them the task of making optometric investigations on paralyzed people. (The first case of paralysis whom he examined and then asked what he saw in the optometer answered: "The little Jesus." I don't know what Moravcsik will do with this optometric task.)

Enclosed I am sending you a totally unbelievable confirmation of your work on Leonardo.[4] I ask you to return the notice to me next time, which I am unfortunately not permitted to use.

Yesterday I was again in the circle of high school teachers,[5] some of whom are going along very enthusiastically. Unfortunately they are very conceited, don't want to learn, but rather know better immediately and want to found great philosophical systems. One, for instance, wants to reduce analysis to mathematical formulas. One despairs at how rare it is to find a person with honest scientific intentions and scientific modesty. By the same token, there are a whole lot of "talents," who, because of their deficiencies, never amount to anything, however.

Next week I will send you the work on money and coprophilia, with a brief postscript on symbolism for Imago.[6]

Please call to Rank's attention the fact that, if a medical student (Hárnik)[7] sends him papers, a certain censorship might perhaps not be inappropriate. [Hárnik is a very diligent, terribly ambitious, but untalented person; he is psychosexually impotent, which he would like to overcompensate for. Of course, that will remain between us.][8] N.B.: I am treating him somewhat gruffly in order to discourage him from becoming an analyst; but he is stubbornly holding out.

Kind regards,
Ferenczi

Over![9]

A kind of compulsion for completeness causes me to expand my communications about myself. (I seem to place uncommon value on your being well informed and basing your opinion on correct data.) I want to add that the depressive impressions of the latest events are also becoming apparent in Frau G. and that she has up to now not been able to repair the damage without loss. But I don't believe that our relations—reduced to friendship and scientific interests, for the time being—cannot be restored.

Just received your letter with the enclosure; I will have to turn down the maker of the request—he is unsuitable. Am thinking of translating the Three Essays myself this summer and to entrust Everyday Life to a suitable translator whom I can keep under closer watch.[10]

Very much in agreement with Brioni.

Frau G.'s mood goes deeper than I thought but is changing nothing in her noble demeanor.

1. These lectures cannot be identified.

2. This may be a reference to Joszef Brenner (1887–1919), who was working at Ernö Moravcsik's clinic at the time. Brenner, a psychiatrist and writer, was one of the first in Hungary to be interested in Freudian ideas. In 1912 he published his *Tagebuch einer Geistesgestörten* [Diary of a Mentally Disturbed Person] (see Mihály Szajbély, ed., *Egy elmebeteg nö naplója, Csáth Géza ismeretlen orvosi tanulmánya* [Budapest, 1978], pp. 27–221), in which he presented the analysis of a case and a theory that attempted to explain psychic mechanisms in the mentally ill. Ferenczi wrote a review of the book (1912, 101) in *Gyógyászat*, no. 24 (1912). In addition, Brenner published novellas influenced by psychoanalysis under the pseudonym Géza Csáth. He was addicted to morphine and committed suicide in 1919. See Eva Brabant, *Présentation, Silence noir, Nouvelles de Géza Csáth*, (Aix en Provence, 1988), pp. 7–18.

3. Unidentified work about Maurice Maeterlinck, *L'oiseau bleu, Féerie en cinq actes et dix tableaux* (Paris, 1909). Maeterlinck (1862–1949), a Belgian writer whose writings are marked by symbolism, won the Nobel Prize for literature in 1911.

4. This enclosure is missing.

5. Evidently the circle that grew up around the high school teacher Gyula Polgár (see letter 252).

6. "Zur Ontogenie des Geldinteresses" [On the Ontogenesis of an Interest in Money] (1914, 146; C., p. 319), and possibly "Zur Ontogenese der Symbole" [On the Ontogenesis of Symbols] (1913, 125; C., p. 276), which were later published in the *Zeitschrift*.

7. Jenö Hárnik (?–?), a member of the Galileo Society, was later practically and theoretically active as a psychoanalyst. He was in contact with representatives of the Hungarian republic and took part in the psychiatric reform in public hospitals. In 1922 he emigrated to Berlin and became a member of the Society there, and from 1926 on he was a docent at the Berlin Institute. According to Charlotte Balkányi, Hárnik died in the insane asylum in Budapest. See also letters 354 and 356.

8. Enclosed in brackets in the original.

9. The letter ends at the bottom of a page; this postscript is written on the back.

10. Ferenczi's translation of Freud's *Three Essays on the Theory of Sexuality* was published in 1915 with an introduction by Ferenczi. *The Psychopathology of Everyday Life* was translated by Maria Takács (Budapest, 1923).

285

Budapest, March 13, 1912[1]

Dear Professor,

I know, of course, that in your recommendations[2] only the most important ones about technique can find a place, but I think that you should also
include a few lines about the following principles:

One ought not to get into any discussions with the patient. If one does
that one forces him into a fighting position to which, for inner reasons, he
is only too inclined; but if one omits them, then he will soon come forth
by himself with confirmations. I customarily do not respond at all when
contradicted, and if the patient wants to compel a response—then I tell
him that further analysis will show whether I am right or not.[3]

Kind regards,
Ferenczi

1. Sealed postcard.

2. "Recommendations to Physicians Practising Psycho-Analysis" (Freud 1912e).

3. Freud had taken the position that "it is never the aim of discussions like this to
create conviction. They are only intended to bring the repressed complexes into consciousness, to set the conflict going in the field of conscious mental activity and to
facilitate the emergence of fresh material from the unconscious" ("Notes upon a Case of
Obsessional Neurosis" [1909]d, p. 181). Freud returned once again to this theme much
later in "Constructions in Analysis" (1937d).

286

Vienna, March 13, 1912
IX., Berggasse 19

Dear friend,

I was really very pleased with the precious confirmation of Leonardo. I
am enclosing the analysis.

Brioni has put us off until the second half of April. We won't get anything
out of that. I request that we think about another place on the Adriatic. I
would like to stay away from Friday evening until Tuesday, perhaps
Wednesday morning.

I had a little talk with Jung[1] that resulted in a nice concession on his
part. An inclination to be reserved in private relations remains and is being
respected by me, i.e., responded to with a corresponding reserve.

There seems to be real progress with Elma. She has indicated this
through a completely altered demeanor and a few astute thoughts that I
would not have thought her capable of. So give her mother the consolation
that she will at least get her back changed for the better. I would like to

send her home for Easter. Now some new but quite different difficulties have set in. We are really in the narcissistic stage in which she behaves very self-sufficiently and actually refuses help. She is now herself, and I am curious how far I can bring her in these four weeks. She no longer plays the part of the good patient at all. I believe it went so well only because she was so utterly[2] indifferent to me. Now I value her more, naturally, and want to keep a close watch on the danger that is connected with that. When she comes back, I think it makes sense for the both of you to resolve anew to consider everything that has happened before to be extinguished.

It is no longer all right with me that you want to concern yourself with translating the Three Essays. I think you have better things to do; I also don't know whether further translations are desirable.

In a hurry before the session.

Cordially yours,
Freud

1. See *Freud/Jung*, March 3 and 5, 1912, pp. 490–493.
2. "Utterly" is in English in the original.

287

Budapest, March 16, 1912
VII., Erzsébet-körút 54

Dear Professor,

For some time the *question of hypochondria* has been leaving me no peace.[1] I have revised my material and find the source of the evil again and again in anal erotism or its derivatives (desire for coprophagia, smelling); very, very frequently an injury of the *money complex* becomes a precipitating cause in the following way: loss (expenditure) of money—regression to anal erotism—displacement of interest in the excremental onto other bodily organs and functions (naturally with negative sign). [See the expressions: poor in blood, bleed to death, his heart hurts (when he has to spend money), a saying from the Talmud: "A poor man is like a dead man." He should suffocate on his money. You can't get your breath (from giving out money) etc.][2]

Hypochondria from masturbation likewise originates by way of anal erotism. For example, collecting sperm is identified with collecting money (valuables). Hence, prohibition of masturbation. If the prohibition is transgressed (marital compulsion to coitus), then it comes to regression (anal erotism). *Hence the constipation of masturbators.* A part of this anal erotic (coprophilic) increase in libido is, however, displaced onto other bodily organs (hypochondria). The choice of organs onto which displacement oc-

curs is not coincidental: the organ itself must be erotically overemphasized.*

So, the psychic consequences of masturbation have two sources: 1.)
castration anxiety, 2.) regression to anal erotism as a result of the loss of
value during masturbation.

The true hypochondriac is an anal erotist who maniacally projects onto
an external cause (illness) his anal-erotic coprophilic interest which has
been displaced to other bodily organs. [Hypochondriacal projection.] The
entire hypochondriacal delusional system serves as insurance against the
insight of anal-erotic wishes.

The colossal abhorrence of anal erotism makes it so that this kind of
libido is sublimated at all costs, and where that does not succeed—it must
be *projected* as far as possible by the ego. A person still does not feel secured
against its return by simple displacement; hence, the compulsion to delusional rationalization.

There are further intimate connections between anal erotism, homosexuality, hypochondria, and *paranoia*. [See my case[3] described in the Zentralblatt: a man interprets his homosexual anal erotism (operations on the
rectum) first hypochondriacally and feels all kinds of lethal illnesses in
himself; only later is it *detached* by persecution mania. Hypochondria is,
after all, also a persecution mania: only one is being persecuted not by
another person but by the *"illness."*]

The most remarkable confirmation of the conception of hypochondria
as a fermentation product of anal erotism is probably the following case:
A hypochondriac finds his body strangely "abnormal." His hipbone especially displeases him; it is supposedly peculiarly "turned outward"; from
time to time he makes funny, spasmodic movements: at the same time he
feels how the bone is "turned inward." Local findings absolutely negative.—Second delusion: in bed he has to sleep "turned inward" (against the
wall), otherwise he is threatened with severe illness. But sometimes he has
to sleep turned straight outward. Explanation: he has a *proplapsus recti*,[4]
with which he is constantly unconsciously preoccupied, with which he
would like to play, to concern himself continually with its inwardly or
outwardly turned ("rolled," as it is called in Hungarian) condition. Instead
of this he builds himself a grandiose delusional structure—in fact, he gradually feels totally altered and like something special, and he adapts his whole
view of the world to this delusional idea.

Hypochondria's therapeutic intransigence and similarity to paranoia can
be explained by this mechanism; so projection is not easily reversed.

The abhorrence of male homosexuality can also perhaps be explained by
intolerence of anal erotism, which is inseparable from it.

Again and again I get an insight into how large a part of human civilization has arisen on account of anal erotism, and how it originates in each

individual. The vicissitudes and transformations of anal-erotic libido can be traced in the normal as well as in the pathological.

Anal erotism + (coprophilia) {
I. *Unaltered* (perverse) use [stool erotism etc.]
II. *Anaclisis on other perversities:* (stool voyeurism, stool sadism, stool masochism, sadistic coprophemia,[5] its masochistic opposite, pederasty (active and passive).
III. *Sublimation:* capitalism, aestheticism. Optical sublimation (sense for painting). Tactile sublimation (plastic). Acoustic sublimation (music). Gourmandism. Love of perfume.
}

Anal erotism + coprophilia { IV. Neurosis {
1.) *Anxiety hysteria:* anxiety about sudden death, often extreme. Fear of accidents.
2.) *Hysteria:* nausea, shortness of breath (asthma), globus.
3.) A root of many *obsessional neuroses* [through agency of masturbation].
4.) Main root of hypochondria. (Projection.)
5.) Dementia praecox: regression to anal erotism + coprophilia (smearing).
6.) *Paranoia:* projection of homosexual anal erotism.
}

In the case histories that I am now reviewing I find everywhere anal erotism as the main source of the pathological fears and, in fact, both the fear of acute illnesses in anxiety hysteria and anxiety neurosis, as well as in the hypochondriacal system. It usually comes down to anxiety about illness or formation of hypochondria when one of the sublimations (particularly the money complex) is severely injured or destroyed.

There is a peculiar *anal-erotic impotence* in people who want to collect their money (their sperm) and are incapable of making sacrifices for a woman.

I would be very happy if you would share with me your view about these questions (if it is possible in a few sentences), or do we want to reserve that for Easter?

Instead of *Brioni* we should consider:

Venice (too noisy?), Lovrana, Lussin piccolo, *Portorose* near Pola; *Novi* (near Trieste), *Lake Garda*. By the way, I will give you free rein.

I was happy about the more favorable news about Elma. In her last letters she was again revealing some resistance.

Kind regards, also from Frau G.

Yours,
Ferenczi

* or it must be especially suited to the symbolization of excremental functions.

1. See letter 139 and n. 6 and letter 140.
2. Enclosed in brackets in the original, as are all similar remarks throughout the letter.
3. Ferenczi, "Reizung der analen erogenen Zone als auslösende Ursache der Paranoia" [Stimulation of the Anal Erotogenic Zone as a Precipitating Factor in Paranoia] (1911, 77; *Fin.*, p. 295).
4. Prolapse of the entire wall of the rectum.
5. Obscene speech; sexual arousal sought by using "dirty" expressions with women. In his paper "Über obszöne Worte" [On Obscene Words] (1911, 75; *C.*, p. 150; *Schriften* I, 70) Ferenczi had differentiated between this term and coprolalia, the unconscious, compulsive utterance of such words.

288

Vienna, March 18, 1912
IX., Berggasse 19

Dear friend,

Your hypochondria structure is very respectable. I am prepared to discuss it at Easter. What I am writing today is only the confession of my standpoint up to now: I have always felt the darkness in the question of hypochondria to be a great disgrace to our efforts but have come up with nothing but suppositions. The problem seemed to me to be: characterization by means of a particular organ source or a particular process. And, with a view toward obsessional neurosis, I opted for the latter, while you choose the former. With regard to the process, I thought of hypochondria as the third actual neurosis and the somatic basis for paraphrenia, as anxiety neurosis is for hysteria. So I drew the erogenous contributions of the organs, which are annexed to the ego rather than to the libido, but with negative sign, but nothing consistent has come out of this, and I don't want to force anything that doesn't seem ready.

If it's all right with you, let's consider the island of Arbe for our Easter trip. Perhaps you can inquire about the connections that must come out of Fiume. I will do the same here. I already know Lussin, but it was not very interesting.

Things have come to a total halt with Elma; I think I know where, in narcissism. What she had earlier is naturally not lost, but definitively taken care of, as is evidenced by her changed state. A solution to the new snag could arrive any day, but . . . Easter is near, and I don't want to keep her over Easter; I also have three new prospective patients for later on.

Today the clean proofs of Imago arrived, and this week we are still awaiting the publication of the volume, which we want to celebrate with an editorial party. You will not find your excellent contributions to the Recommendations put to use in the Zentralblatt this time. They will come into the next essay on technique, which I have in mind after a suitable interval.[1]

Kind regards,
Freud

1. See letter 304 and n. 1.

289

[Budapest,] March 21, 1912

Dear Professor,
The connection Budapest–Fiume–Arbe is as follows:

Sleeping car
dep. Budapest 7:00 A.M. dep. 6:15 P.M.
arr. Fiume   7:54 P.M. arr. 7:10 A.M.

Sleeping car
dep. Budapest 7:40 P.M.
arr. Fiume   8:50 A.M.

Fiume–Arbe
dep. Fiume Monday A.M. 6:00
arr. Arbe Monday   10:45

dep. Fiume Tuesday 6:35
            Friday
arr. Arbe   2:02 P.M.

dep. Fiume Sunday 7:20 A.M.
arr. Arbe   3:15 P.M.

dep. Fiume Thursday 7:35
arr. Arbe   12:30

After all this it is not possible to make a connection with the early express train. We would have to stay overnight in Fiume—the stretch Vienna–Budapest would cost you another night, or you travel directly with the Southern Railway (sleeping car) to Fiume, where we would meet.
Enclosed is an enticing advertisement for the spa *Porto Rose*.

What would you say to Lovrana?

Many kind regards,
Ferenczi

290

Vienna, March 24, 1912
IX., Berggasse 19

Dear friend,

Arbe is confirmed, room reserved for us in the hotel annex. I hope you are satisfied with it. Arbe is supposed to be the most beautiful and most varied part of Dalmatia, with woods, drinking water, and beach.

You see, your information has made the order of travel from April 1 on out of the question. I will leave here with the Southern Railway at 9:30, and we will, I think, meet in Nabresina; in any case, we will arrive in Fiume early enough to be able to have breakfast (Oli is not home yet!).[1] The ship leaves on *Saturday* at 10:15 and arrives in Arbe at 3:10 and returns on Tuesday. So, very convenient. Let us hope everything will come out well, and we will find in Arbe something of the comfort that we sought in vain in Sicily the last time.

Jung writes today that he has been invited by Fordham University to give a series of lectures starting in September.[2] Since his military service runs from August 22 until September 6, he has set the date for the Congress for August 19/20 in Munich, i.e., he is inquiring with me for that reason and wants to ask the branch societies about it. I asked him by telegram to postpone these inquiries and will write to him that this date is terribly inconvenient for me; it disrupts my vacation; I will be in Karlsbad until August 10. August is also—in addition to being in Munich—not a time for scientific work. It is thus advisable to leave the Congress open this year, which he can motivate very well with his trip to America. The latter is again an encouraging sign.

With Elma things continue to go gloomily. She has brought out several quite surprisingly intelligent insights, but she doesn't want to get into the experience with you and doesn't seem to want to finish with me; i.e, because of the transference she wishes to extend her stay past Easter, which I don't want to do. So I am cooling off noticeably again.

I am very much looking forward to Easter and send kind regards.

Yours truly,
Freud

1. Freud's son Oliver often arranged the schedules for Freud's trips.
2. See letter 318, n. 5.

291

Dear Professor,

I tried in vain to get a berth for the night train of April 5, so I will have to travel through in an overcrowded car. As a reward for this ordeal and in order for me to have recovered from the consequences of the night's journey in the time that we are spending together, I will give myself an additional day of vacation and will travel to Fiume at 4 P.M., will arrive there at 5 A.M., get a good rest, and await you at the station on the morning of April 6.

I will now spare you the psychological description of my emotional state; there will be enough time for that in Arbe.

Today Elma writes to her mother that she would like to speak with me before my departure. I don't consider this advisable, so I am asking you to give Elma an hour on Friday as well.

After the efforts and ψ. shocks of the last few months I am extraordinarily looking forward to the—let us hope sunny—days on the Adriatic.

Regards to your family.

Yours,
Ferenczi

Frau G. greets you cordially.

292

[Budapest,] Thursday, April 4.[1]
Six P.M. [1912][2]

Dear Professor,

The sudden cessation of the belated equinoctial storms has made it superfluous for me to communicate with you, so I will confine myself to telling you that I am just about to depart and will await you on Saturday (morning) at the station in Fiume.

Auf Wiedersehen.

Ferenczi

1. Sealed postcard.

2. These notations are at the end of the page; no address or year is given. The letter has been placed in sequence based on its content.

293

Budapest, April 17, 1912
VII., Erzsébet-körút 54

Dear Professor,

One shouldn't prophesy if one doesn't want to make a fool of oneself. I promised you I would write very soon about the development of things, whereby I understood this to be a decision in a negative sense. Instead of this I must content myself with a situation report that will not be too difficult for you to pass judgment on.

The first encounter went according to plan (namely, as I had intended). I was friendly and kind but reserved. Elma evidently was hoping to be received differently and reacted with a rather strong bad temper. Inwardly I felt the great change that had taken place in me in the course of the last three months and in consequence of what I had learned about Elma: hardly anything remained of the sexual overestimation of that time, and I was and am able to gauge correctly the colossal difference in worth between Elma and Frau G. Certainly the effect of these realizations expressed themselves in the fact that my tenderness, which up to this moment had been noticeably inhibited with respect to Frau G., was once again directed toward her (Frau G.).

My peculiar inclination to unite tenderness and sensuality was again noticeably evident here and may also have contributed to the fact that Elma also appeared less attractive to me as a sexual object than she perhaps deserves.

I then spoke with Elma about the future; I wanted her to understand that the events before the analysis could simply not continue, but rather that everything should begin anew. I also told her candidly that Frau G. is indispensable to me as a friend and co-worker and that I have in her everything that I need, except for the youth which I had to seek in her (Elma).

On the following evenings I was constantly in the company of both of them and was striving to establish the basis for a comfortable and harmonious life together. But Elma seemed inhibited; her inhibition grew even stronger, and yesterday she admitted to me that this situation is disagreeable to her. She was already impatient to enjoy life finally and can adapt herself only with difficulty to waiting until I make up my mind, and to suspending her wishes in the meantime (she didn't say this with these words, but the sense of her intimations could not be misunderstood). Some tendency toward jealousy with respect to Frau G. is also noticeable in her.

The effect of her treatment has certainly been very deep. Elma has complete insight into the infantile complexes that make up her character, and she no longer has the ambition to be more than she can be by nature;

she is much more social than she was before, and she has given up the hunt for her illusions. She has apparently separated from you with strong remnants of transference. Hence, the letter that she wrote to you but that I haven't read.

I cannot describe Frau G.'s behavior to you. I would hardly have considered so much gentleness, insight, love, renunciation, loyalty, understanding possible all together in one person. My tendency toward unification could truly feel satisfied. And still, she says that I cannot do without the one thing that she lacks—youth—, and she is promoting the union with Elma with all the means at her disposal—she promises and wishes that our tender and intellectual relationship should remain unchanged. If *she* gives me to Elma and Elma to me, this marriage would seem to her to be the most beautiful and harmonic solution for the future. (My ignominious flight three months ago was something else.) I had to admit she was right about everything—as much as it hurt me—; but I made it clear to her that the possibility of carrying out this plan depended on two conditions: Elma's suitability—and the fact that she becomes agreeable to *me*. (And on Elma's inclination as well, naturally.)

Self-criticism certainly tells me that I was and am somewhat too impatient with Elma—evidently as a consequence of pangs of conscience with regard to Frau G.—Today, for instance—when I saw her (Elma) in a good mood, I definitely found the paths of association of feeling to the libidinal impulses which existed at the time of the analysis. Naturally, she noticed this immediately and reacted accordingly.

You should understand that I will get to the pleasant recollections of the Robinson [Crusoe] days on Arbe only after I have finished the more urgent communications. You are right: now the whole thing appears to me an illusion. One doesn't believe at all that something so blue, sunny, and carefree could be true.

I am working a great deal and am fully booked up, but in the scientific sphere I am not getting beyond some interesting thoughts. I don't have the composure which is necessary for work.

Kind regards,
Ferenczi

294

April 21, 1912
IX., Berggasse 19

Dear friend,

I am using another late hour on Sunday evening to write to you. Not to reply to you, for the vacillating situation that you are reporting on will not tolerate any interference that is not urgent advice, and I can't make up my mind about that despite a charming letter from Frau G.,[1] to which she desires no response. It is certainly not a lack of interest nor fear of responsibility but rather regard for the rights of another and concern about connecting the fate of our friendship with something else, something indefinable.

The time since our separation has passed for me in hard work accompanied by the impossibility of concentrating, so I don't have anything clever to relate to you. I also have little from the outside except for a newspaper clipping which would certainly be of most interest to you because of the fact that I myself have no knowledge whatsoever of the party in question, who knows me so well.[2] (Please return it.)

I didn't write to Jung again until today. There is better news from Pfister; he seems to be holding his own.[3] The photograph that he has enclosed shows the charming face of a girl, access to whom has of course been closed to him for the time being, because he has promised to postpone the divorce by a half year. Bleuler is *supposed* (according to a report from Binswanger) to have been recommended for Breslau,[4] which naturally could be of the greatest interest for the future of ΨA, but the matter is still not firm. You know that Bonhoeffer[5] from Breslau is going to Berlin as Ziehen's[6] successor. On the whole, I don't have a favorable impression of the external politics of ΨA.

My paper in Imago has already been reprinted twice, in "Pan" and in the Neues Wiener Journal.[7] It is the most lifeless thing I have ever written and can only be excused by my being a beginner and by the article on taboo that follows it. Imago seems to be finding a favorable reception from the public.

I greet you cordially and await further news from you.

Yours,
Freud

1. This letter is missing

2. At a session of the neurological section of the Academy of Medicine on April 4, 1912, Moses Allen Starr (1854–1932), professor of neurology at Columbia University, had declared that he knew Freud well and was of the opinion that psychoanalysis was a result

of Freud's dissipated life; see "Attack on Freud's Theory," *New York Times*, April 5, 1912. Freud's reaction in a letter to Putnam of June 25, 1912, was: "His information about my early years amused me mightily. Would that it had been true!" (Hale, *Putnam*, p. 143).

3. Pfister's position as a pastor had been threatened (see *Freud/Jung*, February 25 and March 10, 1912, pp. 487 and 493).

4. Bleuler was being considered for a professorship in psychiatry in Breslau as Karl Bonhoeffer's successor. Binswanger had visited Bonhoeffer, his former teacher, there and had reported to Freud on the visit in a letter of March 5, 1912 (Binswanger, *Reminiscences*, p. 38).

5. Karl Bonhoeffer (1868–1948) was professor of psychiatry in Breslau and later in Berlin, where the Karl Bonhoeffer Sanatoria, still in existence today, were named after him. He was the father of the theologian Dietrich Bonhoeffer, who was murdered by the SS in 1945.

6. Theodor Ziehen (1862–1950), professor of psychiatry and neurology in Berlin and, from 1917 on, in Halle. Ziehen was the first to coin the term "complex" (see *Freud/Jung*, September 11, 1907, p. 85).

7. The first essay of *Totem and Taboo* (1912–13a), "Über einige Übereinstimmungen im Seelenleben der Wilden und der Neurotiker: Die Inzestscheu" [Some Points of Agreement between the Mental Lives of Savages and Neurotics: The Horror of Incest] (*Imago*, 1 [1912]: 17–33). A slightly abridged version was reprinted in the Viennese weekly *Pan*, April 11 and 18, 1912, and in the daily *Neues Wiener Journal*, April 18, 1912.

295

Budapest, April 23, 1912
VII., Erzsébet-körút 54

Dear Professor,

I understand completely that, in the present state of affairs, you don't wish to meddle in the matter with Elma as long as you see no cause for "urgent advice." I myself feel that I have to make the decision alone in this matter and should not share the responsibility with anyone. Certainly I am not afraid that our friendship will be jeopardized by anything connected with this family romance.

The pendulum swings in my inclination between Frau G. and Elma, between mother and sister, spirit and matter, are continuing—although not with such brisk frequency as before. I see the advantages and deficiencies of both women and will learn how to judge these deficiencies with somewhat more patience. It was becoming quite clear to me that I cannot renounce the tender and cerebral relation with Frau G., but that in additon to that I have erotic needs and a longing for domestic comfort and family that I must satisfy in order not to jeopardize through this lack of satisfaction Frau G.'s friendship, which is so valuable to me. I have the assurance that Frau G. will remain true to me even in the case of a union with Elma.

Her capacity for love and sacrifice is simply boundless; only now have I really learned to appreciate her—when one is very much in love, one cannot actually judge the value of one's love object so objectively.

I am not amenable to the idea of a "housekeeper," probably because that would preclude the founding of a family. Thus, the marriage union with Elma would remain only an expedient, provided that she can fulfill the conditions for it. I have already gotten away from demanding the impossible (impossible for her) from her. I now know the extent of her narcissism, her lack of objective interest in people and things. Accordingly, my enthusiasm for her has cooled off considerably. On the other hand, her tender, loving attitude with respect to me has not lost its effect on me, and at times I have the impression that she could fulfill my—to be sure, dashed—expectations as wife and mother—if she only sees reason and tolerates the unaltered continuation of my emotional and intellectual relations with her mother. I spoke with her about this, and she seems to want to accept it—but I don't know what kind of a role her pressing desire for ultimate marriage plays in this. Other open questions: Will I be able to maintain my attitude toward her without getting impatient; will not my tendency toward unification assert itself again later? Will the life-style that I want to lead and that offers little to a young creature desperate to be liked be sufficient for Elma in the long run? Will *I* be able to accommodate myself to a certain extent without being disturbed in my studies?

As far as external matters are concerned, there is not much to report. I am spending my evenings with Frau G. and Elma and am attempting to live together experimentally, in a threesome, as it were. Elma is showing me her newly acquired mastery in the art of cooking and is using every opportunity that comes along to be tender toward me; I am also friendly and loving toward her. I am conversing with Frau G. about scientific matters—Elma also listens, seems interested, and now and then makes some quite good remarks—of course, without that enthusiastic joy of recognition that Frau G. typifies.

So, the matter is such that I no longer feel driven by that irresistible urge for Elma; I am judging her and the situation more coolly and am considering possible marriage to her as a *mariage de raison*.[1] I am hesitating only because I am not convinced whether it would be really reasonable [*raisonnable*] to trade the relative peace of my present existence for the risk of this marriage.

April 25

I let myself be hindered in closing this letter by all kinds of little disturbances, evidently because I felt that I still have to wait if I want to communicate more than these generalities. In the meantime, however, something has taken place that brought matters forward in a specific (albeit still alternative) direction. You may have surmised from the content of my letters that I was of a mind to conclude the marriage with Elma. I was pleased to see my relationship to Frau G. secured for the future, was happy about Elma's tenderness, and fantasized about familial bliss. I thought that consideration for Frau G. was the only thing hindering me in making a decision.—But while, after hard inner struggles, I was striving to become at one with myself, I rather neglected to interest myself in Elma's mental life. I took her as she presented herself and as I knew her from what you said, even though I was instructed by you that she knew precisely how to salvage the relationship to me intact from the crucible of analysis. Today, finally, I turned my attention to her mental life and observed a very strong inhibition in her: she was obviously making an effort to admit to herself and to me only the most pleasant thoughts about our planned union. So I suggested to her that we continue the analysis for a while, to which she agreed rather easily. But the first hour, which we had today, showed her to be so colossally inhibited that I am getting myself prepared for a rather long span of time. I feel myself to be much freer with respect to her than in the earlier analysis—despite the willingness which I exhibited at the beginning for a possible union with her—, and it didn't take much sacrifice on my part to demand and to get from her an agreement to break off unconditionally all relations (with the exception of medical ones) for the duration of the treatment. That depressed her rather strongly, to be sure, but it made no impression on me. She has to decide to speak with me freely and uninhibitedly, to admit her resistances. If she doesn't do that, then I am firmly resolved finally to give her up. From a rational standpoint I cannot act in any other way. Of course, I will conduct myself in a polite and friendly manner with her, as is also my duty as a physician, so it cannot be excluded that, if the results of the analysis do not hamper the plan's realization, something will still come out of the matter in the end. I am not now afraid that sexual overestimation will impede me in the analysis. That will soon be evident, by the way.

In the meantime, I am working from morning until evening [analysis][2] and I hope *finally* also to be able to work on something. That should now become my place of refuge.

I am enclosing the American bluff.[3] Have all kinds of lies and slander against analysis been exhausted? In the end, the prosecuting attorney and confiscation will still come!—But all this does nothing at all to the ideas; they are spreading like an infection from all the scattered hearths, inexorably.

Foerster from Zurich was recently lecturing here; he was also talking about "Christianity and Modern Psychotherapy." According to the newspaper reports, he held the view that the Christian cleric, teacher, and father—like modern psychotherapy—should also be striving to investigate *the dark sides of mental life* and to educate the ministry to *self-knowledge.* So he actually has learned something from Pfister.[4]

The Society for Psychical Research requests that I write an article for the Proceedings. I want to deliver to them a paper on "A New Conception of Hypnotism and Suggestion."[5]

I thank you for the reprint of the paper on incest.[6] Everyone here who has seen it likes *Imago.*

I greet you all cordially.

Yours,
Ferenczi

April 26, 1912
My letter takes on more and more gigantic dimensions and more and more the form of a diary. As a postscript I still have to think about the enclosed letter from Prof. Putnam, which I didn't want to respond to without getting your advice. I think the book by Kollarits (really insignificant in and of itself) had such a strong effect on our valiant Putnam only because it aroused his own repressed doubts.[7] I want to enlighten him (in accord with the facts) on the lack of significance and on the maliciousness of the Jendrassik[8]-Kollarits clan.

My decision of yesterday to educate Elma to freedom of speech with the aid of analysis is being implemented.—She visited me today and seemed honestly to want to go into that. I don't want to carry out the analysis too long (perhaps only a few weeks—provided that she gives up her resistance.

Kind regards—this time really as an *adieu!*

F.

1. A marriage of convenience.
2. Enclosed in brackets in the original.
3. See letter 294 and n. 2.
4. See letter 84 and n. 3 as well as letter 96 and n. 2.
5. Ferenczi's article was later rejected by the Society for Psychical Research (see letter 333).
6. See letter 294 and n. 7.
7. Putnam had asked Ferenczi about the credibility of Jenö Kollarits and his book *Charakter und Nervosität* (see letter 173 and n. 4). For Putnam's letter and Ferenczi's reply, see Hale, *Putnam,* pp. 311–313.

8. Ernö Jendrassik (1858–1921), since 1903 professor of neuropathology, from 1908 on head of the Second Clinic for Internal Disease in Budapest; he was Kollarits's superior. As an opponent of psychoanalysis he tried unsuccessfully in 1919 to prevent Ferenczi's appointment as the first full professor of psychoanalysis at the University of Budapest.

296

Vienna, April 28, 1912
IX., Berggasse 19

Dear friend,

I am replying to you immediately because of your enclosed letter by Putnam. Our good friend has forgotten that lying and swindle found their way over the ocean to Europe a long time ago. Remind him of that and dip the paintbrush in deep in order to paint broadly.

You are otherwise too pessimistic about the persecutions. The only strange thing is that I am not being challenged by any of our friends over there on account of Allen Starr.[1]

I am in great suspense as I devour your news about the course of your family affair. I received a letter from Elma simultaneously with yours. It is very amicable, requests no reply, and will be taken care of by your being so kind as to convey my thanks to her. Of all your misgivings, one has made an impression on me: whether your daily schedule and life-style have room for a young woman who is in love with life and not deeply interested in your work.

A letter from Dr. Margarete Stegmann[2] contains the discouraging news about the miserable course of her marriage, which is now about to break up. That is certainly no sign in her favor. Stegmann has acted unbelievably crazy and counted on something quite unfulfillable.

I have so much work I can't budge; I can't find any time at all to finish the taboo thing. In order to force myself, I have announced it as a lecture in the Society.[3]

Everything is well today at home. Emden is still here.[4]

Kindest regards,
Freud

1. See letter 294, n. 2.
2. Margarete Stegmann (?–?), member of the Berlin Society from 1912. Freud had written to Jung about her and her husband (see letter 64 and n. 5): "One should honour an old woman, but not marry her; really, love is for the young" (Freud/Jung, November 30, 1911, p. 469).
3. See letter 298 and n. 1.
4. Jan van Emden (see letter 223 and n. 8) was again in Vienna for a few weeks (Freud/Jung, April 21, 1912, p. 499).

297

Vienna, May 10, 1912[1]

always welcome also prefer noon—Freud

1. Telegram.

298

Vienna, May 16, 1912
IX., Berggasse 19

Dear friend,

Yesterday I turned loose the lecture on taboo.[1] The reading took three hours and caused several deaths.

On the same day I was surprised by the nice shipment of glass, which gives me an opportunity to thank Frau G. kindly for her interest and effort. Unfortunately I don't know how much I owe for it. By way of an apology I am enclosing your ambiguous coupon.[2]

Today I received a funny collection of typographical errors from a docent in physics[3] who confesses to having been produced by Maeder.

I also want to tell you that we will *very* probably be able to put your beautiful essay on Oedipus in issue three of Imago,[4] if it gets into the hands of the editors very soon.

Kind regards from your at present tired

Freud

1. "The Taboo," in *Minutes* IV, 102 n.
2. Allusion unclear.
3. Unidentified.
4. Ferenczi's essay "Symbolische Darstellung des Lust- und Realitätsprinzips im Oedipus-Mythos" [Symbolic Representation of the Pleasure and Reality Principles in the Oedipus Myth] (1912, 92; *C.*, p. 253) was subsequently also published in *Imago* 1 (pp. 276–284).

299

[Budapest, ca.
May 17–20, 1912][1]

Dear Professor,

This time I want to keep silent about personal matters; I am waiting until I can report in summary.

I will *definitely* send the paper on Oedipus in a few days. I have already notified Rank.

Enclosed is a small communication about a case of *déjà vu*.[2] If you can use it, then do so for the fourth edition of Everyday Life.[3] If not, please hand it over to Stekel for the Zentralblatt.

Frau Gisela asks if you find the price of the little glass collection *(thirty-five crowns)* appropriate. We want to know that so that we will be oriented in the event of further opportunities.

Kind regards,
Ferenczi

1. Balint dates this letter to the beginning of 1912, but its content suggests its placement here.

2. Ferenczi, "Ein Fall von 'déjà vu'" [A case of *déjà vu*] (1912, 86; *Fin.*, p. 319), *Zentralblatt* 2 (1911–12): 648f.

3. Freud 1901b, 4th ed. (Berlin, 1912).

300

Vienna, May 21, 1912
IX., Berggasse 19

Dear friend,

Unfortunately, the fourth edition of Everyday Life has already gone off. I handed over your observation to Stekel.

I ask you to tell Frau Gisela that this time she certainly did not buy dearly. In general, however, one should buy only quite flawless glasses.

Kind regards,
Freud

301

Budapest, May 27, 1912
VII., Erzsébet-körút 54

Dear Professor,

You shouldn't take offense at my stubborn silence. Only certain points of respite are suitable for summarizing and reporting in the changeable battle that I must wage simultaneously with three opponents: with Elma, Frau G., and—myself. Such a state of equilibrium exists at the present moment, for instance, and my first thought was, of course, you and my duty to report to you. (Not as if this duty had not occurred to me countless times in the interim.)

I see more and more clearly that in complicated mental confusion one can count on only a single reliable guide, analysis, and I don't want to conceal from you how very grateful I am to you for this mentor.

It was certainly not easy for me to resist the urging of the passions and to regain the coolness of the intellect; I also don't know how long this feeling of dominance will last. For the time being, however, I think that I am on the right path, on which the decision will have to come by itself.

One event that Elma had to report to me about two weeks ago certainly contributed considerably to my enlightenment. She was accosted on the street by one of her youthful admirers (the Parisian, Lorschy.)[1] She brushed him off and fled from him into a one-horse carriage, but the young man got into the carriage with her. She was very frightened and—very energetically—dismissed him from the carriage.

From the manner in which she reported the incident, however, I saw that she cannot admit to me and to herself everything that is going on in her. Having rapidly made up my mind, I explained that to her on the following day and told her emphatically that there can be no talk of engagement as long as she doesn't commit herself to open (analytic) discourse. If she can't do that, then I will cease all further attempts and consider the matter settled.—After a brief depression and some weeping she declared herself ready for this, but essentially changed nothing in her tactics: she didn't want to yield anything which could have harmed the marriage's coming into being; she wanted to apply the old means of battle (tenderness).—But I remained steadfast, even though I had to withstand very hard inner struggles.—And now, finally, her long-suppressed resentment, with all the negative things that she feels against me and marriage, is beginning to find expression in symptoms, thoughts—even in conscious affects.—If the marriage had gone as planned, she would have had to live all that out in actions, in acts of revenge!—But in this way I am (for the moment) master of the situation and want patiently to continue the analysis, which should then bring about for her and for me a clarification of the situation necessary to make a decision. It is possible that *she* will lose patience and give up the treatment along with her intentions to get engaged. If it comes to that, then I will be comforted by the awareness that a break is preferable to an inauspicious union.

It is possible, however, that this belated analysis—as I am already beginning to notice—will bring to light new material from Elma's ucs.; as soon as she ventures forth with her repressed antisocial affects, genuinely feminine traits, which could not be seen up to now on account of the inhibition from all sides, will immediately become apparent. She is beginning to feel sorry for her mother, and at the same time the infantile sources of her sexual attraction to her mother (homosexuality) are beginning to manifest themselves.

If I were successful in educating her to be ruthlessly honest with me and with respect to herself, I would then have a certain guarantee that she will be reliable in marriage and not the plaything of dark drives, and then something could still come of the matter, provided that she wants it even when she has achieved her complete self-sufficiency in making a decision. But if only one of these stipulations is missing, I will drop the plan.—

Meanwhile, self-analysis daily proves to me that I will, on the one hand, not be able to do without the intellectual communion with Frau G., even after the possible marriage to Elma, but on the other hand, I cannot find erotic satisfaction (especially in the act) with her. So if the plan to marry Elma is dashed, then I will have to look around for a replacement that will not disrupt my tender and intellectual coexistence with Frau G.

In the meantime, dear, good Frau G. is loving and suffering unspeakably. From time to time she gets impatient, has probably withdrawn a part of her libido into her ego and allowed it to regress to various earlier love objects (brothers and sisters), but she also feels how she has coalesced with me and will bow to the inevitable, in order not to lose everything.

Inter arma silent musae.[2] I am not working at all—except for the analyses; the plans for the summer are also floating in air.—

I heard from some Swiss (Constance) that they were expecting you there for Whitsun.[3] Were you there?

Please give me news soon about science, propaganda, personal matters (Jung)—it will positively refresh me.

I hope you have forgiven my long silence, and I am lovingly

Yours truly,
Ferenczi

1. A patient. See letters 217 and 219.
2. "In the din of battle the arts are silent"; derived from "Silent leges inter arma" (Cicero, *Oration for Milo*, 4.10).
3. At Whitsun, from May 25 to 28, 1912, Freud visited Binswanger in Kreuzlingen, after the latter's cancer operation; (see Binswanger, *Reminiscences*, pp. 38–43, and *Freud/Jung*, May 23, 1912, et seq., pp. 508ff. See also letter 316 and n. 2.

302

Vienna, May 30, 1912
IX., Berggasse 19

Dear friend,

I think you have now found the only correct technique, and I am very happy about that.

I should also give you news from the remaining areas of human interest.

Yes, I was really in Constance from Saturday noon until Monday noon. I had been promising Binswanger a visit for a long time, was received like the dear Lord, also saw Stockmayer[1] and a couple of younger doctors, was in the festive company of the Queen Widow,[2] who sits enthroned on Estate Brunegg above Kreuzlingen. The next estate, ten minutes farther up, is Zeppelin's.[3] I saw Arenenberg, where Napoleon the Third spent his youth,[4] on a nice, long automobile trip with Binswanger and Stockmayer on the afternoon of Whitsun, which slowly brightened up. The area around the lake is a garden, Constance is magically, beautifully situated, really at the point on Lake Constance where the Rhine flows out; Hohentwiel, known from Ekkehard,[5] the tower of Radolfzell,[6] the island of Reichenau; everything comes together there.

Of course you know Binswanger to be highly respectable, serious, and honest; he has little talent, knows it, and is very modest. He read aloud to me part of a paper of his, in which ΨA is compared with clinical psychiatry and which is based on good points of view. We also talked about Jung, and he informed me that, although he is close to him as a pupil, he never expects anything from him in the way of personal affection. He [Jung] is not a leader of men, strongly attracts men and then repels them with his coldness and lack of consideration. But he is also irreplaceable.

The three days were very good for me, despite two nights on the train and constant strain there. From now on I am also cutting down on my work somewhat and ceasing science altogether. In Munich, where I stayed from 10 to 12 at night, I even frightened old Privy Councillor Löwenfeld[7] out of his sleep, but was actually happier with his splendid wife, Babette. When I returned, I found requests for treatment from patients from Bolzano and Baku, and, if they come, I can do something for Reitler,[8] to whom I can also transfer a young woman from St. Petersburg from my practice for continuation with him. A letter from Riklin that I found made a painful impression. He writes that, as a consequence of the last newspaper campaign,[9] they lost ground in the city, so that he has little to do, and even Jung has experienced a letdown. I was also asked to send patients to Zurich, should the opportunity arise. I would really need threefold influence in the world to take care of all the necessities. Meanwhile, I am being avoided in Vienna more than ever. Heller relates that he doesn't trust himself to recommend Imago in his Viennese circle because he would lose customers. The subscriptions in Vienna are negligible compared to those in Germany; by the way, the child is doing very well; we have 194 subscribers, and that after the first issue. The Zentralblatt is not far from 500.

I don't think they have behaved adroitly in Zurich. Jung has been letting things slip there in the skill department, and that's probably the reason why he has also written so little about it.

Even before my departure Jokes[10] and the second Collection[11] were published in new editions, unchanged, and that's why I'm not sending you a copy. In Jokes there are a few minor insertions, mostly from Brill's paper.[12] Emden left at the same time as I, and on Monday I am expecting Oberholzer[13] from Schaffhausen for treatment. The Society was closed yesterday, but will convene unofficially every other Wednesday, and, when Jones is here,[14] it will hold its customary summer festival. Before Whitsun there was another ugly scene between Tausk, who is a wild beast, and Stekel, which had all kinds of epilogues as a consequence.[15] Stekel has become negligent in attendance lately, evidently doesn't feel comfortable, and, since he is still in contact with Adler, surprises seem to me to be not out of the question. So, good and bad are mixing together.

Our summer (to Karlsbad and Lovrana) is still quite uncertain. My mother is still ill with a severe neuritis with herpes zoster,[16] although it is hardly serious. I have run dry for today and now greet you cordially in expectation of news from you.

Yours truly,
Freud

1. Wolf Stockmayer (1881–1933), Robert Gaupp's assistant at the University Clinic in Tübingen and member of the Swiss Society; a personal friend of Jung's. He was in Berlin from the end of 1913 on (*Freud/Abraham*, November 4, 1913, p. 154); later active as an analytical psychologist in Stuttgart.

2. Nickname of Binswanger's mother-in-law, who lived on the family estate (Jones II, 92).

3. Count Ferdinand von Zeppelin (1838–1917), builder of the airship named after him.

4. Napoleon III (1808–1873) was president of the Second French Republic (1852–1870). His mother, Hortense (née Beauharnais), fleeing with her children, had finally settled in the castle of Arenenberg after staying in various places.

5. Hohentwiel is both a volcanic peak in the Hegau and a castle named after it, first occupied in the tenth century. It is the setting for Joseph Victor von Scheffel's (1826–1886) principal work *Ekkehard, Eine Geschichte aus dem zehnten Jahrhundert*, a novel published in 1855. Scheffel, who wrote mainly historical fiction, was one of the most widely read authors of the nineteenth century.

6. The so-called Hell Tower, a medieval fortified tower.

7. Leopold Löwenfeld (1847–1924), psychiatrist in Munich. In 1895 Freud had been involved in a scientific controversy with him over the sexual etiology of anxiety neurosis which ended "in our becoming friends and we have remained so to this day" (Freud 1916–17a, p. 245).

8. Rudolf Reitler (1865–1917), Viennese physician, founding member of the Wednesday Society.

9. See letter 275 and n. 6.

10. Freud, *Der Witz und seine Beziehung zum Unbewussten* (1905c), 2d ed. (Vienna, 1912).

11. The second edition of the *Sammlung kleiner Schriften zur Neurosenlehre (2. Folge)* (Leipzig, 1912).

12. Freud had taken a few examples in foreign languages (1905c, pp. 21f, 31, 33) from

an article by Brill, "Freud's Theory of Wit," *Journal of Abnormal Psychology* 6 (1911): 279–316.

13. Emil Oberholzer (1883–1958), a member of the Zurich group. After Jung's split he became the co-founder, in 1919, of the Swiss Society for Psychoanalysis, which is still in existence today, serving as its first president until 1927. In that year he founded his own purely medical psychoanalytic group, which dissolved after his emigration in 1938. He moved with his wife, the child analyst Mira Gincburg (1887–1949), to New York, where he became a member of the Society there.

14. Jones spent the summer in Vienna with his mistress Loe Kann, who was analyzed by Freud (Jones II, 93, and Jones, *Associations*, p. 197).

15. Victor Tausk (1879–1919) became a lawyer and judge in Croatia after studying law in Vienna; from 1906 to 1908 he was active as a writer and journalist in Berlin. In 1908 he went to Vienna, where he studied medicine and eventually became a psychiatrist (1914). Tausk is considered a pioneer in the psychoanalytic investigation of psychoses; see e.g., his essay "Über die Entstehung des 'Beeinflussungsapparates' in der Schizophrenie," *Zeitschrift* 5 (1919): 1–33. For the relations between him, Freud, and Lou Andreas-Salomé (see letter 325, n. 3) and the motives for his suicide, see Paul Roazen, *Brother Animal: The Story of Freud and Tausk* (New York, 1969), and Kurt R. Eissler, *Talent and Genius* (New York, 1971). Tausk was to have taken over the discussion section of the *Zentralblatt*, but Stekel declared that "he would never allow Dr. Tausk to write in *his* journal" (letter 332; see also Jones II, p. 136). According to a version of the story presented by Freud and Federn in 1929 (*Protokolle der Wiener Psychoanalytischen Vereiningung* [Frankfurt, 1976–1981], IV, 108f), Stekel provoked this incident in order to force Freud out of the *Zentralblatt* and to be able to take it over himself. There is no such statement in the English edition *(Minutes)* [Trans.].

16. Inflammation of the nerves and shingles.

303

Budapest, June 5, 1912
VII., Erzsébet-körút 54

Dear Professor,

Many thanks for your interesting information; I am pleased that you spent the Whitsun holiday so pleasantly.

I have been shaken by a kind of scientific fever. I read a little book by *Otto te Kloot* about "The Thinking Horses" (Hans, Muhammed, and Zarif) (ed. Berlin, Wilh. Borngraeber),[1] in which remarkable mathematical achievements of these horses are described (deriving square and cube roots, division, subtraction of large numbers). I am convinced that in these (in my view, flawlessly correct) experiments, *induction* plays the main role. That would be a proof of the correctness of my supposition that animals and primitive people, in which the cs. did not hypertrophy at the expense of the instincts, are better instructed about events in their surroundings than we are. (*Prof. Edinger's*[2] attempt at an explanation touches on the possibility of induction.) The ucs. Ψ. is an organ for physiological qualities, i.e., for *physical* quantities, just as the cs. is an organ for ucs. ψ. qualities.

So, there are two ways to learn new things about the psyche and about nature:

1. An individual with a developed cs. organ (combinatory talent) observes and organizes manifestations of lifeless and instinctive beings (of crystals, plants, mediums, soothsayers, mythmakers, neurotics, savages, animals, etc.), or

2. An individual unites in himself the instinctive and the cs. in high development.

That would be the "genius."

Even if this theory is false: this much (in the event that the experiments on horses prove to be well founded) remains firm, that these animals possess the capacity for induction in an enormously heightened fashion. We humans can only activate the rudiments of it.

Let us first give up the hope of learning more about *nature* with the help of *animals* than we were capable of with our one-sidedly hypertrophied psyche; we can certainly learn very much from them about the activity of the ucs. Ψ itself!

It is obviously high time to go public with the induction experiments. Otherwise someone will get ahead of me, and without using the analytic points of view!

Shouldn't I write a volume on it for the "Schriften zur angewandten Seelenkunde"?

I would be happy to be free of this responsibility so that I can return to psychoanalysis undisturbed by outside problems.

Perhaps I will take a week's vacation to visit the Pythia in Berlin,[3] as well as the Elberfeld horses, before I write up the transference experiments. It would certainly be awkward for me to review the vast occultistic literature. It is certain that the ψ.α. point of view has not yet been expressed there.

I envision the work as consisting of four chapters:

1.) The exact description of the experiments. 2.) The analytic attempts at explanation, at the same time confirmation of analytic assumptions about the nature of the ucs. 3.) Conditions for the success of such experiments (unfortunately, I don't know very much about that). 4.) Attempt at forming a theory.[4]

Kind regards,
Ferenczi

1. Otto te Kloot, *Die denkenden Pferde; Hans, Muhammad, und Zariff* (Berlin, 1912). The Shetland pony Hänschen and the horses Mohammed and Zarif, which could supposedly solve mathematical problems, were attracting attention in Germany at the time.

See also Krall, *Denkende Tiere* (Leipzig, 1912), and H. V. Buttel-Reepen, *Meine Erfahrung mit "denkenden" Pferden* (Jena, 1913).

2. Ludwig Edinger (1855–1918), professor of neurology at the University of Frankfurt and author with Edouarde Claparède (see letter 360, n. 2) of *Über Tierpsychologie* (Leipzig, 1909).

3. Frau Seidler (see letter 73 and n. 2).

4. No such work by Ferenczi could be confirmed. But see Dr. W. B., "Gibt es denkende Pferde?" *Zentralblatt* 3 (1912–13): 629–630.

304

Vienna, June 6, 1912
IX., Berggasse 19

Dear friend,

I like it very much. I also don't want to hold you back any longer. But don't take only a week's vacation, take two weeks; study everything you need and write the volume for me, publication of which I will expedite as quickly as possible. What do you think of the title: The Ucs. and Thought Transference? The term induction is not well enough known by the public. I don't know what you think about the necessity of reaching an agreement with Jung before publication. I believe you promised that; it also means no further influence on his part.

Just yesterday I got out your suggestions for the second edition of the "Recommendations." I will have to open the new volume with an essay of that sort.[1]

Maybe when you go on your trip your path will take you to Vienna for an evening.

There is probably some connection between your scientific plan and your silence about family matters.

In a hurry, so that you won't be held up by waiting for my reply,

With kind regards,
Freud

1. See letter 285 and n. 2. Freud had originally intended to publish his second treatise on the recommended techniques of psychoanalysis ("On Beginning the Treatment," 1913c), as well as the first (1912e), in the *Zentralblatt*. Because of the conflict with Stekel, who thereafter continued to publish the *Zentralblatt* alone (see letter 332 and n. 1), Freud launched the newly founded *Internationale Zeitschrift für ärztliche Psychoanalyse* with his essay in 1913.

305

Budapest, June 10, 1912
VII., Erzsébet-körút 54

Dear Professor,

You have correctly interpreted my scientific enthusiasm. At the moment of writing the letter I didn't know it yet, but soon thereafter it became clear to me that displacements in my libidinal cathexis are in process. The analysis with Elma is going very, very slowly; she is clearly forcing herself to do it and is using (mostly ucs.) every opportunity for obstruction. In the last few days she suddenly started talking about "feelings of regret" (with respect to her mother); of course, I knew immediately that she has become tired of the thing and that the marriage does, in fact, not mean as much to her as the analysis is painful. A fantasy of being abandoned *by me* confirmed my supposition. Accordingly, I am inwardly taking (and have already ucs. taken) measures to organize myself without her and without marriage.—My tender relationship with Frau G. is in part regaining its value, and my scientific interest is increasing.—In today's hour Elma was quite ill; she didn't say a word; I think she is struggling inwardly but doesn't have the courage to make a decision. She would obviously prefer to have me send her away, but I won't do that, in her interest. She should at least profit from the affair to the extent that she comes to an independent decision; otherwise a "feeling of inferiority" would be left behind. But it is even now not *completely* out of the question that a change will take place in her at the last minute; were that to happen, then I would naturally still consider whether I should build my house on such a shaky foundation. For me, personally, this year of trial has also not been without lasting value; I have learned how little one is capable on one's own of evaluating one's theoretical knowledge about mental processes and one's practical experiences with third persons, if one doesn't analyze oneself just as methodically.

June 14

This letter seemed to characterize my mood of the moment, but not the total condition of my inner self; for that reason I didn't mail it. In the meantime the following occurred: Frau G., who has difficulty bearing her daughter's suffering in analysis, talked her into accepting the invitation of a lady of her acquaintance who wants to take her to England with her. Elma said *no*, but seemed to want to make the decision dependent on me. I refused, of course, to make the decision, and explained to her that she had to do that herself. At the same time I spoke with her about my trip to Berlin and about the fact that (since the analysis is going very slowly and certainly has to be continued in the fall] I want to take the fall trip with you [which I actually intend to do, as long as you are in agreement].[1] It was a great effort for me to maintain my composure in the face of the despair which she subsequently fell into. If I had wavered, the scene of the engagement would have had to be repeated. But I remained strong, even though I had to feel that it is still very difficult to renounce her and the thoughts about marriage. In retrospect, however, I am glad I acted as I did. It will soon (?) have to become apparent whether Elma can now decide to work properly on her analysis or whether she decides to give it up altogether. If she holds fast to her policy of obstruction, then I will, in fact, be forced to end the matter once and for all.

I am working a great deal. Eight hours of analysis, two sets of office hours (Health Service and private hours). In the evenings I am usually too tired to work, especially since the hours with Elma take their toll on me.

I am now working on a retort to Putnam's philosophical article. The reply will be very polite and in part appreciative, but basically it will be decidedly negative.[2]

I intend to take the trip to Berlin around June 26; I want to be there about ten days; I will certainly reserve an evening for Vienna and am very much looking forward to our meeting. I will write Jung a short letter only after Berlin.

In anticipation of news from you, I am

Yours,
Ferenczi

1. Enclosed in brackets in the original.
2. James Putnam, "Über die Bedeutung philosophischer Anschauungen und Aus- bildung für die weitere Entwicklung der psychoanalytischen Bewegung," *Imago* 1 (1912): 101–118; Ferenczi, "Philosophie und Psychoanalyse" [Philosophy and Psycho-Analysis] (1912, 93; *Fin.*, p. 326; *Imago* 1 [1912]: 519–526).

306

Budapest [undated,
presumably summer 1912][1]
VII., Erzsébet-körút 54

Dear Professor,

I feel obliged to report on events within me and around me. In general, I had some more insight into illness, with respect to both present as well as past events.

First, I must confirm that my cruelty and severity toward Frau G. could be infantile revenge against my mother. My mother was, up to my father's death, strict and, according to the way I felt at the time and as I do now, often unjust. I have conscious recollections of "fantasies of being abandoned" and bitter fantasies of revenge from my seventh to eighth year.— Poor Frau G. has to atone for everything.—I totally appreciate *consciously* her noble, magnanimous, self-sacrificing behavior in this, the most difficult time of her life—but my inner emotion remains absent or manifests itself only negligibly. With me it is as with so many people who cannot weep at the death of their father or mother. I am glad if I can squeeze out a tear with great effort or if, as was the case when I read G.'s especially touching letter of farewell—some sadness and the feeling of severe loss is stirred up in me.—Along with this infantile desire for revenge, however, my behavior may also in part be influenced by the fact that in the last four years, since I have been testing myself analytically, I have actually been carrying on a continuing struggle for liberation against my maternal fixation. During this time I have constantly sought to come to grips with painful insights that have to do with Frau G.'s age and the sexual intercourse with her that is not entirely satisfying physically. Thus, I have only distributed the pain that I am now missing over a longer period of time, but I have not been spared it altogether.

I have up to now conscientiously carried out the plan that originated in the Türkenschanzpark.[2] Monday evening I gave a lecture. Frau G. and Elma were present. Elma was very disconcerted and was prepared for something bad when I told her she was not allowed to come to me on Tuesday but should expect a visit from me. On Tuesday there was a passionate farewell scene; I released Elma, but told her that I would perhaps return in a few months. On Wednesday I received a letter from her that reads as follows: [I translated the entire letter so that you will get to know Elma better.][3] "Tuesday night. I promise you, Sándor, that I won't write to you anymore, not even on Sundays [allusion], never. Only today do I still want to speak to you. I understand completely that it had to come to this. I am writing you today because I feel that I will no longer be as close to you as I am today, and out of this closeness I would like to tell you what I am feeling. I don't know what my feelings mean. You probably know it better than I, and that is why you wanted us to part. I know quite certainly that you will not come to get me. And yet I have such a terrible anxiety about it. This being alone that now awaits me will be stronger than I; I feel almost as if everything will freeze inside me. I will remain reasonable, but it will be so cold in me, I will freeze so much that I will also have to hate this last refuge, reason.

"I am considering the following: if you were sure of yourself and myself, you would not have done what you did now. Therefore you want something to change in yourself or in me. Isn't that right? So, things are not good the way they are. You want to wait until something changes in us. Perhaps you even prefer that I forget you (even if you love me); you would perhaps rather suffer a little than warm up to the idea that we should stay together. You are so very right! It would be a pity for your life and your future if all your hopes were not fulfilled. You know me, of course, and you know that there is no relying on me. I even think a little bit that you would perhaps not be sorry if I estranged myself from you spiritually; that would be a kind of relief for you. Or maybe not? Perhaps you will be able to forget me without pangs of conscience—as soon as I am no longer suffering?! Or did you push through the divorce[4] because you still love Mother, very much, in fact, and suddenly you can't do without her? Believe me, if it were only a matter of me and not just of you and Mother, I wouldn't be able to bear it. I told you how terribly impatient I am, how I burn with desire. It is a very, very good thing for me to be with you; I don't think there could be anything better. If you will just accept from me the fact that I could live for you, even then I will not be able to show you how much I would like to be to you. I am even very much afraid of that. I love you differently than anybody else who has been close to me up to now. I also feel really a little like your child, so much do I wish to be led by you. Only if we had our child could I feel as if I were your wife. I long for this time very much, but I don't believe it will ever come. Now that you are leaving me, I don't believe it. For that proves to me that you want to change what we are now. I can do no more than give you my body and soul. I know that I can think independently and should judge our situation critically. Perhaps, far away from you, I will gain the self-sufficiency that I lost completely with respect to you but can't do without at all. What do you think, will it be good if I now consciously settle accounts with every little thing, take care of every- thing—and in the meantime the greatest part of my devotion crumbles— which is the main thing anyway? Or can both tendencies be brought into harmony?

"Why did you leave me now? I was afraid of it—and still I didn't believe that it would ever come. I thought, you know me, you see into me so far, so that you know that I can't live alone. If I am alone, I will cease to exist. If that also happens now with respect to you, then I will experience the greatest misfortune that can strike me from within. I thought to myself: you know all that and will not leave me, in order that that doesn't happen. If it doesn't come to that, then no one will be happier than I, and I will wait for you as long as I want—I will not even feel that this time is a time of waiting. But if I stand there with empty hands, with an empty soul after a few weeks—I will not be able to survive this one thing. And yet I know that you don't want to know anything but whether this comes true or not, and you are making our fate dependent upon it. Or am I deceiving myself?

"Why subject myself to the danger that this test will exceed my strength? Do you wish that, perhaps? Or are you also afraid of it?

"Talk about yourself, for once; up to now you have been talking only about me!

[Now comes the story that Elma had a talk with her mother. This arouses her conscience, and she asks me to leave her be and return to her mother, who shouldn't be condemned to staying with her father for the rest of her life.]

"Look, Sándor—there's no harm done to me; I will go to Rome [to her aunts] or to Liebautal [to her previous fiancé]—or wherever; you will marry Mother, forget this episode in your life, and you will live whole and without regret. I don't believe Mother when she says you don't love her anymore.

"Write to me once, one single time, honestly, the way one speaks to an adult, and tell me what you really feel. You'll do that, won't you; then I will be able to live much more in peace. I always want to be with Mother. All inhibition between us must disappear. I want to learn how to speak for her sake—she has no one but me. Unfortunately, with talk one can mitigate only feelings, not facts.

"I don't want to write any empty phrases at the end. I only want to say to you that I pity you if you are suffering. You are suffering because of desolation and because of Mother—and not because of me. Isn't that right?

"Tell me: do you think I could ever bring you happiness?

"It is so terrible to take leave of you now. I won't write to you anymore, since I know that you don't want me to.

"Reply today. Write about yourself.

"And I thank you for everything; I often cannot talk because I have the feeling that I am living in you; everything that I am revolves around you."

I replied tenderly to Elma, but I held fast to my resolve, told her about countertransference and about the necessity to wait and see whether my love for her (—which I hope—) will conquer the distance in space and time, and only then can I build our future on it.—

Three days passed in the meantime. I felt calmed—not at all passionate. I was even astounded by this and thought to myself whether my ucs. didn't just use this whole setup in order to get free of Frau G. "respectably"?—But the matter actually doesn't seem to be so simple. The days of crisis are over, and I catch myself more and more often in fantasies about being married to Elma.

Frau G. is still urging me, a little, to hurry, but she is—as always—friendly, despite her great pain.

Kind regards and

Thankfully yours,
Ferenczi

1. This letter was found in the photostat folder at the end of the year 1912, along with the following note (in English) from Balint: "Without date. Possibly about summer 1912." It was difficult to place it in sequence with certainty, because, on the one hand, several factors in letters 258, 259, and 306 (such as Freud's thanks for the "detailed communication," the "test" for the girl, the plan in the Türkenschanzpark, etc.) speak in favor of a significantly earlier placement, namely between letters 257 and 258 (mid-December 1911); on the other hand, Freud's remark about keeping the relationship between Frau G. and Ferenczi quiet (in letter 259), for instance, do not agree with some of Elma's statements in the letter which Ferenczi translated. Stationery, ink, and pen do not give any indication as to the correct date. After careful consideration (and in order to avoid confusion in the numbering with regard to the French edition, already published) the editor and transcriber have decided to keep this letter in its present position.

2. A park in Währing, a district adjacent to Freud's home district, Alsergrund.

3. Enclosed in brackets in the original, as are similar remarks throughout the letter.

4. Gizella's divorce from her husband.

307

Vienna, June 23, 1912
IX., Berggasse 19

Dear friend,

These last two weeks were the most work all year. Even on Sunday, not a trace of freedom. This only as an excuse.

I am very eager to hear your news and also which evening you want to spend with us. It remains firm that we will travel together in September, if you don't have anything better to do. Brill also wants to visit us around this time and will probably join us for a while. But where are we going?

I approve very much in spirit of your paper against Putnam. You remain the one who wants to put the bell around the cat's neck. But recently I energetically came to your defense against Bleuler.[1]

The news here is the presence of Pfister and Jones, both of whom also participated in the evening on the Konstantinhügel. Pfister was asked by my grand patient[2] to help for a week with a withdrawal process. He is worthy, as always; his love story[3] is not going well, also something like the situation where the girl doesn't really know her feelings. He knew little of an intimate nature about Zurich because he is not being taken into confidence much there, but even according to his information, there is no doubt about the independence movement there. Jones brought me his wife[4] for preliminary treatment, for which he has finally obtained her agreement;

he will stay here with her for the three weeks. She is an extremely intelligent, deeply neurotic Jewess, whose case history is very easy to read. I will be very pleased to be able to expend much libido for her. Jones has also estranged himself from Jung, since he got no replies to his letters to him. I spoke openly with both of them—Pfister and Jones—about the affair, but I think that's enough for now.

Jung's summons to America[5] shouldn't be anything good. A little, unknown *Catholic* university run by Jesuits, which Jones had turned down. Jones holds it against him that he gave up the Congress because of that and calls me to account about why I haven't taken over the direction of the Congress in his stead. I hadn't thought about it and later came up with the response that such a suggestion could only have come from Jung himself.—

Science is naturally quiescent in me; I am happy that I have stood up so well to daily work. In three weeks I will be in Karlsbad with my wife, where I will again find the company of van Emden and wife. A single thought[6] that will amuse you was that the introductory scene in Lear must mean the same as the selection scene in the Merchant of Venice. Three caskets are the same as three women, three sisters. The third is always the correct choice. But this third one is peculiar, she doesn't speak, or she hides (Cinderella!), she is mute. Do you remember the words of the song of Paris in "Beautiful Helena"?

> And the third—yes, the third—
> stood beside them and remained mute.
> I must give her the apple.
> You, oh Kalchas, you know why.[7]

So, the motif of the choice between three sisters, the third of whom is mute. With a few associations I came out with the idea that they are the three—sisters of destiny, the Fates, the third of whom is mute, because she—symbolizes death (Stekel).[8] The *compulsion* of fate is transformed into the motif of *selection*. Cordelia, who loves and is silent, is thus actually death. The situation of Lear with Cordelia's corpse in his arms should be reversed, the old man in the arms of the Fate of death. The three Fates are woman in her three principal manifestations: the one who gives birth, the one who gives pleasure, and the one who spoils; or mother, lover, and Mother Earth = death. Later I got out the fact that the Trinity is derived from the *horae*,[9] i.e., from the seasons, of which the ancients at first only distinguished three. Thus, transferred from vegetation onto the destiny of man.

Kind regards,
Freud

1. Bleuler had criticized Ferenczi on May 5, 1912, in a letter to Freud (Library of Congress). Ferenczi's theories of homosexuality and his hostile criticism of Bleuler on the question of alcohol (see letter 245 and n. 4) caused the latter to doubt whether Ferenczi was capable of observing objectively.

2. Frau Hirschfeld (see letter 269, n. 2).

3. See letter 280 and n. 3.

4. Jones's morphine-addicted mistress, Loe Kann (?–1945), who used his name although they were not married (Jones, *Associations*, pp. 139f). Freud and Jones subsequently corresponded about her analysis; the letters were published in part in Brome, *Jones*.

5. See letter 318, n. 5.

6. Freud published an essay developing this idea a year later under the title "The Theme of the Three Caskets" (1913f).

7. "Und die dritte—ja, die dritte— / stand daneben und blieb stumm. / Ihr musst ich den Apfel geben / Du, oh Kalchas, weisst warum." From the libretto by Meilhac and Halévy to Offenbach's operetta *La Belle Hélène*, act 1, sc. 7.

8. Wilhelm Stekel, *Die Sprache des Traumes* (Vienna, 1911), p. 351.

9. Latin for "hours," the designation for hourly prayers in the Catholic church; the term also connotes natural divisions of time or seasons [Trans.].

308

Berlin, July 3, 1912[1]

Dear Professor,

After complete failure of the induction experiments with Frau Seidler (she didn't want to place herself at my disposal at all), I am traveling immediately to *Freising* (Bavaria) to Prof. Staudenmayer[2] and then home by way of Vienna.

Kind regards,
Ferenczi

1. Picture postcard; the caption reads "Berlin Sieges-Allee."

2. Ludwig Staudenmaier (1865–1933), German chemist; author of works on "experimental magic"; see *Minutes* III, 74 and 128–130 (November 30, 1910, and January 18, 1911).

309

Vienna, July 4, 1912
IX., Berggasse 19

Dear friend,

I imagine that you are at work and will soon have better things to note down. Nothing much new from here. Rank's book on incest[1] was published, very impressive and, I think, very good. In the last two weeks I have had one and a half hours' less work per day, but I am not any more productive.

Everything that comes from Zurich or reports about it speaks of a bad situation there. Oberholzer, Pfister, Binswanger are meeting under the sign of Jung's rebellion, which makes the future very uncertain. He hasn't written back to me for two weeks. Now he is preaching against the analytic activity of laymen, after he himself led Pfister to analysis.

Many thanks to your brother from all of us.[2]

I submitted your paper against Putnam to Rank unaltered. You can still insert some moderation in the proofs that you send to Putnam prior to publication.

When you see Abraham give him my best, but do *not* remind him of his prophecy, "That man in his ambition will yet ruin everything."[3]

I wish you the most astonishing success and await news from you.

Yours truly,
Freud

1. Otto Rank, *Das Inzest-Motiv in Dichtung und Sage, Grundzüge einer Psychologie des dichterischen Schaffens* (Leipzig, 1912).

2. The reason for this remark is unclear.

3. Evidently an allusion to Jung, whom Abraham had on several occasions described to Freud as ambitious; see e.g., *Freud/Abraham*, July 16, 1908, and August 9, 1912, pp. 44f and 121. This particular quotation does not come from the published correspondence, however.

310

Budapest, July 12, 1912
VII., Erzsébet-körút 54

Dear Professor,

It's no use! I will already have to accept the year 1911/12 as a critical one, and for the time being I will have to give up dedicating my time to pursuits other than solving my intricate personal affairs.—The most recent events are as follows: The letter which I mentioned to you in Vienna and in which Frau G. wrote to me, among other things, that, even though she has lost me, she will eternally remain true to you and the cause should already have made me suspect something bad. But it was not until the day before yesterday that the matter became clear to me, when I had a rather long talk with Frau G.—It came out that I expected too much from her when I (tacitly) condemned her to wait quietly for what will come out of Elma's analysis, and made both their fates dependent on it.—Now, she told me herself that she had overestimated her strength when she thought she could reconcile herself to the possibility that in future perhaps only the spiritual and tender component of our relationship would be maintained; she had decided she would rather renounce everything and make a clean sweep of things. Evidently this plan had been brewing in her for a long time, until it was voiced the day before yesterday. The next result was a distressing scene between the both of us which ended with her decision to come again tomorrow (Saturday). It became rather clear to us that the ties that bind us are too strong to tear apart as a result of a conscious willful decision.—I think that Frau G.—and this shouldn't be held against her—accepted the blow and the humiliation that she suffered then all too gracefully, and that the repression at the time is to blame for the fact that she is now losing patience; this is happening at a time when I was and am on the best path of allowing myself not to be forced into any unthinking action, but rather of judging Elma's case with medical detachment, whereby the chances of a final return to Frau G. are significantly improved.—

In the meantime, it is also coming out more and more in Elma's analysis that Frau G., especially during my absence, was hinting that Elma should break off the analysis because I don't love her the way she wishes. I am firmly convinced that Frau G. did not act in this out of consciously egoistic motives, but rather that she is keeping her daughter's welfare in mind. But she could also have thought that I was of a mind to take her welfare into consideration as well, and she should have proceeded in concert with me.—As a result of these innuendos, the relationship between mother and daughter is tense: Elma doesn't dare to talk about me in front of her mother, but because of that, of course, a general inhibition has set in between both of them.—Meanwhile, the analysis is going (more correctly, was going) rather normally; Elma began to tell me more honestly about her sexual fantasies and dreams, but without bringing in anything basically new. I maintained the proper medical posture with respect to her, was hoping gradually to deepen the analysis, which had progressed so favorably in Vienna, and in the meantime also to make up my mind about the future.—

The intermezzo with Frau G. is complicating the situation to a certain extent. I certainly hope that I will be successful in getting my way with her in that she will not only give up her intention of breaking with me but will also continue to be helpful with the analysis of Elma.

In the meantime I also have to watch myself so that I don't allow myself to be forced into some unthinking action. My premature decision to marry Elma could become just as fateful to me as my temporarily insincere breaking off of relations with her—or with both women, for that matter! You see, matters have come to a head, and the word now is to watch out until the coast is clear.—

The accumulated upsets and stimulations of the last few days have produced in me an almost disagreeable increase in sexual libido. After long vacillation, I decided to get relief by the normal way of prostitution. I also succeeded in overcoming my inhibitions to it, and—despite all the disgust that went along with it—I must say that since then I am thinking and acting more coolly and with less passion.

I just received the news from Fräulein Minna[1] about your summer plans. I am very much in agreement with everything!

Best regards,
Dr. Ferenczi

1. This letter from Minna Bernays is missing; for the travel plans, see letter 312 and n. 9.

311

[Karlsbad,] July 16, 1912[1]

Dear friend,

Letter received. Best regards to Mrs.[2] G.—

Arrived yesterday, started cure today, expecting interesting visitor from Hamburg tomorrow.[3]

Cordially,
Freud

1. Picture postcard; the caption reads: "Karlsbad, Etbl. Freundschaftssaal [Friendship Hall]."
2. "Mrs." is written in English in the original [Trans.].
3. A visit from Max Halberstadt (1882–1940), fiancé of Freud's daughter Sophie (1893–1920).

312

Budapest, July 18, 1912
VII., Erzsébet-körút 54

Dear Professor,

On the assumption that the establishment "Freundschaftssaal" on your picture postcard signifies your place of residence, I am sending this letter to that address; sending it by registered mail will compensate for my uncertainty about it.

Now, on to personal matters.

The discussion with Frau G. led to the result that what Elma said about her mother's resentful statements about the analysis were grossly exaggerated, and had been placed into the service of her own resistances toward analysis. Evidently *she* (Elma) doesn't want the analysis, but would like that not she herself but I or Frau G. should be responsible for stopping the treatment.—I put that to her, and she finally admitted that she (Elma) was beginning to lose patience; I told her that nothing could be changed in the method; *c'est à prendre ou à laisser.*[1] At the same time I told her that she had never worked properly since her return from Vienna, but had tried to apply her old arts of seduction and wanted to realize the decision to marry. She had been obstructive the whole time. I frankly admitted having made big mistakes in the last analysis (before Vienna) by accepting her mostly neurotic advances as real, but that *now* I was quite sure of myself, so that she finally had to give up "seducing" me away from the proper analytic path for the second time.

All this has had a shattering effect on her, but it really couldn't have been avoided. The impression of the first (technically incorrect) analysis could only be mitigated in this somewhat brutal manner, that is, through a second *experience.*—

Oddly, she reacted to it with the admission that she had in part only feigned her interest in psychoanalysis, but was still inwardly dominated by a strong sexual aversion. There is a hint here of a way toward further progress in analysis.—

But it is questionable whether it will come to that; possibly her defiance will win the day and she will achieve her goal of breaking off the analysis, wrathful and insulted. I would be sorry about that. I would rather we could part good friends; which, by the way, is not entirely out of the question.—

As far as I am concerned, the matter stands as follows:

I am (especially in the ucs.) not yet free of longingly libidinous feelings with respect to Elma, but I have this inclination under strict control; she, incidentally, expresses herself only at times, especially when I have to hurt her and bring her to tears. Afterwards I am always glad that I remained firm. I see otherwise more and more clearly how unreasonable I was when I thoughtlessly wanted to marry her; I see her weaknesses more and more clearly since my sexual overestimation has diminished in intensity. By the same token, Frau G.'s really rare qualities again become more valuable to me, even though I have learned to do without things that I can't have from her.

Analytic signs speak in favor of the fact that what attracted me to Elma was not only the possibility of founding a family but that, ucs., her coquetry and ill temper (which was complex-determined in her) had an effect on me and thus also played the role of the one who brings death, who spoils. In puberty, the thought of death, which I had evidently strongly invested with libido, was on my mind night after night.

I have been letting the question of induction rest since the failed Berlin trip. The works of *Lotze* came into my hands by coincidence, and—despite the purely speculative mode of treatment—some remarkable points of agreement with the theory of repression appear in them. A few passages are positively stunning. I will quote you a few of them:

(Grundzüge der Psychologie, Vorträge im Wintersemester 1880/81)[2] "On the disappearance of ideas from the ucs." "... Two views opposed each other here. *Earlier* one considered the disappearance to be natural and believed the opposite, that one had to explain *memory. Now* one follows the analogy of the physicalistic law of inertia and believes that one has to explain *forgetting* ...

"... The mind finds itself in various states, according to whether it imagines *a,* or *b,* or nothing at all. It would therefore be conceivable that it works back against every impression imposed upon it, whereby it never, to be sure, totally annuls it, but could still perhaps transform it from a conscious feeling into an unconscious state ...

"... An idea of greater content by no means always represses one of smaller content; on the contrary, the latter is even capable of occasionally suppressing the sensation of external stimuli.—But now ideas never occur in a mind which does nothing else besides; but rather, every impression, besides being connected with what is *imagined* as a result of it, is also connected with a *feeling of value* which it has for the physical and mental well-being of the percipient. *These feelings of pleasure and unpleasure* are obviously just as capable of gradation as pure ideation is incapable of it.*) Now, according to the magnitude of this *portion of feeling,* which, incidentally, is extraordinarily changeable, according to the diversity of the total condition which the mind is in at the moment, or briefly said, according to the degree of *interest* which an idea may arouse for various reasons at every moment, its larger or lesser power directs itself at *repression* [*Verdrängung*] (sic!) of other ideas."—

In conclusion, Lotze says:

"These points of view can only be alleged in general. It is impossible, on the other hand, to form a theory from them that goes into particulars; and it is just as impossible in a particular case to really ascertain the reasons that have actually led to the course of our thoughts, which often seems so capricious."—

* This sentence, which seems rather unclear, relates to other chapters of Lotze's book.[3]

When I have the opportunity I want to write a little paper about the empirical confirmation of Lotze's suppositions by psychoanalysis.[4]

The little Rooster-Man recently produced something new. For some time he has shown unusual interest in *elderly Jews,* but ones that *have to be from the Temple.* He shows longing for them and at the same time terrible anxiety. Recently he wouldn't rest until they let such a man (a Jew with a beard) into the house; shyly and excitedly he danced around him (at some distance from him), didn't dare touch him, but cried when he went away.[5]

The "Society"[6] in London is urging me about my promised paper on Hypnosis.[7] I will write it one of these days.—

In reading Lotze's logic[8] I arrived at the view that what the logicians call *errors in thinking* are the *forms of thinking of the ucs..* I am now watching my neurotics and collecting examples.—

I hope the guest from Hamburg will leave behind favorable impressions; presumably the decision to cancel your stay in Italy[9] (which Fräulein Minna informed me about) relates to these events.

Please give my regards to your wife as well as to Herr and Frau van Emden, who are presumably already in Karlsbad.

Kind regards,
Ferenczi

1. French for "Take it or leave it."

2. Rudolf Hermann Lotze (1817–1881), German philosopher and physician, was a professor of philosophy at Göttingen (from 1844) and Berlin (1881). His philosophy sought to combine research in natural science with speculative and religious goals. Ferenczi is referring to Lotze's *Grundzüge der Psychologie, Dictate aus den Vorlesungen* (Leipzig, 1881). The quotations are from chapter 2, "Über den Verlauf der Vorstellungen" [On the Course of Ideas], in the fourth edition (1889), pp. 21f, 24f, 23.

3. Ibid., chap. 6, "Von den Gefühlen" [On Feelings].

4. Ferenczi, "Aus der 'Psychologie' von Hermann Lotze" (1913, 108).

5. See "Ein kleiner Hahnemann" [A Little Chanticleer] (1913, 114; *C.*, p. 251), *Schriften* I, 170f.

6. Written in English in the original [Trans.].

7. See letter 295 and n. 5.

8. Hermann Lotze, *Logik, Drei Bücher vom Denken, vom Untersuchen und vom Erkennen* (Leipzig, 1874).

9. After giving up his intention of spending his vacation in Italy, Freud planned to travel with Ferenczi and Rank to London for a week in the fall and then with Ferenczi

to Scotland for an additional week (see Jessie Taft, *Otto Rank* [New York, 1958], p. 65, and letter 320); but he got to spend his vacation in the South Tyrol and Rome after all (see letter 323 n. 2).

313

Karslbad, July 20, 1912

Dear friend,

We are living here in the *"Goldener Schlüssel"* [Golden Key]. "Freund-schaftssaal" is our breakfast room. The young man's visit naturally ended with an acknowledgment of the engagement, which is supposed to be made public on the 28th of this month in the *Neue Presse*. There you have an at-the-time unintended overdetermination to the motif of the "three sisters" or three daughters.[1]

I am very glad to hear that you have remained consistently firm against Elma and have thwarted her tricks. It can only work in that way, if it works at all. It was a strong step on your part to get beyond the infantile confines.

ΨA lies far behind me in an unreal glow, although conversations with Emden promise to arouse it from its sleep. This time the cure has had no bad general effects as in the previous year, but I am completely closed off intellectually. The Emdens thank you for your greeting; they are, as always, charming company. We are very amused by the reports about the meeting of the Dutch neurologists on the 3rd of this month,[2] in which he appeared for the first time as a beginner. The presenter Boumann[3] was half convinced, by the way. I have news from Brill. He can be here in September, but he will not be able to stay with us for the entire three weeks of the trip. I would not like to leave beautiful Lake Caldonazzo before September 10, and I expect that, if traveling doesn't bother you any more than before, you will also come see us there.

I have been hearing here, by way of Emden, about the book on thinking animals, and I have the impression that there is not yet a need for thought transference here. The intelligence of animals fits in splendidly with our views on cs. and ucs.

I have received no reply or other news from Jung for about five weeks, but I will also continue to maintain a passive attitude. I send kind regards in expectation of news from you.

Yours truly,
Freud

1. See letter 307 and n. 6.
2. The annual meeting of the Dutch Association for Neurology and Psychiatry on July 3, 1912. See the essay by A. S. (August Stärcke) in *Zeitschrift* 2 (1914): 188–191.
3. K. Herman Bouman (?–1947), professor of psychiatry and neurology at the University

of Amsterdam and director of the Wilhelmina Gasthuis Clinic there. He was a founding member (1917) of the Dutch Psychoanalytic Society.

314

Karlsbad, July 23, 1912[1]

Dear friend,

We are making a concerned inquiry about how you are holding out in the isolation of your hot city. You see, all of Budapest is here.

Yours truly,
Freud

[In Martha Freud's handwriting:]

Yes, indeed, we will soon be able to speak Hungarian, you have sent so many representatives of your beautiful idiom to us. Best regards.

Yours truly,
Martha Freud

[In other handwritings:]

Kind regards, Yours truly, *J. v. Emden.* And Frau v. *Emden.*

1. Postcard.

315

Budapest, July 26, 1912
VII., Erzsébet-körút 54

Dear Professor,

I have just (11:30 P.M.) returned to my lonely home from a solitary walk. On the way out my thoughts were really gloomy. I have reviewed the events of the previous year, occupied myself with the list of casualties, and had to conclude that giving up my (almost realized) fantasy with Elma and the analytic executioner's work with which I had to put this fantasy to death by myself still gives me considerable pain, which I have to make conscious at times. I saw the way back to Frau G. if not closed by the unavoidable consequences of my unfaithfulness and by the painful insight into the loosening of my feelings, then at least no longer accessible in the old sense.

It appears as if my walk of today was a symptomatic act. On the way back (which perhaps symbolized the way back into the old track), I began to consider the events somewhat more philosophically. I thought about the misfortune that I may be saving myself by renunciation; about science, which will certainly further unite me with Frau G.; about the gain in self-reliance and freedom of thought that I owe to these experiences. To be sure, I was not able to answer the question as to whether a lonely life without plans for the future will give me enough motivation for work.

The more assuredly I show Elma that I am treating her only as a patient, the more richly things come to the fore in her which she has hitherto carefully held back. The mistakes that I made in the first analysis have been more or less corrected; in fact—they had to be overcorrected to a certain extent, so that the impact becomes eradicated; certainly the continuation of the analysis will be made significantly more difficult thereby; poor Elma really gets no satisfaction from it, and it is questionable whether she will keep it up for long.

I want to supplement my little paper on hypnosis with a few small novelties.[1] I want to trace the *symptomatology of hypnosis* to the reawakening of capabilities which the child still has but the adult no longer has to the same degree. One can still bring the child to master individual *reflexes* (to regulate the release of urine and stool); if it had been socially necessary, then one would also probably have been able to bring other reflexes under the control of its will. And that is what the hypnotist does in hypnosis. The child learns to "bear" *pain* (= not feel); hypnotic anesthesia corresponds to that. It learns to direct its attention toward certain (outer and inner) impressions (hyperesthesia, hypermnesia). One also learns how to master vasomotor processes in youth (e.g., blushing); the hypnotic analogy to this is the abundance or lack of blood in individual parts of the body, produced by suggestion. Hypnotic *displays of strength* correspond to the exertions children make in order to please their parents (see the wonderful achievements of circus children). From this analogy I want to draw the conclusion that, when infantile complexes (thoughts and contents of feelings) get the upper hand in hypnosis, the neuropsychic system's infantile mode of functioning, especially *infantile teachability,* is once again aroused. This conception does, to be sure, take a large portion of the mystical and miraculous away from hypnotic experiments.—It is more or less comparable to Cohnheim's[2] theory of embryonic cells in cancer: scattered embryonic cells, when they become active, eat up the adult individual; embryonic complexes in hypnosis come to dominate the psyche of the adult and make its already atrophied mechanisms *temporarily plastic* and pliant again.

I am very much looking forward to the fall trip; I hope I can also come to Lake Caldonazzo.

Best regards to my Karlsbad acquaintances. I don't mean my many countrymen there—I didn't send them.

Yours truly,
Ferenczi

1. Ferenczi did not integrate the ideas he mentions here into any work published at the time; he did not expand on them until much later. See e.g., "Notes and Fragments," 1920–1933, 308; *Fin.*, p. 216; "The Dream of the Clever Baby," 1923, 257; *F.C.*, p. 349; *Thalassa: A Theory of Genitality*, 1924, 268; *Psychoanalytic Quarterly*, 2 (1933–34): 361, and 2 (1933–34): 1, 200; and *The Clinical Diary of Sándor Ferenczi*, 1990 (1932).

2. Julius Cohnheim (1839–1884), professor of pathological anatomy in Leipzig. He wrote works on general pathology, embolisms, and inflammation.

316

Karlsbad, July 28, 1912

Dear friend,

I am following with interest all reports about the events in your most intimate life, but I still think that my only duty as a friend is to leave you in peace.

—Sophie's engagement has been concluded in the meantime, is already in the Hamburg papers, and is supposed to be made public today in Vienna. He is a particularly fine and serious person. We easily recognized that much in him in Karlsbad. I think she will have it very good with him.

We are actually very well here. Only today it is supposed to be rather too hot. I can't work at all; everything drowns in hot saltwater.

It is now quite clear with Jung. I received the following letter from him after five weeks' interruption:

"Z. K.[1]   July 18, 1912   Dear Professor,
Until now I didn't know what to say to your letter. Now I can only say: I understand the Kreuzlingen gesture. Whether your policy is the right one will become apparent from the success or failure of my future work. I have always kept my distance, and this will guard against any imitation of Adler's disloyalty.
Yours sincerely, Jung"

This letter seems to me to be a flat refusal, despite some incomprehensible things—for what does he mean by the Kreuzlingen gesture?[2] What is the policy supposed to be that will be proven by the success of his work? Binswanger, to whom I have sent a copy because he alone has been oriented toward the "Kreuzlingen gesture," has the same impression. I will not reply right away; I can also give myself weeks' time and do absolutely nothing, which will facilitate a formal break. We can just see.

Otherwise the following has taken place: several days ago a letter came from Riklin with a paper by him in a Swiss review, "Oedipus and ΨA."[3] Nicely written, but conciliatory to the point of uncertainty and dishonesty toward the public. A new tone has been struck in it, symbolism instead of reality, which I don't like at all. In addition, a mollifying letter from Riklin. I shouldn't worry about them in Zurich. They are working seriously and [are] not paranoid, to which I replied with some praise and much honest criticism. I gather the true content from Binswanger's report about a conversation with Maeder, who was with him for a visit.[4] They are now doubting the influence of infantile complexes and are at the point of already appealing to racial difference in order to explain the theoretical disparity. Those must be pretty shallow experiences to make such doubts possible. The fact that, once again, it is a matter of the "path for traveling salesmen" [*Weg für Handlungsreisende*][5] is evident from a statement of Jung's reported by Oberholzer to the effect that it is not necessary in analysis to go into the details of the experiences; one can be content with uncovering the "tendencies"!

Jung must now be in a florid neurosis. However this turns out, my intention of amalgamating Jews and goyim in the service of ΨA seems now to have gone awry. They are separating like oil and water.

You would probably be very satisfied with the manner in which I am taking all this. I am emotionally quite uninvolved and intellectually above it all.

With deference to your work intentions, do now what you can. You should also celebrate during your vacation. Since we want to be in Caldonazzo before September 1 and don't want to leave before the 6th–8th–10th, I will definitely count on your being there. Give my kind regards to Frau G. and don't take anything too hard. One doesn't learn until later what was misfortune or happiness.

Cordially,
Freud

1. Zurich-Küsnach, Jung's place of residence.
2. Jung had been of the opinion that Freud had not informed him in a timely fashion about his visit of May 25–28, 1912, with Binswanger in Kreuzlingen—which is not far from Zurich—which Jung interpreted as the "Kreuzlingen gesture." In fact he had not been at home when Freud's letter of May 23 arrived (at that time it usually took one day for a letter to reach Zurich from Vienna). See also letter 349.
3. Franz Riklin, "Ödipus und Psychoanalyse," *Wissen und Leben* 5, no. 20 (1912): 20ff. See the review in the *Korrespondenzblatt* (*Zentralblatt*, 3 [1912–13]: 109).
4. Freud's reply to Binswanger is excerpted in Binswanger, *Reminiscences*, p. 46.
5. Freud again applied this expression, which was evidently familiar to Ferenczi, much later, to the work *Entwicklungsziele der Psychoanalyse* [*The Development of Psychoanalysis*, 1924, 204] (Leipzig, 1924), which was written jointly by Ferenczi and Rank.

Regarding this expression, see also André Haynal, *Controversies in Scientific Method: From Freud and Ferenczi to Michael Balint* (New York, 1989), p. 54.

317

Budapest, August 6, 1912
VII., Erzsébet-körút 54

Dear Professor,

After all that I knew about Jung's attitude, his open declaration of war saddened but did not surprise me. The only thing that troubles me is the fate of the "Jahrbuch"; this could do great harm to the cause (if placed tendentiously into the service of "asexual analysis"). But I hope that you (and Bleuler?), if necessary, will intervene more energetically in the editorial affairs of the Jahrbuch.

The "Kreuzlingen gesture" and the "policy" for which Jung reproaches you are obviously on the order of fantasies by which Jung wants to justify his actions and thus appease his conscience. He handles psychoanalysis as though it were a personal affair between the both of you and not something objective and scientific. The other Swiss are all too much under the influence of his suggestion, and they are all a bunch of anti-Semites.

It has never been so clear to me as now what a psychic advantage there is in having been born a Jew and having remained protected in childhood from this atavistic nonsense. Even *Putnam* can easily relapse; you must always keep an eye on *Jones* and cut off his line of retreat.

I am very glad that you are taking Jung's break so easily. That proves to me that you have finally given up the frantic effort to appoint a personal successor and have left the cause of analysis to its fate, after you have done everything in your power to serve it.

My practice is also not resting at present, even in this burning heat. "Better people" are now beginning to report to me as patients, and I have finally instituted the higher fee per hour (twenty crowns) for newcomers.

Elma was recently absent for several days. I have nothing new to report in this matter for now.

Kind regards,
Ferenczi

318

Karlsbad, August 8, 1912

Dear friend,

I haven't heard anything from you for a long time.

Above all, accept my thanks for your congratulatory telegram[1] and direct them also to that lady highly esteemed by you,[2] who customarily makes a direct reply on my part impossible and who this time understood how to write in such a particularly moving way.

Our stay is nearing its end. On Friday we are going to Munich–Bolzano; on the 15th there will be a family gathering before the trip to Karersee. Our state of health here was excellent, and I am expecting a long-lasting good effect. Correspondences and answers to wishes have taken up much time. In the last few days the isolation could no longer be maintained. Frau Stegmann was here yesterday, and Jekels is expected today.

I wasn't able to do anything here but finish my contribution to the debate on masturbation.[3] I received the best confirmations of my totem hypothesis from the book by Robertson Smith on Religion of the Semites.[4]

Yesterday I got a letter from Jung that made it possible for me to reply. He wrote about Bleuler's taking over the Jahrbuch for as long as he is absent,[5] about Rank's book,[6] to which he connected his critique of incest, and he remarked that he would put his presidency up for discussion at the next Congress, so that it can decide whether "deviations" are permitted. In addition, he gives renewed assurance that it doesn't occur to him to overcome the father in the manner of Adler. I replied,[7] while matter-of-factly dropping the friendly form of address, that it was no compliment to the Congress if he did that. The right to divergent views is unquestionable. If the divergence went as far as it did with Adler (elimination of the ucs., repression, infantile sexuality), then he should ask himself in any event what sense it would make to sail under the same flag. Nothing would justify the assumption that his modifications involve such an estrangement from our basic views; his words are in direct opposition to that. Even in Adler's case, the dissolution of our association didn't originate with me but with him. We kept in abeyance until a later date the problem of why such modifications have to take place amid storms of affect and with the loss of human relations. And then I wished him luck for the journey.

I greet you cordially and await news from you.

Yours,
Freud

1. On Sophie Freud's engagement; this telegram is missing.
2. Gizella Pálos.

3. See Freud's "Concluding Remarks" (1912f) to the discussions on masturbation in the Vienna Society.

4. William Robertson Smith, *Lectures on the Religion of the Semites* (London, 1889); used by Freud for the last essay of *Totem and Taboo* (1912–13a). The Scot Smith (1846–1894) is considered the founder of the comparative sociology of religion.

5. On September 7 Jung went to New York to lecture at Fordham University. He had asked Bleuler to take over the editorship of the second half-volume of the *Jahrbuch* in his absence (*Freud/Jung*, August 2, 1912, p. 512). Jung used these lectures as an opportunity to present his views of psychoanalysis, which diverged from Freud's.

6. See letter 309, n. 1.

7. This letter of Freud's is missing in *Freud/Jung* letters.

319

Budapest, August 8, 1912
VII., Erzsébet-körút 54

Dear Professor,

I could have reported in my last letter (August 7)[1] about the events that I want to share with you now, but only in the form of a postscript. The fact that I didn't do it may spring from an ucs. tendency which would like to undo them.—I have given up Elma's analysis and in so doing severed the last thread of the connection between us.—

I wrote to you that she was absent for a few (—three—) days; she was with acquaintances at the Plattensee and felt very well, unpressured, and healthy there, and, as she was reporting to me about this, it became quite clear to me that she is subjecting herself to analysis against her will, solely because of her hoped-for and impatiently anticipated marriage, and her tendency is to withhold from analysis everything that might impede this plan. I explained that to her, and she admitted everything and pressed for a decision. I relied on a basic rule of ΨA. and had no other choice but to explain to her that under these circumstances, analysis was pointless. At the same time I made it comprehensible to her that the affective relations between doctor and patient usually fall victim to the analysis, so that the prospects for a marital union between us were minimal, even in the event that the analysis should continue. I told her at the same time that, if she comes to me as a *patient*, I will always gladly be at her disposal.—

I did this with somnambulistic certainty, paying no heed to the painful uproar inside me.

Elma was in despair; I accompanied her home and handed her over to her mother. Since then I haven't seen her; yesterday I heard from Frau G. that she had not yet recovered and is affirming her unchanged predilection for me. In the winter she wants to go away from Budapest and does *not* want to take the planned trip to Venice-Lido with her mother.

I felt calm—except for occasional mild depression; only last night did my unrest and dreams reveal that these events have shaken me deeply. Frau G. is as kind as ever. Her loyalty and forbearance know no bounds.

My work is dormant. I get out into society a lot and take my mind off things.

Kind regards,
Ferenczi

1. No letter of August 7 is extant; perhaps letter 317, dated August 6, was not mailed until August 7.

320

Karlsbad, August 12, 1912

Dear friend,

Thank you kindly for your news. A sentence from my reading of Voltaire has stayed in my memory:

En cas de doute abstiens-toi.[1]

Regarding the near future, I just want to inform you that I have had Jones reserve lodgings for the both of us, as he offered to do. Further, I have invited Rank to share the week in London with us.[2] It is questionable whether he will accept, since he has worries about examinations. I don't know anything about Brill. We will probably be alone on the trip to Scotland and the return.

From the realm of science, ΨA allows us to recognize two primal stages of human organization: the father horde and the brother clan. The latter develops the first religion, totemism, which is, however, *retrospective obedience [nachträglicher Gehorsam]*[3] to the commandments from the first phase. Thus, the father was overcome first, but since the united brothers gradually became fathers themselves, he returned, probably this time as a god.[4]

I won't write you again from here. We are leaving Wednesday morning. The stay has done us a world of good. I am not tired of being lazy by a long shot. The Emdens left today, and they also want us to stay with them for a day in The Hague.

Best regards also to Frau G.

Yours,
Freud

In London you will probably feel the effects of a conversation that you had with Jones about the formation of a *secret* committee for overseeing the development of ΨA.[5]

1. "In case of doubt, abstain," a Persian rule attributed to Zoroaster (660–583 B.C.); often cited in France in its Latin form, "In dubio, abstine!" Freud had had this sentence, which his friend Ernst von Fleischl-Marxow had told him came from Saint Augustine, engraved by Martha, then his fiancée, on a "votive panel" and hung over his desk in the Vienna General Hospital in 1883. He did the same with a saying of Voltaire's, "Travailler sans raisonner" ("work without judging," that is to say, speculating), from *Candide* (chap. 30); see Jones I, 66, and Clark, *Freud*, p. 70.

2. On the previous day Freud had written to Rank: "I am inquiring of you whether your compulsory study would prevent you from staying with us in London for eight to ten days. I would ask you to be my guest there." Freud repeated his offer on August 18 and termed it "thanks for your last, excellent book." In Freud's view the trip would also "serve the purpose of bringing about a more intimate union between you [Rank] and Ferenczi" (unpublished letters of Freud to Rank of August 11, 18, and 25, 1912).

3. Strachey translates this as "deferred obedience"; see n. 4 and also letter 177 and n. 5 [Trans.].

4. In the last part of *Totem and Taboo* (published in 1913), Freud writes: "Totemic religion arose from the filial sense of guilt, in an attempt to allay that feeling and to appease the father by deferred obedience to him. All later religions are seen to be attempts at solving the same problem" (1912–13a, p. 145).

5. Against the background of the conflicts with Adler and Stekel and the tense situation with Jung, Jones, who had accompanied Loe Kann to Vienna for her analysis with Freud, had spoken with Ferenczi about countermeasures for the future. Ferenczi thought it would be ideal, Jones reports, "for a number of men who had been thoroughly analyzed by Freud personally to be stationed in different centers or countries. There seemed to be no prospect of this, however, so I proposed that in the meantime we form a small group of trustworthy analysts as a sort of 'Old Guard' around Freud" (Jones II, 152). On July 30 Jones wrote to Freud about the plan, which "took hold of [his] imagination immediately." The latter added that the Committee would have to remain "*strictly secret* in its existence and in its actions" (ibid., p. 153). The original members of the Committee were, in addition to Ferenczi and Jones, Rank, Sachs, and Abraham; in 1919 Eitingon joined, on Freud's recommendation. In May 1913 Freud presented each member with an antique Greek intaglio set in a gold ring.

321

Budapest, August[1] 20, 1912
VII., Erzsébet-körút 54

Dear Professor,

I wish you much satisfaction and good weather for your stay in the Tyrolean Alps. For me, the time is now also coming closer for real relaxation, which I need this time more than ever. To be sure, I feel quite fresh mentally and physically, since I have worked very little in the last month, but emotionally the past year has brought me too much stimulation and depression. I hope to be able to arrive in Caldonazzo on September 1. Now I must ask you to give me the address of the anticipated lodgings there, so that I can make an arrangement with the owner of the hotel. Rank writes me that he hopes to be able to travel with us. I am especially looking forward to becoming more closely acquainted with this dear and estimable person. I am very pleased with his book on incest;[2] in certain passages I found his serene wisdom and the fineness of his remarks—especially considering the author's youth—quite astonishing. The third issue of Imago has also been *very* successful. It is a pleasure to work with such editors.[3] *Hellmuth* especially distinguished herself.[4]—

I think your idea about the retrospective obedience of the brother clan as the source of religiosity is excellent. By the way, already last year in Klobenstein you said: "Religion is what the son has."[5]

The separation from Elma is absolute; Frau G. visits me once or twice a week. I intend to report to you personally later about the details of my emotional constitution (which is generally satisfactory).

Don't you think it might be too cold in Scotland in the second half of September?

Kind regards,
Ferenczi

I still hope to get news from you and be able to reply to it before I leave.

1. In the original the month is given as "7" (July), apparently in error. Freud's letter of August 22 (letter 322) is clearly a response to this one.
2. See letter 309, n. 1.
3. Otto Rank and Hanns Sachs.
4. Hermine von Hug-Hellmuth, "Vom wahren Wesen der Kinderseele," *Imago* 1 (1912): 285–298. Hug-Hellmuth (1871–1924), Ph.D., was a teacher and the founder of child analysis. She was the editor of the *Tagebuch eines halbwüchsigen Mädchens* (Leipzig, 1919; rpt. Frankfurt, 1987), the authenticity of which has been disputed; and she was director of the advisory board of the Vienna Psychoanalytic Outpatient Clinic (1923). She was murdered by her nephew, the observation of whom provided material for many of her works. See Wolfgang Huber, "Die erste Kinderanalytikerin," in *Psychoanalyse als Herausforderung*, ed. Heimo Gastager et al. (Vienna, 1980), pp. 125–134; and George MacLean and Ulrich Rappen, *Hermine Hug-Hellmuth: Her Life and Work* (New York, 1991).
5. See Ferenczi's postscript to letter 252: "I remain a 'son' / Have religion."

322

Karersee, August 22, 1912

Dear friend,

I am glad I heard from you today. I was just about to write to you. We are staying here until Friday, the 30th of the month, then a stop in Bolzano and then on September 2 in the *Hotel Seehof, S. Cristoforo* near *Caldonazzo Valsugana, Tyrol*. Only register there without delay and with reference to us; it is supposed to be very crowded. Come to us in Bolzano on September 1 at the well-known Posthotel Erzherzog Heinrich and make the journey with us.

You have certainly earned a vacation and relaxation, now more than ever. I will try to bring along a good mood; Karlsbad, I think, has taken a lot out of me, but I am sufficiently restored physically, still quite inactive intellectually. There is no hint at all of the previous year's lift, the plethora of ideas after the cure; it is absent altogether.

It is quite all right with me that you are so prepared to accept Rank's company; he really deserves everyone's high opinion. One such as he is doubly valuable in these times. I have no news from Brill, however, so his participation is becoming doubtful. Abraham is quite adamant that we should visit him in Berlin at the end of the trip.

If traveling in Scotland turns out to be inadvisable, we can certainly do anything else that occurs to us, maybe Stonehenge, Stratford-upon-Avon, or something else romantic or idyllic. There will be no lack of stimulation with both Joneses.[1]

I am probably in a good mood, extravagant, after all, because of my daughter's engagement to a very nice, trustworthy man, who is now with us; I am being compensated again in place of the thankless people around me, etc. I would like to be improved intellectually when I meet with you.

Give my kind regards to the much-tested Frau G., and don't hesitate to write me several times before you leave.

Yours truly,
Freud

1. Loe Kann and Ernest Jones (see letter 307 and n. 4).

323

Budapest,
August 28, 1911 [1912][1]
VII., Erzsébet-körút 54

Dear Professor,

I already have news from the Hotel Seehof in Caldonazzo; they promised me that they will reserve an appropriate room for me.

So, it remains firm: I will depart on the 31st and will arrive at noon on September 1 in Bolzano, where I have likewise reserved a room for myself at the Archduke Heinrich.

Today I bought the volume "Great Britain" by Baedeker; perhaps you will take it upon yourself to get the volume "London and Its Environs" in Bolzano (likewise by Bädeker [sic]).

The imminence of our seeing each other again spares me the necessity of more detailed communication—I will save everything for our personal talks.[2]

Frau G. also sends kind regards.

Yours truly,
Ferenczi

1. The content of the letter suggests that Ferenczi simply made a mistake, writing 1911 rather than 1912.

2. On August 30 the Freud family traveled to Bolzano, where Ferenczi met them. They had planned to go on to San Cristoforo, in the vicinity of Trent. But when Mathilde fell ill in Vienna, Freud and Ferenczi went to her. As soon as she recovered, they caught up with Freud's family in San Cristoforo. Instead of going on to Great Britain, as they had originally planned, the two men opted for a stay in Rome (Jones II, 94–96).

324

Budapest, October 2, 1912
VII., Erzsébet-körút 54

Dear Professor,

I didn't want to write to you until I could communicate something definite about the state of my health. Now, this is the situation: the whole story seems to have been the consequence of (latent) hemorrhoidal conditions, and is very much on the wane. The matter would probably have been in order much earlier if I had not been overly curious and had not examined myself too often. I had ample opportunity to gather personal experiences about hypochondriacal mental states. Behind this nosophobia[1] there lies, evidently, the apparently missing reaction to the final break with Elma.— The "self-examinations" may have been hidden organ-erotisms.—I found among my notes a dream from the time *before* the departure for the Tyrol, in which, after a scene between myself, Elma, and Frau G., I am climbing a mountain alone, when I discover in myself a syphilitic hardening in an inguinal gland.—

There is still not much to do. A few of my old patients feel so well that they haven't been coming now. Today I threw one out (perhaps somewhat precipitously): a doubting obsessive-compulsive who made me lose my composure.—How does one treat such people?!!—A new patient is coming on the 10th.—In the meantime I have much to do in court. In the evenings I read and note down a number of things about "fetal" sleep theory.[2] So, there is always enough to do.—

Rome, with all its magnificence, has been transformed into vague, nebulous images.—Its aftereffects are being expressed more in the fact that I find conditions, as well as people, here barbaric.—So quickly does one inwardly become a Roman!

I hope you continue to be healthy and in a good mood. Please let me hear from you soon and give my regards to all your family individually.

Frau G. is not coming until this evening. I have been all alone in the meantime.

Many thanks for the countless large and small favors that you did for me during the trip.

Yours truly,
Ferenczi

1. Fear of being or becoming ill.
2. See letter 155.

325

Vienna, October 2, 1912
IX., Berggasse 19

Dear friend,

The beautiful days, etc.[1]

Hardly had I returned home when I fell ill with the influenza which is rampant here, but which was able to damage only the outside of poor Konrad. I am almost back to my old self and deep in work. The neuroses look just the same as they did before the Zurich enlightenment. Jones is here and will probably write to you in order to conjure you up on Sunday.

Two small events have befallen me which have value as omens, one of which is probably a certain sign of success. Kraus in Berlin is—and I have this on good authority—preparing a new Encyclopedia of Internal Medicine and already offered me hysteria or obsession a long time ago. I think I already told you about that. At the time I replied that it would have to be both, and didn't place much expectation on the matter. Yesterday I received the contract for both essays, due April 1, 1915.[2] With that, ΨA has become official, extremely official. Nothing should be said about it for the present, however.

The second augury is an announcement from Frau Lou Salomé Andreas,[3] who wants to come to Vienna for months just to learn ΨA.

Jones brought me the papers by Bleuler, Maeder, and Adler which were distributed at the Zurich Congress and which I am sending to you with the request that you send them back or bring them with you. Three regrettable misunderstandings and oversimplifications of our ΨA. Maeder, for example, forgets that for us the dream is only a special form of expression, takes it in the popular sense, and ascribes to it all kinds of functions which naturally belong to the preconscious day's residues and in that capacity contain nothing new or enlightening. The only function of the dream remains that of guarding sleep. Bleuler doesn't get beyond the superficially descriptive differentiation of cs. and ucs. Adler is well enough known.[4]

A war plan of mine is connected with this impression. I am thinking of offering resistance. I never wanted to avoid inner discussion, and since Jung will unhesitatingly make use of the Jahrbuch to represent himself, I am considering taking the Zentralblatt as my organ. The Zentralblatt is obligated to review all publications and has, up to now, grossly neglected this duty with respect to the Jahrbuch. Now, I want to inspire these critiques myself. But I can't write them myself, and I should select people here, perhaps Reitler, Hitschmann, Tausk, who are prepared to delineate my views.[5] It should not be a secret that I am behind it. But I am counting on you as the general staff in this internal campaign. I don't need to inspire you, so I am asking you directly whether you want to participate in these critical papers about the Jahrbuch. If so, then I will make sure that a *pars leonina*[6] remains reserved for you.

I haven't seen anybody here except Stekel, who is graciously disposed and is reporting a few astounding, as well as incautious, things while he is at it, in the Zentralblatt, which came out today.[7] My wife wants to go to Hamburg with Sophie at the end of the week. Oli is thinking about taking up technology in Berlin, but he doesn't know if he will be able to overcome the difficulties of the local study regimen. Ernst enjoyed Venice very much and wants to learn Italian. My eldest is again quite well; the bad dream has been forgotten.[8]

I greet you kindly and hope to hear from you before you come.

Yours truly,
Freud

1. "The beautiful days in Aranjuez are now at an end," from the beginning of the play *Don Carlos* (1787) by Friedrich Schiller.

2. The story of this project, which never came to fruition, is described in detail by

Jones (II, 248–249). The work, Friedrich Kraus and Theodor Brugsch, eds., *Spezielle Pathologie und Therapie innerer Krankheiten*, 11 vols. (Berlin, 1919–1927), was published after the war without any contributions on psychoanalysis.

3. Lou Andreas-Salomé (1861–1937) was born in St. Petersburg and married the Orientalist Friedrich Carl Andreas (1846–1930). She was a writer, champion of women's rights, and later a psychoanalyst in Göttingen; she became known primarily through her friendships with Friedrich Nietzsche and Rainer Maria Rilke. After she had participated in the Weimar Congress in September 1911, she decided to study psychoanalysis in Vienna. Her notes were published in 1958 (see the reprint, *In der Schule bei Freud, Tagebuch eines Jahres [1912/13]* [Frankfurt, 1983]). Her correspondence with Freud was published in an abridged version (Frankfurt, 1966).

4. The Third Annual Meeting of the International Society for Medical Psychology and Psychotherapy was held on September 8 and 9, 1912, in Zurich. Bleuler, the chairman, spoke about the unconscious, Adler on the organic substrate of the psychoneuroses, and Maeder on the teleological functions of the unconscious. In his presentation Maeder ascribed two functions to dreams: first, their cathartic effect, and second, their attempting solutions which are "preliminary exercises to acts of liberation." Additional lectures were given by Hans Wolfgang Maier, Jones, and Leonhard Seif. Reports on the Congress were written by Franz Riklin (*Zentralblatt* 3 [1912–13]: 119f) and Seif (*Zeitschrift* 1 [1913]: 95–99).

5. A week later Freud submitted a similar request to the regular general meeting of the Vienna Society. Members of the review board at the time were Paul Federn, Eduard Hitschmann, Rudolf Reitler, and Victor Tausk; Ferenczi was not mentioned in Rank's minutes (*Minutes* IV, 103). See letter 327.

6. "The lion's share"; derived from Aesop's fable in which the lion, after hunting with the ass and the fox, appropriates the entire spoils for himself.

7. Wilhelm Stekel, "Fortschritte der Traumdeutung," *Zentralblatt* 3 (1912–13): 154–158.

8. See letter 323, n. 2.

326

Budapest, October 4, 1912[1]

Dear Professor,

I am arriving in Vienna Saturday evening (10 o'clock), will meet with Jones on the same evening, and will visit you Sunday morning. Staying at Hotel Regina.

Kind regards,
Ferenczi

1. Postcard.

327

Vienna, October 17, 1912
IX., Berggasse 19

Dear friend,

A negative proof of thought transference. The day before yesterday I wanted to write to you since I hadn't heard from you for so long, and from this intention I came to the conclusion that you were just then occupied with [writing] a letter to me, so I postponed my action so that the letters wouldn't cross each other. But the assumption proved to be false, at least on superficial examination.

Now for some news: I have written a small paper on technique[1] for the Zentralblatt, a continuation of your suggestions, and I have promised five more for this volume. Since then I have been working on Animism (Omnipotence)[2] and am furious about Wundt.[3] It is a harsh punishment to have to read this rubbish in the evening after eleven hours of work.

I have invited a review board here on Sunday, consisting of Reitler, Hitschmann, Tausk, and Federn. I have made it known that you are an external member of it. I will ask to have the papers about the last Jahrbuch in after exactly a month and ask you also to adhere to this deadline for the most vital piece, your paper on Jung's work on Libido.[4] So, we will open hostilities. The best defense is a good offense.

A long letter from Maeder about our differences, very friendly, open, and decent; no attempt at all to gloss over Jung's behavior, but otherwise full of slanted views and clear anti-Semitic stirrings. You will receive it as soon as it has been responded to (on Sunday); I can't let him wait too long for an answer.

Stekel is a swine and is incessantly inventing new unpleasantness, petty jealousies, and insults. The "Writers' Dreams"[5] are miserable trash; but he always wants to be praised. A valiant book by Marcinowsky, which is a dignified attempt to find favor with the public, has likewise been published ("The Courage to Be Oneself").[6]

Last Wednesday was not good. Sachs has botched things greatly with his methodology of the theory of instinct.[7] According to my mood, I would sooner compare myself with the historical Moses than with the one by Michelangelo, which I interpreted.[8]

Everything well at home. Work up to my ears. Kind regards to you and Frau G.

Yours,
Freud

1. See letter 304 and n. 1.

2. "Animism, Magic, and the Omnipotence of Thoughts", the third essay of *Totem and Taboo* (1912–13a).

3. Wilhelm Wundt (1832–1920), since 1875 professor of philosophy in Leipzig, where he founded the first institute for experimental psychology (1879), in which he sought to investigate empirically elements and laws of the process of consciousness. For that reason Wundt is often termed the father of scientific psychology in German-speaking countries. Freud is referring to Wundt's ethnological works, which he used in writing *Totem and Taboo*: they are *Mythus und Religion*, pt. 2, vol. 2 of *Völkerpsychologie* (Leipzig, 1906), and *Elemente der Völkerpsychologie* (Leipzig, 1912).

4. Ferenczi's critique (1913, 124) of Jung's "Wandlung und Symbole der Libido" was later published in *Zeitschrift* 1 (1913): 391–403.

5. Wilhelm Stekel, *Die Träume der Dichter, Eine vergleichende Untersuchung der unbewussten Triebkräfte bei Dichtern, Neurotikern und Verbrechern* (Wiesbaden, 1912).

6. Jaroslaw Marcinowsky, *Der Mut zu sich selbst, Das Seelenleben des Nervösen und seine Heilung* (Berlin, 1912).

7. Hanns Sachs had delivered a lecture, "Zur Methodik der Trieblehre," on October 16. It was not reproduced in the *Minutes*, since it was to have been published in the *Jahrbuch*; this did not occur, however. In the discussion Freud had criticized Sachs's view "that the instincts have acquired their ambivalence with the choice of an object" (*Minutes* IV, 104).

8. During his stay in Rome in September, Freud had visited Michelangelo's statue of Moses daily and had planned to write an essay about it, which he did not begin, however, until fall 1913 ("The Moses of Michelangelo" [1914b]). According to Freud's view, the historical Moses "had a hasty temper and was subject to fits of passion," whereas Michelangelo's *Moses* "becomes only a concrete expression of the highest mental achievementent that is possible in a man, that of struggling successfully against an inward passion for the sake of a cause to which he has devoted himself" (p. 233).

328

Budapest, [undated][1]
VII., Erzsébet-körút 54

Now, something personal.

My long silence was caused by cares and depressions, which I didn't want to burden you with. Now the matters have been settled, so, I can share them with you.—

My state of ill health, which I told you about on the trip home, has had another consequence that I didn't tell you about in Vienna. I had a rather painful gland in the right inguinal region; later, however, other glands and lymphatic vessels began to swell up, especially in the thigh. Naturally I was convinced that it was syphilis—especially since a doctor gave it a dubious look. Two blood tests yielded *negative* results, but I remained pessimistic in spite of them. I explained everything to Frau G., in order to forestall trouble. She proved to be infinitely good and considerate. Thereupon, relief. The glands soon began to shrink, and now (with exception of

the inguinal gland) they have returned almost completely to normal.—
Syphilis can be eliminated with virtual certainty, the doctors say with
absolute certainty.—Now, however, other hypochondriacal conceptions
came up about the nature of that one large swelling.—

Now I see clearly that my ucs. has still not compensated me for renouncing my wish for a family and wants to regress to infantile scenes of illness,
where much love was given me by my mother, who was normally harsh.
The somatic conditions (which were really present) were the stimulus for
this. Additional overdeterminations: I want to make myself sick in order
to make up for the difference in age between myself and Frau G; with me
as a despised syphilitic, her love would have to appear to me to be the
greatest possible happiness.—

Nonetheless, the case of Elma has been completely settled. I politely but
firmly rejected her attempted advances. Even though I long for youth and
beauty, I still see very clearly what kinds of dangers I have to look forward
to with her. She also no longer attracts me personally.

So, the fact remains: I will resign myself to an intellectual and emotional
union with Frau G., on which I can always build—you and science will
have to share the libido that is left over. I hope I will be able to hold its
regressions in check.

Cordially,
Ferenczi

1. The beginning of this letter is missing. In Balint's transcription the letter contains
the remark, "possibly 4th February 1912—this is very likely correct" [in English in the
original; Trans.]. But in terms of content the letter seems to fit better into this sequence
(the "long silence"; the fear of syphilis, which Freud discusses in his letter of October
20). The missing first pages may have contained the news about the "Rooster-Man"
mentioned by Freud (see letter 329).

329

Vienna, October 20, 1912
IX., Berggasse 19

Dear friend,

Thought transference has held up after all. I accept your new reports
about the Rooster-Man and will probably ask you to publish him as soon
as I have finished "Magic and Omnipotence,"[1] so that I am no longer
separated from totemism by an intermediary.

Your pseudo-syphilis has captured my interest completely; of course I
didn't believe in it for a moment, but what actually was the physical
determinant? I don't see it clearly.

Today's communication contains a letter from Brill, who gives an encouraging and unambiguous explanation of his position.[2] But the serious-
ness of the whole matter is growing; it seems to be a fortunate circumstance that, in his obsessiveness, Jung, through his behavior, is alienating
most people who could become his adherents. Stekel is also causing new
difficulties with his impudence here which indicate he has something up
his sleeve. Perhaps he will let it come down to a test of strength in the
Zentralblatt, which I certainly will not shrink from. Few sacrifices would
be too great for me to get rid of him.

I answered the letter from Maeder, as sharply and honestly as possible,
and I am curious about the effect. You see, I am not expecting anything in
the way of concessions and compromises. All these things are secondary,
of course, and the completion of our work remains the important thing.
But these struggles are good for that; they keep one in suspense. Success
is always something crippling; but the uproar on all sides produces favorable conditions similar to those of my earlier isolation.

If this situation continues, then I will probably have to get a copybook
so that I can record what I have replied.

Soon I am supposed to get the English book about Moses.[3]

Wife and daughter came back today. I am expecting the review board this
afternoon.

I greet you cordially and now hope for correspondence that doesn't cross.

Yours,
Freud

1. See letter 327 and n. 2.

2. Probably Brill's position with regard to the divergent views that Jung presented in
his New York lectures (see letter 318, n. 5).

3. Probably W. Watkiss Lloyd, *The Moses of Michael Angelo* (London, 1863), cited
extensively by Freud in his essay on Moses (1914b, pp. 234ff).

330

Budapest, October 21, 1912
VII., Erzsébet-körút 54

Dear Professor,

First, I would like to give you a report on how I am. The physical
determinant is quite unclear. It is most probably a small periurethral abscess with subsequent creeping infection of the neighboring lymph vessels
and nodes. The symptoms (pain, swelling of the nodes) are gradually sub-
siding; the small joints, which were sensitive for several days, are no longer
painful. Hypochondriacal thoughts come rarely.

I now hope to be able to carry out the work plans that I made. I organized the material for an essay on sleep (fetal regression) and began to read Jung's libido paper.[1] His errors already strike me in the first part. He doesn't know the unconscious! He *identifies* the unconscious with the pleasure principle ("fantastic thinking") and consciousness with the reality principle ("directed thinking"). He thinks that the ucs. mode of working is operable only in the dream, in neurosis, etc., and he doesn't suspect that behind the most intelligent and most moral conscious thoughts of the normal waking person a substructure of drives, fantasies, can be discovered, without which that thought would never have come into being. But he also doesn't know the *preconscious,* and for that reason he is surprised that finished thoughts emerge from the ucs. [pcs!].[2] *That* is the great marvel from which he and Maeder derive the great novelty of *progressive* ucs. thought work. (As if you hadn't done that a long time ago!) These people don't know that a progressive increase of accomplishment and raising of standards is a phylogenetic product of adaptation to reality, make a *virtue* out of a *necessity,* and assume, as it were, a certain moral drive that impels one to adaptation and the achievement of renunciation, etc., whereas in reality all that occurs out of egoism. In Part I Jung still writes rather correct things about symbolism that are well known to us. So I will be able to refute Part II by citing Part I. Here (in Part I) he still takes ucs. fantasies to be *real* and considers their conscious derivatives (e.g., the myths) as symbols. In Part II he seems to turn the proposition around and terms the *Oedipus complex* (the ucs.) an irreal symbol of love in general. But the proposition of the symbol can't be turned around. The snake can be a symbol of the penis, but what motive would force one symbolically to put a *penis* in place of the snake (or *incest* in place of "love")?! The actual thing is always the more despised; *censorship* forces one to symbolic reduction.[3]

In Part I he still talks about the fact that the cases of sodomy that occur today and the paragraphs of the law that are necessary against them speak for the reality of these tendencies in us. In Part II he takes the whole matter quite differently.

As you see, I am beginning to get into the critique of Jung. But I don't consider this task a personal one; I only want to be the exponent of our common efforts; for that reason I ask you to review my remarks, which I will share with you from time to time, and to make your views known to me as the situation warrants. [You see, you should know that I long ago overcame that stage of "refusing outside help," which manifested itself in that significant scene in Palermo.]

The news about Jung's behavior in America (which I must call outright fraudulent) also facilitates my task of criticism. I must also not spare him in any way; he doesn't deserve it, and it would also serve no useful purpose. I will lay bare the total emptiness and confusion that characterize his work; of course, in so doing I want to remain thoroughly matter-of-fact, but the *facts* will naturally speak against him.—

I share your view completely: you, alone, or with a few reliable adherents, can accomplish much more than if you have to take all this nonsense into consideration just in order to (—apparently!—) increase the number of adherents. If we followed that logic we would also have to count Strohmayer, Frank,[4] and all the wild analysts among ourselves.

Kind regards!

Yours,
Ferenczi

Jung will fall to earth between two chairs. People will understand him as little as they do Adler.

On the 30th of this month *I* will open the lecture series of the "Free School" with a lecture on the pleasure and the reality principles.[5]

The case of "crossed correspondence"[6] gets even nicer if you consider the fact that I also began the letter a day earlier, interrupted it, and didn't end it until later.

1. See letter 327 and n. 4.
2. Enclosed in brackets in the original as is the bracketed sentence later in the letter.
3. See Ferenczi's review of Jung's work (1913, 124; *Bausteine* I, 248) as well as "Entwicklungsstufen des Wirklichkeitssinnes" [Stages in the Development of the Sense of Reality] (1913, 111; *C.,* p. 227f; *Schriften* I, 156f); "Zur Augensymbolik" [On Eye Symbolism] (1913, 112; *C.,* p. 275; *Bausteine* II, 268f); "Zur Ontogenese der Symbole" [On the Ontogenesis of Symbols] (1913, 125; *C.,* p. 276); and letter 344.
4. See letter 131 and n. 5.
5. See letter 339 and n. 4.
6. Written in English in the original.

331

Budapest, October 25, 1912
VII., Erzsébet-körút 54

Dear Professor,

I can't help interrupting my reading of Part I of the libido paper in order to tell you what a depressing impression this reading evokes in me. I now see how all too benevolently we once judged this work as "not particularly successful," and I am astonished at how it was possible that we were able to leave unnoticed the purely paranoid thought processes in it. At every moment he [Jung] slides off the tracks of observational science and becomes the founder of a religion. His main concern is not *libido theory* but the salvation of the Christian community. He identifies confession with psychoanalysis and evidently doesn't know that the confession of sins is the lesser task of ψα. therapy: the greater one is the *demolition of the father imago*,[1] which is completely absent in confession. Evidently Jung *never* wanted (and was not able) to let himself be demolished by a patient. So he has *never* analyzed, but to his patients has always remained the *savior* who suns himself in his Godlike nature!

He doesn't want to renounce his hidden homosexuality (Christian community) by making it clear to himself; he prefers to "despise" sexuality, praises the "progressive function of the ucs.," etc. and in its place enjoys praying and being prayed to in the "Christian community."

He is stuck in an incurable complex-mythological confusion; he identifies the concept of imago with the "autonomous complex" of the insane, etc., etc. It is frightful that our president is unmasking himself in this fashion!

I am still not in order. Still no trace of syphilis, but painful swellings in the inguinal and femoral region (inflamed veins?) are still forcing me to move about as little as possible.

Best regards,
Ferenczi
also from Frau G.

1. See also Ferenczi, "Die Bedeutung der Psychoanalyse für Rechtswesen und Gesellschaft" [On Psycho-Analysis and its Judicial and Sociological Significance: A Lecture for Judges and Barristers] (1913, 103; *F.C.*, p. 433; *Unbewusstes*, p. 216).

332

Vienna, October 27, 1912
IX., Berggasse 19

Dear friend,

Superfluous to say that your remarks about Jung are totally clear to me, only a piece of the criticism has to be directed elsewhere. One can't reproach anyone for the fact that he doesn't accept the preconscious, but one can call to his attention the difficulties and obscurities which he will get into by rejecting it.

I ask you to send both letters from Brill and Maeder to Rank, who will forward them to Sachs.

In the meantime, some things have been happening here. There is now a prospect that we will get rid of Stekel, which is already worth a sacrifice.[1] You know that I have been frightfully tolerant and kind toward him since our last reconciliation. In the summer he began with insults and jealousies; first because of you; then he announced he would take up the fight against Imago. Finally, the following occurred. After I had instituted the review board that was supposed to correct his inadequacy in getting papers for the Zentralblatt, he suddenly declared—I will cut short the preliminaries—that he would never concede to having Dr. Tausk write in *his* journal. My answer was, it was not *his* journal, but the organ of the I. ψα A., and it was quite out of the question to exclude a member of it from collaboration because of a personal quarrel with the editor. Then, sulking. In the course of the following week he had me informed from three different quarters that he would separate, make his journal independent, and open it up to *everyone.* So, he considers the situation favorable for committing treason.

Thereupon, my *first* action. I wrote to him that I was withdrawing my latest conribution on technique until the differences between us are settled. I went to Bergmann[2] (Oct. 22)—in whom I have no trust—with the question whether, in the event of a conflict, he would give up me or Stekel.

Only today came a reply from Bergmann to the effect that he would come back to the content of the letter in a few days. Stekel is silent, so things are being planned and prepared. Hence, today my second step. I requested from Stekel that he declare himself, after I heard about his intentions by way of several intermediaries.

I don't yet know what he wants to do. But my next steps have been planned. If no complete capitulation comes from him, and if Bergmann's response is doubtful, then I will immediately resign as director of the journal, request all of our friends by means of a circular to withdraw their names and collaboration from the journal, and I will proceed unhesitatingly to found a new one, which could be called something like ΨA Monatsschrift [Monthly]. The letter to the Berlin publisher Reiss,[3] who offered himself to me in June as a "fanatical adherent," has already been written but not yet mailed. I would like to bring out the new periodical already in January, would prefer to try it as a bimonthly, and begin to store up material for it starting now. The question of the editor remains.

I am vacillating between two people: Abraham and you. What speaks against Abraham is the fact that he is extremely busy; what speaks in his favor is the location, where the publisher also lives. Abraham has not yet been notified. Everything speaks in favor of you, with the exception of your remote place of residence. You see, I hope you won't refuse the offer in the interests of our cause. The publication at two-month intervals will facilitate your work and compensate for the disadvantage of Budapest's geographical location. Either at the next Congress or even beforehand, we will see to it that the Zentralblatt is stripped of its official character. My next intention is to make quick decisions.—

My lecture yesterday began in front of an audience of fifty to sixty. Andreas-Salomé was already there. On Wednesday, in the Society, I am giving a polemical lecture which is connected to a case of illness.[4] Otherwise, my work is going from 8–9 o'clock in the evening. Mrs. Jones is doing very well and has given up the first half of her dose of morphine without difficulty.[5] My more serious works are suffering somewhat from my being too busy. The English book about Moses has arrived; I am now seeking admittance to the museum of the Academy of Fine Arts,[6] where there is a large plaster cast of him.

I am enclosing for you today the uncorrected proof of the paper on technique,[7] and I seek your comments. Your suggestion to discuss the incompatibility with other treatments is yet to be taken into consideration.[8]

So, enough work.

Kind regards,
Freud

1. The break between Stekel and Freud is described from the latter's point of view by, among others, Jones (II, 136f), Clark (*Freud*, p. 357), and Gay (*Freud*, p. 232). See also Freud's letter to Abraham of November 3, 1912 (*Letters*, p. 125). Stekel's version can be found in his autobiography ([New York, 1950], pp. 142ff), in which he presumes that Jung had worked with Freud against him. His resignation from the Society was announced on November 6 (see *Minutes* IV, 103, and letter 302, n. 15, in which the views of Freud and Federn are also cited, and *Zeitschrift* 1 [1913]: 112). Freud founded the *Internationale Zeitschrift für ärztliche Psychoanalyse* as the new official organ of the IPA; he was the director, and Ferenczi, Rank, and Jones were the editors. It was published six times a year, beginning in January 1913. The *Zentralblatt* continued to exist under Stekel's sole leadership until September 1914, when it folded.
2. J. F. Bergmann, publisher of the *Zentralblatt*.
3. Erich Reiss (1887–1951), German publisher of the journals *Zukunft* and *Schaubühne*. He was interned in 1937, and, after his release, emigrated to Sweden, England, and eventually New York, where he lived until his death.
4. Freud's lecture of October 30, 1912, "Eine kasuistische Mitteilung mit polemischen Bemerkungen" [Communication about a Case, Combined with Some Polemical Observations], was directed against Adler's theorem of "masculine protest" (*Minutes* IV, 108ff); see letter 336.
5. Loe Kann, who was addicted to morphine.
6. In Vienna. See also Freud 1914b, p. 226n.
7. To the left of this paragraph, written diagonally, are the words "Special Shipment!"
8. "Combined treatments for neurotic disorders which have a powerful organic basis are nearly always impracticable. The patients withdraw their interest from analysis as soon as they are shown more than one path that promises to lead them to health." (Freud, 1913c, p. 137). At the same time, incidentally, Freud, uncertain as to whether Loe Kann's condition might have been organically determined, had her urine tested.

333

Budapest, October 28, 1912
VII., Erzsébet-körút 54

Dear Professor,

I am returning herewith Brill's and Maeder's letters. Also a letter from Putnam, which I answered very cordially,[1] and the just-received note from Miss Johnson, which contains a polite rejection of my paper on hypnosis by the Society for Psychical Research. So, English prudery even finds something offensive in very temperate communications.—Do you think that I should give the article to the "Psycho-Medical Society"[2] (which is completely unknown to me)? I think it would be foolish to pretend that I am insulted—What we have here is clearly a psychologically understandable symptom of resistance. Or do you think that we should use the occasion to have an educational effect on England?—The question concerns the propaganda of ΨA., and for that reason I don't want to settle it on my own.

My health is now finally *much better*. The local manifestations (pain, light swelling in the inguinal region) have almost completely gone.* The presumed "incubation period" expires today. The psychic roots of the depression are daily becoming clearer to me. I wanted (ucs.) to restore the old situation of satisfaction with regard to Frau G. by devaluing *myself* and forcing her to show herself to me in the full goodness and magnitude of soul of the mother who forgives *everything*. I actually succeeded in this, in part (thanks to Frau G.'s incomparable capacity for sacrifice and kindness of heart). On the other hand, I *really* want to learn gradually how to renounce some things consciously and to be contented with what I actually have in her.

* It *Probably* has to do with resorption phenomena, consequences of a recurring *fissura ani*.[3]

———————

I want to tell you briefly about the ideas that I shared with you about the individual stages of development of the "organ of reality" (lack of need = omnipotence, magic of gestures, magic of words, sense of reality)—with an indication of their significance for symbolism, hysteria, and obsessional neurosis,[4] so that you can refer to them. But first I will wait for a report from you as to whether you still hold to this intention of yours.

Kind regards,
Dr. Ferenczi

1. Putnam's letter is missing. Ferenczi's reply of October 17, 1910, is in Hale, *Putnam,*

pp. 314f. The letters had to do with the discussion by both men of psychoanalysis and philosophy in *Imago* (see letter 305 and n. 2).

2. See letter 336. The attitude of the Psycho-Medical Society toward psychoanalysis was, as Jones wrote to Freud in a letter of August 8, 1913, one of "fair play" (see Clark, *Freud*, p. 412).

3. Anal crevice; a very painful ulceration in the anal region.

4. See Ferenczi, "Entwicklungsstufen des Wirklichkeitssinnes" [Stages in the Development of the Sense of Reality] (1913, 111; *C.*, p. 213).

334

Budapest, October 28, 1912
VII., Erzsébet-körút 54

(postscript)

Dear Professor,

Just received your letter. Naturally, I will put myself at your disposal and that of the cause without hesitation, and I am prepared to assume the editorship, in which I am naturally counting on your support. But if for any reason you transfer the editorial duties to someone else, I will support him to the best of my ability.

I have no doubt that Stekel will fail miserably in his attempt to publish the Zentralblatt alone, but I think he will reconsider and eat crow. Bergmann will also probably reconsider before he decides in favor of Stekel.

I feel freer and more battle-ready since we have begun to set aside the many precautions which the "semi-adherents" have forced us to make.

The article on technique is very nice, its tone superior, free: one notices that you are speaking the plain truth, unconcerned about the interests of others. In the end, the loss of our "friends" will signify the beginning of a scientific blossoming of psychoanalysis. Too long have we allowed ourselves to be duped by the phrase "free expression of opinion"; it finally came to the point where Jung, Adler, and Stekel were proliferating things in our organs that completely contradict the spirit of ΨA.—The new editorship will be much stricter and, if necessary, let harsh criticism reign!

I thank you for your critical remark about my view of Jung's libido paper, and I will endeavor to make the discussion come out as objective as possible, with all necessary harshness.

Kind regards! Request news soon.

Ferenczi

335

Budapest, October 30, 1912
VII., Erzsébet-körút 54

Dear Professor,

I am writing in order to prevent renewed crossing of the correspondence[1] and in order to tell you once again that I have been quite well now for three days. With the exception of slight and occasional reminders along the lymph vessels which run from the perineum to the thigh and to the inguinal glands, I am again quite well. An internist, my friend Dr. Lévy, has examined and reassured me. The surgeon (Docent Dr. Schächter)[2] agrees with Dr. Lévy that it was a case of resorption phenomena; the source of the infection could have been the fissura ani (possibly a small abscess in the urethra).

The six weeks have taken their toll on me to a certain extent (especially since, as you know, I have also suffered psychically); I have lost some weight. I am otherwise quite well, however, and completely capable of accomplishment. On Sunday I went to Érsekuyvár[3] on a matter pertaining to the court, and today I am opening the lecture season of the Free School with a lecture.[4]—

I congratulate you from the bottom of my heart for energetically shaking off Stekel. A small but reliable squad will accomplish much more than the entire following of fools and ruthless egoists. The era of the strong hand will rebuff the doubters and spur on the convinced.

Greetings and thanks from

Ferenczi

1. "Crossing of the correspondence" is in English in original.
2. Ferenczi's friend Miksa Schächter; see letter 111, n. 4.
3. A town in northern Hungary.
4. Probably "Suggestion und Psychoanalyse" [The Psycho-Analysis of Suggestion and Hypnosis] (1912, 94; F.C., p. 55), a lecture at the Free School of Social Sciences in Budapest.

336

Vienna, October 31, 1912
IX., Berggasse 19

Dear friend,

I thank you for your preparedness. My support will certainly be serious, and I also know who will support you in Budapest. For the time being I am awaiting a reply from Reiss in Berlin. In the most extreme exigency, Heller will take the journal and couple it with Imago.

The news about your health sounds reassuring.

I am returning the two letters to you today. I think you should accept the offer. The Ψmed. Society recently put out an excellent article on dreams by Eder.[1]

Yesterday in a lecture I made an energetic advance against the Adlerian rubbish by tracing the "masculine protest" to castration anxiety and penis envy. Andreas-Salomé was there, a woman of dangerous intelligence.—

I have already set up a dossier for our new organ and am gathering material wherever I can get it, to date a treatise and a communication. After Rank's examination (on November 5)[2] the actions which should cost the Zentralblatt its collaborators will begin. Stekel was not present on Wednesday, a real relief.

Hitschmann has come up with the following joke: In Adler's book there are a lot of para-noivelties.

Kind regards,
Freud

1. Montague David Eder, "Freud's Theory of Dreams," *Transactions of the Psycho-Medical Society* 3 (1912): 1–20. Eder (1866–1936) was a founding member (1913) and secretary of the London Society. He later sympathized with Jung's theories, whereupon Jones dissolved the London group and founded it anew as the British Psycho-Analytical Society with another secretary. In the early 1920s, however, Eder returned to Freud's camp and was analyzed by Ferenczi.

2. The final examination for Rank's university study for the Doctor of Philosophy degree, which he had undertaken at Freud's urging and with his support; see also letter 342.

337

Budapest, October 31, 1912
VII., Erzsébet-körút 54

Dear Professor,

Let us hope my dispatches will not cause anything unpleasant with Federn or with his patient.[1]—

I am writing to prepare you for the fact that *Elma*, who went to Vienna today in order to stay there for some time, wants to see you. I encouraged her when she expressed the wish to do so. She probably wants to speak with you about the matter of marriage to the Viennese industrialist Grätz. She is evidently inwardly prepared and only wants your permission; she already has mine.—Elma will come not as a patient but as a *visitor* to one of your office hours. (She asked me if she should pay; I told her no.)

You will certainly strike the right chord with her.

I am waiting in suspense for news in the Society and in your correspondence with the publishers.

Kind regards,
Ferenczi

I told Elma that I would write to you beforehand and ask you whether her visit is desired by you and when she should come.

1. The reference is unclear.

338

Vienna, November 3, 1912
IX., Berggasse 19

Dear friend,

Elma should certainly come and will be sure of a friendly reception, now more than before. Mo., Wed., Fri., 3–4 o'clock.

Still not much new from the theater of war. Reiss has requested a few issues of the Zentralblatt before he notifies us of his decision. Heller is very eagerly courting the unborn child and promises to become a good foster father to it. I will not bring him in before Reiss and then Deuticke have been dispensed with.

Stekel has resigned from the Society. He will probably seek admittance in Munich.

I am working further on Moses, of whom there is also a plaster cast here. Jones has sent me photos of statues by Donatello from Florence which have shattered my conception somewhat.[1]

I am suffocating in work.

Kind regards for you and Frau G.

Yours,
Freud

1. These photographs "opened the possibility of the reason for the pose being a purely artistic one without any special ideational significance" (Jones II, 365).

339

Budapest, November 3, 1912
VII., Erzsébet-körút 54

Dear Professor,

I am sending you herewith a paper by *Jones*,[1] which he had sent to me (evidently in honest observance of the Vienna accords) through Seif, the translator.—In my personal opinion this work is rather untimely, especially at a time when we have to defend the *basic principles* of analysis against attack. The separation of the processes that are only psychologically comprehensible from the actual neuroses is precisely one of those basic principles which have proven themselves to be especially valuable. One ought not to abandon this distinction without compelling reason. But Jones does that in this paper, which attempts to blur these distinctions without bringing in new facts to support this step—purely and simply on the basis of unclear speculations and analogies.—Some points are simply erroneous, as is the idea that *hysteria*, because it has abstinence (impotence) as a consequence, must produce *anxiety neurosis* along the way. Jones forgets that psychoneurosis is not only a hindrance to normal sexual satisfaction but is itself a form of sexual satisfaction, so only that part of the repressed libido that cannot gain expression in psychoneurotic symptoms *must* be transformed into anxiety.—*You* (and not Stekel) have already emphasized the other instance (in which a psychoneurosis can be built up around the nucleus of anxiety). But one should not always belabor the marginal cases that show the differences in a blurred fashion, but rather place the emphasis on the *pure* cases, from which one can learn the essence of the symptomatology in question.—Jung and Maeder also forgot the real meaning of the dream inasmuch as, in some dreams, the preconscious, in other words, the tendency to awaken, plays a large role.—Yesterday Jones wrote me a card; he is evidently awaiting a critique of his paper from me. Would you please give me your view about Jones's paper and about the way in which I should respond to him?

I, too, believe that you are putting an annihilating statement into the fray against Adler when you trace the power fantasies of neurotics to penis envy and fear of castration.—I now have a case in which the feeling of inferiority can be assessed genealogically.—As a child the patient was pampered, masturbated diligently, felt *omnipotent* (conscious memories!); *renunciation* began with object love (he wanted to masturbate on his grown sister's leg), breakdown *(repression)* of the ideas of omnipotence, feeling of inferiority; later an attempt to overcompensate for the inferiority and to regain the omnipotence by altering reality. *Aim* of the whole desire to be powerful, however, is in the unconscious: to conquer all women, even mother and sister, and to regain that unbounded sexual satisfaction that he indulged in during the time of autoerotism.

"Inferiority" is therefore only a reaction to the injury to the feeling of *omnipotence.*[2] Ideas about the lack of a penis and fear of castration are probably the most significant shocks that could befall an omnipotently thinking child.

I must also still report about my poor Konrad. The weight loss (five kilograms) and general fatigue is probably the reason for the fact that my heart is also not behaving quite properly. Dr. Lévy, a *very* reliable internist, can't find any organic change, only a "laziness" of the left ventricle. He is ordering ample nourishment, exercise, sleep, and massage for me, but he thinks it could take a few days before I recover.—Locally (right inguinal glands) still *some* sensitivity to pain, otherwise everything back to normal.

Sachs wrote me that I should become better acquainted with the Viennese. He is certainly quite right there. Up to now I have been all too reserved and preferred being alone to participating in the life of the Society. I have also been somewhat unjust and impatient with those who are half informed.

Things will be different from now on.

Yours,
Ferenczi

I wanted to go to Vienna Sunday to confer with you but preferred instead to get a good rest. Maybe I will come next Sunday. The *Temesvár*[3] Society of Physicians has invited me to give a lecture. I postponed this, too, until December.—Your two principles have made a big impression here (in the lecture).[4]

1. Jones's lecture at the Congress in Zurich (see letter 325, n. 4), "Die Beziehung zwischen Angstneurose und Angsthysterie," in which he presented the view that infantile conflicts, as they form the basis for hysterical phobias, for instance, often lead to "an absolute or relative inability of the person to satisfy himself sexually," which may then "bring about an anxiety neurosis, just like the lack of physical satisfaction." He then added this qualification, perhaps as a result of Ferenczi's critique: "although the psychoneurotic symptom itself makes a kind of hidden satisfaction and a certain relaxation of tension possible." See *Zeitschrift* 1 (1913): 12.

2. See Ferenczi, "Entwicklungsstufen des Wirklichkeitssinnes" [Stages in the Development of the Sense of Reality] (1913, 111; C., p. 231; *Schriften* I, 159), and "Zur Augensymbolik" [On Eye Symbolism] (1913, 112; C, p. 271; *Bausteine* II, 265).

3. Timisoara, a city in what is now Romania.

4. Ferenczi, "Symbolische Darstellung des Lust- und Realitätsprinzips im Oedipus-

Mythos" [Symbolic Representation of the Pleasure and Reality Principles in the Oedipus Myth] (1912, 92; *C.*, p. 253).

340

[Budapest,] November 5, 1912[1]

Dear Professor,

Illness and work [have proved to be?][2] incompatible. I had to go [to] bed—I hope not for a long time. Diagnosis rather unclear. Slight increases in temperature (morning 36.9, afternoon 37.1). I am firmly resolved to get well and to collaborate diligently; I would not like to give up the editorship! Elma will probably soon come to see you. Please make it clear to her that it is actually *her* wish to get married and that she wants to do it (neurotically) in the form of a sacrificial act.

Kind regards,
Ferenczi

1. Postcard.
2. In the first four lines a few words are missing and others are garbled where the stamp has been cut out. Only what could not be unambiguously reconstructed has been enclosed in brackets.

341

[Budapest,] November 6, 1912[1]

Dear Professor,

I have finally succeeded in locating the source of the infection in the right Cowper's gland.[2] The one-day's bed rest has lowered the temperature almost to normal. Subjective state good. There is hope that I will recover in a few days and will be able to begin to realize my work plans. Secondary gain of the illness: analysis showed no trace of albumin in the urine, so that with me it is possibly only a case of "orthostatic" albuminuria.—

I wrote to Jones along the lines suggested by you[3] and told him about Stekel's resignation and the crisis of the Zentralblatt.

Kind regards,
Ferenczi

1. Postcard.
2. The Cowper's glands are two pea-sized glands under the tip of the prostate, the secretions of which are mixed with the semen.
3. A letter from Freud seems to be missing.

342

Vienna, November 7, 1912
IX., Berggasse 19

Dear friend,

Very happy to be enlightened about your malady. I also believe you will soon be restored to health, and I see that one ought to be mistrustful toward your chronic illnesses.

Still no answer from Berlin (hardly possible); meanwhile, arguing with Deuticke, who is making difficulties as usual, but we ought to be able to get him.

Very kind offer from Abraham; he wants to take over the editorship with or without you, or step aside in favor of you. In brief, the way it should be among respectable people. From Seif, who had already been approached by Stekel, unconditional acceptance, along with his sending in Stekel's letter.

Tomorrow evening a little supper at our house in honor of Rank, who has his examination behind him and is therefore virtually a Ph.D.

I am very well, but I don't get to work because of business and practice.

Elma is coming tomorrow, isn't she? I now have office hours only on Mo., Wed., Fri.

Kind regards in your convalescence.

Yours,
Freud

343

Budapest, November 8, 1912[1]

Dear Professor,

Today I am already out of bed, almost free of fever (37.1), able to do things. In suspense, awaiting news.

Kind regards,
Ferenczi

1. Postcard.

344

Budapest, November 10, 1912
VII., Erzsébet-körút 54

Dear Professor,

My—otherwise unedifying—reading of the *Jung*ian work has the advantage of forcing me to do some thinking. That is especially the case with *symbolism*, about which Jung—in a motley mélange—heaps together true and false, important and minor things. One can't make sense out of the confusion of his presentation.

Now, the following idea occurred to me, which might help to clarify the question:

In symbolism (both in the life of the individual as well as in phylogenetic life) one must distinguish two stages from each other: symbolism *before* and *after* repression. I would like to call the first step *phanerosymbolism*, the second *cryptosymbolism*.

Before repression (of the individual, as well as of the species), the sexual (next to the self-preservative instinct) is the most important. It is so important that one hopes to rediscover it in every experience; for that reason the child seeks (and sees) his mother's breast in every object that jumps in front of him, and for that reason the (somewhat older) child sees in every similar object a penis and in every hole an anus or a vagina; similarly, the Indian mystics quite openly call fire boring an act of fertilization [see Jung's work, pt. 2, p. 193],[1] the pieces of wood that are used for it *two testicles,* etc. That is the stage of phanerosymbolism: the desire to rediscover the sexual in all objects, on the basis of the most remote similarity.

It can be assumed that the millennia-long practice of this interest-toned equation of the sexual organs and functions with objects and processes of the outside world [which certainly relates to animism] brought about a firm associative connection between the sexual and those objects: hence the fact, which has also been proved by our philologist,[2] that all words (thing designations) originate from the sexual.

Now, in repression the interest in the sexual is forcefully suppressed; but a part of the affect which is suppressed in the process still finds its way to being realized, and in fact does so in the form of interest (affect) displacement onto things that were sexualized earlier on the basis of their similarity. These things acquire an inadequate affective value, *which is no longer explicable* to the individual himself; they become *cryptosymbols.*

The (now ucs.) phanerosymbolism, when it views the world, would now like to exclaim at every moment: "That is [like] a penis, an anus," etc., and derive pleasure therefrom. But repression prohibits this, so one has to be satisfied with standing enraptured in front of a magnificent *tree,* looking down with horror into a deep *chasm,* and, especially, inexplicably feeling holy terror about things that move and enlarge, without being permitted to divine the cause of these inadequate impulses of feeling.

Cryptosymbolism already seems to be *organized* to a large degree: thus, one can possess cryptosymbols whose phanerosymbolic preliminary stage is to be sought not in one's own individual life but in that of one's ancestors. But *very many* cryptosymbols certainly have their *individual* prehistory [personal symbols].

Perhaps you can express yourself about this idea in your next letter. Of course I know that such constructions don't properly fit into the critique of Jung's work and have to be presented in a different context.

I am very pleased that the plans for the founding are turning out so favorably.—I am eagerly corresponding with Sachs and Rank, and I have written to Jones (along the lines you suggested).—

I would like to pay my next visit to Vienna on an evening of the Society, perhaps give a lecture on the developmental stages of the *ego*.[3] I must, after all, keep up my association with my Viennese colleagues—something which Sachs has rightly called to my attention.

Kind regards,
Ferenczi

State of health satisfactory. Minimal albuminuria is, to be sure, evident, but nephritis improbable. Local symptoms less severe.

1. Enclosed in brackets in the original, as are all similar remarks throughout the letter.
2. H. Sperber, "Über den Einfluss sexueller Momente auf Entstehung und Entwicklung der Sprache," *Imago* 1 (1912): 405–454; cited by Ferenczi in "Entwicklungsstufen des Wirklichkeitssinnes" [Stages in the Development of the Sense of Reality] (*C.*, p. 229; *Schriften* I, 157) and by Freud in the *Lectures* (1916–17a, p. 167).
3. Ferenczi apparently did not give any such lecture.

345

[Vienna,] November 11, 1912[1]

Dear friend,

Too much to do. Still nothing definite to tell you. Read your response to Putnam with great enjoyment, didn't understand his.[2] Am happy that you are well again. A reply to your theoretical stimulations next time.

Cordially,
Freud

1. Postcard.
2. See letter 305, n. 2.

346

Vienna, November 14, 1912
IX., Berggasse 19

Dear friend,

Finally! The journal will be called:

Internationale Zeitschrift
für
ärztliche Psychoanalyse

Publisher, *Heller* in Vienna, editors, *Ferenczi* and *Rank*. It is supposed to come out for the first time on January 15, 1913, bimonthly from then on, but in total size it will approximate one volume of the Zentralblatt. Some of the manuscripts for the first issue have been prepared, some (Jones, Seif)[1] have yet to be received. We have lured away as many as we could from Stekel. Agreements to move came from all sides; the only reservation came from Silberer.

Heller has promised to get a new, reliable printer. He will produce a package deal with Imago whereby he will allow subscriptions to both journals together for 25 marks. Rank will handle relations with the publisher and the Vienna Society. The scientific direction will be yours. We would like, of course, for you to be already represented in no. 1 with a significant contribution, perhaps with your study of Jung's paper?

In the next few days we will also ask you to visit Vienna for the formal takeover and for straightening out all details. This Sunday will still be too early. Heller will not yet have a printer by then. But next week he certainly will, and before Sunday; time is pressing.

Jung is back and has sent the enclosed letter.[2] He is so-so, but in any case makes continuing relations possible. I am sorry that I am not in the habit of copying my replies like a businessman.

Your health is holding out all right, isn't it?

Cordially wishing you luck in your new activity and thanking you on behalf of the cause and myself for your willingness to serve, I will only say: See you again soon.

Yours,
Freud

1. These were the lectures given by Jones (see letter 339, n. 1) and Seif ("Zur Psychopathologie der Angst," *Zeitschrift* 1 [1913]: 18–28) at the Zurich Congress for Medical Psychology; see letter 325, n. 4.

2. In his letter of November 11, 1912, Jung reported on his trip to America, during which he "made room for those of my views which deviate in places from the hitherto existing conceptions, particularly in regard to the libido theory" (*Freud/Jung*, p. 515).

347

Budapest, November 15, [1912]
VII., Erzsébet-körút 54

Dear Professor,

I congratulate you from the bottom of my heart on the new founding, and I am just now in the process of putting together a paper for the new journal (what is it called?). Since Stekel's departure one feels as though one has been freed from a nightmare. I am convinced that we will do it better; one also has much more desire to write if one doesn't have to deal with such an impossible person for an editor as this Stekel is (as talented as he is in some things notwithstanding).

I am also well physically, so I can handle much more work. This year is beginning badly; I have only two to three analyses a day—and one of those is almost at an end—, new ones won't come. But I don't mind; I want to dedicate my free time (which I have filled up to now with illnesses) to science.

Elma was pleased about the friendly reception in the Berggasse. How did *you* find her? I hope that when she comes home she will no longer play the role of the "outcast." Of course, the best thing would be to get her married; but she is being difficult.—

Everything is well with you, I hope. Has Oli decided to go to Berlin? I hear from my friend Dr. Alcsuti[1] that Ernst is in Vienna; so, he didn't go to Munich to study.—

Kind regards,
Ferenczi

1. Alcsuti was the Magyarized name of Gizella Pálos's brother (b. Altschul).

348

[Budapest,] November 17, 1912[1]

Dear Professor,

I am arriving at the Hotel Regina on Wednesday evening around 7 o'clock; Rank has been advised of this. Session on editorship before or (preferably) after the meeting of the Society.

Cordially,
Ferenczi

1. Postcard.

349

Vienna, November 26, 1912
IX., Berggasse 19

Dear friend,

I can finally report to you about the Council in Munich.[1] Extremely satisfactory, more so than I had expected. Result, the personal as well as intellectual bonds will hold firm for years; hence, no talk of separation, defection, and the like. Adler and Stekel are manufactured puppets in Vienna.

Altogether there were, besides me, Jung, Riklin, Seif, Abraham, Jones, and Ophuijsen,[2] representing Maeder. They treated our cause with an almost exaggerated obligingness. Jung from the outset wanted the matter to be considered a fait accompli and only asked to hear suggestions as to how we should get out of the situation with the publisher. I refused, but did give a pragmatic presentation, which culminated in the two suggestions that we divest the Zentralblatt of its official character and bestow it on the new organ. In the end Jung wanted to close the discussion without my having received any answer about it, and when I reminded him of that, he stated that he thought I had felt sure of their tacit agreement. In the course of the debate on practical regulations, Abraham had the idea that the president should travel personally to Wiesbaden in order to settle the matter with Bergmann, and Jung thanked him for the suggestion and promised to do so at the end of the week. Everything is in order, and the friendliness was certainly genuine, albeit purposely so. As soon as the matter has been straightened out with Bergmann, the International Journal will take over all the functions of the Zentralblatt. Both editors and publishers have turned out to be congenial.

Now to the personal background. Riklin thrashed around with arms and legs to protest against an attack by Adler. Seif was charmingly kind, and he asked me to tell you that he has now received, in the way of self-punishment, an abscess of the prostate, the organic cause of which goes back many (over fourteen) years; I then told him that something similar has happened with you. You of course know Abraham to be unshakably loyal. Jones accompanied him to the train station; he came back beaming and seems to have recruited him. Jones, who almost didn't meet us because in his letter Jung had named the 25th as the day of the Council,[3] is outwardly almost unrecognizable, distorted by a thick, black full beard with sideburns; but otherwise, naturally, he is the same. It was very gratifying to me.

Now to Jung. After the session, at 11 o'clock, we took our appointed walk for the purpose of having a talk. I asked him directly what was the matter with him and what his harping on the "Kreuzlingen gesture" meant.

Now he came up with the complaint that I had gone to his enemies Binswanger and Häberlin and had prevented him from seeing me by not informing him of the visit until I had already returned. "What would you say if I wrote you after the fact that I had been in Wiener Neustadt?" I admitted that that would be mean of him, but that had not been the case with me; on Thursday evening before Whitsun I had written to him and Binswanger simultaneously about my trip, so both could have known about it on Saturday morning. I arrived in Constance Saturday at noon and Binswanger was expecting me, so he [Jung] could also have known about it around this time if he had wanted to. No, he didn't get my card until Monday morning, when it was already too late (since I departed at noon on Monday). I remained firm, and then something quite unbelievable and unexpected happened. He suddenly said, meekly: "I was away Saturday and Sunday, sailing, and came back Monday morning." Now the ball was in my court, and I made proper use of it. I asked him whether it didn't occur to him to look at the postmark on the card or to ask his wife before he raised the objection that I had purposely let him know too late? How would he react to a patient who couldn't base his suspicion on anything else? He was absolutely crushed, ashamed, and then admitted everything: that he had already feared for a long time that intimacy with me or with others would damage his independence, and for that reason he had decided to withdraw; that he had certainly construed me according to his father complex and had been afraid about what I would say about his modifications, about his particular manner of expressing himself; that he was certainly wrong in being mistrustful; that it hurt him to be judged a complex fool, etc. I spared him nothing at all, told him calmly that a friendship with him couldn't be maintained, that he himself gave rise to the intimacy which he then so cruelly broke off; that things were not at all in order in his relations with men, not just with me but with others as well. He repels them all after a while. All those who are now with me have turned away from him because he threw them out. His referring to his sad experience with Honegger reminded me of homosexuals or anti-Semites who become manifest after a disappointment with a woman or a Jew. He was behaving like a drunkard who cries unremittingly: "Don't think for a minute that I'm drunk" and was under the influence of an unmistakable neurotic reaction. I had deceived myself on one point, in that I had considered him to be a born leader who by means of his authority could spare others many errors; he was not that, he was immature himself and in need of supervision, etc. He totally ceased contradicting me and admitted everything. I think it did him good. If he were a person on whom impressions stick, I would believe in a lasting change. But there is a kernel of dishonesty in his being that will allow him to slough off the impressions again. The construction of the Kreuzlingen gesture already has this character. Another proof is as follows: already in the year of the Salzburg Congress, in a sudden fit that later subsided, he swore by all that is holy that he had not been angry about me. "What all will people say; if I believed everything they tell me about you!" Later in the evening I talked to Jones, who assured me that he himself had heard the very same talk from Jung.

Jung said goodbye at 5 o'clock with the words: "You will find me completely with the cause." We stayed together until the time of departure. Unfortunately, I didn't have a good day. Tired from the events of the week and a sleepless night in the railroad car, I got a similar anxiety attack at the table as I did that time in the Essighaus in Bremen; I wanted to get up, and for a moment I felt faint.[4] But I got myself up and still felt nauseated for some time; in the evening the nausea subsided with headache and yawning, a rudiment of my condition during the summer. Overnight, on the way to Vienna, I slept fine and arrived here quite well.—

Our dossier is getting full. I hope you are very healthy and are looking forward to the work ahead.

I greet you and Frau G. cordially.

Yours,
Freud

1. The conference of heads of the local psychoanalytic societies met on November 24, 1912, in Munich, where it was agreed to leave the *Zentralblatt* to Stekel and to found the *Zeitschrift* as the official organ of the association. Descriptions of the meeting are in, among others, Jones (II, 145ff), Clark (*Freud*, pp. 370ff), Gay (*Freud*, p. 233), and *Freud/Jung* (editorial remark after letter 327, pp. 521f).

2. Johan H. W. Ophuijsen (1882–1950), Dutch psychiatrist, at the Burghölzli from 1903 to 1913; co-founder (1917) of the Dutch Society. In 1934 he emigrated to New York.

3. See Jones, *Associations*, p. 221, and Jones II, 145.

4. Freud, Ferenczi, and Jung had eaten lunch at this restaurant on the day before their departure for the United States. Freud's fainting spell there was interpreted as a reaction to Jung's stories about bodies on the moors or traced to the fact that Freud and Ferenczi had talked Jung into giving up his abstinence and drinking a glass of wine with them. Freud had also described the incident in letters to Jones, Binswanger, and Jung (*Freud/Jung*, November 29, 1912, p. 524). In all three he spoke about the fact that he had had similar spells four and six years earlier. Freud told Jones that "the final quarrel with Fliess took place in the same room" (Jones I, 317). Schur (*Freud*, pp. 264–272) gives a comprehensive picture and an analysis of Freud's fainting spells.

350

Budapest, November 28, 1912
VII., Erzsébet-körút 54

Dear Professor,

As I almost always do, I also now have to begin with a word of thanks, this time for the detailed report that I so eagerly awaited and read with satisfaction.—It really looks as if you have finally assured more peaceful times with the newest victorious campaign, at least for a time. Your energetic appearance in Vienna may also have made an impression in Zurich and contributed to a turnaround; Jung's bad conscience and the anxious doubts on the part of the other Swiss (Maeder, Riklin) did the rest. The main thing is, certainly, that collaboration with the Zurichers should remain undisturbed for some time; that is in the interest of the cause, and I, along with you, think that that will be possible. Much tact and caution will be necessary on our part if we want to secure the situation. On the one hand, we will have to cultivate personal relations with the Swiss; on the other, we ought not to refrain from critically observing and discussing their activity [in the Monatsschrift[1]];[2] it has now become evident that they take that better than they do mildly forbearing civility. Of course, the *tone* on our part must be friendly, but at least scientifically objective.

I consider your interpretation of Jung's attitude to be correct; the kernel of dishonesty which you talk about in him could also be the kernel of his neurosis.—

We should count the others, Jones, Abraham, among the unshakable; even Seif is very docile and now inclines toward our side. I read the speeches that he made at the Swiss Congress:[3] he likes to fight; perhaps a case of exemplariness of his name[4] (Leonhard).

I don't know how I got onto this, but the fact is that lately I was thinking about whether your malaise at Bremen wouldn't perhaps be repeated in Munich. (At that time we interpreted it as a reaction to Jung's apostasy from antialcoholism).

I wrote a number of reviews for the first issue, discussed a lot of foreign works, so the Monatsschrift will look downright "international."[5]

Besides the Rooster-Man and the paper on reality, I have a complete essay on homosexuality (the lecture in Weimar); it was intended for the Jahrbuch. Should I send it to Jung—in order to keep up the friendship with him and to document our right to the Jahrbuch—, or should I rather reserve it for our Monatsschrift?[6]

As for my health, the matter stands as follows: the trip to Vienna was responsible for a mild relapse of the infection; since then I have *slight* increases in temperature (at the moment 37.3 [in the afternoons]). My doctor has reassured me; I am also calm and able to work.

Frau G. thanks you for your greeting and returns it.

Yours truly,
Ferenczi

1. The *Internationale Zeitschrift für ärztliche Psychoanalyse* [Trans.].
2. Enclosed in brackets in the original, as is the similar phrase later in the letter.
3. See letter 346, n. 1.
4. An allusion to papers by Stekel ("Die Verpflichtung des Namens"; see letter 144, n.

4) and Abraham ("Über die determinierende Kraft des Namens" [On the Determining Power of Names], *Zentralblatt* 2 [1911–12]: 133f).

5. Ferenczi finally published twelve discussions (1913, 126–134c) on works by Jones, Maeder, Brill, Prince, and Frink in *Zeitschrift* 1 (1913): 93f, and 180ff.

6. Ferenczi, "Entwicklungsstufen des Wirklichkeitssinnes" [Stages in the Development of the Sense of Reality] (1913, 111; *C.*, p. 213) and "Ein kleiner Hahnemann" [A Little Chanticleer] (1913, 114; *C.*, p. 240) were published in the first volume of the *Zeitschrift* (pp. 124–138 and pp. 240–246). "Zur Nosologie der männlichen Homosexualität (Homoerotik)" [On the Nosology of Male Homosexuality] (1914, 136; *C.*, p. 296) appeared in the second volume (pp. 131–142).

351

Vienna, November 29, 1912
IX., Berggasse 19

Dear friend,

I subscribe to every word of your program. We will act accordingly. Your critical study of Jung's paper on libido[1] should be a model for that. Enclosed is Jung's last letter,[2] which supports my view. But you know it won't last. Today I received a letter from Brill, who reports on his[3] actions in America, which conform to his questionable and certainly incorrect innovations.

I am finally very tired this week, and I still am not managing to fulfill all my obligations.

Naturally I am very unhappy about the fact that your trip to Vienna has caused a worsening of your condition.

Rank is very enthusiastic. I am discussing with him what he wants to know. The dossier is rich and will certainly have something left over for the next issue.

Good luck!

Yours,
Freud

1. See letter 327 and n. 4.

2. Jung had written: "I hope the insight I have at last gained will guide my conduct from now on" (*Freud/Jung*, November 26, 1912, p. 522).

3. I.e., Jung's.

352

Budapest, December 7, 1912
VII., Erzsébet-körút 54

Dear Professor,

My long silence was due to illness; I didn't want to disturb you with it. Now I am much better again, so I want to report to you in detail about it, at least after the fact. The case history has gone through many developments and complications; in retrospect it can now be presented as follows:

The local symptoms (infection of the Cowper's glands and infiltration of the regional lymph glands (especially in the right inguinal and retroperitoneal))[1] made me and also a specialist think it was syphilis. Thereupon deep depression, several sleepless nights with heart palpitations (tachycardia), weight loss, muscle weakness. The syphilis anxiety later proved to be groundless, but the aftereffects remained. A few days of bed rest brought improvement; but then a new symptom appeared: every time I fell asleep, my breathing became shallow, my pulse got bad, and after three to four hours' sleep I awoke (without anxiety) with a strange breathing, reminiscent of Cheyne-Stokes,[2] which lasted for a time beyond my waking state. My first thought was nephritis. Repeated examinations proved, however, that I am only suffering from orthostatic albuminuria. Then new symptoms were added: hoarseness and general muscle weakness, which could be interpreted as a kind of "myasthenia."[3] Finally, a few days ago I was able to determine that I am breathing badly while lying and sleeping because my *breathing through the nose* is insufficient. It has already been that way for a long time, but it manifested itself *now* because of the partly psychically determined muscle weakness and weight loss. The nose specialist—Zwillinger![4]—in fact diagnosed a *relative* stenosis[5] of both nasal meati and applied cocaine and menthol, whereupon breathing became easier and I had my first good night after weeks of sleeplessness. The rhinologist advised an operation (removal of a part of the nasal septum).

That's the way things now stand. The period of serious diagnoses appears to have been overcome. In the meantime my local condition (in the Cowper's and lymph glands) is improving, and from now on I intend patiently to await the Christmas holidays, when I will go either to Vienna, to subject myself to a rhinological intervention, or to a spa to convalesce. (Semmering? Or Abbazia?)

If something psychic was responsible for the pathogenesis of my illness, and if it was its aim to bring Frau G. closer to me, then the illness did its duty. So much natural kindness, understanding, and forgiving everything completely disarms one, and in the end I will really have to apologize to her for causing her so much suffering. Her nursing has also made me more receptive again toward "maternal" love.

I completely approve of your decision about my essay[6] and would be pleased if you would make a few critical remarks about its content, which I will still perhaps be able to evaluate before it goes to press. *Rank* was so kind as to call my attention to some points; I will be able to take up all his suggestions.

Jung just sent me his paper on libido.[7] I will thank him for it and ask him to collaborate on the Zeitschrift. I am enclosing his letters here.

I hope that I will gradually be able to report more about science and less about being ill.

In a few cases of obsessional neurosis I was able to resolve the ambivalence of impulses of feeling in such a way that the patients (in their aggressive thoughts and symbolic actions) fantasized themselves *first* into the role of the father who punished them for sexual transgression and *afterwards* into that of the punished child—or in reverse sequence. If the one tendency emerged, then the other compulsively came on its heels. Explanation: as children they had two quite equally strong, albeit contradictory, "opinions" about their father: he made an impression on them when he punished them, and they fantasized about one day doing the same with *their* sons; at the same time they hated him and wished him "away" (death wish), since, of course, the punishment affected them. The aggressive tendency now breaks through in obsessive thoughts with an aggressive content; the identification with the victim of their own aggression makes them, in contrast, overly good and scrupulous.

Awaiting news from you.

Cordially yours,
Ferenczi

1. Behind the peritoneum, i.e., in front of the spinal column. The parentheses within parentheses are in the original.

2. Breathing in which the breaths, after a long pause, become gradually deeper and then shallower again; associated with diseases of the heart and brain.

3. Weakness of the muscles.

4. Unidentified.

5. Constriction.

6. Freud had evidently asked Ferenczi, in a communication that is missing, to withdraw a paper of his (possibly "Zur Nosologie der männlichen Homosexualität") in favor of a work by Federn, probably "Beiträge zur Analyse des Sadismus und Masochismus, I. Die Quellen des männlichen Sadismus," *Zeitschrift* 1 (1913): 28ff; see letter 353.

7. Jung's "Wandlungen und Symbole der Libido" had also been published as a book in 1912. (rpt. Munich, 1991); in English, *The Psychology of the Unconscious, CW* Supp. Vol. B.

353

Vienna, December 9, 1912
IX., Berggasse 19

Dear friend,

I already thought you were ill, as your letters indicated. I don't believe for a moment in your syphilis; I would soon have correctly diagnosed your Cheyne-Stokes here. A hypochondriacal trait is unmistakable in the case history. I am egoistic enough just now to wish you a speedy recovery.

I advised you to withdraw your paper after you had transferred the decision to me because Federn would otherwise have felt insulted, while you, as editor, are not allowed to. You should have a prominent place in the second issue with a critical study of Jung's Libido.

Jung has straightened things out well with Bergmann. We will pay 652 marks in damages and are free of him. Today I got confirmation from Bergmann that from now on (January) the Zentralblatt will no longer bear the title of an official organ of the International Association. The Association treasury will pay half, and I will pay the other half. I don't want the membership to be burdened in any way. That is worth 300 marks to me.

Otherwise, Jung is crazy [meschugge]; his letters are vacillating between tenderness and arrogant presumption, and all reports (Jones, Brill) show that he considers his little mistakes to be great discoveries.

Abraham is coming on the 20th of the month and will stay for three to four days. It would be nice if your condition would permit a trip to see us by then.

I am again very capable of work, have settled well analytically my dizzy spell in Munich, and even begun work on the long-delayed third Point of Agreement.[1] All these attacks point to the significance of cases of death experienced early in life (in my case it was a brother who died very young, when I was a little more than a year old).[2] The war mood[3] dominates our daily life; it has not affected my practice yet, but it could turn out that I have three sons on the battlefield at the same time.

I ask you for further news soon and greet you cordially.

Yours,
Freud

1. The third part of *Totem and Taboo* (1912–13a). The reference here is to the work's subtitle, *Some Points of Agreement Between the Mental Lives of Savages and Neurotics* [Trans.].

2. Freud was in fact almost two years old when his brother Julius (b. 1857) died on April 15, 1858.

3. In reaction to the First Balkan War (see letter 384, n. 2.) Austria-Hungary had not joined England, France, and Russia in their November 4 declaration of neutrality in the Balkan question. On December 5 the monarchy renewed the Triple Alliance with Ger-

many and Italy and recognized the territorial changes in Italy after the Italian-Turkish War—all of which was a sign that Austria-Hungary might intervene in the Balkan crisis.

354

Vienna, December 16, 1912
IX., Berggasse 19

Dear friend,

You are well again, aren't you?

_____

Abraham will be with me from Saturday until Christmas. Do you want to come?

_____

Hárnik is applying for acceptance into the Society. I am asking you for a report about him since you are the only one who knows him. If you write a few quick words about him I will still be able to evaluate him on Wednesday.

_____

Zurich suggests that we call our journal:
International Journal for *Therapeutic* ΨA. What do you think about it? I don't like it.

_____

Think about how much of your work should be in the second issue (actually the first with new material).

_____

I am completely absorbed in the Omnipotence of Thoughts,[1] which will come out very concise.

Finally, I greet you cordially, before I start writing again.

Yours,
Freud

1. See letter 353, n. 1.

355

[Budapest,] December 17, 1912

Dear Professor,

This is my first official letter to you! The circular[1] is done by Rank and me together; we didn't want to bother you with it. I sent it to all the branch societies today and am waiting for responses.—

The proofs for the first issue are increasing in number; the journal is becoming more and more impressive. It will be a pleasure to be an editor!

Healthwise: After a long postponement the *faintest* attempt at a local treatment (massage). Thereupon, a relapse!—but not a very serious one.

Even so, I still don't know whether I wouldn't rather rest than travel over Christmas. I will let you know soon about that.—

Now I am in a hurry. I still have to write a few editorial letters.

Kind regards!
Ferenczi

1. This circular is missing. It probably concerned the newly founded *Journal*.

356

Budapest,[1]
December 18, [1912][2]

harnik diligent but psychically impotent pathologically vain person would be unsuitable should be diverted to different career motivation for rejection constitution of local budapest group he turned to me embarrassing reason for rejection don't tell viennese title word therapeutic bad regards

1. Telegram.
2. The year is indicated by the content (see letters 354 and 357).

357

[Budapest,] December 20, 1912

Dear Professor,

At the eleventh hour I am permitting myself to make suggestions regarding the *title* of our journal.

Therapeutic is certainly bad; too *narrow* for the aims of the journal.

"Medical" [*ärztlich*] not only doesn't sound good but is also too one-sided. We want to have other readers besides physicians, or at least not scare them away directly.—

If there should be something limiting in the title, then I think "medicinal" [*medizinisch*] would be a concept with greater scope. Medical is almost identical to therapeutic.

The best thing would be to leave out the adjective altogether and to say simply: *International Journal for Psychoanalysis*. All the more so since we are the official organ of the *whole* International Association, therefore also of the *nonphysicians* who are its members.

The word *journal* [*Zeitschrift*] distinguishes it sufficiently from the "Jahrbuch," which usually doesn't mean something on the order of an archive but rather an organ for briefer communications. The *medical* should then be underscored somewhat more in the *brochure*.—An additional advantage would be that the title would be shortened somewhat as a result. Four long words are rather too much!

My doctors advise me not to travel. Localized hot compresses should accelerate the process: produce either resorption or colliquation.[1] I am beginning to get impatient, but I am forcing myself.—

The reviews about the works in the Jahrbuch are very good, especially Tausk's paper (also Reitler's).[2] The type is definitely too small (tiring!).

How did you settle the matter of Hárnik? I finally have (besides the aforementioned Dr. Radó) another reliable man, *Dr. Hollós*,[3] who was analyzed by *Federn*. All the rest are vain fools who all want to have their own cannons.[4] I will ignore them and be satisfied with the small number. Once there are four of us, I will found the local group.

Kind regards,
Ferenczi

1. Absorption or fusion, that is, liquefaction.

2. Tausk's review of Jan Nelken, "Analytische Beobachtungen über Phantasien eines Schizophrenen," *Zeitschrift* 1 (1913): 84ff, and one by Reitler on Eugen Bleuler, "Das autistische Denken," ibid., p. 169.

3. István Hollós (Heszlein) (1872–1957), psychiatrist, a friend of Ferenczi's and clinical director at the asylum of Lipótmező, where he was the first to introduce psychoanalytic methods of treatment into institutional psychiatry. He was a founding member of the Hungarian Society (1913) and first author of the book *Zur Psychoanalyse der paralytischen Geistesstörung* (Leipzig, 1922), written in collaboration with Ferenczi (1922, 239; *Fin.*, p. 351). In 1925 he was removed from his position because he was Jewish. He described his clinic experiences in *Hinter der gelben Mauer* (Budapest, 1926), a classic of humanistically inspired reform in psychiatry. After Ferenczi's death, Hollós became president of the Hungarian Society until its dissolution in 1944. During the winter of 1944–45 he escaped from the Arrow Cross (the Hungarian Fascists) in the company of a hundred other Jews, through the intervention of the Swedish diplomat Raoul Wallenberg. See "Brief eines Entronnenen" [Letter of an Escapee], from István Hollós to Paul Federn, February 17, 1946, in *Psyche* 28 (1974): 266–268.

4. An allusion to a joke told by Freud: "Itzig had been declared fit for service in the artillery. He was clearly an intelligent lad, but intractable and without any interest in the service. One of his superior officers, who was friendlily disposed toward him, took him aside and said to him: 'Itzig, you're no use to us. I'll give you a piece of advice: buy yourself a cannon and make yourself independent'" (1905c, p. 56).

358

INTERNATIONALE ZEITSCHRIFT FÜR
ÄRZTLICHE PSYCHOANALYSE
Herausgegeben von Professor Dr Sigm. Freud
Schriftleitung: Dr. S. Ferenczi, Budapest, VII. Elisabethring 54
Dr. Otto Rank, Wien IX/4, Simondenkgasse 8
Verlag Hugo Heller & Co, Wien, I. Bauernmarkt No 3
Abonnementspreis: ganzjährig (6 Hefte, 36–40 Bogen) K 21.60 = Mk. 18.[1]

Budapest, December 22, 1912

Dear Professor,

I have been advised by Rank about all details of the events in the local group, and I am also accustomed to telling him about my (certainly mostly posthumous and superfluous) remarks about the journal, so that I can for the most part spare you these things.—In general, I also want to tell you now that I am deeply troubled by the impediment to my trip to Vienna. Precisely in these stormy days, when we have to defend ourselves against open attacks and surreptitious hostilities from all sides, a personal talk with the defender would be indispensable. In addition, for me personally a meeting with you always means encouragement for work, clarification of ripening and unripened thoughts, new insights, and fresh courage.—Instead of this I now have to spend Christmas in my room and torment my poor Konrad with hot compresses.

I intend to be patient with myself for about another week. If nothing changes in the meantime, I will go to Vienna and consult Dr. Zuckerkandl.[2] Also, in the—unfortunately not very likely—event that the matter takes a turn for the better in the meantime, I will come to Vienna around New Year's Eve, if I know you will be home then.

My illness is only a psychic hindrance to work; only sitting (and writing) is also difficult. I do the analyses in a half-reclining position.

My observation that three severe neurotics whom I know were *born prematurely* agrees with our thesis that neuroses are determined by fixations in the developmental "stages of omnipotence."[3] The premature interruption of their state of carefree satisfaction forced these individuals, who did not repeat the complete development of humanity *in utero,* to come into the world still as *savages* and to adapt to *civilization.* At some point I will call this question to the attention of our readers and ask them to review their material in light of this.[4]

I wish you and every individual member of your family a merry Christmas.

Yours,
Ferenczi

Frau G. is going to Vienna for Christmas to visit Elma, who doesn't know anything about it. She will visit you sometime.

1. Preprinted letterhead.

2. Otto Zuckerkandl (1861–1921); an anatomist and surgeon, he was most active as a specialist in diseases of the urethra, bladder, and prostate. A lecturer at the University of Vienna, he was the brother of the famous anatomist and professor Emil Zuckerkandl (1849–1910).

3. See Ferenczi, "Entwicklungsstufen des Wirklichkeitssinnes" [Stages in the Development of the Sense of Reality] (1913, 111; C., p. 213), and the third part of Freud's *Totem and Taboo* (1912–13a, pp. 75–99).

4. Ferenczi's suggestion was not taken up until much later, by István Hollós, with his work "Die Psychoneurose eines Frühgeborenen," *Zeitschrift* 10 (1924): 423–433.

359

INTERNATIONALE ZEITSCHRIFT FÜR
ÄRZTLICHE PSYCHOANALYSE
Herausgegeben von Professor Dr Sigm. Freud
Schriftleitung: Dr. S. Ferenczi, Budapest, VII. Elisabethring 54
Dr. Otto Rank, Wien IX/4, Simondenkgasse 8
Verlag Hugo Heller & Co, Wien, I. Bauernmarkt No 3
Abonnementspreis: ganzjährig (6 Hefte, 36–40 Bogen) K 21.60 = Mk. 18.

Vienna, December 23, 1912

Dear friend,

I am also giving myself the pleasure of writing the Christmas greeting on our stationery. You can imagine that I have no more urgent wish for you than recovery from the boring business. We were quite in agreement but also regretted very much that you didn't come here while Abraham was present. Rank, who is day by day becoming more indispensable, has sounded you out as to whether you want visitors. To tell you honestly, your refusal was all right with me because I am in the greatest rush with the third Point of Agreement.[1]

Your suggestions about the name change have unfortunately been taken care of by the situation. The profit would not have been enough to justify the trouble with the publisher about announcements and printed forms. Incidentally, I had "*Medizinisch*" first, but rejected it on account of the pedagogues.

The embarrassing sensation of the moment is the enclosed letter from Jung,[2] which Rank and Sachs also know about, since I overcame my shame about it. I really must say, he is downright impudent. As prior history I note that he wrote recently that he had the intention of writing a critique of Adler. I responded it would be good, because in Vienna word is stubbornly being spread around that he was once again swinging over to Adler. Whereupon he said: "Even Adler's cronies don't regard me as one of *yours*." Then I asked him if he was objective enough to consider this slip without anger, and now, thereupon, his letter.

My reaction to this is difficult. He is obviously disposed to provoke me so that the responsibility for the break will fall to me and he can say that I can't tolerate analysis. On the other hand, if I respond calmly and moderately and treat him like one of our patients when he gets into a fit of cursing, he will think I am afraid and will get more audacious; or I can continue to treat him, undaunted. In such an awkward situation I will postpone reacting, especially until our journal is secure, and I will send the namby-pamby [*lammherzig*] draft of my reply to you instead of to him.[3]

He has already forgotten the lectures he got in Munich. With deference to my neurosis, I hope I will master it all right. But he is behaving like a florid fool and the brutal fellow that he is. The master who analyzed him could only have been Fräulein Molzer,[4] and he is so foolish as to be proud of this work of a woman with whom he is having an affair. She is probably the one who got him worked up immediately upon his return to Zurich.

My construction of the totem meal is proving to have practical applications. The "brothers" are attacking me from all sides, especially the "founders of religion." A patient recently failed to bring up anything for a whole week because he couldn't allow himself the cruelty of reminding me that a brother or uncle of mine had been executed for larceny and murder.[5] A Dr. Birstein[6] from Odessa, who had come to Vienna as an enthusiastic Adlerian, wanted forcibly to bring a patient of mine to Adler and told him I was so ambitious because I was the son of a *Schames*[7] and was suffering from agoraphobia, etc., etc. Similar kind things are coming out of Zurich. There is something nice and patterned about this thing, but it requires a strong stomach.

I have notified Hárnik entirely along the lines that you advocated, but I did not bring the recommendation before the whole group but rather settled it in committee. The insult to him will further the fulfillment of your intentions. He will certainly find his way to Adler.

In the present crisis I am especially averse to jeopardizing the existence of our organs. But I think Jung is afraid of the eventuality of the Association's demise more than we are and now wants to soak me up from within the Association. I will remain very reserved, but will very gladly take your—cooled—suggestions to heart.

Kind regards and wishes for the quick end to your purely somatic symptoms.

Yours,
Freud

1. See letter 353, n. 1.

2. In his letter of December 18, 1912, Jung had reproached Freud for, among other things, "treating [his] pupils like patients," although he (Freud) had failed to "come out of his neurosis" with his self-analysis. Jung, by contrast, was "not in the least neurotic—touch wood! I have submitted *lege artis et tout humblement* [according to the rules of the art and in all modesty] to analysis" (*Freud/Jung*, p. 535).

3. In the unsent draft of his reply of December 22, 1912, Freud declined to make a judgment about the reproach that he had "misuse[d] psychoanalysis to keep [his] students in a state of infantile dependency," but remarked that "in Vienna [he had] become accustomed to the opposite approach, to wit, that [he] concern[ed] himself too little with the analysis of [his] 'students'" (*Freud/Jung*, p. 537).

4. Maria Moltzer (1874–1944), daughter of the owner of the Dutch distillery Bols, became a nurse in protest against the abuse of alcohol. She was trained by Jung as a psychotherapist and from 1913 on worked as an analytical psychologist. No indication could be found as to whether she had analyzed Jung or not.

5. A similar situation resulted in the analysis of the "Rat-Man," who, according to Freud, had claimed to know "that a great misfortune had once befallen my family. A brother of mine, who was a waiter, had committed a murder in Budapest and been executed for it. I asked him with a laugh how he knew that, whereupon his whole affect collapsed" (Freud 1955a [1907–8], p. 285). The reference is to a railway murder committed by a man named Leopold Freud, no relation to Sigmund Freud (ibid.).

6. Possibly J. Birstein, author of "Ein psychologischer Beitrag zur Frage des Alkoholismus," *Zentralblatt* 3 (1912–13): 501–508.

7. A caretaker in a synagogue.

360

Internationale Zeitschrift
für ärztl. Psychoanalyse
Herausgegeben von Professor
Dr. Sigm. Freud
Schriftleitung: Dr. S. Ferenczi, Budapest,
VII. Elisabethring 54, Dr. Otto Rank, Wien,
IX/4, Simondenkgasse 8
Verlag Hugo Heller & Cie., Wien, I.
Bauernmarkt 3[1]

[Budapest,] Christmas, 1912

Dear Professor,

In a hurry, only to the extent that I would like to answer the enclosed card of *Claparède's*[2] in a positive vein, for which I request your authorization.

Cordially,
Ferenczi

1. Postcard with preprinted letterhead.

2. Edouard Claparède (1873–1940), Swiss psychologist and pedagogue; participant in the First Psychoanalytic Congress in Salzburg (1908) and positively disposed toward psychoanalysis. Founder of the "Institut J.-J. Rousseau" in Geneva (1912); with Théodore Flournoy, editor of the *Archives de psychologie*; like Freud, an honorary member of the American Psychopathological Association. The card from him is missing.

361

Vienna, December 25, 1912
IX., Berggasse 19

Dear friend,

But, of course. Trust in your own power and decide with Rank the way you want.

In the meantime you should have received my long letter. I am in the process of marshaling a very reserved attitude toward Zurich, but there will no longer be any trace of courting. The technical correspondence with Jung, e.g., whether you will be able to put "official organ" on the first issue,[1] will get to you. Meanwhile, we still have to await a reply from New York[2] and then a draft of the contract.

I wish you patience with your illness, to be rid of it soon.

I know that Frau G. is in the Hotel Regina.

Kind regards,
Freud

1. Of the *Zeitschrift*.
2. Evidently the agreement to make the *Zeitschrift*, instead of the *Zentralblatt*, the official organ of the IPA was still pending.

362

INTERNATIONALE ZEITSCHRIFT FÜR
ÄRZTLICHE PSYCHOANALYSE[1]

Budapest, December 26, 1912

Dear Professor,

I thank you for your detailed letter. Jung's behavior is uncommonly impudent. He forgets that it was *he* who demanded the "analytic community" of students and treating students like patients. But as soon as it has to do with him, he doesn't want this rule to be valid anymore. *Mutual analysis* is nonsense, also an impossibility. Everyone must be able to tolerate an authority over himself from whom he accepts analytic correction. You are probably the only one who can permit himself to do without an analyst; but that is actually no *advantage* for you, i.e., for your analysis, but a necessity: you have no peer or even superior analyst at your disposal because you have been doing analysis fifteen year longer than *all* others and have accumulated experiences which we others still lack.—Despite all the deficiencies of self-analysis (which is certainly lengthier and more difficult than being analyzed), we have to expect of you the ability to keep your symptoms in check. If you had the strength to overcome in yourself, without a leader *(for the first time in the history of mankind)*, the resistances which all humanity brings to bear on the results of analysis, then we must expect of you the strength to dispense with your lesser symptoms.—The facts speak decidedly in favor of this.

But what is valid for *you* is not valid for the rest of us. Jung has not achieved the same self-mastery as you. He got the results ready-made and accepted them lock, stock, and barrel, without testing them out on himself. (I don't consider being analyzed by Fräulein Molzer to be a fully adequate analysis.)—For better or for worse: in future you also have to content yourself with self-analysis, from which such a rich harvest has grown for the benefit of science; the rest of us, however, have to consider ourselves fortunate if you help us to control our affects in the only effective, i.e., analytically legitimate way, and give us hints that call our attention to the weak points of our psychic organization.—I, too, went through a period of rebellion against your "treatment." Now I have become insightful and find that you were right in everything, and that you could have done me no other service than allowing yourself, in my "education," to be guided not always by feeling but often by analytic insight.—

Jung is the typical instigator and founder of religion. The *father* plays almost no role in his new work; the *Christian community of brothers* takes up all the more room in it.—His book[2] has a frightfully repellent effect on me; I loathe its content and its form; its superfluous slyness, superficiality, and cloyingly poeticizing tone make me hate it. Imagine—I still haven't finished reading it.

Your response to Jung's letter is quite appropriate, I think. I would change the expression "I am sorry"; it sounds like an apology.[3]

Now on to myself.—I am also a case in need of treatment—but there has been undeniable progress to the extent that I am conscious of that fact. It was and is my intention, if you can grant me time (hours), to go into analysis with you—perhaps two weeks (maybe three), for now.—The following data may serve to orient you about me:

The local process (a Cowperitis) is gradually getting better, since I have been regularly sitting on an air pillow and making hot compresses. The swelling is going down in the regional glands, and the pain is lessening (it was, incidentally, never excessive).

In contrast, there remains a peculiar symptom complex, which I would like to describe briefly. I wake up around 4–4:30 in the morning *usually* without anxiety, with a peculiar disturbance in breathing: I notice that my breathing is very shallow, and my breaths are also very infrequent; my pulse is *very weak* and *slow*; my whole body is cold (the thermometer recently showed 35.5° C), my belly inflated, meteoristic,[4] my nose more or less stuffy (usually only on one side). Then I can't go to sleep anymore, unless I consume something. This morning, e. g., I was naturally washed out, depressed, and weak. Diligent muscular exercise *increases* both my pulse and temperature.

Now, I think I am not justified in judging these symptoms exclusively from the standpoint of an internist. (I did that thoroughly and went through a series of severe illnesses in my mind.) The psychic secondary manifestations (depression, occasional tearfulness), the rapid change of mood, disturbance of work, etc. speak in favor of the likelihood that these symptoms are in large part neurotic. Two dreams that I had during the last few days speak in favor of this:

I. I wake up (this time with anxiety) from the following dream:

"A little black cat is jumping on me every moment, bites me and hangs onto me tightly: I grab it and throw it forcefully onto the floor; but it jumps back again and again. I throw it more and more energetically to the floor (at the same time I have something like pangs of conscience about the fact that I am mistreating the little animal): Finally, the little animal *smashes to bits* on the floor and a *poisonous snake* raises its head (from the cat's blood? its entrails?). Everything jumps away—the snake could bite you in the calves. [(Indistinct) A woman stands on a table and protects herself from the snake by tightly pressing on her dress.]⁵ *You* and your sister-in-law play a role in this dream; (next to it: Italy, a four-poster bed in the following shape: [sketch]. [I can't draw it correctly]

I don't know any more about this part of the dream.—

II. Today I awoke with *some* anxiety from a dream from which I was able to retain the following fragments:

"On a saucer a cut-off—somewhat small and frail but firmly erect—male member is brought in, next to it some kinds of objects (eating utensils?). My younger brother⁶ has just cut off his penis in order to perform coitus (!). I think something like: that is not necessary, a condom would have been sufficient! . . ."

In another piece of the dream there is talk about family resemblance; several members of the family are sitting around a table. One (I?) has a crooked back. The other (indistinct) looks a little better (fatter) in the face than usual.—(The penis has been *flayed*, its skin had been pulled off so that the corpora cavernosa⁷ were laid bare. The power of the erection was striking.)

On dream I

The bodily stimulation that precipitated this dream was obviously the strong meteorism which always wanted to wake me up, but I always wanted to shake off (in the form of a little black cat). (Corresponding to the method of projection that *Federn* describes.)⁸

Little black cat. Memories of small sadisms. I was once very shocked when I threw an apple at my little sister *Gisela's*⁹ head so that her eye swelled up and I thought I had blinded her.—Six to eight years ago I had a *white dog*, with which I played in a similar manner; I teased him by letting him jump after my gloves for a long time. One time I discovered with some trepidation that his torments were too much fun for me. I like dogs very much—I have some fear of cats (of the female sexual animal?). As a young medical student I examined my landlady's pug in Vienna; the animal got an erection and rubbed his member on my hand. I was "astonished" at the strength of his sexual aggressiveness. (I must have been somewhat *aroused* at the time, because afterwards I *threw the animal to the floor* with excessive disgust.) The animal was able to bare his teeth horribly. It also occurs to me that I once dreamed about Elma that she was tearing up my papers like a mad dog.—

I don't (for the sake of resistances?) want to believe that I now want to treat Frau *Gisela* in a similarly bad way as I once did my sister Gisela, with whom I was caught by the cook at the age of about three (maybe even earlier) in mutual touching and (after having been reported to my mother?) threatened with a kitchen knife (obviously a threat of castration). But I *actually* did treat Frau G. badly during the Elma affair. Her touching devotion would correspond to that of the cat which is constantly being shaken off but keeps on coming back. (I must note that since the development of my illness I am again able to feel very warm toward Frau G., so that my aggressiveness toward her has to be lived out in *dream* and *neurosis*.) So, I hate Frau G. because I was threatened with castration on account of my sister G. I actually don't like my sister G., even though our mother claims that we got along well as children. She is one year older than I, and as a child (of twelve years) she had hysterical pains, on account of which I despised her. Now, since her husband was ruined, she has been living with our mother and makes her life difficult by being unable to adapt to the bad situation. I show less sympathy toward her than is commensurate with the state of affairs.

"*Finally, the little animal smashes to bits on the floor etc.*" Instead of *smashes* [*zerschellt*], I wanted to write *shatters* [*zerspringt*]. My sister's eye could have "shattered." In the dream it was like an explosion. (Projection of my meteorism?) Shattering with anger: even with all her kindheartedness, *Frau G.* is sometimes hard on servants, for instance. Certainly, intentions of death (murder) are hidden behind letting the cat "shatter." As a small boy I had a colossal un. . . . . rage against my mother, who was too strict with me; the fantasy of murder (which I don't remember with certainty) was immediately turned toward my own person.—[The word with the periods after it (an adjective with which I wanted to express my inability, my being bound, my inhibited will) won't come to my mind in German! In Hungarian the word is "*tehetetlen*," which at the same time also means *impotent*. So: "my *impotent* rage against my mother." But the German word still escapes me! Substitute words: without result, gagged, lost labour[10] (?), Love's Labours Lost. A king can be incapable. My father wasn't. He produced thirteen children.][11] It is possible that my mother's strict treatment (and my father's mildness) had the result in me of a displacement of the Oedipus complex: [mother's death, father's love]; i.e., a strengthening of homosexuality.—But that must not have come until quite a bit later, at a time when I had already decided in favor of the female sex.—I often accused women of egoism and desire for profit; "they keep to that which offers them more (greater potency, more money)."—I envied a young (albeit a year older than I) playmate because of his bravery: his penis was larger, was "nice and brown" and had blue veins. When I was about five years old he tempted me into allowing him to put his penis into my mouth. I remember the feeling of disgust that that produced in me. [I was afraid he had urinated into my mouth.] I didn't permit him a second time.—But the punctuated word still escapes me! Fresh substitute thoughts: raging, Orlando furioso, *hurler*,[12] *"hörögni"* [Hungarian = groaning], whore. (At the age of fourteen I was terribly shocked to hear that my father, unsuspecting of my presence, told my mother that so-and-so had married a *whore*.) I now deduce that these words (groaning, whore) can be associated with forgotten infantile ideas about parents' coitus.—My fear of impotence must have been responsible for the strong repression of this word. Before my first coitus: great fear that it wouldn't work; masturbatory stimulation of my member in order to *ensure* an erection. But I never had actual impotence (failure). Only about a year ago, when I brought Elma to Vienna for analysis and came back with Frau G., I wanted (without desire, deeply depressed) to make an attempt which failed. With the dangerous coitus in September this year in Vienna (from which I was expecting syphilis) I was—despite unpleasure and anxiety—quite potent.—There must now be unusually much libido stored up in me. Had coitus at least five times since the beginning of September of this year. The local disease process required care.—*Before* September, in the summer, strong libidinal excitations, a great deal of interest in women on the street, coitus a few times with *puellis*.[13] Now (despite abstinence), there is little noticeable from all that. All of my libido must have been converted to illness and anxiety.—Now, possibly, I ucs. hate Frau G. because she (as earlier the cook and my mother) prevented marriage with Elma (earlier touching my sister). I can also impute to her the threat of cutting off my penis—yes! and now it occurs to me that a few times *she really threatened me in jest!* So, I am not permitted to love a young girl, otherwise my penis will be cut off. That agrees with the fact that after the cat's death the *snake* (the penis) raises its head [if she dies, then I can do what I want]. The mischief that I made when I wanted to marry Elma has to be punished by cutting off my penis; *for that reason* I am exposing myself to the danger of syphilis (syphilis eats up the penis). Or: in intercourse with the person with whom I risked infection I wanted simultaneously to do what is forbidden and get punished for it. [In the dream I kill the black cat, let "the snake raise its head"—but as a punishment the snake is poisonous (= life-threatening cutting off of penis, = syphilis).]

The last, muddled part of the dream is mysterious. I interpret that as a kind of defiant apology: (father, after all, did something similar with mother). Only you have moved to the position of father, your sister-in-law to that of mother. [Father also said [= acted =] "whore". = You once took a trip to *Italy* with your sister-in-law *(voyage de lit-à-lit)*[14] (naturally, only an infantile thought!).][15] The infantile "wish fulfillment" of the dream would thus be as follows: "I satisfy my forbidden sexual desires; they won't cut off my penis after all, since 'adults' are just as 'bad' as 'children.'"

The woman with the fear of snakes in the dream reminds me of a scene (or is the condensation of several memories) from the little pleasure house in our vineyard, when once during the wine harvest all the guests, about forty people, had to stay overnight in two rooms and in the hayloft because a thunderstorm had made going home impossible. (I don't know why I chose precisely *this* translation for the Hungarian word "winehouse"! Probably because of the *pleasure* that takes place there.) I must have thought about how the ladies and gentlemen lay beside one another; I thought especially about a beautiful lady friend of my mother's. My mother's beautiful lady friends in general had to bear the brunt of all the suspicions that I spared my mother.—In that "pleasure house" there were many *mice,* and my unconscious must have correctly interpreted the women's *fear of mice.* Confirmation of the interpretation: the *snake* in the dream raised its head like a *rocket* after the bursting of the shell casing. (At the wine harvest there were always fireworks, among them a form of rocket known as a "snake.")

The were no *four-poster beds* at our house; only my newborn sister's *cradle* had a shape like the bed in the dream. (Allusion to the blessing of children in our family.)

———————

Now, I don't know how much of the *neurotic symptoms* in me is *dependent* on the organic substrate, and how much that is apparently organic is psychogenic. (I would like to be instructed by you about that.) I picture the connection as follows:

The game with the danger of syphilis was a *vengeance* turned against my own person because of the hindrances that made marriage to Elma impossible. My ucs. placed the responsibility for it in your and Frau G.'s hands. When a doctor *(in reality)* diagnosed syphilis in me (albeit with reservation)—I had to regressively live out the *anxiety* that I once went through while being threatened with having my penis cut off. (The motor force of neurosis was (is)[16] the large quantity of unsatisfied libido.) The local malady (at the base of my penis) was a constant stimulus to maintain this anxiety, which then degenerated at night into unconscious fantasies of bleeding to death and dying (deceleration of the pulse, cooling, weakness of the pulse, pauses in breathing, general weakness); during the day I was tormented by hypochondriacal ideas about incurable diseases. The meteorism (which came on because of my unhealthy life-style) completed the vicious circle with its consequences. Meteorism can, however, also have anal-erotic roots: my practice has not been going at all for several months. I am living only on old cases; no patient has been coming to me for weeks. [Similar rumors are circulating here about me as about you in Vienna.]

I won't analyze the second dream in detail now. I think it confirms the interpretation of the first (which had not or had barely been undertaken before the dream). "My younger brother" (= I, myself) had *cut off my penis* instead of using a condom.

Postscript:

Today (on December 27) I feel *significantly* better. Hard to say whether my awareness of an improvement in my physical condition or this analysis was of more use.—

Please forgive this *gratis analysis,* which I have gotten from you by sheer obstinacy (if only in writing)!

Yours, recovering,
Ferenczi

1. Preprinted letterhead.

2. Ferenczi means "Wandlungen und Symbole der Libido," published in the *Jahrbuch* (1911 and 1912).

3. In the draft of his reply of December 22, 1912, Freud had written: "I am sorry my reference to your slip annoyed you so" (*Freud/Jung,* p. 537).

4. Inflated by gas.

5. Enclosed in brackets in the original, as are similar remarks by Ferenczi throughout the letter.

6. Either Moritz Károly (1877–?) or Lajos (1879–?).

7. Erectile tissue.

8. See Federn's lecture "Über die Flugsensation im Traume" [On the Sensation of Flying in Dreams] in the Vienna Society on January 31, 1912 (*Minutes* IV, 28–34).

9. Gizella (1872–?), married to Frigges Fleiszner, owner of an iron and household goods concern. The couple had a son.

10. "Lost labour" is in English in the original.

11. The names of only twelve children are known.

12. French for "howl," or "scream."

13. *Puella,* Latin for "girl"; i.e., prostitutes.

14. Journey from bed to bed.

15. An attempt was made by Peter Swales, in "Freud, Minna Bernays, and the Conquest of Rome," *New American Review* (Spring/Summer 1982): 1–22, to verify Jung's claim that Freud and Minna Bernays had had an intimate relationship. See also John M. Billinsky, "Jung and Freud (The End of a Romance)," *Andover Newton Quarterly* 10 (1969): 39–43.

16. Enclosed in parentheses in the original.

363

INTERNATIONALE ZEITSCHRIFT FÜR
ÄRZTLICHE PSYCHOANALYSE

Budapest, December 29, 1912

Dear Professor,

Even after your last letter I didn't know for sure whether you really wanted to come to Budapest yourself.[1] For that reason I didn't mention anything about it in my reply. I only learned for sure from a card from Frau G. that this was the case, and I have to tell you honestly that I am egoistic enough to regret that this plan was not realized. Too bad Rank didn't tell me that! You certainly would have lost a day of work, but not only would you have given me great pleasure, you could probably also have been of medical assistance. My turning down Rank naturally applied only to him, toward whom I would have felt obligated to play host, whereas I would have been able to speak my mind completely in front of you. Too bad!

Just now the last passage of my autoanalytic letter occurred to me *("gratis analysis gotten by sheer obstinacy")*, and I find that this was a very successful condensation of anal-characteristic motives. I wrote the sentence down without thinking.

Yesterday it was suggested to me by a reliable source that I should apply for the position of chief physician at the newly built state Workers' Hospital (3,000 crowns starting salary). But I declined, since I would have had to sacrifice at least two hours a day—and at the same time occupy myself exclusively with organic-traumatic neurological cases and also with administrative agendas. The only thing that spoke in favor of acceptance was the increase in assured income.

It is interesting that with my refusal I smoothed the way for an obsessional neurotic patient (Dr. Lévy,[2] whom you know). That will result in bad complications for his cure.

As soon as I am better I want to get moving again: give some lectures for physicians and laymen, write in Budapest medical journals. Otherwise they will think that my silence means a turnabout on my part.—My getting loud is all the more necessary, since an Adlerian (high school teacher)[3] has been preaching the conquest of "Freudism" on all possible occasions.

Shouldn't I react to *Vogt's* paper (Deutsche Zeitschrift für Nervenheilkunde, no. 44)?[4]

Cordially,
Ferenczi

1. See letter 364.
2. See letter 89, n. 2.
3. Sándor Varjas; see letter 135 and n. 3.

4. An essay by the German neurologist and professor Heinrich Vogt (1875-?), "Kritik der psychotherapeutischen Methoden," *Deutsche Zeitschrift für Nervenheilkunde,* August 12, 1912, pp. 428–473.

364

Vienna, December 30, 1912
IX., Berggasse 19

Dear friend,

Even though tired of writing, I don't want to leave you without a New Year's greeting and a reply to both of your letters. So, cheers to what can be expected to be a difficult 1913!

Rank knew nothing about my intention to accompany him to Budapest. I am also egoistic enough to be just as glad that you turned him down, for only in that way could I do a quick and dirty job of finishing the essay on omnipotence,[1] which has been weighing terribly heavily on me. I could also have reproached myself for not having gone to England for my brother's[2] *eightieth* birthday.

I hope the news about your recovery will not turn out to be "greatly exaggerated" this time.[3] Will you believe or be angry about the fact that I have read your autoanalytic letter, but I have not studied it as I should have? In so doing I have half frustrated your neurotic intention. So, get something from me by sheer obstinacy!

I have just been totally omnipotence, totally a savage. That's the way one must keep it if one wants to get done with something.

Meynert[4] was dictating his psychiatry[5] to a (today †)[6] colleague when the latter informed him of his planned absence the next day on account of his father-in-law's 70th birthday. The answer was: Kill your father-in-law and come![7]

The letter to Jung has not been sent and will not be replaced by another.[8] He can go jump in the lake; I don't need him and his friendship any more than I need his falsehoods.

I just came from Don Juan (because of a cancellation from my evening patient). At the point during the dinner scene: "This music seems extraordinarily familiar to me"[9] I found a good application to the present situation. Yes, this music also seems very familiar to me. I experienced all this already before 1906, the same objections, the same prophecies, the same proclamations, so I am now done with them. Things went differently. It won't surprise me if things go differently now that the storm is blowing not from outside but from inside and the resistance of the so-called analysts will subside by itself. If four to five helpers remain to me, I will defy him just as well as I withstood him that other time, alone.

It was very sensible of you to turn down the position that was offered to you. Your practice will pick up suddenly. A half year ago there was also such a slump in Zurich.

I don't know the paper by Vogt, but I would advise you against reacting to it without looking at it. Let us continue to work. Perhaps the critique of the Zurichers is too much. But, of course, we have to do it; they asked for it, but they won't fail to get angry about it.

Frau G. still won't give up her favorite plan;[10] she thinks it would have been the best thing. I finally allowed myself to reply to her that I was not of that opinion. Unfortunately, she was with us for only a short time.

Sophie's fiancé has been spending the last few days with us and will stay through New Year's Eve. They are quietly happy with each other.

Kindest regards,
Freud

1. The third part of *Totem and Taboo* (1912–13a).

2. Freud's half-brother Emanuel (1833–1914).

3. An allusion to Mark Twain's telegram to a newspaper that had reported his death: "The reports of my death are greatly exaggerated." Freud loved Mark Twain's books and had attended one of his readings in Vienna. He had quoted the same anecdote only a few days earlier in a letter to Binswanger in connection with his fainting spell in Munich (Binswanger, *Reminiscences*, pp. 48f), and he also used it in *On the History of the Psychoanalytic Movement* (1914d, p. 35).

4. Theodor Meynert (1833–1892), professor of psychiatry at the University of Vienna from 1873; famous brain anatomist. He was Freud's teacher, furthered the latter's neuroanatomical studies, and even wanted to hand over his lectures to him (Freud, 1925d, p. 11), but he criticized Freud's theory of hysteria.

5. Theodor Meynert, *Psychiatrie, Klinik der Erkrankungen des Vorderhirns begründet auf dessen Bau, Leistungen und Ernährung* (Vienna, 1884).

6. In his letters Freud indicated by a cross that the person in question was deceased.

7. A similar story is told by Freud himself. When he was in the United States, a patient who was dependent on his father was introduced to him by Stanley Hall, who asked what could be done for the poor man. Freud's answer: "Kill his father" (Jones II, 58).

8. Freud did send a second letter to Jung on January 3, 1913, in which he in part repeated the content of the one he did not send (*Freud/Jung*, pp. 538f).

9. Leporello's exclamation in *Don Giovanni*, act 2, sc. 13. At this point Mozart quotes a melody from his earlier opera *The Marriage of Figaro*.

10. A marriage between Elma and Ferenczi.

365

INTERNATIONALE ZEITSCHRIFT FÜR
ÄRZTLICHE PSYCHOANALYSE

Budapest, January 3, 1913

Dear Professor,

I intended to spend the double holiday in Vienna, but then I thought about the matter and decided to wait another week; in the meantime the—progressively less severe—local manifestations will, I hope, have subsided completely. Yesterday, strangely, a (slight) swelling of the left parotid gland appeared. Milder swellings of this gland, incidentally, have also occurred earlier from time to time (about three and five years ago).

I was pleased about the good mood expressed in your last letter. You actually do feel best when you can be independent of the whole world.— But right now you are in this enviable position.

With regard to editorial matters, I will get in touch directly with Rank, who will probably report everything to you.

Kind regards from me and Frau G.

Yours,
Ferenczi

366

Vienna, January 5, 1913
IX., Berggasse 19

Dear friend,

I am pleased that you are well, now that we need you so urgently. I suggest that you postpone coming here until Jones is here, since a trip doesn't seem quite risk free for you. He is supposed to come on the 9th.

I will share with you the fact that I found a few good, polite, but unambiguous sentences to put an end to my private relations with Jung.[1] The letter was sent the day before yesterday (the one I sent you was not sent, as you know). He wrote again today,[2] but I don't need to reply any further. His behavior is neurotic and puerile. If he were in treatment with me and were paying for it, I would naturally have to put up with his utterances, but this way I can dispense with them and use my strength for other things.

I don't consider the errors of the Zurichers to be rectifiable, and I think that in two to three years we will cease to understand each other, as two completely different movements. So we don't need to direct our polemics toward convincing our opponents, but rather we will be able to criticize coolly and politely from a lofty position. In the meantime, the seeds of ΨA should be carried further; that was Zurich's function. A portion of the new recruits will always come over to us, i.e., possess the rigor to admit the ucs. and repression. Others will seek a retreat to superficiality and will end up God knows where. You will be convinced of the sterility of all these attempts at flight.

The best means of protecting oneself from bitterness remains an attitude which expects nothing at all, i.e., the worst. I advise you to adopt it as well. We will fulfill our destiny by continuing the work, unconcerned about the noise, like the goldsmith of Ephesus.[3]

I greet you cordially and hope to hear good things about your recovery.

Yours,
Freud

1. Freud had written, among other things, "It is a convention among us analysts that none of us need feel ashamed of his own bit of neurosis. But one who while behaving abnormally keeps shouting that he is normal gives ground for the suspicion that he lacks insight into his illness. Accordingly, I propose that we abandon our personal relations entirely" (*Freud/Jung*, January 3, 1913, p. 539).

2. In his letter, which crossed Freud's, Jung had offered to treat him "with the same analytical consideration which you extend to me from time to time" (ibid., January 3, 1913, p. 540).

3. In Goethe's poem "Gross ist die Diana der Epheser" [Great Is Diana of the Ephesians] (*Sophienausgabe* II, 195f), he tells of the ancient goldsmith who, unconcerned about the gain in strength of the new Christian religion, continues to work on statues of his goddess Diana. See also Freud's essay of the same name (1911f).

367

INTERNATIONALE ZEITSCHRIFT FÜR
ÄRZTLICHE PSYCHOANALYSE[1]

[Vienna,] January 6, 1913

Dear friend,

Under the title "Collection," I will now send you more frequently such experiences from my practice,[2] which are suitable for being singled out and which I myself ask to be put in order, i.e., occasionally matched up with similar things. You do the same, and if others follow our lead, then with time we will put together a nice ψα picture book.

Cordially,
Freud

1. Postcard with preprinted return address but without addressee, therefore mailed as a letter.

2. Presumably some of Freud's short contributions published in *Zeitschrift* 1 (1913):

377–382, under the title "Observations and Examples from Analytic Practice" (1913h). See also letter, 387.

368

INTERNATIONALE ZEITSCHRIFT FÜR ÄRZTLICHE PSYCHOANALYSE

Budapest, January 9, 1913

Dear Professor,

I feel restored to the extent that I am daring to undertake the trip to Vienna without risking anything. Tomorrow, *Friday evening*, I am arriving in the "Regina" and request that you leave word for me there as to whether I can see you on the same evening, and if so, at what time.—I will stay in Vienna on Saturday and Sunday and want to make good use of the time. Besides the conferences with Jones and Rank, I also want to consult an internist (Salomon?)[1] and Prof. Zuckerkandl.

Looking forward to the pleasure of seeing you soon.

Yours,
Ferenczi

Frau G. sends kind regards.

1. Hugo Salomon (1872–1954) qualified to teach internal medicine at the University of Vienna, where he was a lecturer from 1913 on.

369

Vienna, January 10, 1913
IX., Berggasse 19

Dear friend,

Jones is picking me up today at 9:30 in the evening. We can be with you around 10. Seif is coming tomorrow morning. Eder is here. We all want to spend Sunday on the Kobenzl.[1] You must eat lunch with us on Saturday (alone).

Kind regards,
Freud

1. A mountain near Vienna.

370

Internationale Zeitschrift für
Ärztliche Psychoanalyse

Budapest, January 25, 1913

Dear Professor,

Much happiness for today's great event in your family![1] "Don't take the loss of such a dear member of your family too much to heart," I would say, if I didn't have reason to presume that you (who checks your ucs. daily) have already had your "Sophie" complex in the works for a long time, so that you certainly won't confront the event unprepared.—Frau G. also sends kindest regards by way of me and takes this opportunity to wish you all good things imaginable.

My health is quite good. No pain since Salomon. Moderate complaints with the unaccustomed cuisine—otherwise, gradual disappearance of the symptoms of convalescence.—

I am in an enthusiastic correspondence with Rank, so I can spare you my letters, which will contribute somewhat to the reduction of your uncommonly increased correspondence.

This time I won't talk or ask you about any more serious things; I think today you have other concerns.

Once again, kind regards and congratulations.

Yours,
Ferenczi

1. The marriage of Freud's daughter Sophie to the Hamburg photographer Max Halberstadt (1882–1940). According to Jones (II, 98), the wedding took place on January 14, which is improbable in view of this letter and Abraham's letter of January 29, 1913 (*Freud/Abraham*, p. 132).

371

Vienna, January 27, 1913
IX., Berggasse 19

Dear friend,

Many thanks from us all for your manifold participation in the wedding celebration with gift, telegram, and letter. You will have an echo of the event in Budapest. My Max's brother, Rudolf Halberstadt, pediatrician, will see or will have already seen you at your home.

The change in your state of health is just as desired as it is—instructive. The first issue of our journal came in today, a happy day. I know the ones that follow will show the marks of your activity more and more clearly.

I am naturally somewhat depleted by the festivities and the farewell. There are also lots of things going on with the adopted children,[1] which is not a matter of indifference to me. Maybe now I am having a stupider time of it altogether.

I hope that our letter writing will not lie completely dormant beneath your professional correspondence, and I am counting on seeing you again at a session in February.

Thank Frau G. kindly for me.

Regards,
Freud

1. The members of the Committee; see also letter 373.

372

INTERNATIONALE ZEITSCHRIFT FÜR
ÄRZTLICHE PSYCHOANALYSE

[Budapest][1]

Dear Professor,

I can't write in my own hand[2] because I am lying here, sometimes with chattering teeth, sometimes feverish.—The influenza that is tormenting me started the day before yesterday—I hope it will not last much longer.—I received the enclosed letter[3] from Jung yesterday. I can edit a reply to him commensurate with your possible suggestions. I hope I will soon be able to bring better news about myself. What was that again about the adopted children?

Cordially yours,
Ferenczi

Kind regards from Frau G.
January 31, [1913]

1. The day, without location or year (which can be inferred from the context), is given at the end of the letter.
2. The letter is entirely in Gizella Pálos's handwriting.
3. This letter is missing.

373

Vienna, February 2, 1913
IX., Berggasse 19

Dear friend,

Your influenza, now I hope overcome, probably had only one meaning, and that was to allow me to get an entire letter from Frau G. for once. In my case it would now make no sense at all, so I intend to withdraw from the epidemic that is going around.

Jung's letter sounds somewhat elegiac; perhaps his Egeria[1] has already left him. She should go to America to bring Rockefeller's daughter[2] to Zurich. It is, of course, a pose, like every other one. Brill also writes that he [Jung] is now making efforts to woo him. (Brill seems *not* to have resigned the presidency of his group.[3] He now has difficulties with the English publisher, who wants to leave out a whole series of dreams because of the impropriety of the material.)[4]

Jung's letter is probably also meant to inform me indirectly. Since you had the idea of involving me in the editing of your letter, I will throw a few sentences on paper which you can use or not, as you see fit. I notice that I informed him of your critique of his work. I wrote him on business during the last few days, and yesterday I received a matter-of-fact reply. He also asks if September 7/8 is appropriate as a date for the Munich Congress.[5] A remark about a "bad reception" of his work.

So, my suggestions.

You know how busy he is. But the impression that the Zurichers, he in particular, don't care about the Viennese journals, is very easy to avoid. Any signs of interest are welcome—[you] would like to believe that he doesn't want a separation. All signs point to the fact that such is also not intended from the other side. You know that it was particularly important for F (me) to show that scientific differences within the framework of the organiztion are borne without difficulty, as long as personal behavior, like that of Stekel and Adler, does not make it impossible. You regret the breaking-off of private relations between F. and him, but, according to the information you have received, you think it is for the best. You had heard from me that he considers all personal relations disturbing to his scientific freedom and that he repeated this in his letter. Then there is nothing else left. F. (I) claim that he (J.) was not in order in his relations with men. You certainly must admit from your own experience that you have had no special difficulties in getting along with F. (me). You would gladly withhold criticism as to which side the greater abnormality is presumed to be on. You think that after things have developed further to a certain extent, a rapprochement will again be possible.

Your critique of his work. Reservations regarding his anticipated lectures in New York.[6] You know the difficulties connected with a theoretical agreement on the libido question. You hope that some results or other with respect to the clinical material will facilitate taking a position. If nothing changes with respect to him regarding analytic technique, then an unresolved issue of dispute could remain. If the opposite occurs, then one would have the opportunity to compare and judge for oneself.

You are surprised that he says that the nature of the dream is so unclear to him. Does he no longer acknowledge the ucs. or repression? You and others are in reasonable agreement as to the significance of both of these factors in the dream. Symbols are still enigmatic for all of us; they can probably be understood historically, from the development of thinking and speaking, etc., etc.

I am looking forward to a quiet Sunday, after the demands of the previous one. For this afternoon I have invited only Frau Lou Andreas-Salomé.[7] As soon as I have taken care of the next little tasks, I will take up totemism. I hope to be able to quote your Rooster-Man soon.[8]

Jones left yesterday for Canada. There was transitory discord between him and his wife, in which the wife, especially, behaved charmingly.[9] I am now altogether satisfied with my adopted children.

Our journal is generally well liked. In my next paper I will now treat the question of what one first says to the patient, and the mechanism of treatment.[10]

Kind regards from all of us and see you soon!

Yours,
Freud

P.S. In the Society we now want to settle the question about the theme for the next round of discussions. I would suggest the social role of neuroses.[11] *Qu'en dites-vous?*[12]

1. A nymph; lover and adviser of the legendary Roman king Numa Pompilius, who owed his rule to her wisdom. Freud's ironic remark may refer to Maria Moltzer (see letter 359 and n. 4).

2. Edith Rockefeller McCormick (1872–1932), daughter of the founder of the Rockefeller dynasty and wife of Harold Fowler McCormick (see letter 121 and n. 2). She was analyzed by Jung in 1915, and in 1916 she founded the Psychological Club in Zurich, a center for Jungian psychology.

3. Before the founding of the American Psychoanalytic Association (APA) on May 9, 1911, which had been promulgated by Jones, Brill had founded the New York Psychoanalytic Society on February 12 of the same year. In contrast to the APA, it accepted only

physicians as members and affiliated itself directly with the IPA. The independence of both American associations was confirmed in September 1911 at the Weimar Congress.

4. Brill was just working on the translation of Freud's *Interpretation of Dreams* (1900a), which was published in London in May 1913 (see letter 395).

5. The Fourth Psychoanalytic Congress took place in Munich on September 7.

6. Jung's New York lectures, in which he had introduced his divergent concept of libido, were published in German under the title "Versuch einer Darstellung der psychoanalytischen Theorie," Jahrbuch 5, 1st half–volume (1913): 307–441.

7. Lou Andreas-Salomé described this visit in her diary; see *The Freud Journal of Lou Andreas-Salomé* (London, 1965), pp. 88–90.

8. Ferenczi's essay "Ein kleiner Hahnemann" was published in the third issue of the *Zeitschrift* (1 [1913]: 240–246) and was cited in detail by Freud in the last essay of *Totem and Taboo*, "The Return of Totemism in Childhood" (1912–13a, pp. 129–131 and 153n.).

9. According to Vincent Brome, who had the Freud-Jones correspondence at his disposal, during Loe Kann's analysis with Freud, Jones had slept with her nurse and companion, Lina. As Brome elaborates further, Kann was able to work this issue out analytically. Freud wrote to Jones that psychoanalysis was able to derive a gain from such episodes, and that he had Jones to thank for a nonetheless dangerous experiment (Brome, *Jones*, pp. 86f).

10. Freud's essay "Zur Einleitung der Behandlung" ("Weitere Ratschläge zur Technik der Psychoanalyse," I) [On Beginning the Treatment (Further Recommendations on the Technique of Psychoanalysis, I)] (1913c) was published in two parts; the first appeared under this title in the January volume of the *Zeitschrift* (1 [1913]: 1–10), the second, supplemented by the formulation "Die Frage der ersten Mitteilungen—Die Dynamik der Heilung" [The Question of the First Communications—The Dynamics of the Cure], was published in March (ibid., pp. 139–146).

11. Freud is referring to the series of writings *Diskussionen des Wiener Psychoanalytischen Vereins*, which was edited by the leadership of the Society and published by Bergmann, and in which volumes about the suicide of students (1910) and masturbation (1912) had been published. Four lectures were subsequently given in the Vienna Society from February to May 1913 under the title "Gesellschaft und Neurose." They were not published separately, however.

12. *French for* "What do you say to that?"

374

Internationale Zeitschrift für
Ärztliche Psychoanalyse

Budapest, February 8, 1913

Dear Professor,

Frau G. was quite astonished by the fact that the reply that you advised me to give corresponded almost word for word with the one that I had been thinking of giving Jung anyway. Now I have sent him our concurring reply (only in my own name, of course); I scarcely believe that he will respond to it; perhaps he will write to me that he recognized you as the guiding spirit of my reply. But that is improbable.—Now, "we can wait;"[1] we are now in the comfortable position of the courted suitor;[2] this situation seems to suit the Zurichers better. As long as one treats them as well as the way *you* did until recently, they will play the recalcitrant ones; their secret (certainly specifically Christian) feeling of guilt (i.e., of the ucs. Oedipus fantasy which is dammed up and repressed especially strongly in them) does not permit them to believe someone who treats them well, i.e., doesn't want to punish them for their sins. But they recognize as their master every person who treats them contemptuously, repellingly, or even coolly. The lay accusations of the Zurich journalists[3] have sufficed to fill them with the greatest anxiety. Maybe they will also grow suspicious when they get to hear nasty things from you and your Jewish adherents.

The first issue of the Zeitschrift was very well liked here. The layout is respectable, serious. I am full of confidence in the future of our newborn child. Would you please tell me briefly *by return mail* whether you will permit me to translate your article on technique into Hungarian with reference to the "Zeitschrift" and to publish it in a local medical journal?[4] (N.B.: Half has already been translated.)

My influenza has abated, and I am also feeling better in other respects, even better than before my acute illness. My illness caused me to ponder about the subject of "neurasthenia." The modern term "vagotonia"[5] naturally says nothing about the nature of the illness; at most it shows the *way* in which the (certainly sexual-chemical) noxa works. I arrived at the supposition that the *biological analysis of neurasthenia* and of anxiety neurosis will at some time lead to knowledge about the vital processes in the organism that is just as significant as that which psychoanalysis has brought forth with respect to mental life. It will then come out that sexuality (i.e., the chemical substances to which drives are bound) plays the *central* role in the *pathology* as well as in the *physiology* of man and is probably also in a struggle here with substances that are bound to the self-preservation of the organism, of individual organs or parts of organs. The contempt for sexuality has evidently also caused as much mischief in biology as it has in psychology.

As for myself, I am convinced that my poor health [*Kränkeln*], which has lasted over half a year, was a bodily reaction to the failure of the marriage project. My body has "played dead" since it saw itself thwarted in its anticipated satisfaction. This may have resulted in a real increase in my disposition to illness.

My friend (and opponent of analysis) Dr Schächter is going to *Corfu* in March, as he does every year, and his invitation to me to go with him is very tempting. Three weeks on the Adriatic and Greek spring: the idea is simply overpowering. Despite the fact that this year, because of illness, etc., I had much less income than the year before, I am still thinking seriously of indulging in this recuperation. I hardly dare ask you if you would like to come along?! We want to embark in Trieste on March 11 and arrive at the same place on April 2. But if I permit my *body* this recuperation, then I have to postpone the planned *analysis*. I know, of course, that resistance toward being analyzed is partly to blame for this postponement! Please, give me your honest opinion about my travel plan.—I would naturally deliver the "Rooster-Man" and the critique of Jung[6] before my departure.

Cordially,
Ferenczi

1. The reference is unclear.

2. As Ferenczi was aware, Freud had promoted such an attitude on the part of the analyst: "While the patient attaches himself to the physician, the physician is subject to a similar process, that of 'countertransference.' This countertransference must be completely overcome by the analyst; only this will make him master of the psychoanalytic situation; it makes him the perfectly cool object, whom the other person must lovingly woo" (session of the Vienna Society of March 9, 1910, *Minutes* II, 447).

3. See letter 275 and n. 6.

4. Ferenczi is referring to Freud's paper "On Beginning the Treatment" (1913c). Ferenczi's translation appeared in the same year in *Gyógyászat* 53 (1913): 129–133.

5. Vagotonic or vagotropic constitution; increased tonicity of the vagus nerve, producing, for example, a slow, weak pulse and lowering of blood pressure.

6. Ferenczi 1913, 114, and 1913, 124.

375

Vienna, February 10, 1913
IX., Berggasse 19

Dear friend,

In order to establish further "points of agreement,"[1] I will say how very forcefully your assessment of neurasthenia has come home to me. I have always been of the opinion that sexual physiology lies behind the actual neuroses in the same way that ego psychology lies behind the paraphrenias.

Do as you wish with translations.

The temptation to go along with you to Corfu was strong, but brief. Aside from the unpleasantness that goes along with being three, this is not the proper time to dispense with a few thousand crowns on account of one's wretched health. That doesn't apply to you, you are young and independent. More and more I see the necessity of confining myself to anal erotism[2] and am thinking of fulfilling my primary function, i.e., to earn money, as intensively as possible. Actually, I have to go to England very briefly during the Easter holiday—over by way of Holland, back by way of

Hamburg—to visit my 80-year-old brother. But I don't like to think about it, even though it will cost me only a few days beyond the obligatory vacation days. It is very good and proper that you want to finish both papers before your trip.

After this letter I want to write the last page of the second article on technique.[3] In this manner of scribbling [*Schmiererei*] I hope soon to have gained a significant routine. Spielrein writes that Kraus in Berlin recently came out very strongly in favor of ΨA in a lecture; he has acknowledged most of it and has severely scolded our opponents. "Why don't you say that (*scilicet* aloud)?"[4]

Kind regards,
Freud

P.S. Stop! I am not thinking about your analysis in such a way that it should disrupt your vacation. I want to keep some furniture in the room, not have to heat with everything.[5]

1. Freud had originally published the essays collected in *Totem and Taboo* (1912–13a) under the title *Über einige Übereinstimmungen im Seelenleben der Wilden und der Neurotiker* (Some Points of Agreement Between the Mental Lives of Savages and Neurotics). See letter 353 and n. 1.

2. In "Character and Anal Erotism" (1908b) Freud had brought the triad of orderliness, parsimony, and obstinacy "into relation" with sublimation, or "the disappearance of . . . anal erotism" (p. 170).

3. See letter 373 and n. 10.

4. "I have for years heard hundreds of times each day the question: 'Why do you not say it,' the word 'aloud' necessary to complete the sense being omitted"; Schreber, *Memoirs*, p. 70n.

5. On June 5, 1910, Freud had written to Pfister: "Discretion is incompatible with a satisfactory description of an analysis; to provide the latter one would have to be unscrupulous, give away, betray, behave like an artist who buys paints with his wife's housekeeping money or uses the furniture as firewood to warm the studio for his model. Without a trace of that kind of unscrupulousness the job cannot be done" (*Freud/Pfister*, p. 38). Possibly he used a similar analogy with Ferenczi and is alluding to it here.

376

Vienna, February 14, 1913
IX., Berggasse 19

Dear friend,

I would like to suggest a correction to your essay,[1] which seems to me to be the best and most significant one that you have contributed to ΨA: In your sensitive discussion about the choice of neurosis (14) you make the *content* of the neurosis dependent on the phase of development of the libido. Can one say that? Is it really the content? But it is certainly the *kind* of erotism, if that is what you mean.

Then in the next sentence: It is conceivable that the phases of sexual development are inextricably associated with those of ego development—I think the opposite is more probable, the displacement of the phases toward one another, which would be a good reason for variations and dispositions. The whole thing should be more cautious.

On the top of 15, instead of "F's statement" it should probably read "remark."[2]

Hearty congratulations.

Yours,
Freud

1. Ferenczi, "Entwicklungsstufen des Wirklichkeitssinnes" [Stages in the Development of the Sense of Reality] (1913, 111; C., p. 213).
2. See ibid., *Schriften* I, 161f (C., p. 237), and letter 377.

377

INTERNATIONALE ZEITSCHRIFT FÜR
ÄRZTLICHE PSYCHOANALYSE

Budapest, February 15, 1913

Dear Professor,

Thanks for the acknowledgment. I was not quite sure whether you would like the paper.

Of course I meant the "content" of neurosis as you did (kinds of erotism). Regarding the associative connection between stages of development of the ego and of sexuality, I know that it is very loose and subject to displacement. I meant only that this connection takes place between the stage of the ego that prevails in *fixation*—and the stages of the libido.—I have corrected the ambiguous passages.

Here is a letter from Jung and my reply to it.[1] I can, of course, alter it as you wish.—

At the same time I am sending you a brief communication[2] for the *Zeitschrift*, about which I have absolutely no idea whether it is worth the printer's ink. Please don't hesitate to express yourself quite freely about it.

My condition is still variable. I still tire very easily and see that I am in need of recuperation.

Cordially,
Ferenczi

1. These are missing.
2. Unidentified.

378

INTERNATIONALE ZEITSCHRIFT FÜR
ÄRZTLICHE PSYCHOANALYSE

Vienna, February 17, 1913

Dear friend,

Jung's letter (returned, with thanks) contains two precious admissions, first, the recognition of his previously denied relationship with Adler; second, the confession that with his contradiction he wanted to institute a neurotic test of love and power with me, which he now certainly sees as having failed. Of course, worth as an instrument takes precedence; worth as a person has to be earned by means of other achievements. When one is so clearly egoistic and unreliable, one needn't be very disappointed if things don't turn out differently.

Your reply (likewise returned) is excellent. The certainty with which you pass judgment on Adler is unsurpassable, and you also express superior and lucid viewpoints against Jung, which, in the face of his incessant mixing of the personal and the professional, have a liberating effect. I will refrain from suggesting that you change your reaction.

Rank will give you a recent example of Jung's dishonesty, even in unimportant matters.

I was still not able to read your contribution. It looks as if it has undergone much correction.

You very much deserve your excursion to Corfu. Even though I can't join you, I will share in it a great deal. I will probably pick up Anna from Merano at the same time.[1] But I strongly urge you to come to Vienna again beforehand, preferably very soon, because we have to discuss the contract for the International Journal with each other, which doesn't work very well by letter; actually, it doesn't work at all. Not to mention all our other interests.

"Scientia," a respectable international review, published in Milan, has urgently asked me for an article about ΨA.[2] In addition, an introduction to Pfister's book[3] and a preface to a little paper by Steiner[4] as my next works. But the wear and tear on my intellectual mechanisms is so great that next I will have to decide on a typewriter.

A very intelligent and gratifying letter from Brill.

Kind regards,
Freud

1. Anna was staying with one of Mathilde's sisters-in-law in Merano. Freud met her in Bolzano on March 22, and they both went to Venice by way of Verona, from which they returned to Vienna five days later (Jones II, 99); see letter 385.
2. "The Claims of Psycho-Analysis to Scientific Interest" (Freud 1913j), *Scientia* 14 (1913): 240–250, 369–384.

3. Introduction (Freud 1913b) to Oskar Pfister, *Die psychanalytische Methode—erfahrungswissenschaftlich-systematische Darstellung* (Leipzig, 1913).

4. Preface (Freud 1913e) to Maxim Steiner's, *Die psychischen Störungen der männlichen Potenz* (Leipzig, 1913).

379

INTERNATIONALE ZEITSCHRIFT
FÜR ÄRZTL. PSYCHOANALYSE[1]

[Postmark: Budapest,]
February 28, 1913

Dear Professor,

You will be able to see me in and after the lecture on Saturday evening. I want to discuss everything with Rank on Saturday. Sunday morning and afternoon until 4 will be free for our discussions.

Cordially,
Ferenczi

1. Postcard with preprinted letterhead.

380

INTERNATIONALE ZEITSCHRIFT FÜR
ÄRZTLICHE PSYCHOANALYSE

Budapest, February 28, 1913

Dear Professor,

As material for our discussion tomorrow I am sending you a letter[1] and an article of Jung's for the "Zeitschrift,"[2] which has just arrived.

Kind regards,
Ferenczi

1. The letter is missing.

2. Probably Carl Jung, "Eine Bemerkung zur Tauskschen Kritik der Nelkenschen Arbeit" [Comment on Tausk's Criticism of Nelken, A], *Zeitschrift* 1 (1913): 285–287 (*CW* 18).

381

Vienna, March 7, 1913
IX., Berggasse 19

Dear friend,

Only a few words to wish you a nice trip and complete convalescence.

Jung has gone to America again for five weeks, to see a Rockefeller woman, so they say.[1] He had earlier willingly accepted my (that is to say, your) suggestion to specify contractually the obligations of the Central Office.[2] He is behaving quite well in these matters.

I am writing for Scientia and will soon be finished.

I hope, we won't need to send you any proofs to Corfu, which will then be intercepted by a Turkish ship.[3]

Kind regards.

Yours,
Freud

P.S. Hoche's circular has been sent to us by Zurich for publication in the Zeitschrift.[4]

1. It can be assumed from an announcement in *Korrespondenzblatt* 1 (1913): 310, which was appended to the *Zeitschrift*, that on March 27, 1913, Jung gave a lecture on psychoanalysis in the Liberal Club in New York. Regarding the "Rockefeller woman," see letter 373 and n. 2.

2. The agreement of May 2, 1913, between Freud and the IPA, represented by its central office (Jung and Riklin), concerned the editorship of the *Zeitschrift*. The central office obligated itself, in the event of differences of opinion concerning the holders of editorial positions, "to ask Professor Freud . . . to convene . . . the Congress of the I.Ps.A. or the Advisory Council to the Central Office, which represents the Congress between sessions, with a view to settling the differences." The office further obligated itself "to supply the *Bulletin* [*Korrespondenzblatt*] . . . to the editors at least three times a year" (*Freud/Jung*, app. 6, p. 580).

3. An allusion to the crisis in the Balkans; see letter 384, n. 2.

4. Alfred Hoche was preparing a paper in opposition to Bleuler for the annual meeting of the German Society for Psychiatry, which was to take place in Breslau in May. He had sent a circular to his colleagues in order to collect material against psychoanalysis. The circular and a report by Eitingon about the meeting were published in *Zeitschrift* 1 (1913): 199, 409–414.

382

Budapest, March 9, 1913

Dear Professor,

I, too, want to take leave of you—in a few lines. I wish for you that I recover quite soundly in Corfu, so that you will have a more reliable worker in me than I was capable of being during the last year. Naturally, I also wish you many other things besides.—

I would rather have granted you the summons to the Rockefellers. Still— the Americans don't deserve better.

I don't understand the remark about Hoche's circular; I haven't heard anything about it yet.

All editorial matters that may come in will be directed to Rank in my absence.

I did have to postpone my critique of the libido paper. I hope to be able to send it to you from Corfu, where I will otherwise only be lazy and sun myse1f.

Perhaps you will also indulge in a few days of rest at Easter. I think you owe it to yourself and to us all.—

Say hello to all your dear ones for me, and make me happy with a letter; my address is: Dr. F., Corfu, Hotel Angleterre et Belle Venise.

See you again.

Yours
Ferenczi

383

Trieste, March 11, 1913[1]

Very odd, enjoying the sea without you. Actually, no real pleasure.

Cordially,
F.

1. Postcard.

384

Internationale Zeitschrift für
Ärztliche Psychoanalyse

Corfu, March 14, 1913

Dear Professor,

I am doing wonderfully well here in the land of the Phaiacians.[1] Sea route smooth and sunny. Everything is glowing and blooming, it is almost unbelievable. Even poor Konrad feels well here. We saw most of the war[2] near Trieste and Pola: (night maneuvers by about twenty-six Austrian "units"). It is teeming here with Epirotic[3] refugees, so that one has to fill one's pockets with *pendáres* and *dekátes*[4] when one goes out. I photographed an Epirotic woman who had an eye tattooed on her forehead; then I saw about twenty with the same ornamentation. (*Only women* have this ornamentation.)

There are two Greek warships here in the harbor. They are afraid of the Hamidie,[5] which is said to be hanging around here.

Kind regards,
Ferenczi

1. A people known from the *Odyssey*, from whom Odysseus received a cordial reception. From there he returned to Ithaca after ten years of wandering.

2. In 1912 Greece, Serbia, Bulgaria, and Montenegro had defeated Turkey, which lost its European territories in the Treaty of London (May 30, 1913). On July 3, 1913, the Second Balkan War, against Bulgaria, ensued over the division of the former Turkish territories. The allies were Romania, Serbia, and Greece; Turkey joined on July 21. In the Peace of Bucharest (August 10), Bulgaria lost Macedonia to Serbia and Greece, as well as Crete and Epirus to Greece.

3. From Epirus, in what is today northwestern Greece. The island of Corfu, which belongs to Greece, is off the shore of Epirus.

4. Pendares and dekares, Greek coins of small denominations.

5. The *Hamidieh*, a Turkish warship.

385

Internationale Zeitschrift für
Ärztliche Psychoanalyse

Vienna, March 20, 1913

Dear friend,

It is nice that you are so charmed. Let us hope it will have a long, satisfying aftereffect.

This evening I am going to Bolzano to pick up Anna. I want to spend the holidays with her in Verona and Venice. I need a break more than ever. All the work has gone smoothly here. With my last energies I finished the program paper for Scientia and the little thing about the three caskets for Imago.[1]

Frau Lou Salomé wants to spend one to two full days with you after completing her stay in Vienna. Her interests are really of a purely intellectual nature; she is a highly significant woman, even though all the tracks around her go into the lion's den but none come out.[2] So, I am inquiring unofficially *when* you will be home and if such a demanding visitor will be convenient for you in the *first* days after your return. Would you be so kind as to tell me both reply and possible excuse as soon as possible?

She has become very friendly with Tausk and is very vigorously championing his cause, which is becoming difficult for me. If you see her, ask her about it and arrive at your own opinion so that we will have a point of departure as to how we should relate to him.

I greet you cordially and wish you all sunshine, green earth, and blue sea.

Yours truly,
Freud

1. Freud 1913j and 1913f.
2. In one of Aesop's fable's, the lion, who lies ill in his den, asks the fox why he doesn't come closer. The fox replies, "I would certainly come in if I didn't see that so many tracks go in but that none come out."

386

GRAND HOTEL D'ANGLETERRE ET BELLE VENISE
JEAN GAZZI & FRERE[1]

Corfu, March 21, 1913

Dear Professor,

More than half of my stay in Corfu is over, and I think I can affirm from now on that I can successfully take home a quite considerable reinvigoration as well as the conviction that my nightly sleep disturbances will have to be ameliorated by an intervention on the turbinate bones of my nose.

I was naturally much more receptive to the beauties of the island on the days which followed nights on which I slept well. I thought of you countless times and wished I could have enjoyed, in an accustomed manner by your side, the beauties, which reminded me in part of the morning in Selinunt.[2]

The excavated Gorgon[3] is great; it should take its place beside the frieze of Palermo.[4] Dörpfeld,[5] the German archaeologist from Athens, is living in our hotel.

The days pass with lazing around, walking, and punting; we frequently take longer trips by car.

Naturally there is a lot of talk here about the war and the regicide.[6] Five to ten of the Turkish prisoners—about five thousand in Corfu!—are dying daily of dysentery. One is already accustomed to encountering one to two funeral processions on every walk.—The people here are already fed up with the war, but they are afraid that after the Turkish war a second one against Bulgaria will follow.[7]—We are leaving here on the 1st, and we will arrive in Budapest on April 4. Kind regards to all our mutual friends and especially to your family.

Cordially,
Ferenczi

1. Preprinted letterhead.

2. A place visited by Freud and Ferenczi on the occasion of their trip to Sicily, where they saw the Temple of Minerva (Jones II, 82).

3. In the museum at Corfu there is part of the pediment from the Temple of Artemis depicting a Gorgon. The Gorgons were three fearsome sisters named Stheno, Euralye, and Medusa, the daughters of Phorkys and Keto. Previously of exceptional beauty, they were changed into man-hating monsters because of their vanity; the mere sight of them was sufficient to turn the observer to stone. Both Freud and Ferenczi later wrote short sketches about the head of Medusa (Freud 1940c [1922] and Ferenczi 1923, 254; C, p. 360).

4. A fragment of the frieze from the Greek Parthenon in the archaeological museum in Palermo.

5. Wilhelm Dörpfeld (1853–1940), German architectural researcher and archaeologist.

6. The murder of George I, king of Greece (b. 1845).

7. This turned out to be the case; see letter 384, n. 2.

387

INTERNATIONALE ZEITSCHRIFT FÜR
ÄRZTLICHE PSYCHOANALYSE

Vienna, April 10, 1913

Dear friend,

Yesterday I heard with satisfaction from Frau Lou[1] that you have recovered very well and that you are soon coming to Vienna for treatment of your nose.

It was not as nice here as in Corfu; also, not much happened. I have also put together from your and my little notes a first series "Observations and Examples,"[2] with which you can also begin, whatever you want. Rank was very good, as always. Jones is coming on May 27.

I have already started writing the work on totem; it can only go very slowly and will have to extend over a two- to three-month period.

My wife is with Sophie in Hamburg for a few weeks.

Kind regards,
Freud

1. Lou Andreas-Salomé had visited Ferenczi in Budapest from April 7 to 9; see her *Freud Journal*, pp. 135–137, and letter 388.

2. See letter 367 and n. 2.

388

INTERNATIONALE ZEITSCHRIFT FÜR
ÄRZTLICHE PSYCHOANALYSE

Budapest, April 12, 1913

Dear Professor,

Frau Lou's visit was extremely exciting. She compelled me to get out the work plans that had been buried among my papers, and she understood everything right away. On this occasion I noticed that I am finally about to work myself out of the neurasthenic conditions that made all joy in work impossible. I owe this success primarily to the discovery that these conditions were the consequence of severe circulatory disturbances, which appeared again solely as a result of a large paunch. An appropriate abdominal bandage immediately did away with all my intestinal disturbances and improved my breathing and circulation. The only thing that remains is the treatment of my nose, and then—I certainly hope—I will be repaired and capable of work.—To be sure, I already have to give up the idea of criticizing Jung's paper in the 3d issue! The material is certainly ready, but on no account do I want to put this difficult and important work on paper hastily.—Next Sunday (April 20) I am coming to Vienna, this time for only one day; I intend to postpone the nose treatment until the Whitsun holiday.

Since my symptoms of illness have almost disappeared, I again have something more left over for my psychic personality. Frau G. still doesn't want to let go of her old plans (my marriage to Elma); this seems to her to be the only possible solution to my life's problem. Up to now I have carefully avoided taking a step in that direction.

I just read Putnam's "Griselda-Fantasy";[1] it reminds me of Jung's work on libido; both are incomprehensible and mystical.

I tried to find out about Tausk from Frau Lou; I will tell you in Vienna about what little has come out in the process.

Kind regards,
Ferenczi

1. James Jackson Putnam, "Bemerkungen über einen Krankheitsfall mit Griselda-Phantasien," *Zeitschrift* 1 (1913): 205–218.

389

INTERNATIONALE ZEITSCHRIFT
FÜR ÄRZTL. PSYCHOANALYSE[1]

Budapest, April 18, 1913

Dear Professor,
   I am coming already Sunday noon at 12:30 and intend to see you (for a short conference) before your office hours. (I will eat on the way.)

Cordially,
Ferenczi

Friday

1. Postcard with preprinted letterhead.

390

INTERNATIONALE ZEITSCHRIFT FÜR
ÄRZTLICHE PSYCHOANALYSE

Budapest, April 26, 1913

Dear Professor,
   Condition of health very satisfactory.—I am writing this time only in order to prepare you for the fact that a *Dr. Varjas*,[1] a high school teacher, who is interested in psychoanalysis (see the last issue of Stekel's periodical, review section),[2] wants to see you. He is an *Adlerian;* he recently wrote a shabby Hungarian *Interpretation of Dreams*,[3] which was published in the *local* "Reklam"[4] [an excerpt from your book, very popular; at the end he criticizes you by saying: it is not civilization that makes neurosis, but rather neurosis that makes civilization! (or something like that)].[5] Very conceited. Now he wants to do a *mathematical* psychoanalysis: calculate the possible types of insanity and other psychic productions on the basis of probability theory. But he lacks (so he says), on the one hand, the mathematical, on the other, the psychiatric schooling. [Otherwise, nothing!]
   I put up with him for a while. But in a dream that he told me he revealed himself to be an uncommonly vain man and one who is scientifically blinded by his vanity, and I became convinced that it really is that way with him.

I am curious about the impression that *you* will get from him. He obviously wanted a recommendation to you from me, but I advised him to go to you directly.

Cordially,
Ferenczi

1. See letter 135, n. 3.

2. A review by Jenö Hárnik of Sándor Varjas, "Zur Kritik der Freud'schen Theorie," pt. 1, *Huszadik Század* 25, no. 6 (1912): 574–583, was published in *Zentralblatt* 3 (1912–13): 345–348.

3. Sandor Varjas, *Az álomelmélete* [On the Dream: Freud's Theory of Dreams] (Budapest, 1913).

4. The book had been published as part of the Modern Könyvtár [Modern Library] series. *Reclam* was the German publisher of a line of cheap paperback books, especially editions of the classics.

5. Enclosed in brackets in the original, as is the similar remark later in the paragraph.

391

INTERNATIONALE ZEITSCHRIFT FÜR
ÄRZTLICHE PSYCHOANALYSE

Budapest, May 3, 1913

Dear Professor,

Our correspondence has definitely been diminishing in frequency and directness for some time. My illness is responsible for this; I obviously hate to bother you with information about my physical condition when we have for so many years either carried on an objective-scientific exchange of ideas or in our letters worked on eradicating certain psychic hindrances which have stood in the way of my work. But this time I will overcome the resistance and summarize the essentials of my condition.—The operation on my nose has not brought about any significant improvement.—Breathing through my nose is still impeded at times; *warmth* is especially harmful to me. When I get warm, a kind of "capillary paralysis" of my skin ensues. The veins in my arms swell up, the nasal turbinate bones disrupt my breathing. All that seems to go together with the blockages in my colon, because the distension of my belly, which often occurs, may produce the same vasomotor phenomena.—Every night I wake up around 3:30–4 o'clock with heart palpitations, which soon abate after the expulsion of intestinal gases; but usually I can't go to sleep anymore afterwards, and then I am tired during the day and incapable of spontaneous work. I admit that all these symptoms overly occupy my attention and are certainly *in part* of a hypochondriacal nature.—As far as my psychic hygiene is concerned, the matter is as follows: I repeatedly tried to satisfy my erotic needs "outside," but (perhaps because of the inferiority of the material) with the sole result that I quickly returned to Frau G. But Frau G. is, incidentally, working tirelessly on restoring relations between me and Elma. Up to now I have been resisting energetically. Elma herself is behaving well, rationally; according to Frau G. she is secretly longing for me, but remains silent and is "sponsoring" us (me and Frau G.), as it were.

The stay in Corfu has strengthened me to some extent, but I am still sorry that I didn't use the time spent there for a stay in Vienna with combined psychic-somatic treatment instead.—By the way, I haven't entirely given up this idea. This year I could choose the month of *June* for my vacation month and use the time in Vienna for analysis and diet cures. What do you think about that?

I am enclosing a letter from Maeder,[1] and my reply to it, which I ask you please to return (perhaps with suggestions on revision).

My analytic hours are increasing again; I have some very interesting cases, which bring me some ideas; but I lack the strength to work them out.

On the whole, I am quite dissatisfied with myself and sometimes see the future in a gloomy light.

Kind regards,
Ferenczi

1. This letter is missing.

392

INTERNATIONALE ZEITSCHRIFT FÜR
ÄRZTLICHE PSYCHOANALYSE

Vienna, May 4, 1913

Dear friend,

Your letter to Maeder is returned enclosed. It is very worthy and appropriate. Diplomacy will certainly no longer be of use against the anti-Semitism unleashed by our Zurichers. But don't solicit, remain firm.

Our correspondence has essentially been limited only because you are now handling all business matters with Rank. I am always glad to hear about how you are, even if you can't report the best. What consoles me is the extraordinary elevation of your intellectuality right at this time. You write better and better and have the nicest ideas. If I could be of use to you, then everything else would take precedence over that. But I know that four or six weeks of analysis would be much too insufficient. For that reason something else comes into consideration, namely, my dearth of inclination

to expose one of my indispensable helpers to the danger of personal estrangement brought about by the analysis. I don't yet know how Jones will
bear finding out that his wife, as a consequence of the analysis, no longer
wants to remain his wife.[1] Should it turn on the fact that women are more
intelligent than we and are justified in subjecting us to their![2] will?

Now try to get to work again. I don't think that there is anything seriously organically wrong with you.—Häberlin and Binswanger are coming
at the end of May.[3] I will ask you to visit then, since I have very little time
remaining. I am now writing about the totem with the feeling that it is my
greatest, best, and perhaps my last good thing. Inner certainties tell me that
I am right. Unfortunately, I get to work so little that I have to force myself
again and again to get into the proper mood. That harms my style as much
as do my many hours of association with people who speak German badly.

In the Society we are now in the process of setting up a Society hangout
attached to Rank's new home.[4] It is supposed to be the clear expression of
our will to live, independent of Aryan patronage.

Rank and Sachs are always equally loyal and diligent.

I will write to you another time about summer plans. I greet you and
Frau G. cordially and ask you for news soon.

Yours truly,
Freud

1. Loe Kann had fallen in love with a man by the name of Herbert Jones, a poet and
writer (ironically termed "Jones the Second" by Ernest Jones; Brome, *Jones*, p. 88), whom
she was later to marry (see letter 454 and n. 4 and letter 476). On June 3 Jones wrote to
Freud: "The idea of losing my wife has not yet penetrated fully into my mind. I have
difficulty in 'taking it in'. . . It is, of course, worse for me that I know how much I have
contributed to the present situation" (ibid., p. 88).
2. The exclamation point is written over the word "our," which has been crossed out.
3. See letter 396 and n. 4.
4. Rank had moved from Simon Denk-Gasse 8 in the Ninth District to Grünangergasse
3 in the more respectable First District. The new seat of the Society was at Franz-Josef-
Kai 65, likewise in the First District.

393

INTERNATIONALE ZEITSCHRIFT FÜR
ÄRZTLICHE PSYCHOANALYSE

Vienna, May 8, 1913

Dear friend,

Today I am enclosing Maeder's letter, which I forgot. According to reports
from Jones we have bad things to expect from Jung and should brace
ourselves for the collapse of the organization at the Congress. Of course,

everything that strives to get away from our truths has public approval in its favor. It is quite possible that they will really bury us this time, after they have so often sung a dirge for us in vain. It will change much in our fate, nothing in that of science. We are in possession of the truth; I am as sure of that as I was fifteen years ago.

When Jones comes we will decide how to defend ourselves. You will be more involved in that than I, who have never accomplished anything by way of polemics. I am accustomed mutely to reject and to go my own way.

Under these conditions much emphasis will be laid on your critique of Jung's paper on libido. I have already thought about whether I shouldn't perhaps contribute a page that sheds light on the thoughtless misunderstanding of my statement about libido in my paper on Schreber. What do you think about that?

I am working on the last segment of the totem study, which is just now managing to expand the rift by a mile; but reading and revision will take up my time up to June 15th. I haven't written anything with so much conviction since the Interpretation of Dreams; so I can anticipate the fate of the essay.

I would like to hear the best about your health. Our summer plans are as follows: Four of us (the women[1] and Anna) to Marienbad until August 14, then three weeks at S. Martino di Castrozza, then Munich, and a trip with an unknown destination. I have promised my family that this time I will have a period which is free of thoughts. I think it will be necessary, because these upsets destroy one inwardly, even if they don't make one neurotic. But I would like to see you in S. Martino, where it is supposed to be quite beautiful and from which we can then travel to Munich. If you want to, decide soon, for there are not many rooms free there. I greet you and Frau G. cordially, and I enclose a depressing piece of writing, which I received from Abraham.[2]

Yours truly,
Freud

1. Freud's wife, Martha, and his sister-in-law Minna Bernays.
2. Possibly "contradictory stuff" (Freud/Abraham, p. 137) by Bleuler (perhaps "Der Sexualwiderstand," Jahrbuch 5 [1913]: 442–452), which Abraham had sent to Freud on May 5.

394

INTERNATIONALE ZEITSCHRIFT FÜR
ÄRZTLICHE PSYCHOANALYSE

Budapest, May 12, 1913

Dear Professor,

I will reverse the time sequence and answer your second letter first.

The Zurichers will certainly leave no stone unturned in order to destroy the organization. But it is not certain whether they will succeed. The united Viennese, Berliners, and Americans (if care is taken that they show up in large enough numbers) could very easily gain the majority over the Zurichers. If they don't get the vote of the Congress, they may resign. At least we will remain amongst ourselves.

I absolutely do not believe that one can bury psychoanalysis. Perhaps it will come to a depression of one to two years, but in the long run the power of truth cannot be kept down by slogans. In the struggle (which I, too, accept only because necessity forces me to do so) I intend, if it comes to that, to fulfill the tasks that the Committee assigns me. Since it can be useful to lead another reliable local group into the field, I intend to found the Budapest group even before the Congress and to notify Jung that I have done so. (Or should I reserve the announcement for the Congress?) I want to accept only four or five very reliable members and have them come along to Munich. For the time being there are only three of us: Dr. Radó, Dr. Hollós, and I.[1]

Next I want to complete my critique of the Jungian libido paper. Never in my life has a more unpleasant task befallen me! *Nota bene:* I have finally arrived at the most secret meaning of Jung's paper. It is none other than his hidden confession of *occultism* in the guise of science. *Dreams tell the future; neurotics are mantically endowed people who foretell the future of the human race* (progress, repression of sexuality). The unconscious knows the present, past, and future; the fate (i.e., the *"task"*) of humanity is revealed in *"symbols."* All that comes from Jung's *astrological* (?) studies.— The little that he has seen of the "occult" was sufficient to bring down the obviously very shaky edifice of his psychoanalytic knowledge.

I thank you very much for your willingness to help me in this critique. I also share Abraham's view that all Committee members should participate in this important matter. Meanwhile, I will write the critique the way I mean it, will then circulate it to all Committee members, and, as far as possible, take their observations into account. Please tell that to Rank also, when you get the chance.—

I am awaiting your work on totem with the greatest anticipation; when can I get to read it?

Now I will return to your first letter, in which you concern yourself mainly with me.

I am doing much better healthwise. The diagnosis of neurasthenia has been confirmed; to be sure, I have learned to understand something quite different in this word than I did before the illness; when I get the chance I will share my ideas about this with you.

I am convinced that my analysis could only improve relations between us. With Jones the matter is different: his wife, not he, was analyzed. I have already gone through this period, in which you analyzed Elma and I subsequently couldn't marry her; I went through it without alienating myself from you or analysis. I hope, by the way, that Jones will also remain loyal. Frau G. is continuing her ceaseless attempts to win me over to Elma; up to now I have remained firm. It is interesting how the two women "play football" with me: one grants me to the other! I presume that reaction formations to their mutual death wishes are behind this. Frau G. certainly is very, very kind to me; after what has happened between us it is obviously not too difficult for her to sacrifice me and in this way to make amends for her repressed thoughts of revenge (against Elma). Elma is full of neurotic death thoughts against her mother, and so she exaggerates her concern about her welfare and is making an effort not to disturb us.

Kind regards,
Ferenczi

Yesterday I began a four-week-long course for medical students. I accepted about twenty auditors.

1. The founding of the Budapest Branch Society took place on May 19, 1913; besides Ferenczi (president), the members were István Hollós (representative), Lajos Lévy (treasurer), Sándor Radó (secretary), and Hugó Ignotus, the only member without a title.

395

INTERNATIONALE ZEITSCHRIFT FÜR
ÄRZTLICHE PSYCHOANALYSE

Vienna, May 13, 1913

Dear friend,

I can write to you again today because the work on totem was finished yesterday. A terrible migraine (a rarity with me) and the unexpected visit of my 80-year-old brother from Southport[1] threatened to hold up its completion at the last minute. I have the urge to write about it; not since the Interpretation of Dreams (the English translation of which I received yesterday[2] [after fourteen years][3]) have I worked on anything with the same feeling of certainty and elation. The reception will be comparable; a storm of indignation, except among my closest supporters. It comes at a very opportune time in the struggle with Zurich; it will separate us the way an acid does a salt.

Whoever wants to kiss the princess who sleeps inside will certainly have to work through a few thorn hedges of literature and papers.[4] I now have time until June 15 to read and to make improvements. Printing should be completed by July 14. I will send you the proofs from the middle of June on.

I am naturally in very high spirits and confront the dark future with equanimity. When Jones comes, you, as a committee, will be the first to get serious work. I think it is right not to let it come to a personal duel between Jung and me. I have broken off our relations, whether he remains in the Association or not.

Your case is not quite the same as Jones's. Jones has had his wife for seven years, and she is actually a jewel. It is certainly not my fault that he has lost her, and hardly his own either, by the way. They were no longer together for a long time.

If you can found your local group, then do it right away, and before the Congress, not just because of the votes but also because of the position that it bestows on you. The man[5] whom you informed me of by way of a wanted poster didn't come, fortunately.

Aren't you responding to the offer of S. Martino? It is an extremely enticing place to stay. We will be very pleased to meet you there. You know that I wouldn't conceal it if it were otherwise.

Kind regards,
Freud

1. Freud's half-brother Emanuel.
2. See letter 373 and n. 4.
3. Enclosed in brackets in the original.
4. A reference to the fairy tale *Dornröschen* (Sleeping Beauty) by the Brothers Grimm, in which the enchanted princess, along with her royal houshold, sleeps behind a dense hedge of thorns until a prince penetrates it and awakens the princess with a kiss.
5. Sándor Varjas; see letter 390.

396

Dr. Sigmund Freud
Universitätsprofessor für Nervenkrankheiten
IX/₁, Berggasse Nr. 19.
Ord. 3–5.   Telephon 14362[1]

[Vienna,] May 19, 1913

Very good and worthy!

Bad conscience on Maeder's part. We will maintain our reserve at the Congress.[2]

Jung is asking today which lectures are being given in Munich and whether the discussion on dreams should remain.[3] Request reply from you.

Binswanger and Häberlin were here all day yesterday.[4] Very pleasant. Next week (i.e., this), when Jones is here, hope to see you.

Reservations made at S. Martino.

Kind regards.

Yours,
Freud

1. The letter is written on both sides of a sheet from a prescription pad.

2. A communication from Ferenczi is evidently missing. It is not clear whether the reference is actually to Maeder, since the name is abbreviated "M" [Trans.].

3. At the conference of organization heads in Munich it was suggested that the title of the forthcoming Congress be "On the Teleological Function of Dreams." In Jung's circular of invitation (*Freud/Jung*, 354J, June 1913, p. 547) it was given more generally as "The Function of Dreams."

4. See Binswanger, *Reminiscences*, pp. 8f.

397

Internationale Zeitschrift
für ärztl. Psychoanalyse[1]

[Budapest,] May 23, 1913

Dear Professor,

I am arriving tomorrow morning (Saturday) around 7 in the evening, am staying as usual at the Hotel Regina, will stay until Sunday evening (maybe night), am bringing the Critique of Libido along. You could call a meeting of the Committee for Sunday morning, in which I could present the Critique as a lecture and make amendments. I would certainly be happy if, after such a long time, you could also grant me a few hours (one to two) as a "private audience." (Perhaps Sunday afternoon?) If it's all right (and you don't have a card game), the Committee meeting could also take place on Saturday evening.

Kind regards,
Ferenczi

1. Postcard with preprinted letterhead.

398

Vienna, May 24, 1913
IX., Berggasse 19

Dear friend,

I am very satisfied that you are coming already today, but I am of no use on Saturday evening after eleven hours of analytic work and at the end of a week without Sunday; the best thing for me would be to go and play cards.

I request that you come on Sunday morning at 10 o'clock, and I think that we had better spend the morning with each other and invite our friends for 3 in the afternoon. If you don't agree, a reply is still possible. I will eat dinner at home at 9—9: 30 and then I will walk to Königstein so that you can meet me.

You know that Jones is here and is staying at the Pension Washington[1] with his—former—wife.

Very much in suspense about your Critique.

Cordially,
Freud

1. The Pension Washington was at Ebersdorferstrasse 8, in the City Hall quarter of the First District.

399

INTERNATIONALE ZEITSCHRIFT
FÜR ÄRZTL. PSYCHOANALYSE[1]

Budapest, May 28, 1913

Dear Professor,

My friend and member of the local Budapest group, H. Ignotus, man of letters and editor of the review "Nyugat"[2] [= Occident],[3] asks you through me to allow him to go to *Scientia* with the request to allow him to publish your paper[4] in Hungarian right after it comes out. (When will it be published, by the way?) I recommend that you give Ignotus the right to do this.

We have a pressing need for such an authoritative overview, since there is so much nonsense going around here *sub titulo* psychoanalysis.—

Yesterday Frau G. was operated on (without anesthesia).[5] Everything went smoothly.—

My stay in Vienna was very refreshing!

Cordially,

F.

1. Postcard with preprinted letterhead.
2. See letter 135, n. 4.
3. Enclosed in brackets in the original.
4. "The Claims of Psycho-Analysis to Scientific Interest" (Freud 1913j); see letter 378 and n. 2. No translation could be found in *Nyugat*.
5. Details of this operation are unknown.

400

Vienna, June 1, 1913
IX., Berggasse 19

Dear friend,

If you think Ignotus should bring out the, in itself, worthless paper in Hungarian, I am of course in agreement and empower him to make arrangements with Scientia about it. Date of publication is unknown to me.

The impression of health that you made here was very gratifying. Let us hope it will now stay that way.

I will see Jones before he leaves to see you.[1]

Cordially,

Freud

1. Jones went to see Ferenczi in order to undergo a training analysis during June and July (he left Budapest on August 1; see letter 413) of two hours a day (see letter 408), which overlapped with Loe Kann's analysis with Freud. Jones himself recalls a longer duration ("summer and autumn"; *Associations*, p. 199, and Jones II, 127) and is mistaken in his assumption that he had been the first analyst to subject himself to a proper analysis. At least one other, René Spitz, had begun analysis with Freud, in October 1911 (see letter 240).

401

INTERNATIONALE ZEITSCHRIFT FÜR
ÄRZTLICHE PSYCHOANALYSE

Budapest, June 7, 1913

Dear Professor,

Here is a new, very confused epistle from Maeder.[1] I think it would be best not to go into the details of what he has omitted, but rather politely—while repeating what has already been said—withdraw. I solicit your view.—

I think the analysis with Jones will work. At present he is *interpreting* too much and is producing only old material that is already known to him; he has already brought the (positive) transference along into the treatment. He is very keen on honesty (I know that from comparing what he has already said with what I know about him). Otherwise he feels quite well.

The heat is terrible!

Kind regards,
Ferenczi

1. This letter is missing.

402

INTERNATIONALE ZEITSCHRIFT FÜR
ÄRZTLICHE PSYCHOANALYSE

Vienna, June 8,[1] 1913

Dear friend,

I am very pleased that Jones is acquitting himself well. Be strict and tender with him. He is a very good person. Feed the pupa so that a queen can be made out of it.

You are right. Our dear Swiss have gone crazy [*meschugge geworden*]. Maeder is as pontifical as Jung is boastful. For us it is a good opportunity to "treat" them. If you want my opinion, I would respond to Maeder again this time while maintaining the basic tone you have already set. Something like this: On the matter of Adler: regret that he didn't rather reply privately to a private letter instead of exposing us to the danger of bringing rectification from Adler. The true Adlerian essence has nothing to do with ΨA but rather wants to put itself in its place. Inasmuch as ΨA is involved, this is improper and will certainly be disapproved of in the Zeitschrift. As far as "withholding" is concerned, it is no worse than if the Zeitschrift withheld from its readers the results of experimental psychology. On the matter of

Semitism: there are certainly great differences from the Aryan spirit. We can become convinced of that every day. Hence, there will surely be different world views and art here and there. But there should not be a particular Aryan or Jewish science. The results must be identical, and only their presentation may vary. Certainly my remark about the Interpretation of Dreams should be taken in this way. If these differences occur in conceptualizing objective relations in science, then something is wrong. It was our desire not to interfere with their more distant worldview and religion, but we considered ours to be quite favorable for conducting science You had heard that Jung had declared in America that ΨA was not a science but a religion. That would certainly illuminate the whole difference. But there the Jewish spirit regretted not being able to join in.

It couldn't hurt to be somewhat derisive.

—Since knocking off the work on totem I have been light and gay.

Kind regards,
Freud

1. In the original the "8" in the date appears to have been written over and changed from a "7."

403

INTERNATIONALE ZEITSCHRIFT FÜR
ÄRZTLICHE PSYCHOANALYSE

Vienna, June 12, 1913

Dear friend,

Today I sent you the first galleys of Totem. There is nothing in them; they belong to the thorn hedges behind which the princess is sleeping. But interesting passages come later, unfortunately also some among them that are in need of improvement. I have retreated far from my initial high opinion of the work and am, on the whole, dubious about it. I would be very pleased if you could alleviate my difficult task by means of a suggestion or addition: so I will refrain from correcting the later passages in question until you send it back, and I strongly request that you express yourself promptly.

In thirty days I will close up the place. I am already very enthusiastic about the vacation. Glad to hear that I will see you again in June.

Jones seems to be very satisfied.

Cordially,
Freud

404

INTERNATIONALE ZEITSCHRIFT FÜR
ÄRZTLICHE PSYCHOANALYSE

Vienna, June 17, 1913

Dear friend,

Your Jung critique has turned out to be excellent; I didn't like it so well until it was in press. I am completely convinced of the "new tendency's" lack of content.

We usually conclude the year's work with a dinner on the Konstantinhügel. This time I would not like to miss you and Jones there, if you are thinking of coming anyway. We will wait for both of you. Does perhaps Saturday the 28th of the month suit you? Incidentally, any day is all right with us, even during the week.[1]

I am now doing nothing but corrections. The work on totem has still not fully come up to my expectations. It is too uncertain; it would be *too* beautiful. I added a few qualifying sentences and am waiting for your and Jones's remarks, by the way.

The Narcissism,[2] the scientific reckoning with Adler, will probably ripen during the summer.

Things are continuing to go well with Frau Jones. Tell him that, please.

I am fully occupied up to the last day (July 12). From May on is usually my busiest time. Pfister's book,[3] which is thought to be very respectable, can be expected any day.

Kind regards to you and Jones in the hope that you continue to be well physically.

Yours,
Freud

1. After the completion of *Totem and Taboo,* according to Jones, "on June 30, 1913, we celebrated the occasion by giving Freud a dinner, which we called a totemic festival, on the Konstantinhügel in the Prater. Loe Kann presented him with an Egyptian figurine which he adopted as a totem" (Jones II, 355).

2. "On Narcissism: An Introduction" (Freud 1914c).

3. See letter 378, n. 3.

405

INTERNATIONALE ZEITSCHRIFT FÜR
ÄRZTLICHE PSYCHOANALYSE

Budapest, June 17, 1913

Dear Professor,

I have received the first morsels of the totem meal; they aroused great curiosity in me about the continuation—the actual analytic part. Unfortunately, I will very probably not be in a position to correct anything, since the entire field is completely new to me. If I get an idea, anyway, I will share it with you.

Jones is very pleasant as a friend and colleague. His excessive kindness works as a hindrance in the analysis; his dreams are full of mockery and scorn toward me, which he has to admit, without being able really to believe in these hidden characteristics of his.[1] He also seems to fear that I will tell you everything that I experience in the analysis. For that reason I ask you not to mention anything about our correspondence in Frau Jones's presence. I now find Jones in some respects scientifically *much* more valuable to us than before our analytic acquaintance with him.[*] But he is inhibited in *production* by his excess of kindness; he forbids himself any independence, which then avenges itself by means of an inclination toward intrigue and secret triumphs, treachery. I think the weeks here will be useful to him. I already find him to be a little less modest, i.e., more honest (with others and with himself). He is diligently learning German and is making good progress.

As for myself, I am again quite well physically. As a result, naturally, I am again suffering more from being sexually unsatisfied.—

At the Congress I would like to touch on the theme of symbol formation. I think that is probably the most current thing that should be discussed. Do you think the subject is suitable?[2]

Sunday after next, we (Jones and I) are coming to Vienna, and we are both looking forward to seeing you.

Yesterday I made Storfer's[3] acquaintance.

Kind regards to the whole family.

Yours,
Ferenczi

[*] Of course, I don't mean by that that analysis has already changed him, but that I underestimated him somewhat before.

1. On the same day Jones wrote to Freud: "I am doing my best in the analysis and think it is going on satisfactorily. Ferenczi discovers in me very strong aggressive ten-

dencies which I have reacted to by too much suppression and submissiveness and which revenge themselves in various impulsive tendencies" (Brome, *Jones*, p. 86).

2. Ferenczi subsequently delivered a lecture, "Glaube, Unglaube und Überzeugung" [Belief, Disbelief, and Conviction] (1913, 109; *F.C.*, p. 437); on symbol formation, he wrote an essay of his own, "Zur Ontogenese der Symbole" [On the Ontogenesis of Symbols] (1913, 125; *C.*, p. 276). See also letter 413.

3. See letter 188, n. 7.

406

INTERNATIONALE ZEITSCHRIFT FÜR
ÄRZTLICHE PSYCHOANALYSE

Budapest, June 23, 1913

Dear Professor,

My impression of the work on totem was deep—despite the fact that I was already acquainted with most (not all) of its trains of thought. The Oedipus complex really proves here to be the hypomochlion,[1] supported on which one can unravel all the secrets of the soul. We (Jones and I) will come back to a detailed evaluation of individual passages after we have read it together once more, that will be tomorrow or the day after. I hasten, however, to ask you *not to insert any qualification,* but to leave everything the way it is in the proofs of the Totem. The presentation of your case is flawless; there is no room left for doubt.

I am thinking after all that that your subsequent vacillation is actually a displaced *retrospective obedience*[2] with respect to the fathers (and your own father), who in this work are depriving you of the last remnants of your power over the soul of man. Your work is namely also a totem meal; you are the priest of *Mithras,*[3] who singlehandedly kills the father—your students are the audience to this "holy" action.—You yourself compared the significance of the Totem paper with that of the Interpretation of Dreams.—But the latter was the "reaction to [your] father's death"![4] In the Interpretation of Dreams you carried out the struggle against your own father, in the work on Totem, against the ghostly, religious father imagoes.—Hence, the *festive joy* at the work's coming into being (at the sacrificial act), which was then followed by the subsequent *scruples.*

I am firmly convinced the work on Totem will one day become the nodal point of the study of the history of civilization.

I find new and outstanding the idea of transmission by means of *unconscious understanding,*[5] which to a certain extent forces the phylogenetic theories into the background.

Jones is my best and dearest patient; he is competent, clever, obedient, and a really dependable friend at the same time; I think we will be able to build on him.

Kind regards, until we see each other again soon.

Yours,
Ferenczi

The brief period of resistance with Jones has been replaced by sound progress.

Postscript to the Remarks about the Work on Totem

In the Introduction it reads that the psychoanalytic explanation of religion "is [not] claiming . . . that that source is the only one or that it occupies *first place* among the numerous contributory factors."[6]

At the end of the work it says (in contrast to this) that the ψα. explanation can assume *none other than the central place* in the synthesis that makes this institution comprehensible.[7]

The second determination is the correct one, in my opinion, but I believe it stands in contradiction to the introductory statement.

Cordially,
F.

1. Fulcrum of a lever. See letter 129, n. 3.
2. See letter 320 and n. 3, and letter 321.
3. Mithras (Greco-Roman), or Mithra (Persian), god of light or the sun. Since at least the beginning of 1911 Freud had been examining the cult of Mithras (*Freud/Jung*, January 22, 1911, p. 388) and had mentioned it in *Totem and Taboo*: "We may perhaps infer from the sculptures of Mithras slaying a bull that he represented a son who was alone in sacrificing his father and thus redeemed his brothers from their burden of complicity in the deed" (1912-13a, p. 153). In *Moses and Monotheism* he came back to the topic in connection with "tragic guilt" (see also letter 221 and n. 13), suggesting that Mithras may represent the ringleader of the band of brothers who boast of having "rebel[led] against [their] father and kill[ed] him in some shape or other" (1939a [1934–1938], p. 87).
4. "[In this book] I found a portion of my own self-analysis, my reaction to my father's death—that is to say, to the most important event, the most poignant loss, of a man's life"; (see the preface to the second edition, written in 1908, during the vacation Freud spent with Ferenczi in Berchtesgaden (1900a, p. xxvi).
5. Freud had written: "We may safely assume that no generation is able to conceal any of its more important mental processes from its successor. For psycho-analysis has shown us that everyone possesses in his unconscious mental activity an apparatus which enables him to interpret other people's reactions, that is, to undo the distortions which other people have imposed on the expression of their feelings. An unconscious understanding such as this . . . may have made it possible for later generations to take over their heritage of emotion" (1912–13a, p. 159).
6. Freud 1912–13a, p. 100; the emphasis is Ferenczi's.
7. See letter 407 and n. 3.

407

Vienna, June 26, 1913
IX., Berggasse 19

My dear friends,[1]

Despite the prospect of seeing you again so soon, I need to respond beforehand to your remarks about the paper on totem and thus do some preparatory work for our conversations.

I thank you both sincerely and kindly for your elucidations and contributions, all of which I acknowledge. The resolution of my doubts must be well founded, for a large part of my confidence has returned since I received your communications. My critical conscience does not yet want to be completely silenced. I consider the matter on the one hand too beautiful, but on the other hand, times and things are too obscure and to a certain extent beyond the pale of sure assessment.

So, as a consequence of your report, *nothing* will be qualified. Only one sentence was inserted before the two objections in [section] 7. "The high degree of convergence should not blind us to the uncertainty of the premises nor the difficulties of the conclusions. I will discuss two of the latter myself."[2]

I have noted very well the contradiction between the introduction and the "central place," and I have let it stand for correction. It corresponds to a development which took place in the process of writing it down and will be compensated for by a "now, however," or the like.[3]

The suggestions from Jones have to do with extensions, which I don't have much desire to make but which cannot be halted in the face of such suggestions. In order not to write a book instead of an essay, I have broken off everywhere. Some things that Jones brings up are so much his property that I would rather see it developed by him in his own context.

The approval and participation of both of you is thus the first pleasure gain that I can register after completing the work. Otherwise, there is stirring in me—like a general wish to sleep while dreaming—a great lethargy, which wants nothing more than to have done with the thing until July 12. My thoughts are now fleeing from it.

I have learned with interest that I am no longer inaccessible to the judgments of others, as I was earlier. Especially if you are the critics.

Auf Wiedersehen on the Hill of Constantine!

Cordially,
Freud

1. The letter is addressed to Ferenczi and Jones.
2. There is a statement to this effect in Freud 1912–13a, p. 157.
3. See ibid., n. 2.

408

INTERNATIONALE ZEITSCHRIFT FÜR
ÄRZTLICHE PSYCHOANALYSE

Budapest, July 7, 1913

Dear Professor,

I just filled my dry fountain pen and immediately picked up two sheets of stationery, because I had the feeling I had much to write. The occasion is sad enough: today is my *fortieth* birthday. This date seems to have activated much in me, and the affect overcame the writing inhibition—which you must have noticed long ago—and which has prevented me for so long from talking about myself. (At our meetings in Vienna what happens to me is similar to what happens to people in analysis: "Nothing comes to my mind"! In Vienna I usually feel in elevated spirits; the big thing that occupies us scientifically captures me completely, and when you say a few reassuring words in response to my personal communications I feel quite in agreement and am happy to return to our scientific subjects. Here at home I then have the "sentiment d'incomplétude"[1] (to speak French with Jung and Janet)[2]—the feeling "as if"[3] we should have talked much more about me.)

I was *quite honest* when I told you that I am happy to see the matter with Elma settled without me; and yet I was *extraordinarily* saddened when I learned—after my return from Vienna—that the marriage with that American is *really* going to take place.[4]—Then, when on the day before the young man's departure for America Elma still didn't say "yes" to the man (certainly not just out of consideration for me, on whom she is no longer counting, but rather because she was hurt by something or other that the American said); so, when the road was opened for me, the old scruples returned in me, and an inner anxiety about the future restrained me from making any advances—in fact, I immediately found Elma less desirable than at the time when she seemed unattainable to me. This strange condition of love is certainly neurotic.

Meanwhile, Frau G. is tirelessly championing Elma's cause with me; she sees in it the only possible and—as she says—favorable solution for all of us; she claims that Elma loves me now as before. But I—now as before—have become skeptical about her capacity for love, and this thought repels me again and again from her, when (in fantasy) I take measures to approach her.

All these struggles are taking place quietly within me—but they bind all my activity and hinder me in my work; thoughts come, to be sure (albeit not very often)—but I lack the energy to carry them out.

Today I said jokingly that I now, finally, feel about twenty-five years old, that is, I feel that I have come of age; and I am not exaggerating in that. I can discover nothing in me that smacks of the set, quiet ways of a forty-year-old.

This week a few patients finally departed, and from now on I have less to do. The two hours with Jones are passing pleasantly; he is not only good and sensitive but also a very clever person, whose company stimulates one to one's best thoughts.—We are now having calmer sessions, after overcoming certain resistances; progress is, however, steady (albeit not always at a uniform pace).

I am thinking with pleasure about the fact that you are saying goodbye to the reality principle and are diving into the rejuvenating pleasure bath of Maria.[5] I wish (and in the process am hoping for the omnipotence of my thoughts) that you will recuperate soon and thoroughly.

I am very much looking forward to the days in the Tyrol. It would be nice to be present again at the birth of new ideas, as in Berchtesgaden and Klobenstein.

Kind regards,
Ferenczi

1. A concept of Pierre Janet's. Adler saw his concept of the "feeling of inferiority" as a further development of Janet's idea. Alfred Adler, *The Neurotic Constitution* (New York, 1917), p. vi.

2. Enclosed in parentheses in the original.

3. An allusion to the book *Philosophie des Als Ob* [Philosophy of the As If] (Berlin, 1911) by the famous neo-Kantian philosopher Hans Vaihinger (1852–1933), who, independently of Adler, established as generally valid for the human spirit the logic of neuroses postulated by the latter—the emanation of fictions, or as-if constructions. See Adler, *The Neurotic Constitution, passim.*

4. Elma Palós married Hervé Laurvik, a writer of Swedish-American extraction; this marriage ended in divorce not long afterwards.

5. Marienbad; see letter 393.

409

Vienna, July 9, 1913
IX., Berggasse 19

Dear friend,

Really? Can I already congratulate you on your 40th birthday? Your wistful letter has deeply moved me, first and foremost because it reminded me of my own 40th, since which I have several times shed my skin, which, as you know, happens every seven years. At the time (1896) I was at the nadir of desolation, had lost all my old friends, and had not yet acquired any new ones; no one cared about me, and the only thing that kept me going was a bit of defiance and the beginning of the Interpretation of

Dreams. When I look at you now, I have to consider you lucky in many respects, even if my congratulations haven't gotten any louder. You stand there securely oriented, an open road ahead of you, highly esteemed by an unusually distinguished circle of friends, whose spiritual leader you have been designated to become. There is one thing you don't have, the possession of which I already felt sure of then,[1] and I know that one misses most acutely and prizes most highly what one can't attain.

On your 40th birthday I can dispense with all reserve and admit to you that I never forcefully advised you against Elma only because I was afraid that you would still have wanted to go through with it, following neurotic patterns. What do you want to do now? For each of us fate assumes the form of one (or several) women, and your fate has some rare, precious qualities.

You know that I recently turned down the Emdens, pleasant company as they are, in order to live for a few weeks, analysis-free, in Marienbad. My next company will be my little daughter, who is now developing so gratifyingly (you have surely long ago guessed this subjective condition of the "choice of caskets").[2] I hope to be fresh enough in S. Martino to be able to appreciate your company more than I did the year before, when everything and everybody was too much for me. Abraham wants to visit us at the end of August and will probably go with us to Munich. I don't yet know how to support your hope that I will then be able to tell you something new. Good things really happen to me in periods of seven years: in 1891 I began with aphasia, 1898/9 the Interpretation of Dreams, 1904/5 Jokes and the Theory of Sexuality, 1911/12 the Totem thing;[3] so I am probably on the wane and can't count on anything bigger before 1918/19 (if the chain doesn't break before then).

I am very pleased by what you write about Jones. I now feel far less guilty of complicity in the outcome of the process with his wife since I see her blooming so, now that she is free. This Loe has become extraordinarily dear to me, and I have produced with her a very warm feeling with complete sexual inhibition, as has rarely been the case before (probably owing to my age). Unfortunately, this child also causes me great concern, which you should not let him (Ernest Jones) share. The swelling of her feet has not abated, so I finally decided to call in Dr. Kaufmann[4] for her, whom I hold in especially high esteem on account of his outstanding achievement with Sophie. He diagnosed *deep* thromboses of the veins, which could easily have become fatal, but he thinks the danger is past now; but he definitely forbids her to undertake any exertion before the end of July. So the trip to Budapest will not take place and will have to be changed to England. Jones should learn nothing of this. I understand only enough of this piece of internal medicine to know that everything is scary. She is cheerful and frivolous. I don't want to make her too anxious.

Martin has now successfully passed his third state examination with the corresponding oral examination and now has only a small oral examination before him and will be able to graduate at the end of October–November. All three of the boys have been especially diligent and respectable lately.

We will carry on our cause quietly and with superior assurance. I had intended to thank Jung for the feeling that the children are being taken care of, which a Jewish father needs as a matter of life and death; I am now happy that you and our friends are giving it to me.

With a hearty cheer for the next two thirds of your existence,

Amicably yours,
Freud

1. That is, a wife.
2. See "The Theme of the Three Caskets" (Freud 1913f).
3. *On Aphasia* (1891b); *The Interpretation of Dreams* (1900a); *Jokes and Their Relation to the Unconscious* (1905c); *Three Essays on the Theory of Sexuality* (1905d); and *Totem and Taboo* (1912–1913a).
4. Rudolf Kaufmann (1871–1927), Viennese internist, specialist in circulatory diseases.

410

Marienbad, July 19, 1913[1]

Dear friend,

Please call to Jones's attention an article in the British Medical Journal, July 5, 1913 (by Forsyth).[2] A leader[3] is complaining about my incomprehensible style. He is probably the farmer with the spectacles.[4] I hope you have sent Loe back successfully.[5] I am very contented here.

Yours,
Freud

1. Postcard.
2. David Forsyth, "Psychoanalysis," *British Medical Journal* 2 (1913): 13–17. Forsyth (1877–1941) was chief physician at Charing Cross Hospital in London and was among the first members of the London Society. Shortly thereafter, at the Seventeenth International Congress for Medicine in London (August 7–12), he defended Freud's conceptions (Ellenberger, *Unconscious*, p. 818). He was later analyzed by Freud and cited by him in "Dreams and Occultism" ("Forsyth/Foresight," in *New Introductory Lectures on Psychoanalysis* [1933a], pp. 48ff). Forsyth, incidentally, was chosen over Jones at Charing Cross, even though he had been second to Jones in the medical qualifying examinations (Brome, *Jones*, p. 36).
3. The word "leader" is in English in the original; unidentified reference.
4. An allusion to "the story of the peasant at the optician's, trying glass after glass and still not being able to read" (1900a, p. 217).
5. Loe Kann had gone from Vienna to Budapest on July 12 (letter from Ernest Jones to

Freud of July 8, 1913). On July 22 Jones wrote to Freud that Kann had returned safely to Vienna (personal communication from Andrew Paskauskas).

411

Dear Professor,

Your kind and heartfelt congratulations have touched me deeply. I cannot yet answer the question: "What will you do now?" I hope to be able to talk with you in detail about these things in the Tyrol.

I am pleased to hear that—despite the bad weather—you are feeling well. It was a difficult year, the one just past!

Jung's paper in the Jahrbuch[1] is in retrospect justifying my critique most admirably. He is trying to blur the differences; it was good to point them out ruthlessly. I think that you will soon have to concern yourself with the question of whether you should resign as director of the Jahrbuch.—

My mother (Frau Rosa Ferenczi) is now living in Marienbad (Haus Worms) and wants to become acquainted with your family, which I also encouraged her to do. I will let you know her address.

Jones is working diligently; I hope the analysis will be useful to him in every respect; he was still not able to emancipate himself *completely* from his latent tendencies (although he is thinking very optimistically about it).[2]

I may not be able to arrive in the Tyrol until the 18th; I will, of course, notify the hotel manager about this at the proper time.

Cordially,
Ferenczi

1. Carl Jung, "Versuch einer Darstellung der psychoanalytischen Theorie" [The Theory of Psychoanalysis, CW IV, 83–226]; Jahrbuch, 5 (1913): 307–441; (the German text of Jung's lectures in America of September 1912).

2. On the previous day, Jones had reported to Freud that the analysis "gave [him] more self dependence and freedom by diminishing further what was left of [his] father complex . . . It is better to have a therefore permanent attitude of respect and admiration than a kind of veneration which brings with it the dangers of ambivalency" (Brome, *Jones*, p. 89).

412

Dear friend,

I ended my cure yesterday, and my toxic lassitude has gone with it. In addition, a paper came today that I am enclosing for you,[1] a good example of specific Adlerian poison. Now, these are our opponents! I will, of course, not respond at all. It seems to be an attempt at a malicious tease. I don't know the author. The most regrettable thing is that he is right about so much that he says about Jung.

I am now going to read Jung's new paper;[2] it will establish our behavior at the Congress but not change it anymore. I don't know why I should resign from the Jahrbuch. I don't want either to provoke a break or vacate a position that is still good.

Today your mother returned my visit. A fine woman with remarkably clear eyes. We will see her again before she leaves.

We are leaving on Monday the 11th and arrive in S. Martino on the 13th. I know that your lateness will be due to a marriage in the family, but I still pity you.

Marienbad was magnificently beautiful the last five days. But I am already too restless for the easy living here.

I have agreed to make a brief report at the Congress. I will convey to you later what it will be about. A request from Jung and an urgent reminder from Abraham are making me do it, although the freedom of discussion that Jung has set up doesn't suit me.[3] I fear we will come apart worse at the Congress than we intend. But we still want to hold onto these intentions as long as possible.

With kind regards, in the expectation of hearing from you.

Yours truly,
Freud

1. An unidentified essay by Alexander Neuer (1883–1940 or 1941). Neuer, a Doctor of Medicine and Philosophy and a psychiatrist from Lemberg (Lodz), was a student of Adler's. One of his articles, "Wandlungen der Libido," *Zeitschrift für medizinische Psychotherapie und medizinische Psychologie,* 7 (1916), was reviewed by Ferenczi in *General Theory of the Neuroses* (1921, 236); see also letter 413.

2. See letter 411, n. 1.

3. At previous Congresses no allowance had been made for discussion of the lectures.

413

INTERNATIONALE ZEITSCHRIFT FÜR
ÄRZTLICHE PSYCHOANALYSE

Budapest, August 5, 1913

Dear Professor,

I find "Dr. Neuer's" paper (probably actually Adler's work) very pertinent; most of his remarks about the hypocritical way in which Jung reigns as a Bayard[1] of psychoanalysis and attacks you in all essential points (infantile sexuality, the unconscious, fixation, etc.) are proper characterizations.—The Zurichers will soon stand there in isolation and very soon present the mystical side of their being (astrology); that is the only "original" thing in their conception. With that, however, they will make themselves innocuous to the cause of ΨA.

I have suddenly decided (led astray by my reading of Jung's lectures) to give a lecture at the Congress about the psychology of conviction;[2] I have already notified Jung of this.—My lecture will have many points of contact with that of Jones[3] (which has turned out to be excellent), and it will attempt to prove that only proper psychoanalysis, which permits one really to *live out* the different psychic experiences by reviving the memory traces, or (when this is not possible) by means of transference to the present, is suited to allow *convictions* to arise in people; whereas all other psychotherapeutic measures (suggestion, Dubois,[4] Adler, Jung) are unsuited to this. I will use this opportunity to 1.) discuss Jung's false assumption that you *have given up* (and not just expanded) the trauma theory, 2.) to test the psychology of "evidence" [on the basis of experiences with obsessional neurotics with doubting mania].[5] The subject can be formulated on various levels; I will make an effort to be as brief as possible.

I find that you have very pointedly characterized my mother in the single sentence that you wrote about her. She is remarkably fresh, mentally (for her age).

I will not attend the wedding in my family after all. Instead, I will possibly spend two to three days in Vienna to get my nose straightened out before the vacation. I hope to arrive in the Tyrol on the 16th–17th. I am already very much looking forward to being with you, and I have the feeling that the things that are all happening in a rush will have a favorable effect on my productivity.

Jones left me four days ago. I miss him *very much*. We have become intimate friends; I grew to love and treasure him; it was a pleasure to have such an intelligent, fine, and respectable pupil. His convictions were more securely based, his self-reliance increased, and probably also his courage to be somewhat more original. Let us hope he will succeed in mastering his neurotic tendencies from now on—but I will not venture to make a *definite* prognosis on this.[6]

We will certainly not be able to avoid clarifying our position with regard to the Jungian theories at the Congress. Rank's,[7] Jones's, and my lecture will surely be full of critical remarks against Jung. How will the Association be able to stay together under such conditions?! In any event, it will require much tact and diplomacy on your part.

Kind regards,
Ferenczi

A paper by Beaurain (Zakopane) on symbol formation in the child will appear in the September issue of the Zeitschrift.[8] Since it is written very one-sidedly in favor of Jung's and Silberer's position, I permitted myself (in hopes of your retroactive approval) to append to this paper a small essay on the same subject.[9]

1. Pierre du Terrail (1470–1524), Seigneur of Bayard, renowned French warrior-hero; because of his bravery he was called "judge without fear and flaw."

2. See letter 405, n. 2.

3. Jones's lecture was titled "The Position of the Physician to the Current Conflicts."

4. Paul Charles Dubois (1848–1918), professor of neuropathology at the University of Bern, successful and sought-after therapist. According to his conception, neurotic disturbances were a product of the imagination and could be cured by the force of the will in a "rational psychotherapy."

5. Enclosed in brackets in the original.

6. Brome (*Jones*, p. 86) cites a statement of Michael Balint's—with whom Ferenczi had evidently spoken about Jones's analysis—to the effect that in the last sessions the analysis had centered on the fact that Jones's mother had fed him with quack milk preparations, which had led to rickets and other serious side effects. Ferenczi had been of the opinion that Jones, in reaction to the breast that was denied him, his small size, and lowly social origin, had at the beginning of his career developed an "omnipotence complex," which at the time of his analysis yielded to a less domineering, more tactful attitude. Jones himself was of the opinion that the analysis had helped him achieve a much greater inner harmony and had given him an irreplaceable and very direct insight into the ways of the unconscious (*Associations*, p. 199).

7. As co-presenter, Rank introduced "The Function of the Dream" into the day's theme.

8. "Über das Symbol und die psychischen Bedingungen für sein Entstehen beim Kind," *Zeitschrift* 1 (1913): 431–435.

9. Ferenczi, "Zur Ontogenese der Symbole," ibid., pp. 436–438; 1913, 125; C, p. 276.

414

Marienbad, August 5, 1913

Dear friend,

I am unmistakably in a toxic condition similar to the one you saw me in last year, and even more similar to the one I had at the beginning of the first Karlsbad cure. Moody, irritable, tired, but this time no weakness of the heart. Always ruminating over the same dark thoughts, taking little things hard, aversion to food; but after filling my stomach, I regularly brighten up.

In this state of intoxication, the stupid nonsense by Neuer that I sent you has weighed especially heavily on me. I have now read Jung's paper myself and I find it good and innocuous, beyond my expectation. Jones is quite right with his criticism; the errors are palpable, the comparisons slanted; much that he presents in his aggressive tone as discovery is, moreover, congruent with our intellectual property; but the contradictions remain entirely on ΨA's ground. Much toward the end about therapy, transference, etc. is even excellent. What is stupid is his insistence on inertia [*Trägheit*] as an etiological factor, instead of the Oedipus complex. Inertia is a universal law, even more general than the Oedipus complex! On the whole, I have very much overestimated the danger from a distance. The connections to Adler are slight. Only Adler's hawk's-eye view could find a reason to claim priority there. It would be quite right if Adler and Aiglon[1] tore each other up a bit with their beaks on the sidelines. We won't come between them.

Another recent adventure is an impertinent letter from the confidence man Friedländer, whose integrity has been certified by a tribunal, and who wants to sue me because of a statement I made about him to Binswanger.[2] I hope my sources won't leave me in the lurch. You can imagine how much I would *otherwise* make of this affair. So, now I have finished gossiping, without awaiting your reply to my last letter.

Cordially,
Freud

On the *13th* of the month, S. Martino.[3]

1. *Aiglon* is French for young *(Jung)* eagle *(Adler)*. Napoleon II, son of Napoleon I (the "*eagle*") and Marie-Louise of Austria, was also known as "l'aiglon." He failed to fulfill the hopes that his father had placed in him (see also Gay, *Freud*, pp. 235f). *L'Aiglon* (1900) was at that time a much-performed play by Edmond Rostand (1868–1918).

2. Freud had evidently not kept to himself his opinion that Friedländer was a "liar, rogue, and ignoramus" (see letter 138 and *Freud/Abraham*, May 6, 1910, p. 89). According to Jones (II, 117), Friedländer never carried out his threat.

3. Freud, his wife, Martha, Minna Bernays, and Anna arrived on August 11 in San Martino di Castrozza, where Ferenczi met them four days later. Abraham also came to visit for a few days. Freud and Ferenczi then went together to Munich to the "Fourth Private Psychoanalytic Association" (September 7–8, 1913). There Freud delivered a lecture, "On the Problem of Choice of Neurosis," published under the title "The Disposition to Obsessional Neurosis: A Contribution to the Problem of Choice of Neurosis" (1913i). Ferenczi's lecture was titled "On the Psychology of Conviction" ("Glaube, Unglaube und Überzeugung," 1913, 109; *F.C.*, p. 437). The atmosphere of the Congress was especially tense on account of the burgeoning conflict with Jung; on his reelection as president, two fifths of the members abstained from voting (see also the, enclosure to

letter 430). Descriptions of the Congress can be found in, among other sources, Jones II, 101–103; Clark, *Freud*, pp. 331f); Gay, *Freud*, p. 239; and *Freud/Jung*, editor's note after letter 356J, pp. 549f. After the Congress, Freud, along with Minna Bernays, who met him in Bologna, went to Rome, where he remained for seventeen days.

415

Rome, September 11, 1913[1]

Dear friend,

As the last one from the previous formation, you should be the first to receive information from the newest. Nothing has been damaged by the well-known fall, other than the wooden container of the inkwell. Meeting in Bologna went according to plan. After endless trip, arrival in Rome 10 minutes to 12 o'clock. Today hot, very hot, sciroccal; but things will soon change, since it has been this way for three days already. It will disappear and make way for normal brightness and beauty. Herr Nisklwead,[2] the innkeeper, was with Bircher as a *patient*, so he knows me and already knows that the Swiss no longer believe, etc. Haven't yet visited Trevi and Moses.[3]

Kind regards,
Freud

1. Postcard.
2. Spelling uncertain.
3. The Fontana di Trevi (according to tradition, the traveler to Rome who throws a coin into the fountain will return to Rome) and the statue of Moses by Michelangelo (see letter 416).

416

[Rome,] September 13, 1913[1]

[Moses][2]
returns your greeting and is entirely of the same opinion as you about the Congress in Munich.

Yours,
Freud

1. Picture postcard from Rome with Michelangelo's statue of Moses at the Church of San Pietro in Vincoli.
2. The greeting is written on the side of the card with the picture. The date and "Yours, Freud" are written, like inscriptions, on the pedestals to the left and right of the statue; the remaining text is at the base. The arrangement of picture and text should therefore be interpreted in such a way as to suggest that the statue is the subject of the statement. Ferenczi seems also to have understood it as such.

417

Internationale Zeitschrift für
Ärztliche Psychoanalyse

Budapest, September 15, 1913

Dear Professor,

After your departure I remained in Munich another one and a half days and spent the entire time in the company of Lou Salomé. I saw as little of Munich as you did of Budapest that time; her interest in scientific matters is so great that in her company one can't talk or think about anything else. Once, v. Gebsattel[1] was also with us; he was a philosopher up to now, but then he changed *saddles*[2] and became a medical student in order to take up Ψα. His philosophical origin is now manifesting itself in his inclination toward terminological discussions; even "prospective tendency" and "finality"[3] are not completely foreign to him, although he thoroughly disliked the pietistic Swiss lectures.

I would have liked to talk with Dr. Hattingberg,[4] but I didn't meet him; v. Gebsattel told me that he *inclines toward Adler.* (This would fit in with the fact that in his lecture he especially stressed the *biological* side of anal erotism, in places clearly at the expense of the psychological.)—In Vienna I visited my nose doctor, who for the time being has refused to carry out an invasive operation and has satisfied himself with "contused dilatation." I was, of course, pleased about that and rushed home, where I arrived Friday evening. Frau G. was waiting for me at the station. She is well and cordially returns your greetings.—My early arrival gave me two vacation days in Budapest, which I spent very pleasantly with Frau G. The news about Elma—who is beginning to set her mind on the idea of marriage to the Swedish-American writer—obviously loosened hidden threads in me that still bound me to her. I feel cheerful, free, and eager for work—am also getting along with Frau G. much more naturally and uninhibitedly.

Today was the first day of work. My office hours were full; today I have two, day after tomorrow four hours. In my free hours I got the old manuscript of the *Weimar* lecture on homosexuality[5] out of the drawer. Only *now* do I know why I haven't published this work for so long. I certainly felt at the time that you were not in agreement with the explanation that homosexuality = obsessional neurosis.[6] But in S. Martino I heard from you that you recognized in homosexuality one of the essential traits of the obsessive-compulsive constitution. Now, no *prohibition* on your part stands in the way of publication![7]

I am sending the paper to Rank for the next issue of the Zeitschrift; I hope you are in agreement with that. At the same time I finished the two short case histories of paranoia that I told you about in S. Martino (1. Ostwald [patient], 2. the "cured" paranoid—who then went insane).[8]

I thank you kindly for both postcards and was especially honored by the Moses greeting.

I received very pleasant news from your wife, whom I asked how you were; I was genuinely happy with her reply. This summer was really too full of disturbances to health! As far as you are concerned, Professor, I maintain that you should give up the Karlsbad cure. I hear about many cases in which there were similarly unpleasant results as in yours.

I hope that you will recover completely in Rome and in the company of your travel companion, to whom I send kind regards, and that you will easily overcome the somatic and psychic shocks of the last few months.

I close with this wish.

Yours truly,
Ferenczi

The cholera in Budapest seems to be ending. No new cases in four days; up to now there has been a total of only eight to nine genuine cases.

1. Victor Emil Freiherr von Gebsattel (1883–1976), German psychiatrist and member of the Munich Branch Society; originally influenced by Adler and Jung. Gebsattel was later a training analyst at the Berlin Central Institute for Psychotherapy and Depth Psychology. On the basis of his Christian-Catholic view, he closely examined the meaning of existential analysis, phenomenology, and existentialism for psychotherapy and anthropology.

2. A play on words: *Geb-sattel* = give saddle [Trans.].

3. The final viewpoint played a major role in Adler's as well as Jung's thinking. According to Adler, most people strive for a goal that is hidden from them; mental phenomena are directed "straight to the final purpose, to the fictitious goal" and appear as if "constructed as an abstraction which has some future tendency in view" (Adler, *The Neurotic Constitution*, pp. 352, 324).

4. Hans Ritter von Hattingberg (1879–1944), Doctor of Laws and Medicine; member of the Munich Branch Society. He had read a paper, "On the Anal-Erotic Character," at the Congress. Hattingberg later became a member of the Aryanized German General Medical Society for Psychotherapy and the German Institute for Psychological Research and Psychotherapy in Berlin. He was editor, with Niels Kampmann, of the *Zeitschrift für Menschenkunde*.

5. Ferenczi, "Zur Nosologie der männlichen Homosexualität (Homoerotik)" [On the Nosology of Male Homosexuality] (1914, 136; *C.*, p. 296); published in *Zeitschrift* 2 (1914): 131–142.

6. "Object homoerotism . . . is . . . an obsessional neurosis" (ibid., *Schriften* I, 188; *C.*, p. 303).

7. In 1920 Freud nevertheless termed Ferenczi's equation of object homoerotism and obsessional neurosis as "less happily" described (see 1920 addendum in Freud 1905d, p. 147).

8. Ferenczi, "Einige klinische Beobachtungen bei der Paranoia und Paraphrenie, Beitrag zur Psychologie der 'Systembildung'" [Some Clinical Observations on Paranoia and Paraphrenia] (1914, 135; *C.*, p. 282).

418

[Rome,] September 22, 1913[1]

Cordial greetings from our great travel enterprise. All is going well. Narcissism[2] is very much in the works. Unfortunately, I am supposed to be in Vienna in the morning a week from now!

Yours,
Freud

[On the picture side, in a different handwriting:]

Kind regards,
Minna Bernays

1. Picture postcard from Rome; the caption reads: "Tivoli—Panorama."
2. "On Narcissism: An Introduction" (Freud 1914c).

419

IMAGO
ZEITSCHRIFT FÜR ANWENDUNG DER
PSYCHOANALYSE AUF DIE GEISTSWISSENSCHAFTEN
HERAUSGEGBEN VON PROFESSOR DR. SIGM. FREUD
Schriftleitung:

OTTO RANK   DR. HANNS SACHS
IX/4, Simondenkgasse 8   XIX/1, Peter Jordanstraße 76
VERLAG HUGO HELLER & CO., WIEN I. BAUERNMARKT 3
Abonnementspreis ganzjährig (6 Hefte, etwa 30 Bogen) K 18- = Mk. 15.—

Vienna, October 1, 1913

Dear friend,

Only reporting to you that I have arrived, still somewhat drunk from the beauty of the seventeen days in Rome. A stomach ailment today is preparing my transition to everyday life. Today I have four hours, tomorrow five, in a week the prospect of nine. Nothing especially interesting there.

Narcissism is, so to speak, finished. I would like to discuss it with you, that is to say, give a lecture to our friends, if you were here. For the time being I can't send you anything, because not a line has been written "in fair copy." A number of interesting things have come out, e.g., the connection with Silberer's fateful discovery.[1]

Rank has probably already told you that we, along with Heller, have cooked up an idea for "supplements" to the Zeitschrift,[2] in order to be independent of the Jahrbuch in publishing larger works. *Qu'en dites-vous!*

Everything is well at home; actually, very pleasant. Ernst is gearing up for Munich, where he intends to move on the 15th. Anna is insatiable with her education plans. Martin is cheerfully cramming for his last oral exam.[3]

This time there is little to say about the "national gift." My travel companion also expended the sums which had been designated for it.

I got two letters from Maeder, which wanted to maintain the fiction of friendly relations; otherwise, they bear witness to the utmost obstinacy. A letter of mine will come between both of them, which will say a friendly good-bye to him.

We will see what this year brings in the way of basically good things, and we will keep external fate, the chronicle of ΨA, from having a deeper effect on our emotions. I await good news from you.

Cordially,
Freud

1. In "On Narcissism: An Introduction" (1914c, pp. 96f), Freud discusses the connection between the "functional phenomenon" in dreams described by Herbert Silberer ("one of the few indisputably valuable additions to the theory of dreams"; ibid., p. 97) and a self-observing agency in the ego.

2. This plan was realized. The first supplement, Gerbrandus Jelgersma's work *Unbewusstes Geistesleben*, was published in 1914 (see letters 456 ff); other supplements were *Beyond the Pleasure Principle* (Freud 1920g), a *Bericht über die Fortschritte der Psychoanalyse in den Jahren 1914–1919* (1921), *Psychoanalyse und Psychiatrie* (1921) by August Stärcke, and the fifth volume (1922), *Zur Psychoanalyse der paralytischen Geistesstörung* [Psycho-Analysis and the Psychic Disorder of General Paresis] by Hollós and Ferenczi.

3. Ernst went to Munich to study architecture. After her qualifying examination, Anna went into training as an elementary school teacher, and Martin concluded his study of law at the end of 1913 (see letter 409).

420

INTERNATIONALE ZEITSCHRIFT FÜR
ÄRZTLICHE PSYCHOANALYSE

Budapest, October 3, 1913

Dear Professor,

Best wishes for the new analytic year; let us hope the stomach ailment will turn out to be a transitory symptom. We should actually—according to the experiences of the last few years—already be better acquainted with the conditions that at times have an unfavorable influence on your health, and do something about them. For my part, I maintain that Karlsbad and the Karlsbad cure are disadvantageous to you. The toxic effect has always set in promptly; we have never seen any favorable effects.

I am eager to learn something about narcissism, and am ready and willing to come to Vienna on the Sunday after next (October 12).

As you may know, I am very much in favor of the idea of "supplements" to the Zeitschrift, since through them we will become independent of the Jahrbuch. I am especially looking forward to the moment when you have your name stricken from the title page of the Jahrbuch and let Jung bear the responsibility for its content alone.—

Today I received the reprint of "Scientia,"[1] which I read with great pleasure. This work cannot remain completely without effect on thinking people.[2]

1. "The Claims of Psycho-Analysis to Scientific Interest" (Freud 1913j).
2. Letter unfinished; see the first sentence of letter 422.

421

Vienna, October 9, 1913
IX., Berggasse 19

Dear friend,

What is it with you? Why are you silent? Aren't you well, or are you having difficulties with your family problem? Is a larger work consuming you at present? Something else? I am naturally very desirous to learn about it soon.

As for myself, I am already completely booked up and overburdened with corrections and business.

Kind regards,
Freud

422

INTERNATIONALE ZEITSCHRIFT FÜR
ÄRZTLICHE PSYCHOANALYSE

Budapest, October 10, 1913

Dear Professor,

I am sending you here an attachment to the letter dated October 3, which I didn't finish writing only because I had reservations as to whether I can keep my promise to be in Vienna on the 12th of the month. Groundwork, which I am doing in preparation for my docentship[1] (the success of which is actually quite doubtful), necessitates my being here, and I had to postpone the decision from one day to the next. Now it is certain that I am *not* coming to Vienna. *Perhaps* next Sunday (the 19th).

Health satisfactory; family complex quiet; I have become much more sober in this matter. Scientifically, I am being tormented by a few things of a general biological nature, which one has to derive from psychoanalysis (but which have nothing to do with your ideas about organic repression).— There is little to do. Two to three hours a day, sometimes only one.—

Next month will pass with patronage matters (docentship), two lectures, and the publication of the third volume of my (Hungarian) works.[2]

Kind regards,
Ferenczi

Frau G. is in Vienna. She will see you sometime during your office hours.

1. Ferenczi would teach at the university only during the short-lived republic (1919) as the world's first professor of psychoanalysis.
2. Ferenczi, 1914, 149, *Ideges tünetek keletkezése és eltünése és egyéb értekezések a pszichoanalizis köréböl* [Origin and Passing of Nervous Symptoms and Other Essays from the Field of Psychoanalysis], in *Gesammelte Aufsätze,* vol. 3 (Budapest).

423

Budapest, October 11, 1913[1]

Dear Professor,
This card was given to me by a certain Dr. v. Ortvay,[2] who spent the month of September (very bearable!) in Egypt. He thinks one could use this month very well for an Egyptian journey. Maybe we'll do it next year!!

Ferenczi

1. Colored picture postcard; the caption reads: "Intérieur d'un temple."
2. Possibly Rudolf von Ortvay (1885–1954), a physicist from Miskolcz, Ferenczi's birthplace.

424

Vienna, October 12, 1913
IX., Berggasse 19

Dear friend,
I almost had the desire to do with you what other respectable people are accustomed to doing, i.e., after their anxiety has turned out to be unfounded, to get angry about the fact that one has made them anxious. But the matter has still not been completely clarified; the tone of your letter is still somewhat dry, the report about the motives for your long silence still not quite exhaustive. Is Rank in fact right when he recently admitted to me that he feared he put you in a bad mood with a certain suggestion

relating to editorship, and when he also wanted to ascribe a certain influence to the other suggestion, which came from both of us, about where to publish your works? I assured him that your sensitivity was not a factor in our calculations. I also don't need to assure you that Rank is completely without rancor and doesn't bear the slightest hint of any bad intention.

All your news was of interest to me, but not all of it was gratifying. To be sure, I am not concerned about the fact that you now have so little to do. That is extremely episodic. The necessity to seek the patronage of a university is—I remember—, less a matter of indifference, but it is perhaps really worth the effort, if one can achieve something without making too great concessions to the rabble. I had to do it too,[1] and although even now I gnash my teeth at the recollection, I still have to be very satisfied with the results.

I don't really believe your Egyptian source. Think about how it was in Sicily in September! It would, of course, be *very* nice, and we should keep it in mind; that is, if my health doesn't frighten you.

I am certainly ready to give up the drinking cures, to which I owe something, completely normal intestinal functioning, which has been undisturbed for three months now. I just took a first step toward looking after myself; I gave up the hour between 8 and 9 in the morning, i.e., I dismissed the designated patient without replacing him. The loss has been compensated for by raising the fee for an hour of treatment.

If you come to Vienna on Sunday I will get out the Narcissism. I let it lie, first, in order to gain some distance; second, because I have to get to the Interpretation of Dreams, for which I get together with Rank every Friday evening.[2] You will have received the third volume of the *Kleine Schriften*.[3] (It has brought me 1,420 crowns with almost no work.)

I send hearty congratulations on your third volume.[4]

It is not right for Frau G. to visit me during my office hours. Wouldn't it be nicer if she would grant me or us an evening?

I greet you cordially and await news from you before the Sunday on which I am supposed to expect you.

Yours,
Freud

1. Freud had assured his achieving the docentship with the support of Hermann Nothnagel and Theodor Meynert (see Freud's letter to Martha of January 16, 1885, *Letters*, pp. 134f). Here he certainly seems to be referring less to that than to his being named professor, the background of which he described in a letter to Fliess (March 11, 1902, *Fliess Letters*, pp. 455–457).

2. In 1914 the fourth edition of *The Interpretation of Dreams* (1900a) was published, in which Freud added a new section on symbolism (chap. 6, sec. E), and which for the first time (up to the seventh edition [1922]) contained two essays by Otto Rank ("Dream and Poetry" and "Dream and Myth"), whose name also appeared on the title page.

3. Freud, *Sammlung kleiner Schriften zur Neurosenlehre,* 3d ed. (Leipzig, 1913).
4. See letter 422, n. 2.

425

INTERNATIONALE ZEITSCHRIFT FÜR
ÄRZTLICHE PSYCHOANALYSE

Budapest, October 16, 1913

Dear Professor,

I freely admit that the motives which I gave as an explanation for my long silence are not adequate; I myself was and am not satisfied with them, but I didn't and don't know what to add. *Consciously,* sensitivity plays no part in this; as for the unconscious, I can't guarantee anything. When I—at times—look at myself objectively, I notice that things for which all rational explanation is missing often go on in a person. After the two "years of illness"—which were marked psychically and somatically by deep depressions, a kind of rejuvenation seems to have come over me, especially since the, apparently final, settlement of the Elma affair. Increase in libido and potency, cessation of hypochondria, tendency toward sociability and amusements (even of a primitive, infantile nature: theater, cinema, etc.), feeling of physical strength, humor and jocularity: my youthfulness, kept down for so long (and which I had already considered lost), comes to the fore in these symptoms. My attempt to explain it is as follows: When I declared myself for Elma, I tore myself forcefully away from Frau G., and in compensation I had to exaggerate Elma's good qualities. (At the time I was temporarily impotent with Frau G.) Then came the great disappointment with Elma; the path to Frau G. was at that time (inwardly) closed to me; the only remaining way out was to be ill (somatic-neurasthenic disturbances and hypochondria: my fixation points, evidently). Gradually (perhaps also with the aid of diversion through illness, i.e., of autoerotism), the rather stubborn tendency to get back with Elma abated; at the same time, Frau G.'s love and kindness made it possible for me once again to restore intellectual and tender relations with her. When I finally saw that Elma also no longer felt bound, I was inwardly freed of her—but without regaining the old, unconditional, enthusiastic love for Frau G.; what remained in me was more in the nature of friendship, tenderness, intellectual communion with her, which, however, are not entirely free of erotism.

When I review the whole development of these things, I have to come to the conclusion that the effect (thus, probably the purpose) of the whole Elma affair was intended to mitigate my strict adherence to the old love relationship with Frau G., which was dictated to me by piety; hindered by my mother fixation, I was not able to do that consciously and voluntarily;

an external occasion had to come to my aid (—Elma—), as if to excuse me. Elma served as a rationalization of my tendencies toward independence.

My present inner and physical well-being may speak in favor of the fact that my relations to those close to me are at the moment free of every kind of overburdening (exaggeration, lie, etc.). That is, to be sure, only a negative advantage; libido also demands positive activity. The task of insight and of the intellect would now be to sublimate these tendencies and to yoke them in the service of scientific work; but I must admit that since I was a child I have had the tendency to give in to laziness (albeit under constant pangs of conscience) .

I still don't know how all that is connected with my long silence. Perhaps *you* can tell me.—One thought comes to mind: maybe you are for me the representative of those persons of respect who have to pass judgment on my actions; as such, you would have to find fault with my impiety. (I know [consciously],[1] that you won't do that.) I want to provoke your anger through my laziness and in this way still receive my deserved punishment, albeit displaced to a different area. If I were now diligent (in writing and in correspondence), then you could praise me—the naughty boy—, which my conscience, burdened for the above reasons, would not be able to bear.— Retrospective considerations agree quite well with this explanation; as a child I rather ostentatiously made a show of being naughty; now I know that I wanted to have my *secret* sins and fantasies punished. Thus: the uprightness known to us in all matters, with the exception of the sexual.

I will *not* come to Vienna this Sunday. I have only just begun the Sunday lectures for medical students,[2] and I don't want to cut the second hour right away.—I will write to Frau G. that she should visit you.

Cordially,
Ferenczi

INTERNATIONALE ZEITSCHRIFT
FÜR ÄRZTL. PSYCHOANALYSE[3]

Postscript to today's letter:

On the first galley of your paper, The Disposition to Obsessional Neurosis, it says: "The two other psychoneuroses, which I have brought together under the heading of 'paraphrenia'"[4]—under which you understand paranoia and dementia praecox. But in your earlier works it said *paraphrenia* (schizophrenia) *only for dementia praecox.*[5] I don't think you should make any changes in this terminology.

F.

1. Enclosed in brackets in the original.
2. Probably the continuation after the summer break of the course begun in May (see letter 394).

3. Postcard with preprinted letterhead, enclosed with this letter.

4. The wording is the same in the final version (Freud 1913i, p. 318).

5. The group of illnesses brought together under Bleuler's term schizophrenia were earlier called dementia praecox by Bénedict-Augustin Morel and Emil Kraepelin. Freud had suggested "giv[ing] dementia praecox the name of *paraphrenia* . . . [which] would serve to indicate a relationship with paranoia (a name which cannot be changed)" (1911c [1910], p. 76).

426

[Vienna,] October 26, 1913[1]

Dear friend,

Your critique of Bleuler[2] is precious, and well deserved. Your denunciations remind one of Zola's "en attendant toujours quelque chose qui ne venait point."[3] As a consequence of this, Narcissism is resting.

Kind regards, also to Frau G.

Yours,
Freud

1. Postcard.

2. In his review (1914, 150; *Zeitschrift* 2 [1914]: 62–66) of Bleuler's, "Kritik der Freudschen Theorien," Ferenczi had attempted to refute Bleuler's critique point for point and had closed with the remark: "It would certainly correspond to the directly acknowledged negative tendency of *Bleuler's* critique if we, too, emphasized its negative factors in our discussion of it. We thereby also protect Prof. *Bleuler* from a repetition of the wrong that has been done to his theory of schizophrenia, which critics have (according to his own statement) 'viewed as much too *Freud*ian.'"

3. "In constant expectation of something that never happened." The source of the quotation from Emile Zola (1840–1902), one of Freud's favorite writers, has not been established.

427

Vienna, October 30, 1913
IX., Berggasse 19

Dear friend,

I need you urgently in Vienna this Sunday. As a consequence of a letter from Jung,[1] we need to make the most important decisions.

Cordially,
Freud

1. On October 27 Jung had written to Freud that he had learned from Maeder that Freud doubted his "*bona fides*," and that he was therefore "lay[ing] down the editorship of the *Jahrbuch*" (*Freud/Jung*, p. 550).

428

INTERNATIONALE ZEITSCHRIFT FÜR
ÄRZTLICHE PSYCHOANALYSE[1]

[Budapest,] November 3, 1913

Dear Professor,

Just received the enclosed letter from Jung.[2] Also enclosed a draft of my reply; request possible suggestions for changes *(and immediate return)*.

Please don't let go of Deuticke![3] Jung should *not* get the Jahrbuch.

Cordially,
Ferenczi

1. Attached to this letter in the photostat folder is another enclosure, which more likely belongs with Ferenczi's letter of November 6, 1913, and which has been placed there; see letter 430, n. 4.

2. The letter is missing.

3. Franz Deuticke, the publisher of the *Jahrbuch*.

429

Vienna, November 4, 1913
IX., Berggasse 19

Rush

Dear friend,

In few words, many thanks!

I have appended some words to your draft, only to round off my reaction without wanting to influence you. The ψευδος[1] that he is the victim of his independent opinions should not remain unchallenged.

The situation with Deuticke is bad. Heller is scrambling to get the Jahrbuch in its new form.[2] Full information next time.

Cordially,
Freud

1. *Pseudos*, Greek for falsehood.

2. Deuticke would nevertheless still publish the sixth and last volume of the *Jahrbuch* (1914) with the slightly altered title *Jahrbuch der Psychoanalyse, Neue Folge des Jahrbuchs für psychoanalytische und psychopathologische Forshchungen* under the general direction of Freud alone, and edited by Abraham and Hitschmann.

430

INTERNATIONALE ZEITSCHRIFT FÜR
ÄRZTLICHE PSYCHOANALYSE

Budapest, November 6, 1913

Dear Professor,

The letter to Jung was sent with the changes suggested. Besides the expressions "ambiguities" and "insults" I also inserted into the letter the sentences contained on the enclosed sheet of paper.—

I received a letter from Jones, which is, however, still not a reply to the one which was mailed in Vienna. He reports the founding of the London group,[1] which he has already communicated to Jung. We will therefore be able to appear more united against Jung. Jones will certainly first have to finish things up with *Eder*—his present secretary—. *Deuticke's* attitude in the whole affair is very significant. If I were in your place I would punish him by withdrawing his right to publication of all psychoanalytic works.

A brother of Claparède's, who had a Budapester for a wife, died here suddenly a few days ago. This morning I accidentally met Prof. Claparède[2] at breakfast at the Hotel Royal; he came to the funeral. Along with a few friendly words that we exchanged, I got from him the news that upon his recommendation I have been designated as one of the discussants on "hypnosis" for the Congress of the Société internationale de Psychologie (in Bern, September 5—12, 1914).* I didn't turn him down; to be sure, it is questionable if I can be in Bern at that time. The co-discussant is a Norwegian whose name was unfamiliar to me.

My lecture in Vienna on thought transference has been confirmed for the 19th of this month.[3]

I eagerly await your news about the course of negotiations.

Cordially,
Ferenczi

[Enclosure:][4]

"Therefore it is totally incorrect if in that ('bona fide') you see Freud's reaction to your 'own scientific views.' That is so little the case that, despite the ever-widening split, we had decided, on Freud's recommendation, to elect you president once again. We went to Munich with this intention. It was only the absolutely unseemly manner in which you, as leader of the Congress, treated the suggestions that came from our side, the very one-sided and partisan comments of yours that accompanied all the lectures, as well as the personal behavior of your group that caused us to protest with the blank ballots (and this time only mutely)."

* President: Dubois.

1. The London Psychoanalytic Society was founded on October 30, 1913, with Jones as president and David Eder (see letter 336, n. 1) as secretary. Jones's letter is missing.

2. See letter 360 and n. 2.

3. Ferenczi gave a lecture titled "Experiments with Thought Transference" at the Vienna Society on November 19. No transcript is preserved in the *Minutes* (IV, 215).

4. The appended text is on a separate sheet of letterhead stationery *(Internationale Zeitschrift für Ärztliche Psychoanalyse)*, without a date. It was filed with letter 428 (November 3, 1913), but it does not seem to relate to the "draft of [the] reply" mentioned there. More likely it is the "enclosed sheet of paper" Ferenczi refers to in the first paragraph of this letter.

431

INTERNATIONALE ZEITSCHRIFT FÜR
ÄRZTLICHE PSYCHOANALYSE

Budapest, November 8, 1913

Dear Professor,

According to *Jones's* and *Abraham's* elucidations, I don't think we can bring about the dissolution of the International Association. Nothing remains but a *collective resignation* of those members of all groups who are with you.[1] An International Psychoanalytic Association from which you, Abraham, Jones, all Viennese and Budapesters, Brill (perhaps Putnam) have resigned—with Jung at the head—won't count for much. You must immediately set in motion the founding of the new Association. Small local interests of London and Berlin don't count; one can't reckon with those who don't want to come along anyway. The public at large will only surmise Jung's downfall from the event of the resignations; the Zeitschrift will then be able to put the whole story into the proper light. The resignations will also put an end to the unpleasant duty of having to publish the Swiss tirades in the Korrespondenzblatt. Jung's "theopsychology" will stand there isolated and won't be able to hide behind your name. We don't get anything out of the International Association. Its dissolution will be a deliverance.

Returning Jones's letter enclosed.

Cordially,
Ferenczi

1. Abraham *(Freud/Abraham*, November 4, 1913, pp. 153f) and Jones (Jones II, 150) had advised against dissolving the IPA. They were skeptical as to whether the American and Berlin groups would agree to such a decision, and they also feared that Jung would oppose the dissolution and that, in the event of the resignation of the group around Freud, "he [Jung] would be left in possession" (Jones II, 150).

432

Vienna, November 9, 1913
IX., Berggasse 19

Dear friend,

The need for immediate action in matters of the Association has already subsided in Rank and Sachs, and I think that you, too, will not be closed to the arguments from the state of affairs and will wait and see whether the occasion for further steps comes from Zurich and whether our resignation can be avoided. When I think of the shabby behavior of so many people in the action against Stekel, I become wary of the magic of my name and would not like to put it to the test again. The whole action will, incidentally, remain completely in the hands of the Committee.

So, the Jahrbuch is ours. Deuticke has become aware of his hastiness and has definitively come to terms with me. I think we should put out the volume for July 1, the time when Jung's would have been published. Nothing has been settled with him regarding details, e.g., the one-time publication. We will negotiate that on the evening of the 19th. It is an opportunity to put all our forces into action. Fate evidently intends to squeeze us dry, as long as we can still give something of ourselves.

I intend to contribute Narcissism and, in addition, a history of ΨA with frank criticism of Adler and Jung.[1] We still won't give up the idea of our supplements because of this.

The matter with Kraus-Brugsch was favorably decided on the same day. I won't write hysteria and obsession for the compilation, but rather a "Psychoanalytic Presentation of the Neuroses" of equal or larger scope.[2]

At present everything has actually been barricaded for me as well as for Rank by the disgusting preparations for the fourth edition of the Interpretation of Dreams. Reading through all that jumble is a harsh punishment.

I am going to Hamburg to see Sophie over Christmas and will spend half a day in Berlin with Abraham on the way back.

I greet you cordially and am very curious about your presentation on the 19th of the month, to which I brought forth something of a prelude in my lecture yesterday.[3]

Yours,
Freud

P.S. Regards to Frau G.

1. "On the History of the Psycho-Analytic Movement" (Freud 1914d).
2. Nothing came of this plan for a contribution by Freud to the compilation by Friedrich Kraus and Theodore Brugsch (see letter 325 and n. 2). Because of the war, it was not until 1920 that Freud was offered the contract, which he refused, since he had already

made a presentation in the meantime in the *Introductory Lectures on Psycho-Analysis*
(1916–17a [1915–17]); see Jones II, 248f.
   3. Freud's Saturday lecture at the university.

433

Vienna, November 12, 1913[1]

very much in agreement[2] hope it won't come to a standstill in the process
greetings = freud

   1. Telegram
   2. Evidently a communication from Ferenczi is missing.

434

INTERNATIONALE ZEITSCHRIFT FÜR
ÄRZTLICHE PSYCHOANALYSE

Budapest, November 12, 1913

Dear Professor,
   Here is the card from Jung, which was announced by telegram.[1] What is
striking is the forced politeness of his manner of speaking (Christian patience in contrast to Jewish intolerance). I will, of course, leave this card
unanswered.
   I am in complete agreement with the change in tactics. Let's wait for
things to develop.
   My day has filled up all of a sudden (of course, partly only temporary
patients, the well-known birds of passage or seasonal guests). I am actually
sorry, because I have too little time for literary activity. The unavoidable
visits in the matter of my docentship will likewise rob me of much time
in the next few days. The first vote will take place on the 25th of the
month. The whole world is prophesying certain failure.
   I may not be able to finish my paper on thought transference for the
presentation on the 19th, so I will have to confine myself to the demon-
stration and to briefly sharing previous experiences.—We will then have
all the more time left over for editorial and Committee consultations.
   I was very pleased about the unexpected turn of events in the Jahrbuch
affair! The solution to the matter of Kraus-Brugsch is also extremely favorable. Perhaps we are at the beginning of a period of ascendancy for Ψα.
   Frau G. thanks you for your greeting and returns it.

Yours,
Ferenczi

   1. The card is missing.

435

Vienna, November 13, 1913
IX., Berggasse 19

Dear friend,

Nothing at all can be predicted about votes. Although, rationally, I share your prognosis, I am still not sure whether I shouldn't soon congratulate you, which I will do very gladly.

I don't find Jung's style Christian but rather impudent and venomous. As if your judgment couldn't be based on your own observations at the Congress. And then, his mockery of interpretation. Truly ψα!

I find it disappointing that you want to abridge us in your lecture. You should accomplish the same amount, no matter whether you have much or little to do. The times demand it now. The suspense over your lecture is already very great.

Jones, who judges things very soberly, today enclosed a letter for me from Putnam,[1] which will get to you by way of Rank-Sachs. Send it back to Jones. Jones has also suggested a Committee meeting in Vienna for Christmas. But I will be in Hamburg at that time, and I offered to spend Sunday, December 28, from noon until evening in Berlin with him and Abraham. Of course, it would also be very nice if you could be there. I will pay a visit to Abraham, in any event.

You should have received Totem and Taboo. Tomorrow there is an editorial supper with Hitschmann.

I am now devoting every free hour to the Interpretation of Dreams, which is very tedious and annoying. I wouldn't be able to get started without Rank. The reading is too stupid. I intend to be finished by Christmas.

I greet you and Frau G. cordially.

Yours,
Freud

P.S. "Little Meyer" has asked for my biography.[2]

1. In this letter (Hale, *Putnam*, pp. 278f) Putnam commented about, among other things, Ferenczi's review of Jung's "Wandlungen und Symbole der Libido."
2. An article (Freud 1914h), the authorship of which is not entirely certain, appeared unsigned in *Meyers Kleines Konversations-Lexikon*, vol. 7, Supplements and Postscripts (Leipzig, 1914).

436

INTERNATIONALE ZEITSCHRIFT FÜR
ÄRZTLICHE PSYCHOANALYSE

Vienna, November 23, 1913

Dear friend,

Today at 3 P.M. the séance[1] took place at my home in the presence of Rank, Sachs, Hitschmann, their wives, my brother, and my children. It went very miserably, hardly any indication of success. The same thing is supposed to have taken place the day before yesterday at the home of Dr. Weiss.[2] I don't know why that is. I handed Prof. Roth an envelope,[3] to put him in a favorable mood, but the contents were wasted. I naturally refused to give a testimonial of any kind.

I know, of course, that things aren't connected with these people or the experiments with them. But I wouldn't build anything at all on them. Rank and Sachs even think that a system of acoustic aids comes into consideration, and the man can't, in fact, be silenced. He regularly utters sounds when the word is shown him, and in that respect he makes himself very suspicious. Seeing doesn't seem to play any role. Both requirements that he makes, not to put him very far away from his wife and to maintain absolute silence, really speak in favor of what Rank and Sachs think. In the absence of the phenomenon, all our attempts at explanation were, of course, dropped; but I also ask you, who have had more success, to check your experiences with him and not make them the basis of your publication.

Rank also intends to write to you about this. We are all now in favor of reversing our thrust. I still like both of my prophecies and along with them Gisirma (not Vilirma).[4]

Kind regards, in expectation of news from you,

Yours,
Freud

My best to Frau G.

1. The séance was with a Professor Alexander Roth and his wife, whom Ferenczi had brought along four days earlier to the Vienna Society for his "Experiments with Thought Transference" (*Minutes* IV, 215). Anna Freud wrote to Jones about the experiments in Freud's home: "I remember that both my father and I were taken aback by the rough way in which the poor woman was urged, forced and hustled to produce results" (Jones III, 389).

2. Presumably Karl Weiss (1879-?), neurologist from Reichenberg, who worked at the neurological clinic of Lothar von Frankl-Hochwart (1862–1914); see Edoardo Weiss, *Sigmund Freud as a Consultant: Recollections of a Pioneer in Psychoanalysis*, ed. Martin

Grotjahn (New York, 1970), p. 10. Weiss was a member of the Vienna Society from March 6, 1912. He emigrated to England in 1938.

   3. Euphemism for money.

   4. The allusions are unclear.

437

INTERNATIONALE ZEITSCHRIFT FÜR
ÄRZTLICHE PSYCHOANALYSE

Vienna, November 27, 1913

Dear friend,

   I ask you again not to be so sure in the matter of Prof. Alexander Roth; just don't build anything on him. We all have the worst impression of him and don't understand how you can be satisfied with his information. The fact that he can't read and still undertakes such experiments makes him such an idiot that one wouldn't think him capable of any other craftiness. I know that this one case doesn't mean anything, but it is precisely for that reason that this one should be mercilessly eradicated. Just imagine, if it came to a public discussion about the man, who is now referring in Vienna to his successes in the ΨA Society, we would have to leave you in the lurch. I think you ought rather to have it cost you something to get back your testimonial, which was given too incautiously.

   Your failure [to attain the docentship] will have the consequence of my being able to congratulate you one half to a year from now. You will naturally not let yourself be deterred.

   Otherwise, nothing new here; a strangely quiet time, in every respect.

Kind regards,
Freud

438

INTERNATIONALE ZEITSCHRIFT FÜR
ÄRZTLICHE PSYCHOANALYSE

Budapest, November 29, 1913

Dear Professor,

   I freely admit that Alexander—if his experiments don't succeed by honest means—will try to doctor his results. I have often observed such tendencies in him. But I must maintain that there can be no talk of cheating in a long series of successful cases. Under the present circumstances I will refrain from publishing the paper on thought transference, but I can't request back from Alexander that testimonial that I gave him. We could stop the misuse of the testimonial by means of a communiqué in the Zeit-schrift. I am enclosing here a draft of this communication. I don't think that a disavowal on your part would mean that you are "leaving me in the lurch." It has to do here with *facts* about which I was able to be convinced and you were not.

I heartily congratulate Martin for his doctorate and wish him several weeks of pleasant recuperation after the miserable torment of the exami-nations.[1]

Kind regards,
Ferenczi

[Enclosure:]

A Lecture on Thought Transference

On November 19, Dr. S. Ferenczi from Budapest gave a lecture in the Vienna Society on thought transference, in which he shared his experiences on the subject—which were gained by chance and collected in an experi-mental manner. He does not consider these experiences conclusive evi-dence, but he demonstrates a married couple, who, in his opinion, do seem to settle the question of telepathy in a positive sense. The experiments, which were carried out under the observation of the members of the Soci-ety and later repeated, yielded a positive result in only a few instances, so they were not sufficient to convince the members of the Society of the actuality of thought transference.

Dr. Ferenczi concedes that this time the experiments were much less successful than usual, but he does call attention to the fact that, when the experiments—for any reason—do not succeed, such artistes are wont to doctor their results; but he maintains that he has carried out a long series of successful experiments in which any possibility of deception has been eliminated.

---

1. After Martin received his Doctor of Laws degree, Freud procured a position for him at the court in Salzburg, at which Martin remained until the beginning of the Second World War. Martin Freud, *Sigmund Freud,* p. 178.

439

INTERNATIONALE ZEITSCHRIFT FÜR
ÄRZTLICHE PSYCHOANALYSE

Budapest, December 10, 1913

Dear Professor,

I still owe you a whole series of thank-yous: for the magnificent work on taboo, for the third Collection of the *Kleine Schriften,*[1] for the offprint of the "pregenital" paper,[2] and now also for your very successful portrait.

In the last few weeks I have been busy correcting the third Hungarian collection,[3] which may be published in two weeks. In the foreword I couldn't resist reacting to the University's harsh treatment of me with a very strong characterization of today's neurologist and psychiatrist types.

Nothing has crystallized out in the way of work plans. I would like to write a detailed discussion of Bergson's work on *laughing* for Imago.[4] Please tell Rank that I requested the German translation, which was just publish-ed by Diederich, from the publisher for review!—The last issue of the Zeitschrift was very elegant. Its few readers in Budapest congratulated me on it.—I have to forward the congratulations to the right place (Vienna).—

Frau G. is now staying in Vienna; her brother-in-law (Herr Stross, with whom Elma was living) died suddenly.—Elma seems to be quite contented; she is now also officially engaged.—

I think I have finally succeeded in discovering the *real* source of my sleep disturbances in the relative insufficiency of my nasal breathing. So I will probably have to go to Vienna at Christmas to take care of this matter.—Otherwise, I feel strong and well.—

Kind regards to all of you.

Yours,
Ferenczi

I was with my mother in Miskolcz on Sunday; because of that I was unable to use the double holiday for an excursion to Vienna.

1. See letter 424 and n. 3.

2. "The Disposition to Obsessional Neurosis" (Freud 1913i), Freud's lecture at the Munich Congress. In this work Freud spoke for the first time about a "pregenital organi-zation" (p. 321) of the libido.

3. See letter 422 and n. 2.

4. Henri Bergson (1859–1941), at the time probably the most significant French phi-losopher (he won the Nobel Prize in 1927); he was renowned for his theory of the "élan vital." His book *Le rire: Essai sur la signification du comique* (Paris, 1900), published in Hungarian in 1913, was not reviewed by Ferenczi, but references to it can be found in his posthumously published notes; see *"Lachen"* [Laughter] (Posthumous, 300; *Fin.*, p. 177); see also letter 446 and n. 2.

440

Dr. Ferenczi Sandor
Idegorvos, Kir. Törvenyszeki Orvosszakerto
Telefon; 42–46   Budapest
VII., Erzsebet-körut 54.[1]

requests Prof. Freud to permit Dr. S. Radó and Miss Ilona Krasso[2] (both medical students) to attend today's lecture.

1. Preprinted calling card, undated.
2. Unidentified.

441

Budapest,[1]
December 18, [1913][2]

am concerned no news from you for so long reassure me greetings = ferenczi

1. Telegram.
2. The year has been deduced from Freud's reply; see letter 442.

442

Vienna, December 21, 1913
IX., Berggasse 19

Dear friend,

As you learned from my reply to your telegram, I was so intensely preoccupied in the last two weeks, fortunately also capable of working, that I wasn't able to maintain my accustomed correspondence. A strong diminution in my practice will probably follow these feverish days, after I return from Hamburg. I am leaving Wednesday evening, can remain in Berlin from 8 to 8 o'clock, in order to discuss all necessary matters with Abraham, and will then be in Hamburg at 7. On Sunday at 3 I will make the return trip without interruption and will be in Vienna on Monday morning.[1] I expect you will come to Vienna during these holidays because of your nose and Jones, but this time I won't be able to count on seeing you. There are only a few tasks left hanging; I would have been able to share some things with you on scientific matters—masochism,[2] for instance.

I am taking along to Berlin the copy of Abraham's critique,[3] with its many layers of marginalia.

It will get very quiet at home; three lonesome womenfolk. Oli has gone to Paris for two weeks. Maybe Ernst will come over from Munich.

Work for the Jahrbuch will begin with us all after New Year's, when I do hope to see you.

I greet you cordially and ask you to give my best Christmas wishes to Frau G., who is doubtless home again.

Yours,
Freud

1. Freud traveled to Hamburg by way of Berlin—where he met his sister Marie (1861–1942), as well as Abraham and Eitingon—to see his daughter Sophie, who was expecting her first child. He returned December 29.

2. During his visit to Berlin Freud also spoke with Abraham about the genesis of masochism, and in the process he seems to have emphasized the "unconscious impulse and wish to be castrated," as can be surmised from Abraham's letter of January 7, 1914 (*Freud/Abraham*, p. 161). See also Freud's remark about masochism (November 5, 1913) in the Vienna Society (*Minutes* IV, 213).

3. Karl Abraham, "Kritik zu C. G. Jung, 'Versuch einer Darstellung der psychoanalytischen Theorie,'" *Zeitschrift*, 2 (1914): 72–82.

443

[Budapest,] December 21, 1913

Dear Professor,

Since I probably have to go to Vienna on the 25th because of the operation on my nose, I wasn't able to spend this Sunday with you and Jones (to whom I send best regards), and I can only wish you a pleasant holiday and a safe journey in writing.

I hope I will hear pleasant news from Jones (whom I would certainly like to see either in Vienna or in Budapest).

Too bad that this Christmas will pass without our having talked things out about technical and personal matters.

Kind regards,

Yours,
Ferenczi

I also wish all your dear ones a happy holiday.

444

Vienna, January 3, 1914
IX., Berggasse 19

D/Dear[1] friend,

The D/[Dear] ought to show you that I just wrote to Jones. I didn't know anything about his suggestion that you should write an article about symbolism for the Jahrbuch.[2] It occurs to me that you, alone among the great ones, were not represented by an original contribution. The only excuse for such an omission would be the consideration that we shouldn't allow ourselves to be bled dry for the one organ and that the Zeitschrift needs still greater care. But in spite of this, it would make more of an impression if you could appear there as well, with whatever you want, of course. Symbolism has perhaps not gotten properly ripe yet.

I finished Moses,[3] but today I still don't know why you protested so vehemently against my anonymity.[4] The next thing, or things, as the case may be, will be Narcissism and the more subjective history of the ψα Movement,[5] both for the Jahrbuch. I am very well and am working with ease on the usual things.

Let us hope the operation on your nose has done you some good. From today on I am going to work more energetically on Loe.

With a hearty toast to the new year,

Yours,
Freud

1. Freud evidently began writing the salutation in English and then crossed out the first letter [Trans.].

2. See letter 446 and n. 1.

3. "The Moses of Michelangelo" (Freud 1914b); see letter 327 and n. 8.

4. The essay was published anonymously in *Imago* 3 (1914): 15–16, with this note: "The editors have not refused acceptance of this contribution, which is, strictly speaking, not according to plan, because the author, who is known to them, is close to analytic circles, and because his manner of thinking nonetheless shows a certain similarity to the methodology of psychoanalysis." On April 12, 1933, Freud wrote to Edoardo Weiss: "My relationship to this work is something like that to a love child . . . Not until much later did I legitimize this nonanalytic child" (Weiss, *Sigmund Freud as a Consultant*, p. 74).

5. Freud 1914c and 1914d.

445

[Vienna,] January 6, 1914[1]

Dear friend,

Did you get the letter about the Congress from Jung,[2] and what are you considering doing? Tomorrow I am holding a war council with Rank and Sachs.

Is the ψ paper by the Polish lady philosopher[3] usable?

An interesting letter from Putnam[4] is coming to you next, after it makes its rounds.

Kind regards,
Freud

1. Postcard.
2. Jung, still president of the IPA, had inquired about the location of the Congress, which had been planned for September 1914 but was not held on account of the war.
3. Luise von Karpinska (1871–1936), from Zakopane (Poland), later professor of psychology at the University of Lodz; she had been a guest of the Vienna Society in December 1909 and January 1910. The essay, "Über die psychologischen Grundlagen des Freudismus," appeared in *Zeitschrift* 2 (1914): 305–326.
4. In his letter of December 25, 1913 (Hale, *Putnam*, pp. 167–169), Putnam presented his position on Freud and psychoanalysis against the background of the conflict with Jung.

446

Budapest, January 8, 1914

Dear Professor,

I have been quite well since the operation on my nose. Yesterday there was a brief relapse into my sleep disturbances, but they disappeared again today, so I can hope that from now on I will regain my normal ability to do things, even though the possibility cannot be excluded that additional (small) repairs to my turbinate bones will be necessary.—It is possible that I will have to spend this or next Sunday in Vienna (and this time, again, in nasal matters).

I had brief conversations with the members of the Society about Jung's letter, and we decided to recommend *Dresden*. But I will reply to Jung only after receiving your recommendation in regard to this, for we want to go in concert with Vienna, Berlin, and London.

My practice is increasing; now and then new patients are also reporting, which has no longer been the case for months.

I want to work out for the Jahrbuch one of the themata that I have been occupied with.—Symbolism is certainly not suited to this—it is, as you correctly remark, still unripe.—The *General Theory of Neuroses* has been assigned to me for review in the Jahrbuch;[1] a nice, but difficult subject.

My reading of Bergson's essy on laughter gave me occasion to think about laughing in general. I think I have found a significant supplement to your view on laughter developed in "Jokes."[2]—

A similar supplement to your explanation of the rescue fantasy (as a retaliation for birth)[3] is as follows:

The child, who is struggling with the Oedipus fantasy (aggression toward the father—sexual-sadistic aggression toward the mother), feels inhibited in these fantasies by feelings of *gratitude*. In order to be able to succumb to the Oedipus fantasy with less worry, he wants to rid the world of the feeling of being obligated to thank, by also, for his part, saving his parents' lives and "settling accounts" with them.[4]

Kind regards.

Yours,
Ferenczi

1. Ferenczi, "Allgemeine Neurosenlehre" (1914, 148), *Jahrbuch* 6 (1914): 317–328.

2. See "Lachen" [Laughter] (Ferenczi 300; *Bausteine* IV, 191; *Fin.*, p. 182): "(Modification of Freud's definition.) The effect of the comic consists of: (i) laughter; (ii) laughing at (secondary, cultural product, Bergson)."

3. The motive of rescue—the fantasy of saving the parents from danger—had been described by Freud as a derivative of the "parental complex": "When a child hears that he *owes his life* to his parents, or that his mother *gave him life*, his feelings of tenderness unite with impulses which strive at power and independence, and they generate the wish to return this gift to the parents and to repay them with one of equal value" (Freud 1910h, p. 172).

4. "It is as though the boy's defiance were to make him say: 'I want nothing from my father; I will give him back all I have cost him.' He then forms the phantasy of *rescuing his father from danger and saving his life*; in this way he puts his account square with him" (ibid.).

447

Vienna, January 8, 1914
IX., Berggasse 19

Dear friend,

You will have received the request of our esteemed president to express ourselves regarding the location of the next Congress. Again incorrect, since a different decision has been taken with regard to the Congress.[1] What are you thinking of doing? On no account should you respond until you have come to an understanding with us, Berlin, and London. Rank will write to you about further details.

Today Jones sent a letter from Putnam reporting that his youngest, 17-year-old daughter (not Griselda) died of diabetes.

He further claims that in 1909, as a child, she was in our company.[2] I can't remember that *at all*. It would be interesting to know if you can.

This miserable strike[3] is still crippling us.

With kind regards to you and Frau G.

Yours,
Freud[4]

1. "Report on the Fourth Congress of the IPA in Munich on September 7 and 8, 1913," *Zeitschrift* 2 (1914): 407, reads: "For the next site of the Congress Dr. Abraham suggested Schandau bei Dresden, and Heidelberg was suggested by the other side. After a slight majority favored Schandau, it was decided to ask the groups again before the next Congress."

2. Putnam had asked Jones (December 16, 1913; Hale, *Putnam*, pp. 280f) to forward his letter with the news of the death of his daughter Frances Cabot Putnam (1897–1913) to Freud. Freud had become acquainted with the girl, then twelve, during his stay at Putnam's camp in the Adirondacks. On Griselda, see letter 388 and n. 1.

3. A strike, begun on December 27, 1913, as a result of a wage dispute in the printing trades, had shut down the presses. It lasted until January 30, 1914.

4. Diagonally on the remainder of the page, which is otherwise empty, is written, in pencil and in an unidentifiable hand (perhaps Ferenczi's) the word "Kelent" (meaning unknown).

448

INTERNATIONALE ZEITSCHRIFT FÜR
ÄRZTLICHE PSYCHOANALYSE

Budapest, January 10, 1914

Dear Professor,

Abraham writes me that he is in favor of Dresden. We should all come to an agreement on that.—I believe Jung will get a numerical majority with America's aid.—I am sending you the Polish paper enclosed. It is *very good.* The few critical remarks can certainly be easily invalidated; they come from the practical inexperience of the writer. Perhaps I will write a small postscript to it.[1] But we also shouldn't publish the paper without a critique.—

I won't come to Vienna until Sunday after next (the 18th).

Kind regards,
Ferenczi

1. See letter 445, n. 3; no such postscript was published.

449

Vienna, January 12, 1914
IX., Berggasse 19

Dear friend,

I am writing furiously on the "History of the ψα Movement," and I have much to do otherwise. So please accept purely matter-of-fact communications without any afterthoughts.

We will all vote for Dresden. Jones writes me something about it today that is complicated and incomprehensible. But he doesn't come into consideration, he says, because his group hasn't been admitted yet.[1]

I will hardly be able to read Karpinska's paper. Your endorsement is certainly sufficient. Since the Jahrbuch is full, should we perhaps put her into the Zeitschrift?

I hope you will also have time for us when you come on Sunday the 18th. Usual arrangements. Would you like to have Lou over for dinner with us?

Kind regards,
Freud

P.S. Bring along the letter from Brill.

1. "Jung had not yet recognized the British Society, so it could not act" (Jones II, 150).

450

INTERNATIONALE ZEITSCHRIFT FÜR
ÄRZTLICHE PSYCHOANALYSE

Budapest, January 15, 1914

Dear Professor,

I fear that I will not be able to visit on Sunday and partake of your Sunday meal because on *Saturday* and *Sunday* (once each day) I will have to undergo smaller interventions in my much-abused organ of scent. But perhaps I will be sufficiently restored on Sunday evening that I will be able to chat with you for a few hours. I am not considering returning until Monday afternoon—I hope as a healthy person.

My practice is going well. I am fully booked. I just (three days ago) began the analysis of a typical masochist, a very intelligent and worthy man (lawyer), who came to me indirectly on your advice. A lady (young widow), who loves him and whom he also would like to love, once went to you for advice, and you referred the patient to me.—(The lady knew only about his impotence, not about his masochism.)

It is strange how different the complaints and case histories of patients sound according to whether one has been oriented to the situations beforehand or not. We deal with the patients' complaints as we do with material in dreams: one never knows at first whether one should take them in a positive or a negative sense. And yet it happens just as often that the patients relate the opposite of the unconsciously real rather than a piece of actual self-perception. If one knows the structure of a neurosis, one can immediately at the first interview distinguish the wheat (self-perception) from the chaff (reaction formations). If one is still not oriented, one is inclined to believe *absolutely nothing* the patient says.

The masochistic patient begins his story with the fact that he was actually *never in love* with the women with whom he engaged in masochistic manipulation. The woman, for instance, with whom he has had such a relationship for more than ten years now is (emotionally) quite distant from him. He initiates the masochistic action *(oscula ad nates)*[1] *"like an official duty once a week" (ipsissima verba)*[2] and has an ejaculation in the process. But when he really loves a woman, he can't even imagine the masochistic action—instead, he is *absolutely inhibited* with her in intromission and ejaculation (in erection *not* completely). A striking confirmation of your theory of masochism, according to which the masochist is subservient precisely toward the *person whom he doesn't love* (in order to defend against the threat of castration that has come from such a person).—You once told me that in your experience the homosexual masochist was once threatened by his father, the heterosexual by his mother.[3]—But one can conceive of a case (perhaps this is such a one) in which masochistic tendencies can develop with respect to the one, and impotence with respect to the other type *of the same sex.* (If, for instance, a boy experienced friendly advances from one woman and horrible threats from another, he may later become impotent with lovable women and develop masochistic *compulsion* with stern women.)

My patient's second dream brought even more unequivocal confirmation of your assumption. [I don't need to say that I give him absolutely no explanations but let him talk constantly!][4] He dreamt that he was released from my treatment cured and that I and my assistant declared his case to be unique; "it was the first case in which masochism was recognized as (?)." (The word represented by the question mark doesn't come to his mind; there were *two* expressions that he didn't remember. The first thought is *obligatio facendi,* the second *servitut*[5]!!—so, two legal expressions, especially the second of which, which simultaneously means *obedience, servitude,* was up to now characteristic of masochism in *this* sense, but from now on should also be interpreted in the sense of Roman law, namely as *a duty* to *tolerate intrusions of third persons* onto *my property.*)

See you soon.

Yours,
Ferenczi

The Polish work is not kosher for the Jahrbuch, too long for the Zeitschrift, very suitable for Imago.

1. Latin for "kisses on the buttocks."

2. Latin for "his very own words."

3. In his lecture on a "case of foot fetishism" in the Vienna Society on March 11, 1914, however, Freud formulated the relationship the opposite way: "Someone who has been intimidated early by a man has a tendency to be masochistic toward women, and the other way around" (Minutes IV, 245).

4. Enclosed in brackets in the original.

5. Obligatio ad faciendum = "an obligation that consists not in refraining from doing something but in a deed or action, so that he who fails to fulfill this duty commits a criminal offense." Servitut = "limitation of the right to property by means of rights of use to others in the form of subjection (right of way, right of pasture, right to fruits of the soil)." Karl Luggauer, Juristenlatein, 2d ed. (Klagenfurt, 1970).

451

INTERNATIONALE ZEITSCHRIFT FÜR
ÄRZTLICHE PSYCHOANALYSE

Budapest, January 29, 1914

Dear Professor,

I hope that I will hereby initiate a series of letters which will not deal with illness (I mean my own).

As the event most worthy of mention since my return home I can only cite the talk by Prof. Apáthy (the neurofibril Apáthy)[1] against psychoanalysis. He has put himself at the head of the "eugenic movement" and from this position has let loose against psychoanalysis—as a panerotic aberration of the Jewish spirit. A few "liberal" newspapers have reacted to this attack by defending the Jews, pointed to the "kernel of truth" in your theories, and warned about identifying psychoanalysis with Jewry.

In the next few weeks the critiques of my collection[2] will come out; they will sound favorable because I didn't send any review copies to my prospective detractors.—

With the lawyer, the differences between the two types of women actually seem to be fading. His cs. predilection for Jews and his secret aversion to them—I think—has a connection with the castration complex.

I am more and more certain of being able to trace a case of impotence that I have been treating for a year and a half to anal-sadistic constitution. The patient sees (ucs.) in coitus 1.) an act of cruelty, 2.) incontinence (not urethral but anal). He retains sperm the way a normal person retains his stool.—The patient suffered for a long time from incontentia alvi.[3]—He is unusually reserved, doesn't "let himself go" in any way.—

A brother of his has been imprisoned for life on account of a *murder* committed in the heat of passion. Two other brothers are more or less impotent. A cousin (clear anal character) is the same impotent man about whom we once consulted with Stekel.[4]—

I am eager to hear news.

Cordially,
Ferenczi

1. István Apáthy (1863–1922), professor of histology, zoologist, and a poet and features writer. Founding member of the Hungarian Social Science Society, at a meeting of which, on January 24, 1914 (the founding of a section on eugenics), he had attacked "Freud's worm's-eye view of the world" and designated him as a "representative of a Semitic panerotism." Géza Szilágyi responded to Apáthy's attack in the daily *Az Ujság* ("Freud és Apáthy," March 11 and 12). Neurofibrils are the very fine filaments in the cells of the ganglia and their processes.

2. See letter 422, n. 2.

3. Inability to control defecation.

4. See letter 194.

452

Vienna, February 1, 1914
IX., Berggasse 19

Dear friend,

The only good news: the strike[1] is over, things can start up again. Nothing else, other than the fact that I am writing, constantly writing,[2] and don't have any time for it.

Magnus Hirschfeld was here this morning, and at noon we are expecting van Eeden,[3] who gave a lecture here, along with Heller and Rank.

Your boastfulness about your health, and your second edition strike a very agreeable chord.

Cordially, with apologies for my brevity,

Yours,
Freud

1. See letter 447, n. 3.

2. Probably "On the History of the Psycho-Analytic Movement" (1914d).

3. Frederik Willem van Eeden (1860–1932), an old acquaintance of Freud's; Dutch neurologist, poet, and social reformer, founder of the socialist-communist colony Walden in Bussum (1898). According to Jones (II, 368), he and Freud had tried in vain to win him over to psychoanalysis. See also *Minutes* II, 420f, for February 9, 1910.

453

Internationale Zeitschrift für
Ärztliche Psychoanalyse

Budapest, February 9, 1914

Dear Professor,

Despite your request to return to more peaceful work from now on, I couldn't resist reacting correspondingly to the unmatched impudence and conceit of Jung's paper (see Archives de Psychologie). I sent the critique to Rank for the Zeitschrift.[1]—

After the honeymoon that psychonalysis has enjoyed in Budapest, it now seems to be getting more serious resistance. Apáthy's attacks have caused the "Social Science Society" to come back to the idea that was floated last year but rejected by me of letting adherents and opponents of Ψα. have their say in a public discussion. I still owe them a reply, was decidedly in favor of rejecting it again, and would still be, had not* the arguments of my friend Ignotus shaken me to a certain extent. Ignotus thinks that we ought not brusquely refuse the offer of the "Social Science Society" (the only group on which we can count for some support and defense, in the event of brutal attacks). They will take my avoidance as running away, which could harm still more the already bad reputation of Ψα., etc.

Finally, I allowed myself to to be softened up to the extent that I would be ready to agree to the discussion under the following conditions:

I can *a priori* not recognize any of those who are more or less interested in Ψα. as adherents of Freudian psychoanalysis, since I am not aquainted with their views about the details of the questions that interest us. I consider myself today (as long as I am not instructed by a better) the only one here who understands and does psychoanalysis in your sense. So, if they want to discuss *Freudian* psychoanalysis, they should give me the right to react immediately to every individual speech.

Without harboring the illusion that this discussion will serve any purpose *in merito* and convince even one opponent or make him waver, I still don't consider it out of the question that I can take the opponents and half-opponents, the wild and the *tame* psychoanalysts (a new category), by the horns and demonstrate their animal nature and ignorance *coram publico* [publicly], which in the end, after so many years of silence, would do me good.

But I will wait with my reply until you tell me what you think of this plan. I would not like to be forced into any ill-considered action.

Have you written anything new about "déjà vu"?[2] I would be very much interested in hearing it.

I am waiting in suspense for the proofs of Moses, and I hope that my friend Berény will prove his worth as an illustrator better than Heller's protégé.[3]

Kind regards,
Ferenczi

* Subsequent correction [the "not" has been inserted between the lines].

1. Carl Jung, "Contribution à l'étude des types psychologiques (Communication présentée au Congrès de Psychanalyse à Munich 1913)," *Archives des psychologie* 13, no. 52 (December 1913). *CW* 6. Ferenczi's review (1914, 151) was published in *Zeitschrift* 1 (1914): 86f.

2. "'Fausse Reconnaissance' ('déjà raconté') in Psycho-Analytic Treatment" (Freud 1914a).

3. On Berény, see letter 238 and n. 3; Ferenczi refers to the illustration for Freud's analysis of the statue of Moses (1914b, pp. 226f).

454

Vienna, February 11, 1914
IX., Berggasse 19

Dear friend,

Yesterday I had editorial company for supper and learned from Rank that you have already criticized Jung's latest declaration. I was very pleased by your dash. Our critical issue will also be very extensive; unfortunately, it has not yet begun to go to press.

I must approve of your intention for a public discussion for you and for Hungary. Your temperament and your quick-wittedness are a proper guarantee of its success. Public interest in ΨA is probably also abating in Russia, Poland, etc., where they failed to position themselves properly in the first assault wave. Not so in Germany and America.

I would be very pleased if you could move your friend to attempt the two drawings of Moses. The ones by Fräulein Wolf[1] are unsatisfactory. The engraver Max Pollak, who "etched" my portrait "with a needle,"[2] has also promised to deliver these drawings. But that shouldn't hold you back. My doubts have not been overcome, and I will certainly hold up publication if an illustrator doesn't support them effectively, convince me first, so to speak.

I am writing very assiduously on the history of the ψα movement, and I hope to have worked on Jung, and with that have finished it by Sunday. Should I send you the manuscript first? You would then have to send it back to me soon with your remarks, so that it can go by way of the Viennese, through Hitschmann, to Abraham.

Health and practice are now good. Everything mostly in order at home. You should visit us again at the end of the month, when the work is in process. Loe is behaving much better; incidentally, she has been diagnosed with pyelitis sinistra[3] and a portion of genuine pains; mixed case always unpleasant. The presence of her new Jones,[4] whom she is supposed to marry im May, is doing her good.

Kind regards, to Frau G., also.

Yours,
Freud

1. Unidentified.

2. Max Pollak (1886-?), noted Viennese painter and, above all, graphic artist. His etching of Freud, printed in *Sigmund Freud: His Life in Pictures and Words*, ed. Ernst Freud, Lucie Freud, and Ilse Grubrich-Simitis (New York, 1985), p. 202, was described by Karl Kraus: "Max Pollak portrayed the researcher sitting at his desk in his study. The foreground is made strangely lively by the antiques and archaic figurines on the desk. From the half-light of the study rises mightily the cerebral head of the scholar with that reflective gaze turned inward to a certain extent, which characterizes concentrated intellectual creative work." *Die Fackel*, March 28, 1914, p. 57.

3. Inflammation of the renal pelvis on the left-hand side.

4. Loe Kann, who had resumed her analysis with Freud in November of the previous year (Brome, *Jones*, p. 104), and her fiancé, Herbert Jones (see letter 392, n. 1), were guests at the Wednesday session of April 22, 1914 (*Minutes* IV, 256), at which Freud was not present because of illness (see letter 470). Freud went to Budapest for her wedding in early June (see letter 476).

455

Budapest,[1]
February 15, [1914][2]

please send manuscript[3] = regards ferenczi

1. Telegram.

2. This telegram was filed in the Balint folder under 1918, but it would appear to belong here in view of its content and Freud's response (see letter 456). The year 1910 impressed on the telegram form confirms this assumption (later impressions were used after mid-1914).

3. The manuscript of "On the History of the Psycho-Analytic Movement" (Freud 1914d).

456

Vienna, February 15, 1914
IX., Berggasse 19

Dear friend,

Today two pieces of news. I'll begin with the lesser one. I have finished the History of the ψα Movement and am prepared to send it to you as soon as you express the wish to see it. You will then be so kind as to expedite the packet *securely* to Abraham—for I can't write it over again—and then send to me under separate cover your criticisms, reservations, suggestions, so that I can use them in the corrections. It was trying work; you know the first part.

Second: sudden receipt of a paper by Jelgersma,[1] rectorial address on the 339th anniversary of the famous old University of Leyden, called ontgeweten (ucs.) Geestesleven. I am trying to understand it, but I see that it has to do with the Interpretation of Dreams and—is friendly. Next day I received a newspaper from Renterghem[2] with a long excerpt from the paper; then a letter from Abraham, who confirms that Jelgersma has spoken out unreservedly in favor of us and ΨA and has fantasized about translation, etc. Finally, a letter from the author himself, which I am enclosing for you (for the shortest time) and which really confirms the miracle. Imagine, official psychiatrist, rectorial address, ΨA from head to toe! What surprises are yet to come!

Heller wants to write to him and arrange for a German edition of the little paper.

On Friday, the 20th of the month, at my place, there will be an official Moses evening, at which the fate of this experimental piece is supposed to be decided (Heller, Rank, Sachs, Pollak, the artist who has delivered very good drawings to me).[3] Too bad you are in Budapest.

Your telegram requesting the manuscript has just come. So, I will have it sent tomorrow. I want to read Jelgersma's letter in the Society on Wednesday. The paper about déjà vu that you asked about is a piece of junk.

Are you in a mood to undertake something this Easter (April 12)? Perhaps go to Arbe again, which must be very nice later in the season. If everything goes all right in Hamburg, scheduled for mid-March,[4] I am quite ready. Would you like to take the little one[5] along? She is amusing; you know her from the Pordoijoch,[6] of course. She has had a slight fever without visible cause for six weeks now. She doesn't feel well, and I am worried about her.[7]

Kind regards,
Freud

1. Gerbrandus Jelgersma (1859–1942), professor of psychiatry (1899–1930) at the University of Leyden in Holland; the clinic there still bears his name. On February 9, 1914, he had given a rectorial address, "Unconscious Mental Life," at the celebration of the 339th anniversary of the university's founding; the address was published in 1914 as the first supplement to the *Zeitschrift*. In 1920 Jelgersma founded the Leyden Society for Psychoanalysis and Psychopathology, which had friendly relations with the Dutch Psychoanalytic Society.

2. Albert Willem van Renterghem (1845–1939), neurologist and psychiatrist, one of Freud's first adherents in the Netherlands; head of the Institute for Psychotherapy in Amsterdam. Freud mentioned Jelgersma and Renterghem in "On the History of the Psycho-Analytic Movement" (1914d, p. 33).

3. Freud wanted to hear the opinion of an artist on his interpretation of *Moses* (Jones II, 366). See letter 459.

4. The expected birth of Ernst Wolfgang (March 11, 1914), son of Sophie and Max Halberstadt, and Freud's first grandchild; see letter 463 and n. 2.

5. Anna.

6. A mountain pass in the south Tyrol.

7. Shortly before the beginning of the journey (they eventually decided on Brioni, April 9–13, 1914), Anna developed whooping cough, so Rank went along in her place; see letter 468.

457

Budapest, [undated][1]

Most pleasantly surprised by Jelgersma's appearance. On Abraham's recommendation I wrote to Jelgersma already *yesterday* and asked him to release the speech for the Zeitschrift.

More next time.

Ferenczi

1. Written on the back of a preprinted calling card. In the upper right-hand corner, in different ink and (presumably) a different hand, is written "1914." The content justifies placing it in this sequence.

458

Budapest, February 18, 1914

Dear Professor,

Jelgersma's appearance and his letter were great events. I didn't know that Heller wants to get the paper, so, for that reason, I immediately wrote to Jelgersma at Abraham's urging, asking him to release the article for the Zeitschrift. But that shouldn't prevent Heller from publishing it separately.—Enclosed is a genuinely "Zurich" letter on the same subject, by *Ophuijsen*.[1] "Jelgersma *adapted too much*," he thinks, and wants "to push *youth* aside." One can see that the logical consequence of an absolute ego psychology (which denies the role of the libido) leads unerringly to a kind of persecution mania. The Christian religion, which always fears the revenge of the killed father, may be the cause of this obviously epidemic psychosis among the Swiss analysts.—

If you think I should, I will send Ophuijsen's paper back to him. I find it partisan and malicious. The fear of new competition may also play a role in this. I very much like the candidly clear way in which Jelgersma talks about sexuality and even incest; I see in this good indications for his future development.

I would *very much* like to make the Easter journey. We will naturally also take Annerl along. I hope she is again quite well and that we can again look up our Italian friend at the northern end of the island (the one who brewed us that good coffee).

They are talking about us a lot again in Hungary. The newspaper writers are praising my new collection, and our competitors are getting riled up. I will allow the discussion to take place (probably in March).—

I read your manuscript aloud to Frau G. yesterday. We liked the first and third parts *enormously*. The middle one (the somewhat lengthy description of the Congresses) could be shortened. I was pleased by the *complete* agreement of our views with regard to Adler and Jung. I will suggest small changes in the enclosed notes.—What is nice is the analogy of *total rejection*[2] and that of the *cultural overtones!*[3]

Kind regards,
Ferenczi
and from Frau G.—

February 20
P.S. In order not to delay sending off the letter, I am sending you the notes—which I first have to write out in fair copy—later.—

Yesterday I had another talk with the criminalist Dr. Rustem Vámbéry (son of the deceased Orientalist). He asked me to write an article on the possibility of the application of psychoanalysis to criminal psychology for his journal.[4]—

1. The letter is missing.

2. "And yet daily experience with patients had shown that total rejection of analytic knowledge may result whenever a specially strong resistance arises at any depth of the mind" (Freud 1914d, p. 48).

3. On Jung: "The truth is that these people have picked out a few cultural overtones from the symphony of life and have once more failed to hear the mighty and primordial melody of the instincts" (ibid., p. 62).

4. Rustem Vámbéry (1872–1948), lawyer, champion of Hungarian radicalism; member (1918) of the Council of State under Mihály Károlyi. In 1938 he emigrated to London and then to the United States, where he served as Hungary's ambassador. His father was the Orientalist Armin Vámbéry (Hermann Vamberger) (1832–1913). Ferenczi's article (1914, 148a) was published under the title "Büntények lélekelemzése" [Psychoanalysis of Crime] in *Szabad Gondolat*, no. 1 (1914).

459

Vienna, February 23, 1914
IX., Berggasse 19

Dear friend,

Thanks for your notes, which, in addition to those still to be expected, will be taken into consideration. Perhaps we still have an opportunity to deal with them by word of mouth before we go to press. Now the manuscript will probably soon go to Berlin. It will be the first to be typeset for the Jahrbuch.

I completely confirm your judgment about Ophuijsen's critique. You will have a good rationalization for sending it back if you tell him that you want to put out the German translation yourself. But who will translate it? Heller already has his agreement for the German edition. Don't you want to come to an agreement with Heller, so that Jelgersma doesn't get the impression of an unplanned process?

Annerl is better. She no longer has a fever and is very happy to be able to travel with us. But before I write about rooms I suggest that you consider whether we shouldn't rather go to Brioni, which is new to us. We would have to make reservations there very early.

I am in the middle of Narcissism, in which my debt to you[1] will become apparent. It is naturally going very hard, but it has to be done by Easter. The Moses evening ended without any real result. I wanted to hear a proper objection from the artist, but I couldn't get it out of him. It will probably come into being anyway.

Thank the first reader of the historical contribution in my name for her interest and applause! How is she?

Kind regards,
Freud

P.S. Enclosed a letter, critique by Ophuijsen and a letter from me to you.[2]

1. See letter 461 and n. 1.
2. Freud's meaning is not clear here.

460

Budapest, February 26, 1914[1]

in agreement with Brioni = ferenczi

1. Telegram.

461

Vienna, March 4, 1914
IX., Berggasse 19

Dear friend,

We have been accepted in Brioni. I suggest we leave on Thursday evening (Maundy Thursday), so that we arrive on Friday noon.

Heller claims that he sent you the etching of my portrait. I am very curious to know what you think about it. Family is very dissatisfied, while others praise it highly.

Narcissism is progressing and will be finished in March. I will present it to you, also in order that you can indicate in which passages I can refer to your Sense of Reality.[1]

I am in favor of putting Jelgersma's lecture not in the journal but in the form of the first supplement.

On Saturday my wife is going to Hamburg, we hope at the right time.[2]

I greet you cordially in expectation of news from you.

Yours,
Freud

1. Freud 1914c, p. 75. Freud had also asked Abraham to "look out yourself the passage where I have to mention your first (Salzburg) paper" (*Freud/Abraham*, March 16, 1914, p. 167).

2. For Sophie's anticipated delivery; see letter 463 and n. 2.

462

INTERNATIONALE ZEITSCHRIFT FÜR
ÄRZTLICHE PSYCHOANALYSE

Budapest, March 6, 1914

Dear Professor,

First (as almost always), a series of thank-yous: I thank you this time for the favorable settlement of the matter of the Easter trip and for the etching, which I find *excellent*. The engraver doesn't yet seem to be a "modern" one; nevertheless, a somewhat bolder breeze is blowing in his work. I am convinced that this man can also do something in the Moses matter. But it would still be worth the trouble to try out my friend (Berény) as well.

The march of our troops against Zurich in the first issue of the second volume is downright impressive. Eitingon's wonderfully sharp polemic against the murder of the concept of ucs.[1] was a pleasant surprise to me.—

—I am very busy (completely booked up almost every day); therapeutic results can be achieved—albeit with great effort—with sufficient persever-ance on both sides.

In the evenings I am so tired that I don't succeed in doing any other work. I don't deny that psychic factors play a part in this.—Condition of my nose is more satisfactory; sleep not yet. Maybe after Brioni!

Kind regards to you and to all who are at home.

Yours,
Ferenczi

1. Max Eitingon, "Über das Ubw. bei Jung und seine Wendung ins Ethische (aus der Diskussion der Berliner Psychoanalytischen Vereinigung am 17. Januar 1914)," *Zeitschrift* 2 (1914): 99–104.

463

[Vienna,] March 11, 1914[1]

Dear friend,

Tonight (10th/11th) at 3 o' clock a little boy, my first grandchild![2] Very strange! An oldish feeling, respect for the wonders of sexuality! Sophie is very well; she even said over the telephone: "It wasn't so bad."

Kind regards, to Frau G., also.

Yours,
Freud

Jahrbuch and Imago published.

1. Postcard.
2. Ernst Wolfgang Halberstadt (later W. Ernest Freud); today a psychoanalyst in Germany. The *fort-da* game of the one-and-a-half-year-old boy was described and interpreted by Freud in *Beyond the Pleasure Principle* (1920g, pp. 14–17).

464

INTERNATIONALE ZEITSCHRIFT FÜR
ÄRZTLICHE PSYCHOANALYSE

Budapest, March 16, 1914

Dear Professor,

As a postscript to my congratulations I am sending you only the information that I would like to spend next Sunday (March 22) in Vienna, in order to talk out all personal, business, and scientific matters before the Easter trip. I request your kind reply as to whether or not I am coming at an inconvenient time.

Kind regards,
Ferenczi

Regarding Abraham's plan,[1] I am letting you know in advance that I am in favor of waiting to see what the effects of the bombs[2] are and perhaps to proceed only after the Jahrbuch has come out.

1. Abraham's letter of March 16, 1914, has been published only in abridged form, so his plan can only be deduced indirectly from Freud's reference in his reply to "your proposal of aggressive action against Jung" (Freud/Abraham, March 16, 1914, p. 167).

2. The publication of the critical discussions in the Zeitschrift (see letter 470, n. 5) and of Freud's "History of the Psycho-Analytic Movement" in the Jahrbuch.

465

Vienna, March 18, 1914
IX., Berggasse 19

Dear friend,

I desire your visit this Sunday all the more in view of the fact that it is my first work-free Sunday in months. Narcissism has arrived in Berlin after going through all the stops in between. I am not satisfied with it.[1]

I thank Frau G. most cordially for her kind message. Like all ladies, she didn't include her address with the letter.

I am expecting you early in the morning.

Auf Wiedersehen.

Yours,
Freud

1. Freud expressed himself to Abraham with similar dissatisfaction (Freud/Abraham, March 16 and April 6, 1914, pp. 167, and 170f).

466

INTERNATIONALE ZEITSCHRIFT FÜR
ÄRZTLICHE PSYCHOANALYSE

Budapest, March 23, 1914

Dear Professor,

In a big hurry. I just want to tell you that right on the first day I owe the solution to a year-and-a-half-long resistance to your explanation yesterday[1] of the "masculine protest." A patient (engineer) has always been terrified of, among other things, tearing and macerating pieces of meat. (I always interpreted this correctly as castration anxiety.) Today, among other things, he had the following thoughts: 1.) A tooth, broken in half; terribly painful. 2.) Three iron bars, held together by rings and broken in two. 3.) A cooked sausage. When I told him that he is sorry about his penis, i.e., about his masculinity, which he has to sacrifice to my love if he wants to satisfy me *as a woman*, his resistance lifted all of a sudden, his anger ceased, and he began to work properly.[2]

The *enormous* importance of being oriented toward this true essence of masculine protest immediately dawned on me yesterday. I think that *I* would never have hit on it because of my own similar ucs. complexes.

I am happy to be able to send you this confirmation so quickly.

Cordially,
Ferenczi

1. During Ferenczi's visit on Sunday, March 22.

2. This train of thought played a major role in Freud's analysis of the "Wolf-Man" (*From the History of an Infantile Neurosis* [1918b (1914)]), whose treatment, begun in 1910, was just then coming to an end. For example: "It seems, therefore, as though he had identified himself with his castrated mother during the dream, and was now fighting against that fact. 'If you want to be sexually satisfied by Father,' we may perhaps represent him as saying to himself, 'you must allow yourself to be castrated like Mother; but I won't have that.' In short, a clear protest on the part of his masculinity!" (p. 47; see also p. 110).

467

INTERNATIONALE ZEITSCHRIFT FÜR
ÄRZTLICHE PSYCHOANALYSE

Budapest, April 1, 1914

Dear Professor,

I have already reserved a sleeping berth for Thursday (April 9) and will travel not via Fiume but rather—like you—via Pola. To be sure, I already have to leave my sleeping car, which goes on to Venice, very early (in Divacca) and change to your train from Vienna. Perhaps we can meet for breakfast in the dining car (if there is one). I think I understood correctly that you wanted to leave Brioni on *Monday*; my sleeping car ticket for the return also says Monday. If I have made a mistake and you are also inclined to spend Tuesday in Brioni, I ask you to let me know as soon as possible.

As a sign that I am feeling well, I now have all kinds of smaller and larger work plans, which I am in part putting on paper. Perhaps we will be able to talk about them in Brioni—but I hope we won't; our main concern should be the sun and the sea.

Kind regards to all.

Yours,
Ferenczi

468

Vienna, April 5, 1914
IX., Berggasse 19

Dear friend,

I wasn't able to get a sleeping car ticket anymore, so I will have to risk it as it is. I can't decide on the return trip now. I have canceled my patients until Wednesday morning, but I am prepared to leave Brioni perhaps Monday and skip work in Vienna on Tuesday. A lot has to do with how pleasant the stay is for us; making a previous commitment also has its disadvantages.

You will be surprised to hear that I am coming in the company of someone else. Annerl has whooping cough and naturally can't come; she has been very good and herself proposed that I take someone else along in her place. Rank has accepted and will therefore share our lodgings. We will be all Zeitschrift.

Since you left I have had a bad time, unmistakable overtiredness and intolerance to tobacco. I have also not worked on anything since.

These last few days were overshadowed by a small scare, which I hope will turn out to be nothing. The packet with the manuscripts for the Jahrbuch that Abraham sent to Hitschmann on the first of the month hasn't arrived yet. It is hard to think what will happen if it really gets lost. Let's hope it will come tomorrow,[1] but it stands as a warning to have every manuscript copied.

Good news from Hamburg. My wife is coming at the end of the month, and Oli is leaving on Wednesday for his trip to Egypt.

Eder's translation of the little dream[2] came into my hands yesterday. Otherwise, nothing new.

I will bring along a fountain pen with an attached card from Loe for you. Kind regards and *auf Wiedersehen.*

Yours,
Freud

1. It did in fact arrive the next day (*Freud/Abraham*, April 6, 1914, p. 170).
2. *On Dreams* (Freud 1901a), trans. M. D. Eder (London, 1914).

469

INTERNATIONALE ZEITSCHRIFT FÜR
ÄRZTLICHE PSYCHOANALYSE

Budapest, April 18, 1914

Dear Professor,

After a very restless night (I had to change trains three times), I did arrive refreshed in Budapest, full of the most pleasant "engrams" [memories] about the stay in Brioni. Aside from all the other experiences, I owe to this trip my closer acquaintance with Rank, whose valuable personality I became acquainted with, in addition to his kind and pleasant qualities, which were already familiar to me. A real circle of friends is gradually coming out of the "Committee," in which one feels well and secure. But I had to observe not without pain that my position with respect to you, specifically, is still not completely natural, and that your presence arouses inhibitions of various kinds in me that influence, and at times almost paralyze, my actions and even my thinking. I didn't want to disturb your vacation by telling you this—but you probably noticed it anyway.

The next few days will be dedicated to the papers in the Jahrbuch.[1]— Shouldn't I also spruce up my lecture at the Munich Congress[2] (with the little piece of epistemology) for the Jahrbuch—as we had earlier planned? Or will I already be too late for it?

I am thinking back with great pleasure on the rediscovery of fire.[3] It was precious. I still think that the solution you found is correct.

Kind regards,
Ferenczi

1. Ferenczi, "Allgemeine Neurosenlehre" (1914, 148), *Jahrbuch* 6 (1914): 317–328.

2. Ferenczi, "Glaube, Unglaube und Überzeugung" [Belief, Disbelief, and Conviction] (1913, 109; *F.C.*, p. 437); first published in German in *Populäre Vorträge über die Psychoanalyse* (Vienna, 1922).

3. Freud did not publish his thoughts on the acquisition and control of fire (1930a [1929] and 1932a [1931]) until much later; see also letter 470. A few weeks later Otto Rank talked about his intention of writing a paper on fire; see Rank's letters to Freud of June 25 and 26, 1914.

470

Vienna, April 24, 1914
IX., Berggasse 19

Dear friend,

I had certainly noticed in Brioni that you are somehow inhibited, and I connected it with Rank's presence; but I didn't pursue it further because I was suffering from a hypochondriacal withdrawal of libido. Since then a great tracheitis-laryngitis[1] has broken out in me with a clear lifting of the prodromal general symptoms.[2] I haven't stopped working—out of greed and a feeling of obligation—, but I missed last Wednesday, and today I haven't felt well for a long time, neither locally nor generally, and above all I am very incapable of thinking.

Jung's surprising resignation[3] has made our task much easier. He does, in fact, seem to be a part of that power that etc.[4] What goes on in him and what he intends can't be figured out but can only be a matter of indifference to us. Perhaps he has succumbed to the salvo in the Zeitschrift,[5] and the bomb in the Jahrbuch is coming too late. I have immediately begun to feel like a "conference of heads" and have initiated an action about which you, like our other friends, are supposed to be or have already been notified by a letter from Rank.[6]

There is nothing at all left for me about the acquisition of fire. Cultural history is mute on the subject. But I am very curious as to what kind of serious things the both of you will come out with.

The material for the Jahrbuch must, as Hitschmann says, be cut back. For that reason Rank and Sachs have withdrawn their contribution.[7] So, you should save your lecture for another time, or let it ferment as the germ of a new work.

Kind regards to you and Frau G.

Yours truly,
Freud

1. Inflammation of the windpipe and larynx.

2. Symptoms that precede the actual characteristic manifestations of illness.

3. Four days earlier Jung had written to Freud: "Dear Mr. President, The latest developments have convinced me that my views are in such sharp contrast to the views of the majority of the members of our Association that I can no longer consider myself a suitable personality to be president. I therefore tender my resignation to the council of the presidents of the branch societies, with many thanks for the confidence I have enjoyed hitherto. Very truly yours, Dr. C. G. Jung" (Freud/Jung, p. 551).

4. "That power that always wants evil and always creates good"; see letter 35, n. 2.

5. Ferenczi's programmatic critique of Jung's "Wandlungen und Symbole der Libido" (1913, 124; Zeitschrift 1 [1913]: 391–403) and the adversarial discussions of his works by Abraham, Ferenczi, and Jones in the next volume of the Zeitschrift (2 [1914]: 72–87).

6. On April 30 Freud sent letters with the same text to each of the presidents of the

six European branch societies (Berlin, Budapest, London, Munich, Vienna, and Zurich) with the request "to nominate that person among the six eligible presidents of the branch societies whom you wish to entrust with the leadership of the Association until the election of a president, whereby you do not need to exclude yourself . . . I, myself, am inclined to choose Dr. *Abraham* as the provisional head of the Association, because from his place of residence he can most easily make preparations for the Congress, which will take place in Dresden." Freud's suggestion was accepted.

7. Unidentified.

471

Internationale Zeitschrift für Ärztliche Psychoanalyse

Budapest, May 6, 1914

Dear Professor,

The past week has been like a state of war for me. I moved from the second to the third floor (my address remains otherwise unchanged: Elisabethring 54); at the same time I rearranged the furniture. I had to make all these changes—which, by the way, are not yet completely finished—without disrupting the work of analysis, which I just about managed to do. The books are still all over the place—and right now I had to write the paper for the Jahrbuch; I did it from memory and only afterwards had to look up the references. But Hitschmann seems to be satisfied with the paper.

Jung's resignation had a very pleasant effect on me. I don't think you need from me any "official" assent to your suggestions, with which I am in total agreement.

Dr. Jászy (university docent at the law school and leader of the radical youth)[1] didn't let me rest until I agreed to the plan for a detailed symposium on psychoanalysis. We have agreed that two lectures on psychoanalysis will be held in the fall of this year; I am supposed to speak on the status of psychoanalysis today, *Rank and Sachs* (in German) are to talk about the application of psychoanalysis to the social sciences.[2] [Of course, I made out the bill there without the innkeeper, and I don't know whether Rank and Sachs are of a mind to come to Budapest.][3] Jászy wants to ask a number of personalities (including opponents) to take part in the discussion, and he wants to give me the task of responding to them. I think it will be easy for the three of us to disable our antagonists (who are certainly not even oriented to the elements of $\Psi\alpha$.).

I am anticipating with interest your news about the presidents' responses.

Kind regards,
Ferenczi

1. Oszkár Jászi (1875–1957), leading figure in the radical movement in Hungary and, in 1914, head of the Radical party. He was secretary of the Social Science Society, director of the Free School of Social Sciences, and editor in chief of *Huszadik Század* [Twentieth Century]. In 1918 he became a member of the Council of State and minister without portfolio in Károlyi's government. In 1919 he became professor of sociology at the University of Budapest. During the republic under Béla Kun he emigrated to Vienna, and in 1925 he went to the United States, where he taught at Oberlin College in Ohio.

2. Not only were Rank and Sachs editors of *Imago, Zeitschrift für die Anwendung der Psychoanalyse auf die Geisteswissenschaften*, but also they had published a book together, *Die Bedeuting der Psychoanalyse für die Geisteswissenschaften* [The Significance of Psychoanalysis for the Humanities] (Wiesbaden, 1913).

3. Enclosed in brackets in the original.

472

Vienna, May 12, 1914
IX., Berggasse 19

Dear friend,

I didn't write you in the last few days because I didn't know what to write. You remember my discomfort in Brioni. Shortly afterwards my laryngitis broke out, which went as far as my nose, but is almost all better today. At six in the evening, perhaps brought on by an excess of festivities, an acute intestinal condition set in, which Dr. Zweig[1] examined with a proctoscope, and then he congratulated me. He then admitted that I didn't yet have the neoplasm that he suspected, but rather a very acute inflammation of the romanum.[2] So I have been restored to life and can write to you again. I am now, by the way, subjectively better than I was before these illnesses.

The matter of the presidency has been smoothly decided in the meantime, as you know. Abraham will soon get things rolling and will deliver a Korrespondenzblatt to us. I will also correspond with him about the date of the Congress, which would be very inconvenient for me at the beginning of September. He himself is in favor of postponing it until September 20/21; we will get together for a private congress the day before. I will then be able to give the lecture in Leyden[3] on about the 23d and then go to Hamburg. Our summer plans have been completely halted by my illness and uncertainty as to whether Zweig will recommend treatment.

My best wishes for your move! The planned tournament impresses me very much; I will certainly talk Rank and Sachs into going.

I haven't worked *at all* since Brioni. Yesterday I began correcting my "History of the ψα Movement." The next time you come here you will be able to admire a ψα gallery like the one in Worcester.[4] Stanley Hall has gone over to Adler, according to a paper that I received today.[5] I greet you and Frau G. cordially.

Yours, still alive,
Freud

1. Walter Zweig (1872–? [after 1954]), *Privatdozent* in Vienna, specialist for diseases of the stomach and intestines; jokingly referred to by Freud as his *personal* physician [*Leibarzt*] (*Freud/Abraham*, May 13, 1914, p. 176 n. 1).

2. A part of the large intestine.

3. Jelgersma had invited Freud to lecture at the University of Leyden in the fall (Jones II, 105).

4. Possibly an allusion to the photographs in the psychological seminar in Worcester (*Freud/Abraham*, March 9, 1914, p. 166).

5. Unidentified.

473

INTERNATIONALE ZEITSCHRIFT FÜR
ÄRZTLICHE PSYCHOANALYSE

Budapest, May 13, 1914

Dear Professor,

Since Brioni I have been well, physically, which with me goes along with (intellectual) productivity. Stemming from the problem of enuresis, some ideas have occurred to me about the "amphimixis of partial instincts" at the onset of the primacy of the genital zone.[1] This time I set about not to dissipate the matter with epistolary and oral discourse, but to write the matter up and—without regard for possible disgrace—to send it to you as free associations on this theme.

The unanimous outcome of the presidential election surprised me. Is there something malicious behind it?[2]

I received the enclosed card from Dr. Ophuijsen,[3] which I answered in a conciliatory tone, but not without remarking that he could see from the issues of the Zeitschrift that have been published so far that we are not timid about proceeding ruthlessly (if the cause demands it). He can also believe us when we assure him that this time there was no reason to do so.

My practice is going well.

Kind regards,
Ferenczi

1. By *amphimixis* Ferenczi meant "a synthesis of two or more erotisms in a higher unity," for instance, "an integration of anal and urethral erotisms into genital erotism"; see *Thalassa: A Theory of Genitality*, 1924, 268, 3: 369 (*Schriften* II, 325). In this work

Ferenczi discussed in detail these thoughts which had occupied him since 1910 (see letter 155).

2. Ferenczi was surprised by the acquiescence of the two presidents who did not belong to the Committee, Maeder in Zurich and Seif in Munich, to the suggestion of making Abraham interim president. Maeder, as Freud wrote to Abraham, had "agreed in a very gracious fashion, Seif did so laconically" (*Freud/Abraham*, May 7, 1914, p. 174).

3. This card is missing.

474

Budapest,[1]
May 16 [1914][2]

congratulations on recovery request news soon about how you are— ferenczi

1. Telegram.
2. The date 1914 is suggested by the context; see letters 472 and 475.

475

INTERNATIONALE ZEITSCHRIFT FÜR
ÄRZTLICHE PSYCHOANALYSE

Vienna, May 16, 1914

Dear friend,

I am reacting to your kind telegram to tell you that I am the picture of health, completely restored and better than before Brioni. So, nothing this time, yet! I have just been correcting the $\psi\alpha$ Movement and am cognizant of Jones's warning not to tone anything down. Good letters today from him and Sachs. From Putnam a brave defense of sexuality in The Interpretation of Dreams in the Journal of Abnormal Psychology (April-May).[1] Otherwise, only losses: Stanley Hall, as mentioned, total Adlerian; Spielrein, crazy [*meschugge*], writes that I have something against her.[2] Scientia is announcing a paper by Adler about individual psychology.[3] Next he will be called to America to free the world from sexuality and to base it on aggression!

I am eagerly awaiting your fantasy about the amphimixis of partial instincts. Haven't read anything clever in a long time.

Still very unenthusiastic about work.

We could have told Ophuijsen the real truth right away, and we really should do it the next time.

Abraham's first action should already have gotten to you. I am very much in agreement with the 20/21 of September.[4] Then I will give a lecture in

Leyden on or about the 23rd, then on to Hamburg. Summer still quite uncertain.

Yours,
Freud
redivivus

1. James Putnam, "Dream Interpretation and the Theory of Psychoanalysis," *Journal of Abnormal Psychology* 9 (April-May 1914): 36–60.

2. This letter from Sabina Spielrein is missing. She probably had complained that Freud had something against her because he never sent her any patients. Freud's reply of May 15, 1914: "Now you are going crazy yourself, and, what is more, with the same symptoms as your predecessor! One day I, all unsuspecting, received a letter from Frau Jung saying that her husband was convinced I had something against him. That was the beginning; you know the ending. And your argument that I have not yet sent you any patients? Exactly the same thing happened with Adler, who pronounced himself persecuted because I had sent him no patients. Do you recognize the well-known mechanism of unduly magnifying a man in order to hold him responsible?" Aldo Carotenuto, ed., *A Secret Symmetry: Sabina Spielrein between Jung and Freud* (New York, 1982), p. 121.

3. Alfred Adler, "Die Individualpsychologie, ihre Voraussetzungen und Ergebnisse," *Scientia* 16 (1914): 74–87.

4. The date suggested for the planned Congress.

476

Vienna, May 24, 1914[1]

please visit lawyer ernoe neuwirth szabadsagter 5 matter speed up marriage loe kann to herbert jones if possible whitsun rank and I coming as witnesses don't mention ernest's relation to loe otherwise give information and inform us = cordially freud

1. Telegram.

477

INTERNATIONALE ZEITSCHRIFT FÜR
ÄRZTLICHE PSYCHOANALYSE

Budapest, June 4, 1914

Dear Professor,

Just read Narcissism with delight. Haven't had such pleasure in reading in a long time. But I also have to admit to you—and you can take this openness as a sign of the uninhibited inner freedom that is beginning to develop in me—that for years I have actually not been able to read anything thoroughly except your writings. Everything else is basically boring to me;

you have spoiled us greatly, given us too beautiful, powerful things to read, after which nothing else seems to taste good. It is impossible to stress all the passages that I liked, so I will refrain from doing so. In accordance with your request, however, I will designate a few passages which we discussed in part together, and which I have in part referred to in already published works. Of course, you should cite me only when you, too, have the feeling that these things did not originate independently of me. Our work should certainly also be called a "collective" one; each of us must renounce a portion of the satisfaction of our ambition.

1.) I call your attention, for instance, to the trains of thought in the "introjection paper" (Jahrbuch I, 2), where being in love is described as inclusion of objects into the sphere of interest of the originally autoerotic libido. That would correspond roughly to the *emanations* of Narcissism.[1] I described neurosis as an exaggeration of this process.[2]

On p. 430—2nd paragraph—I let the separation of the ego from the outer world originate from the conflicts of the originally unified mental life (through border displacements).[3]—

2.) In the paper "Stages in the Development of the Sense of Reality" I believe I was first to have referred to the *infantile* expressions of omnipotence (magic).[4]

3.) The reference to the idealization of the *criminal* comes, I believe, from me.[5]

———

While I'm at it I think I should call your attention to the fact that it is perhaps not superfluous if you said expressly about the "emanations of the libido" that you understood therein an *intrapsychic* process, i.e., the displacement of libido onto the *perceptual image* of a real object, otherwise someone would think at the end that you mean by that an *"emanation" onto the object itself.*

I can also not refrain from putting your magnificent distinction of sublimation and idealization[6] into the following precise formulation:

The idealizer sublimates functionally.

The sublimator functions ideally.—

Kind regards,
Ferenczi

1. "Thus we form the idea of there being an original libidinal cathexis of the ego, from which some is later given off to objects, but which fundamentally persists and is related to the object-cathexes much as the body of an amoeba is related to the pseudopodia which it puts out . . . All that we noticed were the emanations of this libido—the object-cathexes, which can be sent out and drawn back again" (Freud 1914c, pp. 75f).

2. "The psychoneurotic suffers from a widening . . . of his ego" ("Introjection and Transference," 1909, 67; *C.*, p. 48).

3. Ibid., p. 49.

4. "Stages in the Development of the Sense of Reality" (1913, 111, *C.*, p. 213 passim); cited by Freud in the corresponding section of his work (Freud 1914c, p. 75).

5. "Indeed, even great criminals and humorists, as they are represented in literature, compel our interest by the narcissistic consistency with which they manage to keep away from their ego anything that would diminish it" (Freud 1914c, p. 89).

6. "Sublimation is a process that concerns object-libido and consists in the instinct's directing itself towards an aim other than, and remote from, that of sexual satisfaction . . . Idealization is a process that concerns the *object*; by it that object, without any alteration in its nature, is aggrandized and exalted in the subject's mind . . . In so far as sublimation describes something that has to do with the instinct and idealization something to do with the object, the two concepts are to be distinguished from each other" (ibid., p. 94).

478

Budapest, June 7, 1914

Dear Professor,

I am thinking a great deal about your paper on narcissism, and now and again things occur to me that relate to it. Since you have not yet (I think) finished correcting it, I would like to call your attention to a passage which could be misunderstood, but which can be made unambiguous by changing one single word.

You speak of two kinds of "end of the world" (that of dementia and that of being in love).[1] The *world* actually only gets lost in dementia, while being in love has to do with the *end of the ego,* which can nevertheless bring with it no lesser cataclysms and can be just as revolutionary psychically as the regression to narcissism is in dementia.

This time I will spare you further derivatives of this subject.

Frau G. sends kind regards.

Yours,
Ferenczi

In being in love, the world is not destroyed, but the object of love represents *the whole world* to the lover.

1. "There are two mechanisms of this 'end of the world' idea: in the one case, the whole libidinal cathexis flows off to the loved object; in the other, it all flows back into the ego" (Freud 1914c, p. 76).

479

Internationale Zeitschrift für
ärztliche Psychoanalyse

Budapest, June 19, 1914

Dear Professor,

With regard to the—*very* justified—wish to take up the important relation of the *ambivalence* of savages and of neurotics in my paper,[1] I have already done what is necessary. On the question of the presidential letter,[2] I share the view of Rank and Sachs.—I will naturally assume the task of presenting a paper on the topic of "The International Psychoanalytic Association," but I hope it won't come to that; I wrote to Abraham to that effect; a letter from Abraham to me calls our (the Zeitschrift's) attention to the fact that the works of Morton Prince, Häberlin, and Blüher[3] should not have been published without editorial corrective commentary. I, too, believe we ought not to spare the editorial red ink. Otherwise it will happen to us again that someone quotes a collaborator like Beaurain (whom I did contradict)[4] as a "psychoanalyst" *against* analysis. (See the little piece about the dream in Löwenfeld's collection.)[5]—Just read through Jelgersma's issue;[6] for the most part very good and understandable; he could have spared himself the genteel reserve.—I recently wrote a little paper on neuroses of the age of involution,[7] with points of contact with masturbation, neurasthenia, and—melancholia! I will send it to you; please read it with forbearance; i.e., don't dismiss it right away if it appears incorrect to you. In any case, write to me what you think of it. It is my first reaction to your Narcissism.—Enclosed, a kind letter from Putnam. I will reply in a similarly amicable manner.[8]—Abraham writes to me that he wants to come to Seis.[9] What can you tell *me* about the place? Should I really be breathing down your neck again for the whole of August—or do you want for once to take a rest without me and without psychoanalytic conversations?!

I have nothing else to write.—Regards from Frau G., who was very pleased about your stay here.[10]—We have to be careful with Varjás.—

Cordially,
Ferenczi

1. Ferenczi's essay on "Allgemeine Neurosenlehre" (1914, 148) for the *Jahrbuch*.

2. See letter 470 and n. 6 as well as letter 473 and n. 2.

3. Morton Prince, "Psychopathologie eines Falles von Phobie," *Zeitschrift* 1 (1913): 533–546; Paul Häberlin, "Psychoanalyse und Erziehung," *Zeitschrift* 2 (1914): 213–222; Hans Blüher, "Zur theorie der Inversion," *Zeitschrift* 2 (1914): 223–243, and "Der sogenannte natürliche Beschäftigungstrieb," *Zeitschrift* 2 (1914): 29f.

4. See letter 413 and nn. 8 and 9.

5. Probably Hans Henning, *Der Traum, ein assoziativer Kurzschluss* [The Dream, an

Associative Short-Circuit] (Wiesbaden, 1914). The book was published by the publisher of *Grenzfragen des Nerven- und Seelenlebens,* ed. Leopold Löwenfeld and Hans Kurella, but not in the same series.

6. See letter 456, n. 1.

7. Ferenczi's "Contribution to the Understanding of the Psychoneuroses of the Age of Involution" (posthumous, 303 [*Fin.*, p. 205]), is dated "approx. 1921–1922" in *Bausteine* III, 180, but a comparison of the content with his description in this letter makes it probable that it is the work mentioned here.

8. Putnam's letter is missing. In his reply of June 19 Ferenczi, alluding to Jung's resignation as president, wrote: "It . . . pleases me personally that you are with us in this very unnecessary and unpleasant inner crisis of the International Association . . . In science, compromises ought to be avoided" (Hale, *Putnam*, p. 315).

9. Freud had originally invited Abraham "to spend the whole summer together" (*Freud/Abraham*, July 18, 1914, p. 184). "Freud's summer plans had been to go to Karlsbad for intestinal treatment on July 12, from there to Seis in the southern Dolomites for his holiday proper, then to the Psycho-Analytical Congress Abraham was arranging in Dresden on September 20, and after that to Holland to deliver a lecture at the University of Leyden on September 24. His daughter [Anna] would join him there on her return from England and he would escort her home" (Jones II, 172).

10. For the wedding of Loe Kann and Herbert Jones; see letter 454, n. 4.

480

Vienna, June 22, 1914
IX., Berggasse 19

Dear friend,

We are living under the expectation of the "bomb," which is supposed to be sent out as soon as it comes in. No greater interest, for the time being.

I am likewise eagerly awaiting your contributions or drafts. It seems to me that the Zeitschrift now needs a few powerful accomplishments. In the case of ambivalence, we would especially have to think about Bleuler's paper.[1] Abraham is correct in principle with his remark about the works that have been listed, but it is hardly the proper time to wield the critical red ink, otherwise we won't get any contributions, and one has to allow for a certain multiplicity of views, even an alloy with such-and-such percent nonsense.—Putnam has also written to me in a kinder manner than usual.[2] It could be that after the schism we will keep three of the four American groups.[3]

About the summer, I want to reveal to you that I inevitably need some time to be alone, since I have to do the work for Kraus,[4] which can only be cooked up on quiet walks. Then it depends on when I will be finished with it. Perhaps in as little time as four weeks, so September 4–5. Abraham won't come until before the Congress. Then it would be very nice if we could spend the time from September 18 until Holland or Hamburg together. The time from September 4 to 18 has not yet been scheduled. Perhaps we will stay in Seis; I will report to you on every phase.

You really should take part in the occultist congress.[5] Timewise it can't be combined with our Congress (October 16–24!).

Give my best regards to Frau G.

Incidentally, I am working again like a real beast, 8 in the morning—9:30 in the evening!

Yours,
Freud

a. Putnam
b. Occult.

1. The "apt term" (Freud 1912–13a, p. 29), ambivalence, was introduced by Bleuler in 1910 in a lecture "Über Ambivalenz" (report in *Zentralblatt* 1 [1910–11]: 266–268) and in *Dementia Praecox oder Gruppe der Schizophrenien* (Leipzig, Vienna, 1911).

2. In his letter of June 2 Putnam had praised Freud's study of *Moses* (Freud 1914b) and had shared Freud's view of Adler: "I believe . . . that I am driven by my own complexes to overanxious attempts 'to do justice,' which are really attempts at conciliation" (Hale, *Putnam*, p. 174).

3. The New York Psychoanalytical Society, founded by Brill; the American Psychoanalytic Association, initiated by Jones; the Washington-Baltimore Psychoanalytic Society, founded by William Alanson White (1870–1937); and the Boston Psychoanalytic Society, founded in 1914 with Putnam as president and Isidor Coriat (1875–1943) as secretary. Freud could have feared the defection of the group around White and Smith Ely Jelliffe (1866–1945), who accepted Jung's desexualized concept of libido.

4. The planned "Psychoanalytic Presentation of the Neuroses"; see letter 432 and n. 2.

5. A plan that fell victim to the war.

481

INTERNATIONALE ZEITSCHRIFT FÜR
ÄRZTLICHE PSYCHOANALYSE

Budapest, June 23, 1914

Dear Professor,

Jones recently sent me some offprints with a request to review them for the Zeitschrift, among others, the enclosed article about the "Interrelation of Biogenetic Psychoses."[1] I miss the true psychoanalytic spirit in this paper and find it to be—except for a few telling remarks—unclear and confusing. What is your opinion about this paper, and how should I fulfill my duty as a reviewer in this instance?

Kind regards,
Ferenczi

1. Ernest Jones, "The Inter-Relation of the Biogenetic Psychoses," *American Journal of Insanity* 19 (1914); rpt. in *Papers on Psycho-Analysis* (London, 1920), pp. 466–473.

482

INTERNATIONALE ZEITSCHRIFT FÜR
ÄRZTLICHE PSYCHOANALYSE

Budapest, June 26, 1914

Dear Professor,

I have rarely been so unsure about the worth or worthlessness of a work as I am about the enclosed.[1] You can tell me your opinion without hesitation; I am prepared for the worst. I ask you to consider my courage in presenting it to you anyway as a kind of honesty which does not wish to hide even what is inferior. But I will also not conceal the fact that some of it appears to me to be important and correct in some instances.

I am pleased that I did the right thing with my suggestion to leave you in peace this summer. I can't very well postpone my vacation until September (—you already know, of course, that Budapest is not a proper summer resort in August—); so I will keep to the plan to leave here, where I won't have anything to do, on August 1. I will sound out Jones to see whether he is free at this time, and will possibly go to England, where I haven't been yet.—

I read through the "History of the Psycho-Analytic Movement" again in one sweep. I find it *excellent* and am pleased that you didn't allow yourself to be softened up to make any changes. It can't fail to have an effect, and I am anxiously awaiting news from you.

Tomorrow I am going to the provinces to see my sister, who lives near Nyiregyháza,[2] but I will be back Monday evening.

With kind regards to you and yours,

Ferenczi

A patient who has already been cured of impotence, who now has to live in abstinence owing to gonorrhea, delivered to me an important contribution to the *regression of the genital to the oral*. He has since often been preoccupied with his *teeth*; he constantly has to bite or gnash his teeth. I now think that even *biting* makes a libidinal contribution to the genital (see the analogy of rhythm while biting and during coitus), and that *tooth symbolism* finds its last source therein. So: a prospect for the uncovering of the *organic bases of symbolism*.

1. Probably his "Contribution to the Understanding of the Age of Involution"; see letter 479.
2. See letter 203 and n. 4.

483

Vienna, June 28, 1914
IX., Berggasse 19

Dear friend,

I am writing under the impression of the surprising murder in Sarajevo,[1] the consequences of which cannot be foreseen. It appears to me that personal involvement here is slight.

Now, to our affairs! I think you are too strict with Jones. There was, for instance, still no cause to distinguish between ego libido and object libido, and besides, the paper is meant for a specific audience. I have to concede to you only that he repeatedly says introversion[2] when he means regression. One could also hold that against him. The important thing, the remarks as to how one neurosis can cover another or something severe, are just as new as they are important. If my memory serves me correctly, they come from an "unknown author,"[3] who also told him about the cases in question. But you shouldn't hold that against him, either in print or by word of mouth.

I think you are right in your supposition that your manuscript[4] means something special. This is an experiment which promises much and is in urgent demand. I have been tormenting myself for a good ten years with these problems, but in the absence of reliable observation I haven't taken them up seriously. Now, the observation of climacterics has given you this base of support. I have much to advise and to suggest on the subject, but I can't do it in writing. I am, quite honestly, inwardly much too tired, although to all appearances I have been holding up very well these last few weeks. I think you should come to Vienna once more before I leave, just because we will see each other later this year. We will discuss it then, and I will keep your draft for that reason.

This year I gave up the "evening on the Konstantinhügel"[5] on the advice of friends, so you can choose your day at your discretion.

Nothing has been felt in the way of reaction to the bomb, outside of Vienna, naturally. There are a few here who are enthusiastic; one hears more and more clearly from the others that it is too harsh, and one can imagine what others will yet say about it. I don't think that any further statements, consequences, even trials for defamation of character will do anything to me. I got everything off my chest once and for all—that was worth the effort—and I am still figuring on the dissolution of the untenable relationship with the Zurichers. I certainly won't continue the polemic.

I still have two weeks from 8 in the morning until 9 in the evening to work here. Martin is already at the court in Salzburg.[6] Anna is leaving before us on July 7.[7] It was actually an extraordinarily difficult year.

In expectation of hearing from you soon, or seeing you,

Yours,
Freud

1. The murder of Archduke Franz Ferdinand, successor to the Austrian throne, and his wife on June 28 by Gavrilo Princip and other assassins of the Young Bosnia movement, which set in motion a rapid and furious chain of events leading, finally, to the First World War.

2. Introversion (withdrawal of libido into one's own self) was a concept introduced by Jung.

3. Freud himself had brought up this problem in "On Beginning the Treatment": "Often enough, when one sees a neurosis with hysterical or obsessional symptoms . . . one has to reckon with the possibility that it may be a preliminary stage of what is known as dementia praecox ('schizophrenia,' in Bleuler's terminology; 'paraphrenia,' as I have proposed to call it)" (1913c, p. 124). But Freud could also be referring to remarks that Ferenczi had made with respect to Jones, possibly during his analysis.

4. See letter 482 and n. 1.

5. The traditional farewell gathering of the Vienna Society at the end of the work year.

6. See letter 438, n. 1.

7. To Hamburg. Anna then went on to England on July 15. In August, by which time England was at war with Austria—with Jones's aid and under the protection of the Austrian ambassador—she made the return trip to Vienna via Gibraltar and Genoa.

Works by Freud and Ferenczi
Cited in the Text

Sigmund Freud

1887d   "Bemerkungen über Cocainsucht und Cocainfurcht, Mit Beziehung auf einen Vortrag W. A. Hammonds." *Wiener Medizinische Wochenschrift*, 37 (1887): 929–932.

1887e   "Rezension von: Obersteiner, H[einrich]." *Anleitung beim Studium des Baues der nervösen Centralorgane im gesunden und kranken Zustande.* Leipzig, 1888. *Wiener Medizinische Wochenschrift*, 37 (1887): 1642–44.

1889a   "Review of August Forel's *Hypnotism*." S.E. 1:91–102.

1891a   With Oskar Rie., "Klinische Studie über die halbseitige Cerebrallähmung der Kinder." Volume 3 of *Beiträge zur Kinderheilkunde,* ed. Kassowitz. Vienna.

1891b   *On Aphasia.* London, 1953. Reprinted in part in *S.E.* 14:206–215.

1893c   "Some Points for a Comparative Study of Organic and Hysterical Motor Paralyses." *S.E.* 1:160–172.

1895d   With J. Breuer., *Studies on Hysteria. S.E.* 2.

1895g   "Über Hysterie." Three-part lecture held at the Vienna Medical Doctors' College, October 14, 21, and 28, 1895. *G.W. Nachtragsband,* 352, 354–357.

1896b   "Further Remarks on the Neuro-Psychoses of Defence." *S.E.* 3:162–185.

1900a   *The Interpretation of Dreams. S.E.* 4–5.

1901a   *On Dreams. S.E.* 5:633–686.

1901b   *The Psychopathology of Everyday Life. S.E.* 6.

1905c   *Jokes and Their Relation to the Unconscious. S.E.* 8.

1905d   *Three Essays on the Theory of Sexuality. S.E.* 7:135–243.

1905e [1901]   "Fragment of an Analysis of a Case of Hysteria." *S.E.* 7:7–122.

1907a   *Delusions and Dreams in Jensen's "Gradiva." S.E.* 9:7–93.

1907c	"The Sexual Enlightenment of Children." *S.E.* 9:131–139.
1908b	"Character and Anal Erotism." *S.E.* 9:169–175.
1908c	"On the Sexual Theories of Children." *S.E.* 9:209–226.
1908d	"'Civilized' Sexual Ethics and Modern Nervous Illness." *S.E.* 9:181–204.
1908e	"Creative Writers and Day-Dreaming." *S.E.* 9:143–153.
1908f	"Preface to Stekel's *Nervöse Angstzustände und ihre Behandlung.*" *S.E.* 9:250f.
1909b	"Analysis of a Phobia in a Five-Year-Old Boy." *S.E.* 10:5–147.
1909d	"Notes upon a Case of Obsessional Neurosis." *S.E.* 10:155–249.
1910a [1909]	"Five Lectures on Psycho-Analysis." *S.E.* 11:7–55.
1910b [1909]	"Preface to Ferenczi's *Lélekelemzés: Értekezések a pszichoanalizis köreböl*" [Papers on Psycho-Analysis]. *S.E.* 9:252.
1910c	*Leonardo da Vinci and a Memory of His Childhood. S.E.* 11:63–137.
1910d	"The Future Prospects of Psycho-Analytic Therapy." *S.E.* 11:141–151.
1910e	"The Antithetical Meaning of Primal Words." *S.E.* 11:155–161.
1910g	"Contributions to a Discussion on Suicide." *S.E.* 11:231f.
1910h	"A Special Type of Choice of Object Made by Men." *S.E.* 11:165–175.
1910i	"The Psycho-Analytic View of Psychogenic Disturbance of Vision." *S.E.* 11:211–218.
1910k	"'Wild' Psychoanalysis." *S.E.* 11:221–227.
1910m	"Review of William Neutra's *Letters to Neurotic Women.*" *S.E.* 11:238.
1911b	"Formulations on the Two Principles of Mental Functioning." *S.E.* 12:218–226.
1911c [1910]	"Psycho-Analytic Notes on an Autobiographical Account of a Case of Paranoia (Dementia Paranoides)." *S.E.* 12:9–79.
1911e	"The Handling of Dream-Interpretation in Psycho-Analysis." *S.E.* 12:91–96.
1911f	"'Great Is Diana of the Ephesians.'" *S.E.* 12:342–344.
1911j	Translation with additional footnote of James J. Putnam, "On the Etiology and Treatment of the Psychoneuroses" (*Boston Med. Surg. Journal,* 163 [1910]), under the title "Über Ätiologie und Behandlung der Psychoneurosen." *Zbl. Psychoanaly.,* 1, 137; *S.E.* 17:271f., n. 2 (footnote only).
1912a [1911]	"'Postscript' to the Case of Paranoia." *S.E.* 12:80–82.
1912b	"The Dynamics of Transference." *S.E.* 12:99–108.
1912c	"Types of Onset of Neurosis." *S.E.* 12:231–238.
1912d	"On the Universal Tendency to Debasement in the Sphere of Love." *S.E.* 11:179–90.
1912e	"Recommendations to Physicians Practising Psycho-Analysis." *S.E.* 12:111–120.

1912f	"Contributions to a Discussion on Masturbation." *S.E.* 12:243–254.
1912g	"A Note on the Unconscious in Psycho-Analysis." [In English.] *S.E.* 12:260–266.
1912k	"Postscript to the Second Edition [of *Delusions and Dreams in Jensen's 'Gradiva'*]." *S.E.* 9:94f.
1912–13a	*Totem and Taboo. S.E.* 13:1–161.
1913a	"An Evidential Dream." *S.E.* 12:269–277.
1913b	Introduction to Pfister's *Die Psychanalytische Methode. S.E.* 12:329–331.
1913c	"On Beginning the Treatment (Further Recommendations on the Technique of Psycho-Analysis I)." *S.E.* 12:123–144.
1913e	Preface to Maxim Steiner, *Die psychischen Störungen der männlichen Potenz. S.E.* 12:345f.
1913f	"The Theme of the Three Caskets." *S.E.* 12:291–301.
1913h	"Observations and Examples from Analytic Practice." *S.E.* 13:193–198.
1913i	"The Disposition to Obsessional Neurosis." *S.E.* 12:317–326.
1913j	"The Claims of Psycho-Analysis to Scientific Interest." *S.E.* 13:165–190.
1914a	"Fausse Reconnaissance" ('déjà raconté') in "Psycho-Analytic Treatment." *S.E.* 13:201–207.
1914b	"The Moses of Michelangelo." *S.E.* 13:211–236.
1914c	"On Narcissism: An Introduction." *S.E.* 14:73–102.
1914d	"On the History of the Psycho-Analytic Movement." *S.E.* 14:7–66.
1914g	"Remembering, Repeating, and Working-Through (Further Recommendations on the Technique of Psycho-Analysis II)." *S.E.* 12:147–156.
1914h	"Freud, Sigmund" [unsigned article, authorship uncertain] in *Meyers Kleines Konversations-Lexikon*, vol. 7 *(Ergänzungen und Nachträge)*. Leipzig, 1914.
1915a [1914]	"Observations on Transference-Love (Further Recommendations on the Technique of Psycho-Analysis III)." *S.E.* 12:159–171.
1915e	"The Unconscious." *S.E.* 14:166–204.
1916–17a	*Introductory Lectures on Psycho-Analysis. S.E.* 15, 16.
1918b [1914]	"From the History of an Infantile Neurosis." *S.E.* 17:7–122.
1919h	"The Uncanny." *S.E.* 17:219–256.
1920g	*Beyond the Pleasure Principle. S.E.* 18:7–64.
1925d	*An Autobiographical Study. S.E.* 20:7–70.
1930a [1929]	*Civilization and Its Discontents. S.E.* 21:64–145.
1932a [1931]	"The Acquisition and Control of Fire." *S.E.* 22:187–193.
1933a	*New Introductory Lectures on Psycho-Analysis. S.E.* 22:5–182.
1937d	"Constructions in Analysis." *S.E.* 23:257–269.
1939a [1934–38]	*Moses and Monotheism. S.E.* 23:7–137.

1940c [1922]	"Medusa's Head." *S.E.* 18:273f.
1941d	"Psycho-Analysis and Telepathy." *S.E.* 18:177–193.
1955a [1907–08]	Original Record of the Case of Obsessional Neurosis (the "Rat-Man"). *S.E.* 10: 254f., 259–318.
1958a [1911]	With D. E. Oppenheim. *Dreams in Folklore. S.E.* 12:180–203.
1987h	Four Letters to Paul Häberlin (March 3, 1910; June 4, 1911; June 15, 1911; May 16, 1913) [in French translation, printed in part, with partial facsimile]. *Les bloc-notes de la psychanalyse,* no. 7 (1987): 283–288.

Sándor Ferenczi

1908, 57	"The Effect on Women of Premature Ejaculation in Men." *Fin.* 291–294.
1908, 60	"Actual- and Psycho-Neuroses in the Light of Freud's Investigations and Psycho-Analysis." *F.C.* 30–55.
1908, 61	"Analytical Interpretation and Treatment of Psychosexual Impotence in Men." *C.* 11–34.
1908, 63	"Psychoanalysis and Education." *Fin.* 280–290.
1909, 65	"The Analytic Conception of the Psycho-Neuroses." *F.C.* 15–30.
1909, 66	"On the Psychological Analysis of Dreams." *C.* 94–132.
1909, 67	"Introjection and Transference. *C.* 35–93.
1910, 69	"Zur Organisation der Psychoanalytischen Bewegung." *Bausteine* I:275–289.
1910, 70	*Lélekelemzés. Ertekezések a pszichoanalizis köréböl* [Papers on Psycho-Analysis]. Manó Dick, Budapest.
1911, 75	"On Obscene Words." *C.* 132–153.
1911, 76	"Anatole France as Analyst." *The Psychoanalytic Review,* 4 (1917): 344.
1911, 77	"Stimulation of the Anal Erotogenic Zone as a Precipitating Factor in Paranoia." *Fin.* 295–298.
1911, 78	"The Psycho-Analysis of Wit and the Comical." *F.C.* 332–344.
1911, 79	"On the Organization of the Psycho-Analytic Movement." *Fin.* 299–307.
1911, 80	"On the Part Played by Homosexuality in the Pathogenesis of Paranoia." *C.* 154–186.
1911, 81	"Alkohol und Neurosen. Antwort auf die Kritik von Eugen Bleuler." *Jahrbuch* 3 (1911):853–857.
1911, 81a	"Exploring the Unconscious." *Fin.* 308–312.
1912, 84	"On the Definition of Introjection." *Fin.* 316–318.
1912, 85	"On Transitory Symptom-Constructions during the Analysis." *C.* 193–212.
1912, 86	"A Case of *déjà vu. Fin.* 319–320.

1912, 91	"Dr. S. Lindner; a Forerunner of Freud's in the Theory of Sex." *Fin.* 325.
1912, 92	"Symbolic Representation of the Pleasure and Reality Principles in the Oedipus Myth." *C.* 253–269.
1912, 93	"Philosophy and Psycho-Analysis." *Fin.* 326–344.
1912, 94	"Suggestion and Psycho-Analysis." *F.C.* 55–68.
1912, 98	"Lelki problémak a pszichoanalizis megvilágitásában" [Psychic Problems in the Light of Psychoanalysis]. Manó Dick, Budapest.
1912, 99	"Foreword to S. Freud, 'Pszichoanalyzis' [On Psychoanalysis]." Manó Dick, Budapest.
1912, 100	"On Onanism." *C.* 185–192.
1913, 103	"On Psycho-Analysis and Its Judicial and Sociological Significance. A Lecture for Judges and Barristers." *F.C.* 424–434.
1913, 104	"Taming of a Wild Horse." *Fin.* 336–340.
1913, 105	"To Whom Does One Relate One's Dreams?" *F.C.* 349.
1913, 108	"Aus der 'Psychologie' von Hermann Lotze." *Imago,* 2 (1913): 238–241.
1913, 109	"Belief, Disbelief, and Conviction." *F.C.* 437–450.
1913, 111	"Stages in the Development of the Sense of Reality." *C.* 213–239.
1913, 112	"On Eye Symbolism." *C.* 270–276.
1913, 114	"A Little Chanticleer." *C.* 240–252.
1913, 124	"Kritik der Jungschen 'Wandlungen und Symbole der Libido.'" *Zeitschrift,* 1 (1913): 391–403; *Bausteine* I: 243–268.
1913, 125	"On the Ontogenesis of Symbols." *C.* 276–281.
1913, 126	"Review of Jones, E., 'Papers on Psycho-Analysis.'" *Zeitschrift,* 1 (1913): 93; *Bausteine* IV: 49–51.
1913, 127	"Review of Maeder, A., 'Sur le Mouvement psychanalytique.'" *Zeitschrift,* 1 (1913): 94, *Bausteine* IV: 51–52.
1913, 128	"Review of Brill, A. A., 'Freud's Theory of Compulsion Neurosis.'" *Zeitschrift,* 1 (1913): 180.
1913, 129	"Review of Brill, A. A., 'Psychological Mechanism of Paranoia.'" *Zeitschrift,* 1 (1913): 180.
1913, 130	"Review of Brill, A. A., 'Hysterical Dreamy States, Their Psychological Mechanism.'" *Zeitschrift,* 1 (1913): 180.
1913, 131	"Review of Brill, A. A., 'A Few Remarks on the Technique of Psycho-Analysis.'" *Zeitschrift,* 1 (1913): 180.
1913, 132	"Review of Brill, A. A., 'The Only or Favourite Child in Adult Life.'" *Zeitschrift,* 1 (1913): 180. *Bausteine* IV: 53–54.
1913, 133	"Review of Brill, A. A., 'Analeroticism and Character.'" *Zeitschrift,* 1 (1913): 181. *Bausteine* IV: 52–53.
1913, 134	"Review of Prince, Morton, 'The Meaning of Ideas as Determined by Unconscious Settings.'" *Zeitschrift* 1 (1913): 185–186.

1914, 135	"Some Clinical Observations on Paranoia and Paraphrenia." *C.* 282–295.
1914, 136	"On the Nosology of Male Homosexuality." *C.* 296–318.
1914, 139	"Falling Asleep during the Analysis." *F.C.* 249–250.
1914, 145	"The 'Forgetting' of a Symptom and Its Explanation in a Dream." *F.C.* 412–413.
1914, 146	"On the Ontogenesis of an Interest in Money." *C.* 319–332.
1914, 148	"Allgemeine Neurosenlehre." *Jahrbuch,* 6 (1914): 317–328.
1914, 148a	"Büntények lélekelemzése" [Psychoanalysis of Crime]. *Szabad Gondolat,* no. 1 (1914).
1914, 149	*Ideges tünetek keletkezése és eltünése és egyéb értekezések a pszichoanalizis köréböl* [Origin and Passing of Nervous Symptoms and other Essays from the Field of Psychoanalysis]. *Gesammette Aufsätze,* vol. 3. Budapest.
1914, 150	Review of Bleuler's "Kritik der Freudschen Theorien." *Zeitschrift,* 2 (1914): 62–66; *Bausteine* IV: 54–64.
1914, 151	Review of Jung's "Contribution à l'étude des types psychologiques (Communication présentée au Congrés de Psychanalyse à Munich 1913)." *Zeitschrift,* 2 (1914): 86f. *Bausteine* IV: 64–66.
1915, 160	"The Dream of the Occlusive Pessary." *F.C.* 304.
1917, 192	"Ostwald über die Psychoanalyse." *Zeitschrift,* 4 (1916–17): 146. *Bausteine* IV: 46–48.
1917, 199	"Barátságom Schächter Miksával" [My Friendship with Max Schächter]. *Gyógyászat,* no. 52 (1917).
1921, 236	"General Theory of the Neuroses." *International Journal of Psychoanalysis,* 1 (1920): 294.
1922, 239	(With István Hollós.) *Psycho-Analysis and the Psychic Disorder of General Paresis.* New York: Nervous and Mental Disease Publishing Co., 1925 (pt. 3 in *Fin.,* 351–370).
1922, 241	"A pszichoanalizis és a társadalompolitika" [Psychoanalysis and Social Politics]. *Nyugat,* no. 8 (1922).
1922, 245	"Social Considerations in Some Analyses." *F.C.* 413–418.
1923, 254	"The Symbolism of the Medusa's Head." *F.C.* 360.
1923, 257	"The Dream of the Clever Baby." *F.C.* 349–350.
1924, 264	(With Otto Rank.) *The Development of Psycho-Analysis.* New York: Nervous and Mental Disease Publishing Co., 1925.
1924, 268	*Thalassa: A Theory of Genitality. Psychoanalytic Quarterly* (1934): 2 (1933): 361–403; 3 (1934): 1–29; 3 (1934): 200–222.
1926, 272	"Organ Neuroses and Their Treatment." *Fin.* 22–28.
1928, 283a	"Psychoanalyse und Kriminologie." *Bausteine* III: 399–421.
1931, 292	"Child Analysis in the Analysis of Adults." *Fin.* 126–142.
1934, 296	"Some Thoughts on Trauma." Included in *Notes and Fragments* (1920–33), 308.
1938 [1909], 299	"On the Interpretation of Tunes Which Come into One's Head." *Fin.* 175–176.

Posthumous, 300   "Laughter" (*ca.* 1913). *Fin.* 177–182.

Posthumous, 303   "Contribution to the Understanding of the Psycho-Neuroses of the Age of Involution" (*ca.* 1921–22). *Fin.* 205–211.

1920–33, 308   Notes and Fragments (1920 and 1930–32). *Fin.* 216–279.

1990 [1932]   *The Clinical Diary of Sándor Ferenczi.* Ed. J. du Pont. Trans. M. Balint and N. Zarday-Jackson. Cambridge, Mass.: Harvard University Press, 1990.

Index

Note: Numbers refer to correspondence numbers.